D1766385

Travel and Tropical Medicine Manual

Fifth edition

The Travel and Tropical Medicine Manual

Fifth Edition

CHRISTOPHER A. SANFORD MD, MPH, DTM&H
Associate Professor, Family Medicine
Associate Professor, Global Health
University of Washington
Seattle, WA
USA

PAUL S. POTTINGER MD, DTM&H, FIDSA
Associate Professor, Infectious Diseases Medicine
Associate Director, Infectious Diseases Fellowship Program
Director, Antimicrobial Stewardship Program
University of Washington
Seattle, WA
USA

ELAINE C. JONG MD, FIDSA, FASTMH
Medical Director, University of Washington Campus Health Services
Director Emeritus, University of Washington
Travel and Tropical Medicine Clinic
University of Washington School of Medicine
Seattle, WA
USA

ELSEVIER

Edinburgh   London   New York   Oxford   Philadelphia   St Louis   Sydney   Toronto   2017

ELSEVIER

ISBN: 978-0-323-37506-1

Inkling ISBN: 978-0-323-41743-3

E-Book ISBN: 978-0-323-41742-6

Content Strategist: *Belinda Kuhn*
Content Development Specialist: *Nani Clansey*
Content Coordinator: *Joshua Mearns*
Project Manager: *Srividhya Vidhyashankar*
Design: *Christian Bilbow*
Illustration Manager: *Amy Faith Heyden*

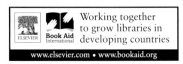

Printed in China
Last digit is the print number: 9 8 7 6 5 4 3 2 1

CONTENTS

SECTION 5: DERMATOLOGY

SECTION 6: SEXUALLY TRANSMITTED DISEASES

SECTION 7: HELMINTHS

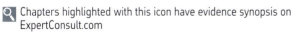 Chapters highlighted with this icon have evidence synopsis on ExpertConsult.com

PREFACE

The world is a book, and those who do not travel, read only a page.
   Augustine of Hippo (354-430)

Since the first edition of this manual was published in 1987, interest in travel medicine and clinical tropical medicine have continued to surge. International arrivals increase each year: in 2014, 1.1 billion people crossed an international border; this is projected to increase to 1.8 billion in 2025. More than 3200 medical providers and others with an interest in travel medicine in more than 90 countries are members of the International Society of Travel Medicine; membership in the American Society of Travel Medicine and Hygiene tops 3600; and more than 4300 registrants attended its 2014 annual meeting.

Our planet is rapidly becoming warmer, more populous, and increasingly urban. Microorganisms are increasingly resistant to existing antimicrobial agents, and the regular appearance of previously unrecognized infectious agents is the rule rather than the exception. Significant inroads on common infectious diseases, including measles and malaria, have been made in recent years, while other diseases, including dengue fever, are increasingly common. Higher rates of migration, tourism, and human encroachment of tropical rainforests are leading to the appearance in temperate regions of illnesses heretofore seen almost exclusively in the tropics. Hence it behooves medical practitioners, regardless of where they practice, to be familiar with illnesses occurring both locally and globally. It is our hope that this manual will serve as a pragmatic tool for medical providers who offer many types of care, including pre-travel and post-travel medicine, care of immigrants and refugees, and working in low-resource settings.

This edition contains several new chapters: Students Traveling Abroad, Travel and Mental Health, Ebola Virus Disease and Viral Hemorrhagic Fevers, Antibiotic-Resistant Bacteria in Returning Travelers, and The Role of Point-of-Care Testing in Travel Medicine.

We are grateful to our colleagues at Elsevier, including Nani Clansey, Belinda Kuhn, Srividhya Vidhyashankar, and Joshua Mearns, for their editorial insights, patience, persistence, and attention to detail. And we are indebted to our respective spouses—Sallie, Julie, and Britt—for their support and forbearance during the lengthy editorial process.

Christopher A. Sanford, MD, MPH, DTM&H
Paul S. Pottinger, MD, DTM&H, FIDSA
Elaine C. Jong, MD, FIDSA, FASTMH

LIST OF CONTRIBUTORS

Susan Anderson, MD
Travel, Tropical, Wilderness
Medicine Consultant
Global Health and Humanitarian Relief
Clinical Associate Professor
Division of Infectious Disease and
Geographic Medicine
Innovation and Global Health
Stanford, CA, USA
CDC/ISTM GeoSentinel Site Director for
Emerging Infectious Disease
Director of Travel Medicine
Travel Medicine and Emergency/Urgent
Care
PAMF
Palo Alto, CA
USA

Vernon Ansdell, MD, FRCP, DTM&H
Associate Clinical Professor
Department of Tropical Medicine
Microbiology and Pharmacology
University of Hawaii
School of Medicine
Honolulu, Hawaii
USA

Paul M. Arguin, MD
Domestic Unit Chief
Centers for Disease Control and
Prevention/Center for Global Health/
Malaria Branch
Atlanta, GA
USA

Howard D. Backer, MD, MPH
Director
California Emergency Medical Services
Authority
Sacramento, CA
USA

Jared Baeten, MD, PhD
Senior Fellow
Department of Medicine
University of Washington
Seattle, WA
USA

Stephen A. Bezruchka, MD, MPH, AM
Departments of Health Services & Global
Health
School of Public Health
University of Washington
Seattle, WA
USA

Micah M. Bhatti, MD, PhD
Clinical Microbiology Fellow
Division of Clinical Microbiology
Department of Laboratory Medicine and
Pathology
Mayo Clinic
Rochester, MN
USA

Andrea K. Boggild, MSc, MD, DTMH, FRCPC
Clinical Director
Tropical Disease Unit, Toronto General
Hospital
Parasitology Lead, Public Health Ontario
Laboratories
Assistant Professor, Dept. of Medicine,
University of Toronto
Toronto, ON
Canada

Frederick S. Buckner, MD
Professor
Department of Medicine, Division of
Allergy & Infectious Diseases
University of Washington
Seattle, WA
USA

Connie Celum, MD, MPH
Professor
Departments of Global Health and
Medicine
Adjunct Professor
Department of Epidemiology
University of Washington
Seattle, WA
USA

Martin S. Cetron, MD
Director, Division of Global Migration
and Quarantine
National Center for Preparedness,
Detection and
Control of Infectious Diseases
Centers for Disease Control and
Prevention (CDC)
Atlanta, GA
USA

Shireesha Dhanireddy, MD
Director
Infectious Disease Clinic
Assistant Director
Madison Clinic
Harborview Medical Center
Associate Professor
Infectious Diseases
University of Washington
Seattle, WA
USA

Julie Dombrowski, MD, MPH
Assistant Professor, Division of Allergy &
Infectious Diseases
University of Washington
Deputy Director for Clinical Services
Public Health - Seattle & King County
HIV/STD Program
Harborview Medical Center
Seattle, WA
USA

Mark Enzler, MD
Assistant Professor of Medicine
Division of Infectious Diseases,
Department of Medicine, Mayo Clinic
Rochester, MN
USA

Charles D. Ericsson, MD
Professor of Medicine and Dr. and Mrs.
Carl V. Vartian Professor of Infectious
Diseases
University of Texas Medical School at
Houston
Houston, TX
USA

Carey Farquhar, MD, MPH
Professor
Department of Medicine, Division of
Allergy and Infectious Diseases
Professor
Department of Global Health and
Department of Epidemiology
University of Washington
Seattle, WA
USA

Brian D. Gushulak, BSc, MD
Migration Health Consultants, Inc.
British Columbia
Canada

James P. Harnisch, MD, FAAD
Clinical Professor of Medicine
University of Washington
Director
Seattle Regional Hansen's Disease Center
Seattle, WA
USA

N. Jean Haulman, MD
Clinical Assistant Professor
Department of Pediatrics
Co-Director
UW Travel Clinic at Hall Health Center,
Travel Medicine
Univesity of Washington
Seattle, WA
USA

Shevin T. Jacob, MD, MPH
Acting Assistant Professor
Division of Allergy and Infectious Diseases
University of Washington
Seattle, WA
USA

**Elaine C. Jong, MD, FIDSA,
FASTMH**
Clinical Professor Emeritus
Department of Medicine, Division of
Allergy and Infectious Diseases
University of Washington School of
Medicine
Seattle, WA
USA

Kevin C. Kain, MD, FRCPC
Professor of Medicine
Department of Medicine
University of Toronto, Canada Research
Chair in Molecular Parasitology
Director, Centre for Travel and Tropical
Medicine
Toronto General Hospital
Toronto, ON
Canada

Andrea Kalus, MD
Associate Professor
University of Washington
Department of Medicine
Division of Dermatology
Seattle, WA
USA

Edmond Kay, MD
Diving Medical Officer
University of Washington
Seattle, WA
USA

Sarah Kohl, MD
Clinical Associate Professor of Pediatrics in
the School of Medicine
Department of Pediatrics
University of Pittsburgh
Pittsburgh, PA
USA

**Saba M. Lambert, MBChB, DTM&H,
PhD**
Clinical Research Fellow
Department of Infectious and Tropical
Diseases
London School of Hygiene and Tropical
Medicine
London
UK

Anne M. Larson, MD
Director, Swedish Liver Center
Swedish Health Services
Seattle, WA
USA

W. Conrad Liles, MD, PhD
Associate Chair and Professor of Medicine
Adjunct Professor, Departments of
Pathology
Pharmacology, and Global Health
University of Washington
Seattle, WA
USA

Poh Lian Lim, MD, MPH
Head & Senior Consultant
Department of Infectious Diseases
Institute of Infectious Diseases
Tan Tock Seng Hospital
Singapore

Andrew M. Luks, MD
Associate Professor
Division of Pulmonary and Critical Care
Medicine
Harborview Medical Center
Seattle, WA
USA

Sheila M. Mackell, MD
Pediatrics & Travel Medicine
Mountain View Pediatrics
Flagstaff, AZ
USA

**Douglas W. MacPherson, MD,
MSc(CTM), FRCPC**
Associate Professor
Department of Pathology and Molecular
Medicine
McMaster Universit
Hamilton, ON
Canada

**Jeanne M. Marrazzo, MD, MPH,
FACP, FIDSA**
Professor of Medicine
Division of Allergy & Infectious Diseases
Adjunct Professor
Department of Global Health
Medical Director
University of Washington STD Prevention
Training Center
University of Washington
Seattle, WA
USA

Robert Martin, MPH, DrPH
Director
Laboratory Systems Development
International Training and Education
Center for Health
Professor
Department of Global Health
University of Washington
Seattle, WA
USA

Susan L.F. McClellan, MD
Associate Professor
Department of Medicine
Division of Infectious Diseases
Director
Travel Clinic, Tulane University
New Orleans, LA
USA

R. Scott McClelland, MD, MPH
Professor of Medicine, Epidemiology, and
Global Health
University of Washington
Seattle, WA
USA

Anna McDonald, MD, MPH, DTMH
Global Health Fellow
Department of Family Medicine
University of Washington
Seattle, WA
USA

Anne C. Moore, MD, PhD
Medical Epidemiologist
Division of Parasitic Diseases
National Center for Zoonotic
Vectorborne and Enteric Diseases
Centers for Disease Control and
Prevention (CDC)
Atlanta, GA
USA

Aliza Monroe-Wise, MD, MSc
Senior Fellow
Department of Medicine, Division of
Allergy & Infectious Diseases
University of Washington
Seattle, WA
USA

Masahiro Narita, MD
Professor
Division of Pulmonary and Critical Care
University of Washington School of
Medicine
Seattle, WA
USA

Michael Noble BA, MD, FRCPC
Professor
Department of Pathology and Laboratory
Medicine
University of British Columbia
Vancouver, BC
Canada
Affiliate Professor
Department of Global Health
University of Washington
Seattle, WA
USA

Prof. Dr. Hans Dieter Nothdurft
Klinikum der LMU
Abt. für Infektions- und Tropenmedizin
Muenchen
Germany

Thomas B. Nutman, MD
Head Clinical Parasitology Section and
Head Helminth Immunology Section
Laboratory of Parasitic Diseases
National Institute of Allergy and Infectious
Diseases
National Institutes of Health
Bethesda, MD
USA

Lucy A. Perrone, BS, MSPH, PhD
Assistant Professor
Department of Global Health
University of Washington
Seattle, WA
USA

Paul S. Pottinger, MD, DTM&H, FIDSA
Associate Professor
Department of Medicine, Division of
Allergy & Infectious Diseases
University of Washington
Seattle, WA
USA

Dr. Camilla Rothe
Universitätsklinikum Hamburg Eppendorf
Abteilung für Tropenmedizin und
Infektiologie
Hamburg
Germany

Christopher A. Sanford, MD, MPH, DTM&H
Associate Professor
Family Medicine, Global Health
University of Washington
Seattle, WA
USA

Eli Schwartz, MD, DTM&H
Medical Director
The Center for Geographic Medicine and
Tropical Diseases
The Chaim Sherba Medical Center
Tel Hashomer
Israel

Christopher Spitters, MD, MPH
Associate Clinical Professor
Division of Allergy & Infectious Diseases
University of Washington School of
Medicine
Seattle, WA
USA

Neil R.H. Stone, MBBS, MRCP, FRCPath, DTMH
Clinical Research Fellow
Institute of Infection and Immunity, St.
George's
University of London
London
UK

Mari C. Sullivan, ARNP
Medical Officer
American Embassy, Kuala Lumpur
US Department of State, Foreign Service
Kuala Lumpur
Malaysia

Kathrine R. Tan, MD, MPH
Medical Officer
Centers for Disease Control and
Prevention/Center for Global Health/
Malaria Branch
Atlanta, GA
USA

Samuel B. Thielman, MD, PhD
Adjunct Associate Professor of Psychiatry
Duke University School of Medicine
Durham, NC
USA

Ellen Thompson, BA
Medical Student
University of Washington School of
Medicine
Seattle, WA
USA

Shawn Vasoo, MD
Associate Consultant
Department of Infectious Diseases
Institute of Infectious Diseases, Tan Tock
Seng Hospital
Singapore

Abinash Virk, MD, DTM&H
Associate Professor of Medicine
Division of Infectious Diseases
Mayo Clinic College of Medicine
Rochester, MN
USA

Stephen L. Walker, PhD, MRCP(UK) DTM&H
Clinical Lecturer and Consultant
Dermatologist
Department of Infectious and Tropical
Diseases
London School of Hygiene and Tropical
Medicine
London
UK

Timothy E. West, MD, MPH
Associate Professor of Medicine
Division of Pulmonary & Critical Care
Medicine
Adjunct Associate Professor of Global
Health
Director
International Respiratory & Severe Illness
Center (INTERSECT)
University of Washington
Seattle, WA
USA

Martin S. Wolfe, MD, FACP, FIDSA, FASTMH
Traveler's Medical Service of Washington
Washington, DC
USA

Yuan Zhou, MD
Senior Infectious Disease Fellow
University of Washington
Seattle, WA
USA

CHAPTER 1

Approach to Travel Medicine and Contents of a Personal Travel Medicine Kit

Elaine C. Jong

 Access evidence synopsis online at ExpertConsult.com.

A new medical specialty, travel medicine, emerged in the 1980s in response to the health needs of increasing numbers of international travelers—a phenomenon resulting from the rapid expansion and growing accessibility of commercial jet transportation. In 1990, the World Tourism Organization (WTO) reported approximately 457 million international arrivals per year. In 2014, the WTO reported 1138 million international arrivals per year, and just under half of these involved countries outside Europe. The upward trend in international travel is projected to continue.

When travel involves geographic translocations of people going from relatively sanitary and industrialized countries in northern temperate zones to destinations in countries with developing economies and tropical environments, potential exposures to exotic diseases and exacerbations of chronic health conditions during travel create unique health concerns for both individuals and societies. Travel medicine is interdisciplinary: it involves a spectrum of knowledge across the health specialties of epidemiology, preventive medicine, primary care, emergency medicine, infectious diseases, tropical medicine, gastroenterology, dermatology, and others. Travel health providers apply a heightened geographic awareness of destination-specific diseases and environmental conditions, as well as considerations of personal safety and well-being to individuals and their journeys.

As international travelers pursue their exploration of the world for recreational, educational, business, religious, and humanitarian purposes, physicians and other healthcare providers need to know how to counsel their traveling patients with regard to a wide variety of health issues. It has been reported that only 1-3.6% of deaths in travelers are due to infectious diseases; however, the risks for acute and chronic morbidity in the individual traveler and the potential for global spread of common as well as exotic human pathogens means that continued attention to transmission, treatment, prevention, and control of communicable diseases are essential considerations for international travelers (Chapters 3-9). Travel health issues involving environmental factors, from time zone changes to air pollution, temperature extremes, and barometric influences at high altitude and undersea are covered in Chapters 2 and 9-11. The psychological and emotional well-being of international travelers is increasingly recognized as a factor contributing to travelers' health (Chapters 2 and 17).

Personal safety has emerged as another important issue in travelers' health. Studies have shown that motor vehicle accidents (25%) and other injuries and accidents (15%, including drownings and falls from height) accounted for more deaths in American travelers than infectious diseases and other illnesses (10%). Heart attacks and other cardiovascular problems in male travelers over 60 years of age accounted for 50% of reported deaths but probably do not represent a preventable consequence of travel. Recommendations for travelers with special needs are given in Chapters 12-19.

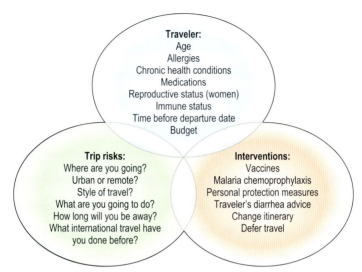

Fig. 1.1 The travel medicine triad.

APPROACH TO TRAVEL MEDICINE

Travel medicine practice involves the "travel medicine triad" consisting of the traveler, the trip, and the proposed health interventions (**Fig. 1.1**). The health status of the traveler is the starting point: the very young and the very old are at increased risk from certain infectious diseases due to age-related changes in the immune system; travelers with underlying medical conditions may need more assistance in the health maintenance strategies during travel and may even need to alter their desired itineraries based on access to healthcare at the destination.

Assessment of trip risks is related to the destination(s), with travel to rural tropical areas, communities with high prevalence or outbreaks of diseases that are not preventable by vaccine, extreme environments, and remote regions presenting more challenges than trips on standard tourist routes. Updated information on outbreaks, epidemics, and health conditions abroad are posted on the websites of the Centers for Disease Control and Prevention (CDC, www.cdc.gov) in Atlanta, Georgia, and the World Health Organization (WHO, www.who.int) in Geneva, Switzerland. In addition to the CDC and WHO, regional health agencies and public and private health information services also issue periodic guidelines and health information for international travelers. However, many guidelines are by necessity very general; the optimal practice of travel medicine calls for individualized recommendations for each traveler and trip based on the travel health assessment described by the "travel medicine triad" above. Whenever possible, international travelers should seek medical advice 4-6 weeks in advance of their departure date. *This allows adequate time for immunizations to be scheduled, for advice and prescriptions to be given, and for special information to be obtained when needed.*

The medical approach to travel becomes even more complex when the traveler plans a long-term trip lasting months to years, often involving multiple destinations. Such travelers may need to start 3 or more months in advance of anticipated trip departure in order to complete vaccine series and other health examinations needed for issuance of visas, permits, school registrations, and other required documents. **Table 1.1** summarizes the steps for pre-travel medical preparation.

TABLE 1.1   Pre-Travel Medical Recommendations

1. Consult personal physician, local Public Health Department, or travel clinic about recommendations for immunizations and malaria chemoprophylaxis after selection of the travel itinerary, preferably 4-6 weeks in advance of departure.
2. Prepare a Traveler's Health History (Table 1.2) and a Traveler's Personal Medical Kit (Table 1.7).
3. Carry a satellite phone or a telephone credit card that can be used for international telephone calls or make sure that the friends or relatives listed in the health history would accept an international collect call in case of an emergency.
4. Make sure to have the telephone number of your personal physician, including office and after-hours numbers and a fax number, if available.
5. Check medical insurance policy or health plan for coverage for illness or accidents occurring outside the country of origin (home country).
6. Specifically inquire if the regular insurance policy or health plan will cover emergency medical evacuation by an air ambulance.
7. Arrange for additional medical insurance coverage or for a line of credit as necessary for a medical emergency situation.

TABLE 1.2   Traveler's Health History

International travelers should assemble the following information in a concise and clearly written form to carry with them:

1. An up-to-date immunization record (preferably the International Certificate of Vaccination).
2. A list of current medications giving both trade names and generic names as well as the dose and dosing schedule.
3. A list of all medical problems, such as hypertension, diabetes, asthma, and heart disease (cardiac patients should carry a copy of the most recent electrocardiogram).
4. A list of known drug allergies and other allergies (e.g., bee stings, peanuts).
5. ABO blood type and Rh factor type.
6. Name and telephone number (and fax number, if available) of the traveler's regular doctor.
7. Name and telephone number of the closest relative or friend in the home country who might assist if the traveler incurs serious illness while out of the country.

All travelers should be advised to assemble the information listed in **Table 1.2** in a concise and clearly written form to carry with them. In addition, travelers should plan to carry a supply of medications adequate to last the duration of the trip in their carry-on (not checked) luggage and an extra pair of eyeglasses even if contact lenses are usually worn, along with a copy of the prescription for the corrective lenses.

Health interventions in travel clinics include health education on the trip risks identified for a particular traveler and trip and, at a minimum, recommendations on immunizations, malaria chemoprophylaxis, management of traveler's diarrhea, and prevention of insect-vectored diseases.

Immunizations for Travel

Travelers going to destinations in tropical and developing countries from countries in North America and Western Europe are exposed to communicable diseases that are infrequently encountered at home due to a generally high standard of sanitation and mandatory childhood immunization programs. For example, adult travelers have acquired measles and chickenpox on trips abroad. Paralytic polio is transmitted outside the Western Hemisphere in countries where sanitary conditions favor oral-fecal transmission and routine immunizations do not reach a high level of coverage among susceptible populations. Thus all travelers should be questioned about their status with regard to the routine immunizations of childhood—tetanus, diphtheria, measles, mumps, rubella, and polio—and a primary series or booster doses of the vaccines should be given as appropriate. Vaccines against *Haemophilus influenzae* type b, hepatitis A, hepatitis B, human papillomavirus, meningococcal disease, pertussis, pneumococcal disease, and varicella are also included in the current childhood and pre-adolescent immunization schedules in the United States. Older children and adult travelers should be up-to-date with age-appropriate booster doses or receive a primary series of these standard immunizations if travel will place them at risk (Chapter 5). Travel immunizations for children are covered in Chapter 12.

The vaccinations administered to travelers should be recorded in a copy of the yellow booklet, the "International Certificate of Vaccination or Prophylaxis," which is recognized by the WHO. This record should be kept in a secure place with the passport, as it becomes a lifelong immunization record. There is a special page for validation of the yellow fever vaccine, which must be done in an official vaccination center, as well as additional pages to record the other vaccines.

Up-to-date information on areas where cholera and yellow fever are reported is best obtained from the CDC (www.cdc.gov/travel) or the WHO (www.who.int) websites. Smallpox and cholera vaccines are no longer required for international travel, according to WHO regulations. Proof of meningococcal vaccine receipt is required for visa applications to Saudi Arabia during the time of the Hajj. In the United States, owing to relatively limited supplies and the fact that it must be given within 1 hour after reconstitution of the vaccine, the yellow fever vaccine is available only from official vaccination centers registered by the Department of Public Health in each state.

Some confusion exists over the difference between *required* vaccinations and *recommended* vaccinations. In the CDC publication *Health Information for International Travel* (commonly called "The Yellow Book"), there is a country-by-country listing of vaccines required for entry. The Yellow Book can be accessed through the CDC website or purchased in printed format. Someone calling a travel clinic to ask which shots are required for a trip to Kenya or Venezuela, for instance, would be told by staff consulting the Yellow Book that yellow fever vaccine is not required for a traveler arriving from North America. Yet if one refers to maps showing where yellow fever is endemic, one can see that Kenya and Venezuela both lie within the endemic zones. Thus, yellow fever vaccine might be *recommended* to a traveler to those countries even though the vaccine is not a requirement for entry, depending on that traveler's intended activities and in-country itinerary.

Other vaccines may be recommended to travelers, depending on their destinations, degree of rural exposure during travel, eating habits, purpose of the trip, and state of health. In this group are the vaccines against hepatitis A, typhoid fever, cholera, meningococcal disease, rabies, Japanese encephalitis, and influenza. Certain travelers, such as healthcare workers, missionaries, Peace Corps volunteers, students, and any person likely to have household or sexual contact with residents in tropical or developing countries should consider immunization against hepatitis B. Persons who are going to tour rural areas or live or work in the People's Republic of China, India, Thailand, Republic of Korea, and other Asian countries need to consider Japanese encephalitis B vaccine. Travel immunizations are considered in detail in Chapter 5.

Malaria Chemoprophylaxis

In addition to travel immunizations, a major consideration for international travelers is whether their travel will take them to an area where malaria is transmitted. Malaria has a worldwide distribution in tropical and subtropical areas. It is reemerging in areas once considered to be free from risk and continues to be a serious problem for the traveler because of the emergence of new drug-resistant strains in areas where the use of chloroquine

TABLE 1.3   Recommendations to Avoid Mosquito Bites

1. Remain in well-screened areas, especially during the hours between dusk and dawn.
2. Sleep under mosquito netting if the room is unscreened.
3. Wear clothing that adequately covers the arms and legs when outdoors.
4. Apply mosquito repellent to exposed areas of skin when outdoors and wear permethrin-treated outer clothing. The most effective mosquito repellents for application to skin surfaces contain *N,N*-diethyl-3-methylbenzamide (DEET) (formerly known as *N,N*-diethyl-m-toluamide), which is also effective against biting flies, chiggers, fleas, and ticks. Clothing as well as mosquito netting can be sprayed with products containing permethrin. Permethrin does not repel insects but works as a contact insecticide that leads to the death of the insect.

phosphate and other antimalarial drugs were formerly highly effective for malaria prevention and treatment.

In Africa, South America, Asia, and the South Pacific, infections with chloroquine-resistant *Plasmodium falciparum* malaria (CRPF) are a significant risk to travelers because falciparum malaria can rapidly progress to serious morbidity and mortality if not promptly diagnosed and treated. Updated information on the risk of CRPF is published in the CDC publication *Morbidity and Mortality Weekly Report*, but the CDC website should be consulted for the most current information on a given travel destination. Chemoprophylaxis, or the taking of drugs to prevent clinical attacks of malaria, is recommended to travelers going to areas of malaria transmission, in addition to personal insect precautions. Drugs currently used for the prevention of chloroquine-resistant malaria include mefloquine (Larium®), doxycycline (Doryx®, Vibramycin®), and atovaquone/proguanil (Malarone®). These and other antimalarial drugs are discussed in Chapters 6 and 20.

Malaria is a protozoan parasite transmitted to humans by nighttime biting female anopheline mosquitoes. Since the risk of infection is related to the number of bites sustained, and since current malaria chemoprophylaxis regimens are not completely protective, all travelers should follow certain simple precautions when visiting or staying in malarious areas (**Tables 1.3** and **1.4**). In addition to preventing bites from mosquitoes spreading malaria, these precautions will help the traveler avoid bites from other mosquito species and insects that spread a variety of diseases in tropical and subtropical areas, for which there are no prophylactic drugs nor vaccines (dengue fever, hemorrhagic fevers, viral encephalitis, leishmaniasis, trypanosomiasis, filariasis, etc.) (**Table 1.5**). In an analysis of travel-associated illnesses among 17,353 returned travelers reporting to a GeoSentinel Site by Freedman and co-authors, vector-borne diseases accounted for almost 40% of the case reports, exceeding respiratory transmitted diseases and food- and water-borne diseases, respectively.

Traveler's Diarrhea

Between 30 and 60% of travelers to tropical countries are affected by traveler's diarrhea. This illness is characterized by sudden onset of four to five movements of watery diarrhea per day, sometimes accompanied by abdominal cramps, malaise, nausea, and vomiting. An attack typically lasts 3-6 days. The pathogens causing gastrointestinal disease are acquired mostly through fecal-oral contamination, and preventive strategies to avoid illness include careful selection of food and water (Chapter 8).

Adequate means for purification of water vary depending on the water source. Bringing water to a boil is probably the most reliable way to kill pathogens up to 20,000 ft above sea level. Water purification tablets are convenient and commercially available, and are almost as effective as boiling when the water is at 68°F (20°C). Portable water purification filters have become a popular alternative employed by many travelers; the devices using iodine–resin technology have proved to be effective against the broadest range of pathogens. Heating, chemical, and filtration methods of water purification are discussed in detail in Chapter 7.

TABLE 1.4   Insect Repellents and Insecticides[a]

Examples of Insect Repellents Containing DEET for Skin Application

Ultra 30™ Lotion Insect Repellent: 30% DEET in a liposome base, up to 12 h protection against mosquitoes; DEET is also effective against ticks, gnats, no-see-ums, sandflies, biting flies, deer flies, stable flies, black flies, chiggers, red bugs, and fleas (Sawyer Products, Safety Harbor, FL; distributed by Recreational Equipment Inc [REI])

Off! Deep Woods™: 23.7% DEET, up to 6 h of protection against mosquitoes and other insects (SC Johnson, Racine, WI)

Off! Skintastic™: 6.65% DEET, up to 3 h of protection against mosquitoes and other insects (SC Johnson)

Sawyer Premium Broad Spectrum Insect Repellent Spray™: contains DEET plus a special fly repellent additive, R-326; use according to package directions (Sawyer Products)

Examples of Permethrin-Containing Insecticides for Application to External Clothing and Mosquito Nets (see **Fig. 1.2**)

Permethrin for Clothing Tick Repellent: contains permethrin in a non-aerosol pump spray can; repels ticks, chiggers, mosquitoes, and other bugs (Sawyer Products). One application lasts 4 weeks or through six washings.

PermaKill Solution: 13.3% permethrin liquid concentrate supplied in 8-oz bottle; can be diluted (1/3 oz permethrin concentrate in 16 oz water) to be used with a manual pump spray bottle or diluted 2 oz in 1 1/2 cups of water to be used to impregnate outer clothing, mosquito nets, and curtains (Sawyer Products). Permethrin impregnation of garments or mosquito netting will achieve protection for up to 1 year or good for 30 launderings.

[a]Brand names are given for identification purposes only and do not constitute an endorsement.

TABLE 1.5   Important Arthropod-Borne Diseases

Arthropod Vector	Biting Characteristics	Disease
Anopheles mosquitoes	Evening and nighttime Indoors and outdoors Mainly rural	Malaria Lymphatic filariasis (Wuchereria *bancrofti*, *Brugia malayi*, *Brugia timori*) Rift Valley fever O'nyong-nyong fever
Aedes mosquitoes	Daytime (dusk, dawn) Usually outdoors Mostly urban	Dengue fever Yellow fever Chikungunya fever Lymphatic filariasis Rift Valley fever Ross River fever Venezuelan equine encephalitis
Culex mosquitoes	Usually evening and nighttime Mostly outdoors Rural and urban	Japanese encephalitis Lymphatic filariasis Venezuelan equine encephalitis St. Louis encephalitis West Nile encephalitis Murray Valley encephalitis Ross River fever Rift Valley fever Chikungunya fever

TABLE 1.5   Important Arthropod-Borne Diseases—cont'd

Arthropod Vector	Biting Characteristics	Disease
Mansonia mosquitoes	Usually nighttime Usually outdoor Rural and urban	Venezuelan equine encephalitis Chikungunya fever Lymphatic filariasis
Fleas	Night or daytime Indoors or outdoors Urban and rural	Plague Endemic (murine or flea-borne) typhus
Body lice	Night or daytime Indoors or outdoors Urban and rural	Trench fever Louse-borne relapsing fever Epidemic (louse-borne) typhus
Ticks	Day and nighttime Outdoors Rural	Mediterranean spotted fever African tick typhus Rocky mountain spotted fever Queensland tick typhus Congo Crimean hemorrhagic fever Omsk hemorrhagic fever Lyme disease Ehrlichiosis Tularemia Babesiosis Tick-borne relapsing fever Tick paralysis
Mites	Day or nighttime Indoors or outdoors Urban or rural	Scrub (mite-borne) typhus Rickettsialpox
Culicoides midges (no-see-ums)	Day or nighttime Usually outdoors Rural	Mansonellosis
Deer and horseflies (Tabanids)	Daytime Outdoors Rural	Loiasis Tularemia
Black flies (*Simulium*)	Daytime Outdoors Rural	Onchocerciasis (river blindness)
Sandflies (*Phlebotomus*, *Lutzomyia*)	Nighttime Usually outdoors Urban and rural	Cutaneous leishmaniasis Visceral leishmaniasis (Kala azar) Bartonellosis (Oroya fever) Sandfly fever
Tsetse flies (*Glossina*)	Daytime Outdoors Rural	African trypanosomiasis (African sleeping sickness)
Triatomine/reduviid bugs	Nighttime Indoors Rural and urban	American trypanosomiasis (Chagas disease)

Source: Vernon Ansdell, personal communication, 2007.

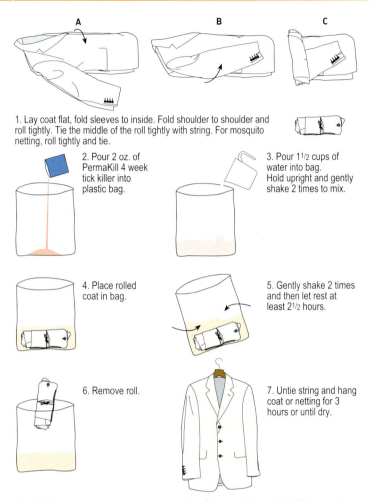

A   B   C

1. Lay coat flat, fold sleeves to inside. Fold shoulder to shoulder and roll tightly. Tie the middle of the roll tightly with string. For mosquito netting, roll tightly and tie.

2. Pour 2 oz. of PermaKill 4 week tick killer into plastic bag.

3. Pour 1½ cups of water into bag. Hold upright and gently shake 2 times to mix.

4. Place rolled coat in bag.

5. Gently shake 2 times and then let rest at least 2½ hours.

6. Remove roll.

7. Untie string and hang coat or netting for 3 hours or until dry.

Fig. 1.2 **How to apply permethrin to your clothing.** (Courtesy of Rose, S.R., 1993. International Travel Health Guide. Travel Medicine, Northampton, MA.)

Owing to widespread publicity in the lay press, many travelers want to know more about the use of antibiotics to prevent diarrhea while traveling. Most travel health experts advise against using drugs as a preventive measure for traveler's diarrhea, the chief objections being the potential for undesirable side effects, allergic reactions, and possible occurrence of antibiotic-associated colitis. However, in selected travelers with time-sensitive mission-critical objectives, prevention of traveler's diarrhea might warrant the use of antibiotic prophylaxis involving daily oral doses of antibiotics for a limited time. Antibiotic prophylaxis and empiric self-treatment of traveler's diarrhea are discussed in detail in Chapter 8.

MEDICAL EMERGENCIES DURING TRAVEL

Emergency medical care abroad is not a subject likely to be broached by the average travel agent, for fear of alarming the potential traveler. Yet all travelers, especially those planning long-term travel (trips of 3 weeks or longer), the very young and the very old, and those with special medical conditions (cardiac, pulmonary, gastrointestinal, or hematologic problems; pregnancy; human immunodeficiency virus [HIV] infection; organ transplant; etc.) need to have a plan in case the need for emergency medical care arises. Even the young traveler in perfect health can break a leg, be involved in a motor vehicle accident, or be bitten by a rabid dog.

People planning trips to exotic places but who will stay in urban, first-class hotels may have relatively easy access to English-speaking physicians with biomedical training at a level seen in high-income nations. However, many places where modern tourists go are far from English-speaking medical practitioners and modern hospitals. At some travel destinations, medications for treatment of certain infections and special medical conditions may not be available under any circumstances. Thus, for such travelers, pre-travel counseling, preparation of the traveler's medical kit, and a medical emergency evacuation plan are of great importance.

Finding a Physician in a Foreign Country

For travelers with specific medical conditions, the treating physician at home will often be able to supply the names of colleagues in foreign countries who could be consulted in case of emergency. Professional associations such as the International Society of Travel Medicine (ISTM, www.istm.org) and the American Society of Tropical Medicine and Hygiene (ASTMH, www.astmh.org) maintain membership directories that include clinical members working in many destination countries. Foreign embassies often have lists of local physicians that have provided care to their staff. University or other teaching hospitals can be relied on to provide quality care and are likely to have staff members who speak English and other languages. The International Association for Medical Assistance to Travellers (IAMAT, www.iamat.org) is another resource for travelers. Among its many services, this nonprofit organization provides to its members names of English-speaking physicians who have agreed to care for travelers in many countries around the world (**Table 1.6**).

Emergency Information Needed

The Traveler's Health History (Table 1.2) and the International Certificate of Vaccination or Prophylaxis should be carried with the passport at all times. Although a medical-alert

TABLE 1.6 Methods for Purification of Water[a]		
Method	**Brand Name**	**Quantity to Be Added to 1 Quart or 1 Liter of Water**
Iodine compound tablets[b]	Potable Aqua®	Two tablets are added to water at 20°C, and the mixture is agitated every 5 min for a total of 30 min.
Chlorine solution, 2-4%	Common laundry bleach	Two to four drops are added to water at 20°C, and after mixing, the solution is kept for 30 min before drinking.
Iodine solution[b]	(2% tincture of iodine)	Five to ten drops of iodine are added to water at 20°C, and after mixing, the solution is kept for 30 min before drinking.
Heat		Water is heated to above 65°C for at least 3 min (at 20,000 ft altitude or 6000 m, water boils at 80°C).

[a]The methods presented here are sufficient to kill *Giardia* cysts in most situations. Heat is the best method when tested in a laboratory situation. (See Chapter 7 for more detailed information.)
[b]Iodine-containing compounds should be used with caution during pregnancy.

bracelet or necklace (available for order in most pharmacies or from Internet vendors) is recommended to travelers with life-threatening allergies or medical conditions, people offering assistance in some countries may not recognize the significance of, or even look for, such identification.

Payment for Services

Coverage for emergency medical services abroad should be verified with the traveler's regular insurance company or healthcare plan before the trip. Medicare will not cover services provided in foreign countries, with the exception of an urgent problem arising en route from the United States to Alaska that requires medical treatment in Canada. Several companies specializing in medical insurance and emergency medical evacuation for travelers are listed in the Appendix. Payment for medical services abroad is customarily due when care is given, but travelers will need to save the receipts for reimbursement by their health coverage plan. Insurance companies are unlikely to pay for procedures or treatments that are experimental or not available in the United States.

Emergency Medical Care en Route

At the time of writing, most international commercial aircraft carry an emergency first-aid kit, with supplies and equipment for a basic life-support response. Advanced life-support equipment and drugs may not be available for passengers with acute cardiac or pulmonary emergencies, although some aircraft do carry automatic external defibrillator units. Generally, oxygen is available only in the event of cabin decompression, although some airlines carry small portable tanks for medical emergencies. Patients with chronic pulmonary conditions requiring supplemental oxygen must make arrangements at the time of reservation for supplies of in-flight portable oxygen tanks. In the event of a serious medical emergency that occurs during flight, most commercial aircraft will reroute and land at the closest commercial airport. Chapter 4 presents further details of air carrier health issues, and Chapter 16 further explores medical issues for travel with chronic medical conditions.

Commercial international cruise ship lines carrying fee-paying passengers are required by maritime law to have a physician on board at sea. The qualifications of the ship's physicians and the availability of advanced life-support equipment and drugs may vary from line to line, so specific inquiries should be made.

Emergency Evacuation Home

Contingency plans for a medical emergency should be discussed openly and the need for special travel insurance coverage considered with all travelers regardless of underlying health. Even a healthy young traveler is at risk for contracting a serious illness or accidental injury during travel.

Some commercial airlines will allow passage of a seriously ill person back to the United States only when that person is accompanied by a licensed physician. Payment of the physician and purchase of his or her round-trip airfare must be provided in such cases. In other cases, emergency evacuation home must proceed by way of specially equipped aircraft (helicopters and fixed-wing aircraft), which usually carry their own teams of medical personnel, including physicians and nurses. Costs for such evacuations can run to tens of thousands of dollars, depending on geographic location, weather conditions, and medical needs.

Emergency evacuation insurance is available; however, prospective subscribers need to read the terms carefully, as some plans provide only for evacuation to the nearest regional medical center, not for transport back to a medical facility in the traveler's home country. Given that very ill people would prefer to receive a customary standard of care, evacuation of a patient to a foreign medical center, where English and other Western languages may be spoken as a second language and where medical protocols are different, may not be as satisfactory as evacuation back to the traveler's country of origin. Names and addresses of organizations arranging international emergency transport services for their members are given in the Appendix.

Emergency Blood Transfusion

The traveler's blood type, if known, should be listed in the Traveler's Health History and/or in the space provided in the International Certificate of Vaccination or Prophylaxis booklet. If an urgent blood transfusion becomes necessary, however, and the blood type is unknown, the traveler's blood can be quickly typed and then tested against the donor's blood. However, in certain parts of the world, certain blood types may not be easily obtainable. For instance, in the People's Republic of China, the predominant blood type is A-positive among the resident population.

Travelers with bleeding conditions or tendencies (e.g., those on anticoagulation therapy or those with a history of bleeding peptic ulcers) should get information before their trip from their local blood bank about resources in the countries to be visited.

WILDERNESS AND ADVENTURE TRAVEL

The more remote from access to established medical care facilities, the more the traveler has to anticipate self-care or peer care for medical problems that might occur. Many of the medical concerns arising during adventure travel are covered throughout this book. However, the treatment of serious injuries and trauma in the wilderness and the approach to survival skills is beyond the scope of this book and are the focus of the Wilderness Medical Society (www.wms.org). Specific training and equipment may be needed for survival in wilderness settings or extreme environments.

The adventure or expedition traveler planning a remote and/or challenging route is advised to get accurate information regarding the physical difficulty and inherent environmental risks associated with the trip itinerary, to carefully review the qualifications and personalities of the trip leader(s) and fellow adventurers, to query the dietary arrangements for the trip, and to verify the possibilities for emergency evacuation. In addition, adventure travelers should acquire advanced first-aid skills and prepare themselves to be in optimal physical condition prior to departure.

THE TRAVELER'S MEDICAL KIT

Table 1.7 presents recommendations for a traveler's medical kit for a short-term international trip. Depending on geographic location(s), type(s) of activities planned, and underlying health, the traveler may augment the kit with regular prescription medications, medication for high-altitude sickness, antifungal preparations, treatment for ectoparasites, and additional antiparasitic drugs. Pulmonary patients may need to make arrangements for portable oxygen supplies and even oxygen concentrator machines, and peritoneal dialysis patients may travel with dialysate fluids and accessories and may need advance reservations for access to dialysis services at the destination (see Chapter 16).

Prescription Medications

At least a few days' supply of necessary medications should be taken in hand-held luggage. Preferably, the entire supply of usual prescription medications, enough to last the whole trip, should be taken in the hand-held luggage. If possible, travelers should not pack their prescription medications in checked luggage, as the baggage could be lost or pilfered in transit. Travelers should not plan to purchase prescription medications abroad as a cost-reducing strategy: expired, improperly stored, and counterfeit drugs are a growing problem worldwide, or the traveler's usual medications may simply not be available.

SUMMARY OF CONSIDERATIONS FOR HEALTH AND TRAVEL

In addition to travel immunizations, malaria chemoprophylaxis, possibility of traveler's diarrhea, and prevention of insect-vectored diseases, travelers need to be counseled about common medical problems of international travel that may be related to the mode of transportation, changes in altitude, changes in time zones, increased exposure to sun, taking of new drugs, and changes in climate and humidity (Chapters 2, 4, 6, and 9-11).

TABLE 1.7   The Traveler's Personal Medical Kit[a]

Below are listed some of the suggested items for the traveler's personal medical kit. Not all of these items are necessary or appropriate for every traveler; items should be selected based on the style of travel and destination(s).

Prescription items[b]

Antibiotics: Antibiotics may be useful for travelers at risk for skin infections, upper respiratory infections (URIs), and/or urinary tract infections (UTIs), as well as for treatment of traveler's diarrhea.

Skin infections
   Mupirocin 2% (Bactroban) topical antibiotic ointment, 15-gm tube or 1-gm foil packets. Apply to infected skin lesions three times a day.

Upper respiratory tract infections (sinusitis, bronchitis):
   Azithromycin, 250-mg tablet. Two tablets PO first dose, followed by one tablet PO q24 h × 4 additional days; or
   Amoxicillin 875 mg/clavulanate 125-mg tablet. One tablet PO q12 hr × 7 days.

Urinary tract infections (uncomplicated):
   TMP/SMX DS tablet: One tablet PO q12 h × 3 days; or
   Ciprofloxacin, 250-mg tablet: One PO q12 h × 3 days.

Antibiotics, Multipurpose: These provide empiric coverage for skin infections, URI, and UTI. (Note that ciprofloxacin and levofloxacin are commonly used for treatment of traveler's diarrhea as well.)
   Amoxicillin 875 mg plus clavulanate 125-mg tablet (Augmentin 875 mg). One tablet PO q12 h × 3-7 days; or
   Ciprofloxacin (Cipro), 500-mg tablet. One tablet PO q12 h × 3-7 days; or
   Levofloxacin (Levaquin), 500-mg tablet. One tablet PO q24 h × 3-7 days.

Allergic Reactions (bee, wasp, or hornet stings; food; etc.):
EpiPen emergency injection of epinephrine:
   Use according to package directions for severe reaction to bee sting or for other allergic reaction causing shortness of breath, wheezing, or swelling of the lips, eyes, or throat. This will give short-acting relief. As soon as the afflicted person can swallow, administer Benadryl tablets as directed below.

Benadryl (diphenhydramine), 25-mg tablet (non-prescription):
   Take two tablets by mouth immediately, then one to two tabs q6 h × 2 days following an allergic reaction. Use Benadryl alone for mild to moderate allergic skin reactions and itching, and take Benadryl following the use of the EpiPen.

Medrol Dosepak (methylprednisolone):
   For use with severe and persistent allergic reactions such as hives (urticaria) and/or angioedema (swelling under the skin). Follow the instructions for the tapering dose schedule in the packet. May be required in addition to Benadryl for severe allergic reactions.

Bronchospasm/asthma: Albuterol or salbutamol inhaler (multidose inhaler):
   Use for asthma attacks or for allergic reactions that cause persistent wheezing. Two puffs 2 minutes apart, each inhaled as deeply as possible into the lungs, up to four times a day.

Cough Suppressant: A small bottle of prescription cough syrup or a few tablets of codeine-containing medication (Tylenol #3 tablets will serve this purpose as well as that of treatment for severe headache or pain).

Diarrhea Treatment: An antimotility drug such as loperamide (Imodium) (non-prescription) plus an antibiotic (e.g., ciprofloxacin, levofloxacin, azithromycin) may be prescribed for self-treatment (see Chapter 8). *Note: Ciprofloxacin and levofloxacin are not licensed for age under 18 years.*

Eyeglasses: If corrective lenses are used, bring along an extra pair of eyeglasses and the prescription.

High-Altitude Illness: Acetazolamide (Diamox) may be prescribed for prophylaxis of high-altitude illness for high-altitude destinations (see Chapter 10).

Jet Lag: In some cases, a short-acting sleeping medication is helpful in treating sleeping problems associated with jet lag (see Chapter 9).

TABLE 1.7   The Traveler's Personal Medical Kit—cont'd

Malaria Pills: As the malaria situation in many countries continues to change, malaria chemoprophylaxis changes as well. Updated information on the malaria situation for specific destination(s) needs to be carefully reviewed, and appropriate medications prescribed (see Chapter 6).

Motion Sickness: Travelers who experience motion sickness may be prescribed a medication for this (Chapter 9) or may purchase over-the-counter medications (Dramamine, Marezine).

Nausea and Vomiting: Compazine (prochlorperazine), 25-mg rectal suppository. This may be helpful when oral medications cannot be tolerated and an injectable antiemetic is not available.

Pain Relief: A modest supply of prescriptive pain medication may be needed for headache, toothache, or musculoskeletal injury, especially for rural travel or extended trips.

Tylenol #3 (acetaminophen with 30 mg codeine) tablets: one to two tablets PO q4-6 h prn severe headache or pain.

Antibiotic Ointment: Triple antibiotic ointment (Neosporin) for topical application on minor cuts and abrasions.

Antifungal Powder or Cream: For travelers prone to athlete's foot and/or other fungal skin problems.

Antifungal Vaginal Cream or Troches: For women prone to yeast vaginitis associated with changes in climate or following antibiotic use (see Chapter 14).

Antihistamine tablets (diphenhydramine, chlorpheniramine, cetirizine, loratadine, etc.): For relief of nasal and skin symptoms due to allergies.

Decongestant Tablets (pseudoephedrine, etc.): For nasal congestion due to colds, allergies, or water sports.

Diarrhea, Traveler's: Bismuth subsalicylate (Pepto-Bismol) or loperamide (Imodium) tablets may be taken to manage symptoms of traveler's diarrhea (see Chapter 8).

Hydrocortisone 1% Cream: For topical relief of itching due to insect bites or sunburn.

Laxative: For relief of "traveler's constipation" due to changes in diet and schedule. Patients with a history of this problem may need to take a fiber supplement and/or stool softener.

Oral Rehydration Salts: WHO-ORS (Jianas Brothers, Kansas City, MO) or CeraLyte (Cera Products, Columbia, MD): packets of balanced oral rehydration salts and sugar to be mixed in purified water safe for drinking for fluid replacement and rehydration during severe diarrhea (see Chapter 8).

Throat Lozenges: For relief of throat irritation due to air pollution or upper respiratory infection.

General health and first-aid supplies

Antiseptic Solution: Topical solution for cleansing of minor cuts and abrasions (Hibiclens, Mölnlycke Health Care, Norcross, GA).

Bandages: Adhesive bandage strips with sterile pad (BandAids), 4 × 4-inch sterile gauze pads, 2-inch roll gauze dressing, 2-inch elastic bandage (Ace wrap).

Blister Pads or Moleskin: For prevention of blisters on feet

Ear Plugs: For ear protection in noisy environments and to aid sleep in the presence of snoring companions or noisy hotel accommodations.

Case (Waterproof): To hold and organize medications and supplies; zipper-lock plastic bags can serve this purpose.

Condoms (Latex): For prevention of sexually transmitted diseases.

Hand Sanitizer (Waterless) or Pre-moistened Towelettes: For hand cleansing on the go.

Insect Repellent (with DEET): For topical application to exposed areas of skin (see Tables 1.3 and 1.4).

Insecticide Spray (with Permethrin): For application to external clothing, mosquito nets, curtains, etc. (see Tables 1.3 and 1.4).

Safety Pins: Rustproof baby diaper pins are useful for all kinds of emergency repairs, pinning room curtains shut, hanging laundry on wire hangers, etc.

Continued

TABLE 1.7   The Traveler's Personal Medical Kit—cont'd

Sanitary Supplies (for Menstruating Women): Tampons and/or sanitary napkins (these may not be readily available in tropical and developing parts of the world). (See Chapter 14 for other useful components of a travel medicine kit for women.)

Scissors: For general use, if not included in pocket knife.

Skin Glue: For repair of minor lacerations, in place of sutures.

Swiss Army Knife, SOG Multi-tool, or Similar: An all-purpose gadget, especially useful if tweezers and scissors are included. (Check airline guidelines for transporting in carry-on or checked bags.)

Sunglasses: With UV light protective lenses.

Sunscreen: Any brand with sun-protective factor (SPF) sufficient to protect against UV-A and UV-B.

Tape, Duct: For general equipment repairs, creating splints, etc.

Tick Pliers: For participants in outdoor activities, to remove ticks safely and completely (see **Fig. 1.3**).

Toilet Paper: Often not available in public rest facilities when one is in desperate need (compact rolls are available in sporting supply stores).

Thermometer, Oral: Very important for assessment of illness while traveling.

Urinary Deflector or Funnel: Device allowing women to urinate from a standing position (see Chapter 14).

Water Disinfection Chemicals: See Table 1.6 and Chapter 7.

Water Disinfection Device, Portable: See Chapter 7.

[a]Trademark names are provided for identification only and do not constitute an endorsement.
[b]Dosage information applies to adults in good health without contraindications to the given drug.
PO, orally; prn, as needed.

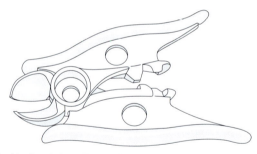

Fig. 1.3   **The tick pliers. A lightweight plastic device for safe and complete removal of ticks.**

It is important to know the female traveler's reproductive plans or if she is possibly pregnant. The physical demands and geographic factors of travel may influence the pregnancy. Additionally, certain required or recommended vaccines may be contraindicated, as may some drugs used for malaria chemoprophylaxis or for the relief of common traveler's ailments (Chapter 14).

Travelers with HIV infection need thoughtful pre-travel counseling on vaccines, potential drug interactions, geographic infectious disease hazards, and access to medical care during travel (Chapter 15). When the traveler has an underlying medical condition, travel arrangements and health recommendations become increasingly important (Chapter 16). Travelers' mental and emotional health may be challenged by being away from home, being among relative strangers, and adaptation to new dietary and cultural customs (Chapters 17-19).

If an extended stay abroad is anticipated (6 months or more), even generally healthy persons should have a routine physical examination, including routine screening laboratory tests, blood typing, and evaluation of tuberculosis status (skin test or screening chest radiograph). The long-term traveler should also have a complete dental examination. Sometimes the form and content of the pre-travel medical evaluation will be dictated by the requirements of the sponsoring employer or agency, the health insurance carrier, or even the application for a foreign student visa, foreign resident status, or a foreign work permit. Requests from foreign governments for pre-travel syphilis serology, HIV serology, examination of a stool specimen for ova and parasites, and chest radiograph are not uncommon when individuals apply for temporary residency (Chapter 18).

Diseases spread by sexual and intimate contact should also be discussed with the international traveler, especially those going abroad for an extended stay. In addition to the sexually transmitted diseases (STDs) frequently seen in Northern temperate climates (gonorrhea, syphilis, chlamydia, hepatitis B, herpes simplex, and HIV), lymphogranuloma venereum, chancroid, and granuloma inguinale are a risk in many tropical and developing countries.

The prevalence of HIV infection is many times higher than the number of acquired immunodeficiency disease syndrome (AIDS) cases reported, and the infection is present in all countries. In Africa and Asia, heterosexual intercourse is a major mode of transmission of HIV. Recent reports suggest that sexual contact with residents of developing countries occurs with surprising frequency among tourists, business travelers, and expatriate workers. International travelers need to be warned of the risk of sexual contact with strangers, regardless of sexual orientation, and particularly of contact with sex-industry workers, in whom HIV infection and other STDs are more prevalent (Chapters 41-44). Travelers who might engage in sex with new partners should be advised to purchase high-quality latex condoms and to use them during intercourse.

Finally, when the traveler returns home with a significant change in health, providers of medical care need to be acquainted with the signs and symptoms of serious tropical diseases. For example, misdiagnosis of a case of *P. falciparum* malaria as the "flu" can lead to tragic consequences for the patient, or an occult infection with *Strongyloides stercoralis* may threaten the health of a patient who has survived organ transplantation but must be maintained on immunosuppressive drugs. A patient passing a large intestinal worm, while usually not facing a life-threatening situation, may still present to an emergency room in a state of extreme anxiety and fright. An appreciation of the geographic distribution of tropical and exotic diseases and the risk factors contributing to the transmission of disease can help the healthcare provider to generate an appropriate differential diagnosis for illness occurring in the returned traveler (Chapters 3 and 20-49). A similar approach is used for the health screening of immigrants, refugees, and international adoptees, because they, too, are members of the population of international travelers (Chapter 19).

Although behavior modification and compliance with travel health recommendations may be just as important in optimizing the health of travelers as receiving travel vaccines and taking the recommended malaria chemoprophylaxis, communicating and motivating desired behavior changes among travelers seeking pre-trip medical advice is one of the biggest challenges facing travel health advisors today.

FURTHER READING

Auerbach, P.S. (Ed.), 2011. Management of Wilderness and Environmental Emergencies, sixth ed. CV Mosby Company, Baltimore.

This textbook is in its sixth edition and remains the ultimate resource for medical information on wilderness and environmental health issues. With ample illustrations and wilderness lore, it also makes fascinating reading for arm-chair adventure travelers.

CDC, 2016. CDC Health Information for International Travel—2014. Oxford University Press, New York.

Also known as "The Yellow Book," the CDC HIFIT is issued every 2 years by the Centers for Disease Control and Prevention and provides authoritative guidance for international travel health from a US public health and regulatory perspective. The Yellow Book may be purchased in print, and the content is also freely accessible at www.cdc.gov/travel and through mobile applications for Android and iOS devices. The website www.cdc.gov is an invaluable source for the latest information on global health emergencies and disease outbreaks and has links to travel and tropical medicine clinic directories maintained by the ASTMH and the ISTM.

Freedman, D.O., Weld, L.H., Kozarsky, P., et al., 2006. Spectrum of disease and relation to place of exposure among ill returned travelers. New Engl. J. Med. 354, 119–130.

Steffen, R., Rickenbach, M., Wilhelm, U., et al., 1987. Health problems after travel to developing countries. J. Infect. Dis. 156, 84–91.

Research on travel-related illnesses is difficult to conduct as travelers are on the move, becoming ill in one location and seeking care in another.

Jong, E.C., Terry, A.C., Marcolongo, T., 2016. The IAMAT Guide to Healthy Travel. International Association for Medical Assistance to Travellers (IAMAT), Toronto.

The IAMAT Guide to Healthy Travel is written to educate the traveler and features a countdown for pre-travel preparations, a check-list for travel medicine kit supplies, and a glossary of common travel ailments along with guidance for self-care. The printed booklet is pocket-sized to be taken on a trip; content may be accessed through the eLibrary at www.iamat.org.

Keystone, J.S., Freedman, D.O., Kozarsky, P. (Eds.), 2013. Travel Medicine: Expert Consult—Online and Print, third ed. Saunders, Philadelphia.

This comprehensive and detailed textbook covers all aspects of travel health and has searchable content and downloadable images at expertconsult.com. It serves as a valuable reference book for clinicians providing pre-travel services including immunizations, malaria chemoprophylaxis, and advice for traveler's diarrhea, as well as other health issues, and for those caring for returned travelers with travel-related illnesses.

Hargarten, S.W., Baker, S.P., 1985. Fatalities in the Peace Corps: a retrospective study: 1962–1983. JAMA 254, 1326–1329.

Hargarten, S.W., Baker, T.D., Guptill, K., 1991. Overseas fatalities of United States citizen travelers: an analysis of deaths related to international travel. Ann. Emerg. Med. 20 (6), 622–626.

Paixao, M.L.T., Dewar, R.D., Cossar, J.H., et al., 1991. What do Scots die of when abroad? Scott. Med. J. 36, 114–116.

Prociv, P., 1995. Deaths of Australian travelers overseas. Med. J. Aust. 163, 27–30.

Data on overseas fatalities are relatively scarce, but the four articles listed above suggest that citizen travelers can succumb to accidental trauma and pre-existing cardiovascular disease.

CHAPTER 2

Urban Medicine: Threats to Travelers to Cities in Low-Income Nations

Christopher A. Sanford

Each year, more than 50 million travelers from industrialized nations visit low-income nations. Whereas many travelers and travel providers associate international travel with rustic and sparsely peopled environments, an increasing proportion of travelers, including students and international business travelers, spend most or all of their time abroad in urban environments. Even tourists whose final destinations are rural and remote must contend with urban settings for at least portions of their trips. Tourists who visit the game reserves of East Africa often fly into Nairobi, population 3 million; travelers to the beaches of southern Thailand usually transit through Bangkok, population 8 million; and trekkers to Machu Picchu, Peru, almost always fly first to Lima, population 9 million. Travelers must survive these urban environments if they are to reach their more rustic final destinations.

During the 20th century the world population almost quadrupled, going from 1.7 billion in 1900 to 6 billion by 2000; it passed the 7 billion mark in 2012 and is projected to reach 9.6 billion in 2050. Despite acquired immune deficiency syndrome (AIDS) and widespread malnutrition, sub-Saharan Africa is anticipated to be the region of fastest growth. A 2014 UNICEF study found that a quarter of the world's children under 18 years of age lived in Africa, and this proportion will reach almost half by 2100. If current population growth continues, Africa's population will increase from 1.1 billion today to 4.2 billion in 2100.

Growth of urban centers is markedly more rapid than that of rural areas. In 2014, 54% of the world's population lived in urban areas; by 2050 this proportion is predicted to rise to 66%. An additional 2.5 billion people will be living in cities by 2050, with almost 90% of this growth anticipated to be in Asia and Africa. The rate of urban growth in the developing world almost strains credulity. As an example, in the six and a half decades between 1931 and 1995, Lagos, Nigeria, grew from 126,000 to more than 10 million inhabitants. At the present time in almost all Latin American countries, between one-quarter and one-third of the population lives in a single city.

These trends—the overall increase in population, almost all of which is occurring in the developing nations, and the increasing urbanization—combine to yield massive and rapid growth in cities. Urban conglomerations with more than 10 million inhabitants are termed "megacities." In 1950, there were two: New York City and Tokyo. By 1995 there were 14, and in 2015, 22, of which the majority are in low- and middle-income nations. If we extend the definition of megacity to include surrounding metropolitan area, there are 36 megacities, 14 of which have populations of at least 20 million (Tokyo, Delhi, Seoul, Shanghai, Mumbai, Mexico City, Beijing, Lagos, Sao Paulo, Jakarta, New York, Karachi, Osaka, and Manila). Regarding this proliferation of megacities, urbanists Peter Hall and Ulrich Pfeiffer wrote, "Humanity has not been down this road before. There are no precedents, no guideposts."

This rapid growth has accentuated a number of health problems of megacity inhabitants. Large peri-urban slums—termed *favelas* in Brazil, *bastis* in India, *pueblos jovenes* in Peru, and elsewhere slums and shantytowns—ring megacities. Generally without basic services such as water, electricity, and controlled sewage, these neighborhoods are ideal for the spread of most infectious diseases, including tuberculosis and those caused by intestinal parasites. Rapid and haphazard urban expansion is also accompanied by poverty, crime, and pollution.

Historically, travel medicine providers have emphasized risks from infectious diseases, including vaccine-preventable diseases, malaria, and traveler's diarrhea. However, only 1-3% of deaths of international travelers are due to infectious diseases. About half of all deaths of international travelers are due to cardiovascular causes, including myocardial infarction and cerebrovascular accidents; these occur primarily in elderly travelers. The remaining deaths among travelers are due to causes that mirror those found in developed countries: motor vehicle crashes, drowning, falls, and homicide.

Travelers' risks from specific threats are certainly affected by the size of the towns in which they stay, but the complex relationships between risk and level of urbanization are only beginning to be studied, described, and elucidated. Western medicine has made impressive progress in establishing links between particular infectious diseases, behaviors that place travelers at risk for those diseases, and interventions during the pre-travel consultation to lower those risks. However, establishing the benefit of interventions for non-infectious hazards, which comprise the most significant threats to the urban traveler, remains a virtually unexplored field.

In this chapter, the particular hazards and stresses that are expected in urban environments, including motor vehicle traffic, air pollution, heat illness, crime, and recreational drug use, will be considered.

INFECTIOUS DISEASES

Morbidity from infectious diseases is common in international travelers, with up to 75% of travelers becoming ill during their time abroad; these illnesses are most often self-limited episodes of diarrhea or upper respiratory illness. Almost every infectious disease for which travelers are at risk is transmitted in the urban setting. Indeed, it is easier to list infectious diseases that are not transmitted in cities than those that are. Japanese encephalitis, and bartonellosis, are among those not commonly spread in cities; however, these diseases are infrequent in travelers regardless of destination. Yellow fever is not currently endemic in urban areas, but its urban vector, the *Aedes aegypti* mosquito, is now present in urban areas of the Americas, and there is concern that yellow fever could erupt in explosive outbreaks from urban transmission cycles.

The vast majority of infectious diseases, including all the more common ones that are transmitted to international travelers, including hepatitis A, tuberculosis, and traveler's diarrhea, are vigorously transmitted in urban regions. Urban malaria is widespread throughout Asia and Africa. Many diseases, including meningococcal meningitis, are particularly associated with crowded living conditions. Zoonotic cutaneous leishmaniasis is expanding into many urban areas, including several cities in Colombia and peri-urban foci in Venezuela. In Brazil the national average dengue incidence rate is 34.5 cases per 100,000 inhabitants; in cities in Brazil the incidence rate of dengue fever can be as high as 268 cases per 100,000 inhabitants. Dengue fever in tourists is well documented. These infectious diseases are discussed in detail elsewhere in this book.

TRAUMA

Motor vehicle crashes are the most common cause of death in non-elderly travelers to the developing world. Travelers between the ages of 15 and 44 years have a two- to three-fold higher rate of death in accidents as compared with the same age group in developed nations. Males are more likely to be involved in both fatal and nonfatal accidents. A study of 309 Canadians who died abroad showed that 25% of deaths were due to accidents; motor vehicle crashes formed the biggest subgroup within the accidental death category. Accidental injury was by far the most common cause of illness and death reported for 801 visitors to Jamaica's northern coast, causing 22.3% of illness and death. Furthermore, tourists may be more likely than indigenous populations to become involved in motor vehicle crashes. In a study of tourists to Bermuda, the rate of motorcycle injuries was found to be 5.7-fold higher among tourists than among the local population. A study at a regional hospital in Corfu, Greece, showed that among residents and Greek tourists, only 15% of accidents were due to motor vehicle crashes, but among foreign tourists, 40% of accidents were due to motor vehicle crashes.

The amount of trauma attributable to driving on the opposite side of the road relative to travelers' home nations is not known but may be significant. In a study of nonfatal motor vehicle crashes in Greece, travelers from left-side-driving countries were more likely to be injured than those from right-side-driving countries. In New Zealand, the failure to drive on the left was found to be a significant factor in nonfatal motor vehicle crashes.

Travel by motor vehicle is markedly more dangerous in the developing world as measured by every metric that has been employed. The number of deaths per one billion vehicle kilometers is 3.7 in Sweden, 7.6 in the United States, and 55.9 in Brazil. Many countries probably have higher rates still, but motor vehicle crash-related mortality statistics are not collected in much of the developing world. A study performed in Ghana demonstrated that reports on fewer than 10% of pedestrian injuries were collected and tallied. An estimated 1.24 million people die each year from traffic injuries, and 25 million are permanently disabled. As bad as these statistics are, they appear to be growing worse rapidly.

The pattern of road traffic fatalities differs between developed and developing countries. In the United States, over 60% of road crash fatalities occur among drivers; in the least motorized countries, fewer than 10% of road crash fatalities occur among drivers. Most road traffic injuries in developing countries occur in urban areas, where approximately 90% of road traffic fatalities occur among passengers, pedestrians, and cyclists. Urban pedestrians alone account for 55-70% of road traffic deaths. Among children under the age of 4 years and between 5 and 14 years, the rate of death from road traffic injuries in low-income countries is six times that found in high-income countries. Those who reside in these countries are often aware of these risks. In Lagos, Nigeria, buses are known as *danfos*, "flying coffins," or *molue*, "moving morgues." A regular commuter on Lagos buses said, "Many of us know most of the buses are death traps but since we can't afford the expensive taxi fares, we have no choice but to use the buses."

A study performed in Accra, the capital of Ghana, investigated alcohol use among drivers. Of 722 drivers who were selected randomly, 21% had a blood alcohol concentration higher than 80 mg/dL, indicating impairment. This rate is significantly higher than the rates of impaired drivers in the developed world, which range from 0.4% in Denmark to 3.4% in France. Alarmingly, 3.7% of bus drivers and 8.0% of truck drivers in this Ghana study had blood alcohol concentrations of ≥80 mg/dL.

Compounding this situation, there are no formal emergency medical systems in most low-income countries. In Ghana, 70% of trauma patients travel to the hospital by taxi or bus, 22% travel by private vehicle, 5% are brought by the police, and 3% travel by ambulance. All the patients who arrived in ambulances were transfers from other hospitals; no trauma patients were brought to the hospital directly from the field by ambulance. The absence of emergency medical services in the field and limited care at medical facilities combine to yield a markedly elevated rate of death following trauma relative to the developed world. In a study by Mock and colleagues (1993), the mortality rate for patients with mid-level injury severity scores, which can be thought of as life-threatening but eminently treatable, was 6% at a level I trauma center in Seattle and 36% in Ghana—a six-fold difference.

Travelers should be advised to use seat belts whenever possible and to avoid riding in motor vehicles at night. Travel by motorcycle is less safe than travel by cars; travelers should avoid riding on motorcycles. Travelers should avoid riding in informal locations on vehicles, such as the roof of a bus or the back of an open truck. Travelers planning to rent bicycles, mopeds, or motorcycles should pack and wear appropriate helmets. Pedestrians should remain vigilant in urban settings and never assume they have the right of way. Additionally, pedestrians should not wear headphones or ear buds in urban settings.

Pre-travel providers should feel free to attempt to rearrange travelers' priorities. When travelers state that their top priority is addressing a particular (often uncommon) infectious disease, the pre-travel provider can reply, "Good question, we'll get to that; first let's discuss seat belts, helmets, and the benefits of assigning a designated driver." Additionally, the benefits of obtaining medical and evacuation insurance prior to international travel should be discussed with every traveler. The information that emergency medical evacuation alone may cost US$50,000-100,000 may motivate travelers to obtain medical and evacuation insurance prior to travel.

AIR POLLUTION

The first attempt to control air pollution occurred in 1306, when England's King Edward I banned the burning of coal in an effort to control the malodorous clouds of coal smoke above London. The ban was not enforced, and London became one of the first cities to suffer from significant air pollution. It is not necessary to memorize which foreign cities have significant air pollution; it is safe to state that virtually all large cities in the developing world have significantly polluted air. According to a 2013 World Health Organization (WHO) index, four of the 10 most polluted cities in the world are in Iran; two are in India.

The number of deaths attributable to air pollution is staggering. WHO estimates that each year ambient (outdoor) air pollution causes 3.7 million premature deaths; indoor pollution is estimated to cause 4.3 million deaths each year. The discussion below will focus on ambient air pollution. The majority of deaths attributable to outdoor air pollution—88%—occur in low- and middle-income countries, with the majority of these occurring in the WHO Western Pacific (including China) and Southeast Asia (including India) regions. Forty percent of deaths due to ambient air pollution are caused by acute lower respiratory infections, 40% to stroke, 11% to chronic obstructive pulmonary disease (COPD), 6% to lung cancer, and 3% to ischemic heart disease.

The US Environmental Protection Agency terms the six principal air pollutants "criteria pollutants"; these are carbon monoxide, nitrogen dioxide, ground-level ozone (not to be confused with "good ozone," which is in the stratosphere at 10-50 km above the earth), particulate matter (air-borne particles <10 μm in diameter), sulfur dioxide, and lead. Some medical writers have tried to compare the level of air pollution in a given city with smoking a certain number of cigarettes per day, but this is an inaccurate analogy; the pollutants and carcinogens are different. Carbon monoxide is formed by the burning of fuels, such as gasoline, oil, or wood. Persons with pulmonary and cardiac disease may develop dyspnea and angina at carboxyhemoglobin (COHB) levels of 3-4%. Exercise in a traffic tunnel will increase the COHB level to 5% within 90 min. Elevated carbon monoxide levels have been found to increase the rates of hospitalization of elderly patients with congestive heart failure.

The effects of air pollution, specifically ozone and particulate matter, on mortality and hospital admissions due to respiratory and cardiopulmonary disease have been demonstrated in both short-term studies, which have investigated day-to-day variations of pollutants, and long-term studies, which have followed cohorts of urban residents over some years. Effects have been found even at very low levels of exposure.

The developing world has no monopoly on polluted air. However, the air of urban centers in high-income nations seems pristine when compared with that of large cities in low-income nations. In high-income nations the average PM_{10} (particulate matter <10 microns), in micrograms per cubic liter, is 26; this compares with a global average of 71, an average in Southeast Asia of 128, and an average in Eastern Mediterranean countries of 208. In Jakarta, Indonesia, due to the use of leaded gasoline in most vehicles, the level of lead in the atmosphere in 2000 was 1.3 $\mu g/m^3$; the WHO's recommended maximum is between 0.5 and 1.0 $\mu g/m^3$. In Bangkok, motorcycles are popular, as they can thread through the ever-present traffic jams. Between 1993 and 2000, the number of registered motorcycles in the Bangkok metropolitan region increased from 1.1 million to 2 million; future growth is projected to be 15% per year. Some 90% of these motorcycles have two-stroke engines, which are the worst offenders with regard to suspended particulate matter and hydrocarbon emissions. The numbers of vehicles in Asian urban areas have grown exponentially over the past two decades; in Delhi and Manila, the number of vehicles has been doubling every 7 years.

Air pollution does not have to be severe to affect children with asthma. In a French study, children with mild to moderate asthma had measurable short-term decrements in pulmonary function tests that correlated with prevailing levels of photo-oxidant and particulate pollution, even though the levels of these pollutants were within those specified by international air standards.

Air polluted with particulate matter causes increased serum concentrations of fibrinogen and platelets, with sequestration of red blood cells in the lungs. Particulate matter also increases the risk of cardiac arrhythmias, but the significance of these changes for cardiovascular events remains unclear. During an exacerbation of air pollution in Augsburg, Germany, in 1985, increases were noted in residents' heart rate, plasma viscosity, and C-reactive protein, all of which can contribute to an increased risk of cardiovascular events.

Multiple studies have linked air pollution to increased mortality. A restriction that reduced the sulfur content of fuel oil utilized by power plants and road vehicles in Hong Kong led to a substantial reduction in deaths from all causes, from respiratory diseases, and from cardiovascular diseases. Long-term exposure to fine particulate air pollution causes increased cardiopulmonary morbidity, including lung cancer. A study of the 1997 "haze disaster" in Indonesia found that over 90% of 543 people interviewed had respiratory symptoms. The elderly and those with a history of asthma had increased symptoms.

Ozone is produced by the effect of sunlight on volatile organic compounds or oxides of nitrogen. In a study of children who performed in outdoor team sports in 12 communities in southern California with varying levels of pollution, ozone was the pollutant most strongly associated with the development of asthma. Ozone triggers inflammation, and animal studies suggest that it causes increased susceptibility to bacterial infection. Great variability among individuals exists regarding the response to ozone, with a minority demonstrating significant responses at only moderate levels. One study showed that for each 50 parts per billion increase in peak ozone levels, hospitalization rates increase by 6-10% for asthma, pneumonia, and COPD.

Children living in Santiago, Chile, were found to have increases in lower respiratory tract illnesses in direct proportion to the levels of particulate matter and ozone. For children 3-15 years of age, the increase in lower respiratory tract symptoms is 3-9% for a 50 $\mu g/m^3$ change in particulate matter and 5% for a 50 parts per billion change in ozone. A study performed in India found that urban children had a higher level of exercise-induced bronchospasm than did children living in rural areas. A recent study performed in southern California found that associations between severity of air pollution and asthma were stronger in asthmatic children not taking anti-inflammatories (inhaled cromolyn, nedocromil sodium, or corticosteroids) than in children who were.

A Denver, Colorado, study found strong associations between rates of childhood cancers including leukemia, and distance of residence from streets with a high density of motor vehicles. In the highest traffic density category, that of close proximity to roads with >20,000 vehicles/day, the odds ratio for all cancers was 5.90, and that for leukemia was 8.28. In Amsterdam, a much higher relative risk of death was found in individuals who lived on main roads, as compared with those who lived away from main roads. Recent epidemiological research indicates that the effects of air pollution on life expectancy are not uniformly distributed throughout populations but are influenced by factors including education level and antioxidant vitamin status. Intriguingly, the use of antioxidant vitamin supplementation has been found to markedly reduce the ozone-induced reduction in pulmonary function in young, healthy, nonsmoking adults.

It is reasonable to assume that long-term visitors to heavily polluted cities will develop many of the same sequelae as do residents. The effects of air pollution on the short-term traveler have not been studied; anecdotally, many develop eye and respiratory irritation. What are the implications for providers of pre-travel medical advice? Patients with COPD should travel with a "rescue cocktail" of three drugs for use during exacerbations: an additional bronchodilator, an oral steroid, and an appropriate antibiotic. Patients with asthma, particularly those with a history of exacerbation in response to air pollution, should carry an additional inhaler and an oral steroid. The possible benefits of placing asthmatic children on an antiinflammatory medication, for example, montelukast sodium (Singulair), just prior to and during their stay in a heavily polluted region should be considered. For elderly travelers, a pre-travel physical examination with pulmonary function tests may be useful in screening for pulmonary disease. Certainly, travelers with diagnosed cardiac or pulmonary disease should have these conditions adequately controlled prior to departure and should be advised to minimize their duration of stay in heavily polluted cities, to avoid heavy exercise while residing therein, and to have a low threshold for seeking medical care should they become dyspneic or develop chest pain (Chapter 16).

HEAT ILLNESS

Like mountains, cities are capable of creating their own weather. Asphalt and concrete absorb light then re-radiate it as infrared radiation, raising the temperature of the air; this is termed the "urban heat island effect." Many cities are 1-6°C warmer than surrounding rural areas; this urban-rural temperature difference is greatest at night. Plants, particularly trees, secrete large amounts of water from their leaves, and the evaporation of this water absorbs significant heat; thus urban heat is compounded both by the presence of asphalt and concrete surfaces and the absence of vegetation.

Every year there are approximately 400 deaths in the United States that are attributed to excessive heat. Multiple studies have shown that the elderly, particularly women, and the mentally ill are at increased risk for serious heat illness, including heat exhaustion, heat stroke, and death. The heightened susceptibility of the elderly is due to dysfunctional thermoregulatory mechanisms, chronic dehydration, medications, and diseases involving the systems that regulate body temperature. Additionally, some individuals may be genetically predisposed to a higher risk of exertional heat illness and malignant hyperthermia. Many drugs, including phenothiazines, anticholinergics, diuretics, beta-blockers, and alcohol, can impair thermoregulation (Chapter 9).

A Spanish study that investigated heat waves in Madrid between 1986 and 1997 found that mortality increased by 28% for every degree Celsius by which the temperature rose above 36.5°C; women above 75 years of age were most heavily affected. Another Spanish study investigated the effect of heat on mortality in Seville, which is known for its hot summers. All-cause mortality increased by up to 51% above the average in those over 75 years of age for each degree Celsius above 41°C. This was more pronounced for cardiovascular diseases than for pulmonary diseases, and, as with the Madrid study, it affected more women than men.

A study on heat-related deaths in London found that mortality due to heat began at a relatively low temperature and that there was a 3.4% increase in deaths for every 1 degree Celsius over 21.5°C. In a case study of six cases of classic heat stroke seen at a Taiwan emergency department, the most frequent co-morbid conditions were hypertension (4/6) and mental illness (3/6). All six patients were middle class and were not socially isolated. Most avoided cool air and avoided staying in air-conditioned rooms.

Mean surface temperatures in the tropics are expected to rise between 1°C and 3°C by 2050. The combination of increasing urbanization and global warming will lead to bigger, hotter cities that will alter the distribution and intensity of both infectious and chronic diseases in their inhabitants.

The combination of increasing urbanization, leading to higher temperatures, and the increasing age of tourists, leading to increased susceptibility, will probably make heat-related illness in urban travelers increasingly common. Travelers should be warned that cities are warmer than surrounding rural regions. Additionally, travelers should know that in humid regions, "sweat doesn't work"; it does not evaporate, and hence does not cause cooling but only leads to fluid loss. Adequate hydration and limiting exposure to the mid-day heat are thought to be protective. Travelers need to be aware that thirst is not always a reliable indicator of hydration status; they should drink sufficient fluids such that urination occurs at normal frequency, and urine is near-colorless. For the elderly or those with chronic pulmonary or cardiac conditions, minimizing the duration of stay in particularly hot cities (e.g., airport transfer only) may be the wiser option.

CRIME AND SECURITY

Personal safety is an often neglected area in pre-travel counseling but is, as Leggat and Klein (2001) state, "one of the most important areas for travel health advisors to cover when giving advice for travelers going to virtually any country." A study that investigated the health problems of medical students at the University of Tasmania, Australia, during overseas rotations concluded that "assaults ... and harassment are of increasing concern, and students need pre-travel counseling on how to avoid getting into dangerous situations." In a study of travel claims made by travelers from Australia, theft and assault combined to make up 12% of all claims, placing crime as the third most common reason for claims, behind "general medical" and "loss." Urban crime is multifactorial; overpopulation and poverty are key factors.

Street crime is common in large cities around the world. Travelers from high-income nations are viewed as relatively wealthy. Travelers should avoid wearing expensive jewelry or watches and to carry no more cash than they need for the day. "Bum bags" or "fanny packs" are thought to be high-risk, as these can represent "one-stop shopping centers" for muggers. Travelers should not accept food or drinks from strangers, as the drug-and-rob strategy is a not uncommon scam. If robbed, travelers should not resist and should report the theft to the local authorities.

Urban travelers should be aware of the "mustard scam" in which a substance is squirted onto the clothes of a traveler; a seemingly helpful local then wipes off the substance while picking the traveler's pockets. As a precaution, valuables can be kept under the clothes in a belt around the traveler's waist or in a safety pouch hung around the neck. Should travelers experience unexpected substances spilled on their clothing, they should walk away and refuse offers of aid in cleaning. Hotel safes are generally secure, and their use for storage of all important documents and other belongings should be encouraged, although travelers should be aware that there is usually a limit to a hotel's liability regarding theft. Particularly valuable items should be left at home.

The slash and grab technique is also common in the urban centers of the developing world; the thief slices a slit in the bottom of a traveler's purse or backpack, then grabs whatever falls out. Some backpackers in cities with a high rate of slash and grab thieves, for example, Rio de Janeiro, take the ungainly but often effective measure of wrapping their backpacks with metal mesh wire.

The global annual homicide rate is 7.6 homicides per 100,000 inhabitants. There is marked variation between countries; respective rates for selected nations are shown in **Table 2.1.**

A study by Hargarten et al. (1991) found that 9% of fatalities among American travelers overseas are due to homicide. A Canadian study found that of a similar percentage of deaths of Canadian travelers who died abroad, 8%, were due to homicide. The US State Depart ment maintains a regularly updated listing of Consular Information Sheets, Travel Warnings, and Public Announcements for all foreign countries at its Bureau of Consular Affairs website (www.travel.state.gov). Travelers should be encouraged to check this site on a regular basis, both prior to and, if possible, during their travels. Travelers should be reminded that war,

TABLE 2.1   Annual Homicide Rate, Selected Countries, per 100,000 Residents

Country	Homicide Rate
Germany	0.8
United Kingdom	1.0
Canada	1.6
United States	4.7
Mexico	21.5
Democratic Republic of Congo	28.3
Jamaica	39.3
Honduras	90.4

major internal strife, and natural disasters are not spectator events; countries with significant turmoil should be avoided. Street demonstrations in many low-income nations can turn violent with little notice; travelers should be advised to not photograph or join protests.

Wearing clothes with a military appearance, for example, camouflage-pattern fatigues, is unwise in low-income nations. Many low-income nations have a history of unwelcome military intervention in their recent past, and travelers dressed in garb that strikes residents as being reminiscent of armed forces may draw unwelcome attention. Tourists should avoid photographing buildings or other subjects with security implications (e.g., police barracks, military maneuvers) in countries with recent or current civil unrest. A good rule of thumb is that if uniformed soldiers or policemen are in sight, the tourist should ask permission prior to taking photographs. If the soldier or policeman says "yes," the tourist may click away with impunity; if "no," the traveler should put the camera away. Photographing sensitive subjects can lead to, at a minimum, impoundment and/or destruction of the camera and its film or digital memory card, if not a several-hour session of answering questions as to why the tourist was taking those particular photos.

Kidnapping of international travelers has recently increased; employees of international and nongovernmental organizations are at higher risk. The use of licensed taxis is preferable to the use of more informal ones. Hotels have a vested interest in their guests not being the victims of crime; asking a hotel to call a taxi, as opposed to hailing one randomly on the street, reduces the risk of robbery and kidnapping. Although tourists are not generally a target for terrorist attacks, the bombing of a tourist bus in Luxor in November 1997, which killed 58 people, was a notable exception.

Travelers should inform family and their local embassy of their arrival and itinerary and carry a mobile phone if possible. A key point to stress to travelers is that crime and accidents are not random; risk can be reduced by cautious strategies. The need for travelers to be informed and wary is increasing, as fewer people are traveling in package tours but are instead creating their own itineraries. Although some strategies employed by criminals, for example, the mustard scam or slash and grab robbery, are associated more with urban centers than with rural areas, the incidence of tourists who are victims of crime in urban areas as opposed to rural regions is unknown.

ILLICIT DRUG USE

The use of illicit psychotropic drugs by travelers is common. Potasman et al. (2000) found that among 2500 long-term young travelers to the tropics, 22.2% used recreational drugs. In the study by Beny et al. (2001) regarding psychiatric problems in returned travelers seen at an Israeli clinic, 8 of 15 patients had used illicit drugs while abroad.

Whereas the link between alcohol and tourist injuries as a result of balcony falls and diving accidents has been documented, there are no studies investigating the impact of illicit drugs on tourist accidents. A study that investigated psychiatric interventions for Japanese nationals in New York, New York, suggested that substance abuse disorders were common in those who required emergency psychiatric care.

Informing travelers of the draconian penalties for possessing illegal drugs in many developing nations may have some deterrence value. One-third of the 2500 US citizens who are arrested overseas each year are arrested for drug offenses. A number of countries, including the Bahamas, the Dominican Republic, Jamaica, Mexico, and the Philippines, have enacted more stringent drug laws that impose mandatory jail sentences for individuals convicted of possessing even small amounts of marijuana or cocaine for personal use. Many European countries, including Austria, France, Greece, Ireland, Luxembourg, and the United Kingdom, may impose a life sentence for narcotic trafficking. The death penalty remains an option in several countries (including Malaysia, Pakistan, and Turkey) for those convicted of smuggling illicit drugs.

CONCLUSION

Cities contain the best and the worst of humankind; they are fascinating in and of themselves, and transiting through urban conglomerations is necessary for visiting many of the remote and sublime regions of the world. The author of this chapter would not recommend that travelers avoid travel therein.

Nor is it the intent of this chapter to trivialize the importance of infectious threats to travelers. These diseases, most notably malaria, traveler's diarrhea, and vaccine-preventable diseases, can cause significant illness and must be addressed with every traveler. However, given that the raison d'être of the pre-travel encounter is risk reduction, pre-travel healthcare providers must attempt to address other major risks to health, including road traffic injuries. It should be stressed that the morbidity and mortality among travelers is not random but can be influenced by a traveler's attention to personal safety and environmental conditions. Appropriate pre-travel advice can increase the odds that travelers to cities in low-income nations will return home with fond memories, enlightenment, and a desire for further travel in the nonwealthy regions of the world.

FURTHER READING

Burkart, K., Khan, M.M., Schneider, A., et al., 2014. The effects of season and meteorology on human mortality in tropical climates: a systematic review. Trans. R. Soc. Trop. Med. Hyg. 100, 393–401.
A cogent discussion of the effects of increasing temperature and urbanization on the burden of disease.

The Economist. Africa's population: can it survive such speedy growth? August 23, 2014. Available at <http://www.economist.com/news/middle-east-and-africa/21613349-end-century-almost-half-worlds-children-may-be-african-can-it>.
This article discusses the current and projected high rate of population growth in Africa.

Geneva Declaration of Armed Violence Report. September 2008, p. 67. Available at <www.genevadeclaration.org> (accessed April 6, 2015).
This document summarizes global armed violence.

The Guardian, 2014. Iran's government steps up efforts to tackle pollution. Available at <http://www.theguardian.com/world/iran-blog/2014/mar/10/irans-government-steps-up-efforts-to-tackle-pollution> (accessed April 6, 2015).
This article notes that sub-standard gasoline for motor vehicles is a major source of Iran's urban air pollution.

Hargarten, S.W., Baker, T.D., Guptill, K., 1991. Overseas fatalities of United States citizen travelers: an analysis of deaths related to international travel. Ann. Emerg. Med. 20, 622–626.
This study of death certificates found that after cerebrovascular accidents, motor vehicle injury was the greatest cause of death of international travelers.

Mock, C.N., Adzotor, K.E., Conklin, E., et al., 1993. Trauma outcomes in the rural developing world: comparison with an urban level I trauma center. J. Trauma 4, 518–523.
This study found that the rate of death for similar levels of injury is markedly higher in Ghana than at a level I trauma center in the United States.

Potasman, I., Beny, A., Seligmann, H., 2000. Neuropsychiatric problems in 2,500 long-term young travelers to the tropics. J. Travel Med. 7, 225–226.
This study found that neuropsychiatric problems are common in young travelers to the tropics.

Stocker, T.F., Qin, D., Plattner, G.-K., et al., 2013. Climate Change 2013: The Physical Science Basis. Intergovernmental Panel on Climate Change, Working Group I Contribution to the IPCC Fifth Assessment Report (ARS). Cambridge University Press, New York.
This report details the extensive evidence for global climate change.

United Nations, 2014. World Urbanization Prospects: The 2014 Revision, Highlights (St/SER.A/352). United Nations DoEaSA; Population Division, New York. Available at <http://esa.un.org/unpd/wup/Highlights/WUP2014-Highlights.pdf>.
This report summarizes the rapid urbanization of recent years, with projections regarding future urban growth.

United Nations Office on Drugs and Crime (UNODC). Global Study on Homicide—Data: UNOCD Homicide Statistics 2013. Available at <http://www.unodc.org/gsh/>.(accessed April 6, 2015).
A detailed report on homicide related to other criminal activities, interpersonal homicide, and socio-political homicide.

WHO. Burden of Disease from Ambient Air Pollution for 2012. Available at <http://www.who.int/phe/health_topics/outdoorair/databases/AAP_BoD_results_March2014.pdf?ua=1>.
This report summarizes the global burden of ambient (outdoor) air pollution.

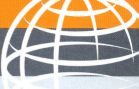

CHAPTER 3

Emerging Infectious Diseases and the International Traveler

Camilla Rothe and Elaine C. Jong

In 1992 a landmark report by the Institute of Medicine titled "Emerging Infections: Microbial Threats to Health in the United States" highlighted the importance of the often underappreciated concept of emerging infectious diseases (EIDs). This report brought EIDs back into scientific discourse; however, the awareness that diseases emerge and periodically reemerge goes back millenia, as Morens and colleagues (2008) highlight in their historical review.

The term "emerging infectious diseases" is broad. It covers newly recognized human diseases caused by pathogens that have recently jumped species as well as older pathogens that have emerged in new populations due to changes in human behavior or modifications to natural habitats. It also encompasses older pathogens that are reemerging in areas once brought under control, often due to microbiological adaptation or breakdown of public health measures. An overview of recent travel-related EIDs in the 21st century is given in **Table 3.1**.

According to a recent comprehensive literature review by Taylor et al. (2001), more than 1400 species of infectious organisms known to be pathogenic to humans were identified. Around 175 pathogenic species were associated with diseases considered to be emerging, and of these, 75% were zoonotic. Causal factors contributing to the emergence of new pathogens include human population growth resulting in human encroachment on wildlife habitats, increased human contact with domestic and wild animals, changes in agricultural practices, and globalization of food markets.

Travelers are an important factor in the global dissemination of EIDs due to the increased frequency and speed of both local and international travel. International travelers may have been in direct or indirect contact with previously isolated, remote populations and ecosystems. The challenge is that travelers returning home may harbor exotic infections that are still in the incubation stage. During the acute stage of illness, nonspecific flu-like clinical signs and symptoms may not suggest the correct diagnosis to local healthcare providers. Thus, infections acquired during travel may be transmitted to others in the community by returned travelers before the diagnosis can be made. In addition to international travelers, imported animals, birds, foods, and insects from abroad, especially from tropical developing countries, can also pose a significant threat to the public health of receiving countries by serving as means of transportation for pathogens into new geographic areas.

APPROACH TO INTERNATIONAL TRAVELERS

The burden of detection of imported infectious diseases among returning travelers is most likely to fall on primary healthcare providers who initially see the ill traveler, and the public health officials to whom they report. In the 21st century, all persons presenting for diagnosis and treatment of an acute illness should be asked, "Where have you traveled?" as part of **27**

TABLE 3.1 Examples of Travel-Associated Emerging and Reemerging Infections in the 21st Century

Year	Travel-Related Emerging Diseases in the 21st Century
2003	Global outbreak of severe acute respiratory syndrome (SARS) caused by a novel coronavirus. SARS was spread by travelers to 30 countries on five continents.
2005-2007	Reemergence of chikungunya fever leads to a large outbreak, affecting the islands in the Indian Ocean and large parts of South and Southeast Asia (1). The spread is facilitated by adaptation of the chikungunya virus (CHIKV) to a new vector, *Aedes albopictus*. Imported cases in Italy and France prompt autochthonous infections in both countries (2). CHIKV infections are confirmed in travelers returning to Europe, Australia, the United Kingdom, and the United States.
2008	First outbreak of Lujo hemorrhagic fever. The novel arenavirus is named after the origin of the index patient, a travel agent from Lusaka who was airlifted to Johannesburg for treatment, causing several further cases through nosocomial spread.
2009-2010	"Swine flu pandemic" caused by influenza A (H1N1). A virulent variant of H1N1 had also caused the Spanish flu in 1918-1919, killing tens of millions of people worldwide.
2011-2012	Outbreak of acute muscular sarcocystosis among international travelers returning from Tioman Island, Malaysia (3).
2012-2013	First recorded outbreak of Middle Eastern respiratory syndrome caused by a novel coronavirus (MERS-CoV).
2012-2014	Outbreak of schistosomiasis in German and Canadian travelers returning from Corsica (France).
2013-2015	First recorded chikungunya outbreak in the Western hemisphere starts from the Caribbean Islands, spreading to the United States, Latin America, and French Polynesia.
2013-2014	Zika virus outbreaks in the Western Pacific and Southeast Asia lead to a number of imported infections in international travelers.
2014	Fatal case of influenza (H5N1) in a Canadian traveler returning from China.
2014	Chikungunya virus imported by a traveler from Cameroon into France leads to 14 autochthonous cases (4).
2014-2015	Large Ebola Zaire outbreak in Guinea, Liberia, and Sierra Leone. A Liberian traveler visiting friends and relatives imports Ebola into the United States, causing two consecutive cases among healthcare workers.
2015	First case of influenza A (H7N9) outside China found in a Chinese traveler to Malaysia.
2015	Zika virus cases documented in South America for the first time.

Sources
1. Burt, F.J., Rolph, M.S., Rulli, N.E., Mahalingam, S., Heise, M.T., 2012. Chikungunya: a re-emerging virus. Lancet 379 (9816), 662–671.
2. Tomasello, D., Schlagenhauf, P., 2013. Chikungunya and dengue autochthonous cases in Europe, 2007-2012. Travel Med. Infect. Dis. 11 (5), 274–284.
3. Esposito, D.H., Stich, A., Epelboin, L., Malvy, D., Han, P.V., Bottieau, E., et al., 2014. Acute muscular sarcocystosis: an international investigation among ill travelers returning from Tioman Island, Malaysia, 2011–2012. Clin. Infect. Dis. 59 (10), 1401–1410.
4. Delisle, E., Rousseau, C., Broche, B., Leparc-Goffart, I., L'Ambert, G., Cochet, A., et al. 2015. Chikungunya outbreak in Montpellier, France, September to October 2014. Euro. Surveill. 20 (17), pii:21108.

the routine medical history, since so many individuals in our global society have traveled to or may have originated in tropical developing areas.

The travel history should be as specific as possible in terms of the cities and areas of each country visited. Activities and exposures, such as swimming in freshwater lakes or rivers, walking barefoot on beaches or muddy trails, receiving many insect bites, eating raw or exotic foods, drinking unsafe water or beverages with ice cubes in countries with low sanitation, and close/intimate contact with new partners should also be subject to inquiry. Since most of the EIDs are specifically discussed in other chapters of this book, the purpose of this chapter is to provide a conceptual framework for their consideration and recognition.

EMERGING AND REEMERGING ZOONOSES

Many factors are responsible for emergence of infectious pathogens that originate in wild animals. These include travel into previously uninhabited areas, changes in land use and demographic patterns with disruption of stable ecosystems, greater contact with previously isolated animal populations, changing agricultural practices that allow transfer of pathogens between wild and domestic animals, and food customs that involve hunting, butchering, and ingesting wild game including nonhuman primates (bush meat).

Two transmission patterns have been described for transmission of pathogens from wild animals to humans. One pattern consists of rare events when direct animal-to-human transmission of an animal pathogen occurs, but then direct human-to-human transmission maintains the infection in the human population for a limited time or permanently. Examples of diseases with this transmission pattern are human immunodeficiency virus (HIV), influenza A, Ebola virus, and severe acute respiratory syndrome (SARS).

The second pattern of transmission is where human infections with animal pathogens result from repeated episodes of direct animal-to-human transmission or repeated vector-mediated animal-to-human transmission, and the infections are not usually propagated by human-to-human transmission. Examples of diseases with this transmission pattern are rabies and other lyssa viruses, Nipah virus, West Nile virus, Hantavirus, Lyme borreliosis, tularemia, leptospirosis, and ehrlichiosis.

VECTOR-BORNE DISEASES

Many emerging infections are vector-borne diseases. When competent vectors such as mosquitoes, ticks, and fleas preexist in a geographic environment, movement of infected human or animal hosts into that area can lead to rapid expansion of transmission.

West Nile Virus

A prime example of an emerging vector-borne disease was the spread of West Nile virus in North America, transmitted from birds to humans and horses by *Culex* mosquito vectors. Following the initial 1999 detection of the agent in Queens, New York, the new pathogen (thought to have been introduced by an infected human traveler or migrant bird) spread rapidly across the continental United States from coast-to-coast within 5 years—affecting human activities, veterinary practices, and blood-banking guidelines in the wake of its spread (**Fig. 3.1**).

Chikungunya Virus

One of the most important emerging vector-borne viruses in the recent years has been chikungunya virus (CHIKV). The alphavirus is transmitted to humans by the bite of infected daytime-biting *Aedes* mosquitos, mainly *Aedes aegypti* and, since more recently, *Ae. albopictus*. The disease has been reported among travelers returning from endemic areas as a cause of acute illness characterized by sudden onset of fever, chills, severe joint pain with or without swelling, lower back pain, and a maculopapular rash, similar to the symptoms of dengue fever. In some CHIKV patients, residual joint pain and impairment persists for months and even years after the acute illness, leading to considerable morbidity.

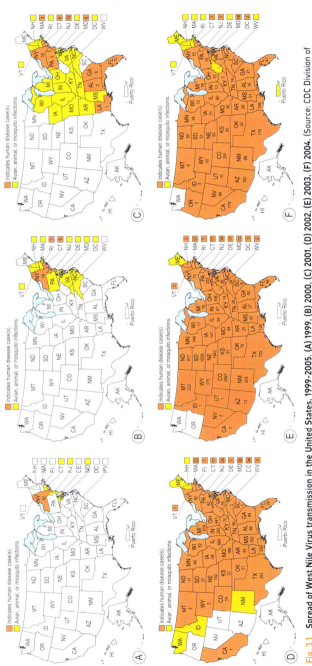

Fig. 3.1 **Spread of West Nile Virus transmission in the United States, 1999-2005.** (A) 1999, (B) 2000, (C) 2001, (D) 2002, (E) 2003, (F) 2004. (Source: CDC Division of Vector-Borne Infectious Diseases. Online. Available at http://www.cdc.gov/ncidod/dvbid/westnile/mapactivity/surv&control.htm#maps. Accessed 03/24/2008.)

As reviewed by Weaver et al. (2015) a large outbreak of chikungunya emerged in 2004 in coastal Kenya; in 2005 it spread to the Indian Ocean islands and subsequently to India and many countries in Southeast Asia, causing several million cases. In 2007 cases of chikungunya were first reported from Europe: infected air travelers imported the disease into France and Italy, which led to local autochthonous transmission. It turned out that the virus had adapted to a new vector, *Aedes albopictus*, facilitating viral spread to an even wider geographic region. Further factors contributing to the magnitude of the outbreak were an increase in air travel to and from affected areas, previous lack of exposure to the virus of the newly involved populations, and spread of *Ae. albopictus* from its native Asia to islands of the Indian Ocean basin and to Southern Europe. In 2013 a further large outbreak originated on the Caribbean island of St. Martin. It rapidly spread through the Caribbean, to the United States, to Latin America, and to French Polynesia, causing several million cases. This was the first time a chikungunya outbreak had officially been recorded in the Western hemisphere.

Zika Virus

Another emerging virus transmitted by *Aedes* spp. is Zika virus (ZIKV). Zika is a flavivirus that causes a clinical picture indistinguishable from chikungunya or dengue. Even though it usually causes a mild illness, the development of subsequent Guillain Barré syndrome has been reported in a number of cases. Zika was known to be endemic in Africa and Southeast Asia. In 2007, an outbreak of Zika virus infection occured on Yap island (Micronesia). These were the first recognized cases outside Africa and Asia. The emergence of ZIKV on the isolated island community showed the potential of the virus to spread through commerce and travel across long distances. An even larger outbreak occurred in 2013-2014 in French Polynesia, causing an estimated 32,000 cases and spreading within the region. In the context of this outbreak, cases related to international travel were reported by Zammarchi et al. (2015) in two Japanese, one Norwegian, and two Italian travelers. A number of further travel-related cases of Zika virus were reported. Interestingly, one scientist returning to the United States from Cameroon with ZIKV later infected his wife, probably by sexual transmission, as discussed by Foy et al. (2011). In 2015, Zika was first detected in Brazil, leading to autochthonous transmission of the virus.

Dengue Virus

Dengue fever virus is the most common arbovirus infection among international travelers to endemic regions (Chapter 21). Its incidence has increased 30-fold in the past 50 years due to international trade and travel as well as failing public health measures. Dengue is also on the rise in formerly non-endemic areas such as Europe and East Asia as a consequence of increasing migration, the tourist industry, international trade, and demographic changes. Quam et al. (2015) show an increasing trend of imported dengue into Italy and project a further fourfold increase by 2020. Recent dengue fever virus outbreaks as reported by Knope et al. (2013) in Australia, China, Japan, France, and Italy were linked to importation of the virus in infected travelers and the presence of *Aedes* mosquitoes in the local environment, which promoted subsequent human-to-human spread in the local populations.

P. knowlesi Malaria

A growing number of travelers from industrialized countries are visiting malaria-endemic areas annually. Nevertheless, the number of malaria cases recorded in international travelers is decreasing. Emerging, however, is the number of cases of *Plasmodium knowlesi* malaria seen in travelers. *P. knowlesi* was first described in the 1920s as a simian malaria parasite, and it was not known to infect humans until the 1960s when it was found in malaria patients in Malaysia. This led to its recognition as the fifth human malaria parasite. In 2006 it first appeared in the context of travel medicine when a Swedish traveler returning from Malaysia was diagnosed with *P. knowlesi* infection. Muller et al. (2014) in their review highlight several reports of imported *P. knowlesi* cases in travelers from all over the world. *P. knowlesi* is not geographically restricted to Malaysia but was also found in Vietnam,

Singapore, Thailand, Cambodia, and the Philippines and may well occur in jungle or forest areas in other countries of the region. On microscopy *P. knowlesi* closely resembles *Plasmodium malariae*. It is therefore not completely clear if the parasite is truly emerging or has rather been misclassified in the past. Travel in or near forested areas is considered a risk factor. Cases are mostly mild, but severe and fatal cases have been reported (Chapter 20).

Artemisinin-Resistant *P. falciparum* Malaria

Emergence of artemisinin resistance among *Plasmodium falciparum* strains has been reported from the Thai-Cambodian border. Few published cases so far document artemisinin-resistant *P. falciparum* malaria in returning travelers, although, interestingly, some are found in travelers returning from Sub-Saharan Africa and not from the known high-risk areas in Southeast Asia, as Van Hong et al. (2014) report.

Lyme Borreliosis

Increased case numbers of Lyme borreliosis (*Borreliaburgdorferi*) in North America have been reported over the past decade. Causal factors include increasing populations of humans as well as animal reservoirs (white-footed mice, white-tailed deer, *Ixodes* ticks) and mutual encroachment on traditional habitats. These have resulted in expanded opportunities for tick-borne transmission of Lyme borreliosis in suburban areas close to human dwellings as well as in the recognized transmission risk areas of grasslands and shrubs at the edge of forests (Chapter 24).

AIR-BORNE DISEASES

Pathogens that are transmitted directly or indirectly through aerosolized droplets have huge potential for rapid global spread. Disease transmission of air-borne pathogens may occur whenever a susceptible person is in close proximity to an infectious person, and wherever large groups of people are crowded together. Additionally, direct inoculation from contaminated fingers to mucosal surfaces of the mouth, nose, and eyes is probably as significant as droplet inhalation in transmission of respiratory viruses. Personal hygiene measures including frequent hand cleansing and respiratory etiquette can help prevent the spread of infections. Continued public health guidance and a legislative framework for implementation of mandatory screening, isolation, and quarantine of travelers meeting infectious case definitions are necessary to prevent transmission and prevent outbreaks.

SARS-CoV

Severe acute respiratory syndrome coronavirus (SARS-CoV), spread by travelers to 30 countries on five continents in 2003, was termed by Heymann et al. (2013) the "first pandemic of the 21st century." The SARS pandemic illustrated the pivotal role of international travelers in the rapid global spread of an air-borne EID and showed the challenges of detecting and detaining infectious individuals. Al-Tawfiq et al. (2014) point out that in addition to significant morbidity and mortality, the SARS pandemic resulted in economic costs of an estimated 100 billion USD.

MERS-CoV

In 2012 another novel virus closely related to SARS was discovered in the Kingdom of Saudi Arabia (KSA) named Middle Eastern respiratory syndrome coronavirus (MERS-CoV).

Great concern arose since the KSA hosts two of the largest mass gatherings worldwide every year, namely the Hajj and Umrah pilgrimages. So far no case of MERS-CoV could be linked to one of these events. However, MERS-CoV was detected in travelers from the Saudi Arabian peninsula to more than a dozen countries in Northern Africa, Europe, Asia, and North America. MERS-CoV is a zoonotic virus and infection primarily occurs through contact with camel or camel products. Embarek et al. (2015) point out that the risk of human-to-human spread is considered low outside healthcare settings, and so far no sustained onward transmission to persons in contact with infected travelers on aircraft has been reported.

Other examples of pathogens in this group are influenza A, including avian influenza (H5N1 and H7N9), measles, and tuberculosis.

FOOD- AND WATER-BORNE DISEASES

Changes in animal production systems and in the food production chain are thought to be among the main factors causing emergence of food-borne zoonoses. The most important food-borne zoonotic pathogens include *Salmonella* spp., *Campylobacter* spp., enterohemorrhagic *Escherichia coli*, *Giardia lamblia*, and *Cryptosporidium parvum*. Whether these pathogens are just common or truly "emerging" in travelers is difficult to assess, since most data from travel-related surveillance networks lack a clear denominator.

New pathogens of fecal origin can lead to water-borne outbreaks when water supplies are contaminated through wildlife or domestic animal feces. If contaminated water supplies are used for agricultural production, transmission of pathogens of zoonotic origin can occur through human ingestion of contaminated fruits and vegetables.

Sarcocystosis

One recent example of an emerging zoonotic food- or water-borne disease is sarcocystosis, caused by an intracellular coccidian parasite of the genus *Sarcocystis*. A large outbreak of acute muscular sarcocystosis occurred in 2011-2012 among tourists on Tioman Island (Malaysia). The travelers who presented with fever and severe myalgias were found to have marked eosinophilia and raised creatine kinase levels. The muscle biopsy from six of the patients was histologically diagnostic for acute muscular sarcocystosis, and DNA of the snake-associated parasite *Sarcocystis nesbitii* could be isolated in one case. Two international travel surveillance programs, GeoSentinel and TropNet, contributed greatly to the investigation of the outbreak, alerting their network members and thereby facilitating the identification of further cases of this otherwise rarely reported zoonotic disease.

Acute muscular sarcocystosis is usually caused by ingestion of sporocyst-containing food or water contaminated with feces from infected carnivorous final hosts (e.g., cats, snakes, humans). The source of infection in the case of the Tioman Island outbreak remained unclear; however, almost all travelers reported potential exposure to untreated water. Another series of cases was suspected in travelers returning to Germany from the same island, as Tappe et al. (2014) report.

Prevention of food-borne and water-borne diseases involves personal precautions and further development and implementation of food safety programs. Individual travelers can reduce their personal risk of exposure by selection of safe foods and beverages (see Chapter 8). Nations can improve the safety of their food and water supplies by adopting integrated approaches to food safety and designating a responsible authority to assure compliance. The Food and Agriculture Organization (FAO)/World Health Organization (WHO) have recently established a new framework of microbiologic risk assessment to guide efforts of member countries in reducing pathogen contamination at relevant points in food production chains.

OTHER

S. haematobium Urinary Schistosomiasis

An outbreak of urinary schistosomiasis was reported in 2013-2014 from a non-endemic area in Corsica (France) affecting several German, French, and Canadian travelers. The parasite, *Schistosoma haematobium*, had presumably been introduced from the African continent by a traveler or migrant (Chapter 48). The species of water snail required to maintain the infection cycle was later found in the Cavu river, where the affected travelers had bathed, as highlighted in a case series from Gautret et al. (2015).

Ebola Virus

See Chapter 28, "Viral Hemorrhagic Fever."

TABLE 3.2   Important Sources in Emerging Travel-Related Diseases: Emerging Diseases, Outbreaks, and Surveillance News

Source	URL
CDC Health Alert Network	http://www2a.cdc.gov/HAN/ArchiveSys/
CDC MMWR Weekly Surveillance and Summaries	http://www.cdc.gov/mmwr
European Centre for Disease Prevention and Control (ECDC)	http://www.ecdc.europa.eu/en/Pages/home.aspx
Eurosurveillance	http://www.eurosurveillance.org/
GeoSentinel Surveillance Network	http://www.geosentinel.org
HealthMap	http://www.healthmap.org
ProMed Mail	http://www.promed.org
UK Health Protection Report	http://www.hpa.org.uk/hpr/
WHO Global Response and Alert	http://www.who.int/csr/en
WHO Global Response and Alert Outbreak News	http://www.who.int/csr/don/en/
WHO Weekly Epidemiological Record	http://www.who.int/wer/

INFORMATION RESOURCES FOR EMERGING INFECTIOUS DISEASES

Numerous EIDs, some of which constitute potential risks to international travelers, are discussed in the journal *Emerging Infectious Diseases*, published by the Centers for Disease Control and Prevention (CDC) in the United States. Several hundred emerging infections have been mentioned in the Federation of American Scientists' Program for Monitoring Emerging Diseases (ProMED), which is a simple bulletin board system that contains the most up-to-date reports of disease outbreaks. Bulletins are sent out via electronic mail, and free subscriptions are available by registering your e-mail address at the website (see **Table 3.2** for these and further sources).

The world is dynamic, and what happens in one area can rapidly affect other areas at great distances. This has enormous implications for travel medicine, since a disease that is endemic in one area can rapidly become epidemic in another area through the movements of global travelers. Those providing pre-travel counseling and post-travel treatment need to be aware of potential hazards and outbreaks in regions in which the traveler will be visiting, or from which the traveler is returning.

REFERENCES AND FURTHER READING

Al-Tawfiq, J.A., Zumla, A., Memish, Z.A., 2014. Travel implications of emerging coronaviruses: SARS and MERS-CoV. Travel Med. Infect. Dis. 12 (5), 422–428.

Embarek, P.K.B., Van Kerhove, M.D., 2015. Middle East Respiratory Syndrome Coronavirus (MERS-CoV): Current Situation 3 Years after the Virus Was First Identified. World Health Organization (WHO), Geneva. May 15, 2015.

Foy, B.D., Kobylinski, K.C., Chilson Foy, J.L., et al., 2011. Probable non-vector-borne transmission of Zika virus, Colorado, USA. Emerg. Infect. Dis. 17 (5), 880–882.

Gautret, P., Mockenhaupt, F.P., von Sonnenburg, F., et al., 2015. Schistosomiasis ex Corsica: local and global implications. Emerg. Infect. Dis. 21 (10), 1865–1868.

Heymann, D.L., Mackenzie, J.S., Peiris, M., 2013. SARS legacy: outbreak reporting is expected and respected. Lancet 381 (9869), 779–781.

Institute of Medicine Committee on Microbial Threats to Health, 1992. Emerging Infections: Microbial Threats to Health in the United States. Washington, DC, National Academy Press, 1–294.

Knope, K., National, A., Malaria Advisory, C., et al., 2013. Increasing notifications of dengue in Australia related to overseas travel, 1991 to 2012. Commun. Dis. Intell. Q. Rep. 37 (1), E55–E59.

Morens, D.M., Folkers, G.K., Fauci, A.S., 2008. Emerging infections: a perpetual challenge. Lancet Infect. Dis. 8 (11), 710–719.

Muller, M., Schlagenhauf, P., 2014. *Plasmodium knowlesi* in travellers, update 2014. Int. J. Infect. Dis. 22, 55–64.

Quam, M.B., Khan, K., Sears, J., et al., 2015. Estimating air travel-associated importations of dengue virus into Italy. J. Travel Med. 22 (3), 186–193.

Tappe, D., Stich, A., Langeheinecke, A., et al., 2014. Suspected new wave of muscular sarcocystosis in travellers returning from Tioman Island, Malaysia, May 2014. Euro. Surveill. 19 (21), article 2.

Taylor, L.H., Latham, S.M., Woolhouse, M.E., 2001. Risk factors for human disease emergence. Philos. Trans. R. Soc. Lond. B. Biol. Sci. 356 (1411), 983–989.

Van Hong, N., Amambua-Ngwa, A., Tuan, N.Q., et al., 2014. Severe malaria not responsive to artemisinin derivatives in man returning from Angola to Vietnam. Emerg. Infect. Dis. 20 (7), 1199–1202.

Weaver, S.C., Lecuit, M., 2015. Chikungunya virus and the global spread of a mosquito-borne disease. N. Engl. J. Med. 372 (13), 1231–1239.

Zammarchi, L., Stella, G., Mantella, A., et al., 2015. Zika virus infections imported to Italy: clinical, immunological and virological findings, and public health implications. Journal of Clinical Virology: The Official Publication of the Pan American Society for Clinical Virology 63, 32–35.

CHAPTER 4

Jet Health

Elaine C. Jong

 Access evidence synopsis online at ExpertConsult.com.

Once onboard a commercial jet aircraft headed to destination, the traveler faces the novel environment of the airplane cabin, in which a passenger's health may be impacted by the air quality and pressurization, among other prevailing conditions. Chronic health concerns may be exacerbated and new health issues may arise after spending hours sitting with limited mobility in the company of strangers and in contact with potentially contaminated surfaces and furnishings. Trauma associated with air turbulence, and syncope due to medication effects or other factors may lead to serious sequelae among aircraft passengers. Mental health issues may arise due to confined surroundings, overindulgence in alcoholic beverages, or taking new travel medications. The purpose of this chapter is to identify potential health risks associated with air travel and to discuss guidelines and optimal approaches to prevention. Over the past decade, enhanced emergency medical kits and automatic external defibrillators (AEDs) onboard some commercial airlines have allowed for successful resuscitation in cases of sudden cardiac death and other in-flight emergencies.

CABIN AIR QUALITY

Regarding cabin air quality, there exist several well-known myths that supposedly contribute to poor air quality, including the beliefs that aircraft ventilation systems cause build-up of contaminants and pathogens and that decreased O_2 levels and increased CO_2 levels in the cabin result in adverse symptoms. These beliefs will be shown to be untrue as the determinants of cabin air quality are reviewed in detail below. **Table 4.1** shows the five variables contributing to cabin air quality. Cabin air quality turns out to be relatively good when aircraft cabin ventilation systems are operating as designed and passengers have no cardiopulmonary co-morbidities.

Pressurization

Without major exception, the cabin environment is kept pressurized to 8000 ft (2400 m) above sea level. This is not an arbitrary flight level. It was chosen through research performed on pilots in early NASA (National Aeronautical and Space Agency, U.S.A.) studies and is felt to be the altitude that most of the general public can tolerate without exhibiting signs or symptoms of altitude sickness. This altitude maintains the average individual on the upper flat part of the oxygen dissociation curve (**Fig. 4.1**).

Most healthy individuals will tolerate this altitude very well. However, literature on altitude sickness reveals a subset of the population who will be symptomatic. While the percentage of O_2 remains the same at normal flight altitude as it does at sea level (21%), the partial pressure of O_2 decreases from 103 mmHg to 69 mmHg at 8000 ft. This pressure will ensure that about 90% of all hemoglobin will be saturated in the healthy individual.

Despite that, those individuals with significant pathology such as chronic obstructive pulmonary disease (COPD), recent myocardial infarction (MI), or unstable angina might

TABLE 4.1   Variables Contributing to Cabin Air Quality

Pressurization
Ventilation
Contamination
Humidity
Temperature

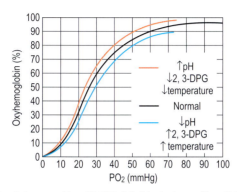

Fig. 4.1   **O₂ dissociation curve.** Note: 2,3-DPG (2,3-diphophoglycerate) in red blood cells facilitates O2 release to tissues; high altitude increases 2,3-DPG, shifting the normal OCD to the right (blue line).

suffer significant decompensation from even minor alterations in their O_2 dissociation curve. It is important for clinicians to consider this before allowing their patients to embark on a long voyage without supplemental oxygen. See the section below "Supplemental Oxygen during Air Travel." It is interesting to note that some of the next generation passenger aircraft, such as the Boeing 787 Dreamliner, are able to operate at the lower cabin altitude of 6000 ft due to the extensive use of composite materials in the fuselage, which are able to tolerate the higher pressurization.

Ventilation

The myth that aircraft ventilation contributes to poor quality of cabin air is completely unfounded. Depending on the type of aircraft, about half of the cabin air is recirculated. The other half is fresh air that is supplied by engine compressors, cooled by air-conditioning packs, and then blended with recirculated air. As a reference point, an office building may recirculate between 65 and 95% of its air. Older aircraft such as the Boeing 727 and McDonald-Douglas DC-9 do not recirculate air. It is only with the fuel crisis in the 1970s that modifications were made to newer aircraft to decrease the amount of fresh air brought into the cabin by the engines, thereby decreasing fuel consumption. It is of note that the fresh air brought into the cabin is virtually sterile.

Despite these modifications to newer aircraft, cabin air is exchanged in its entirety quite frequently. Consider the Boeing 767 used in both domestic and long-haul international versions. The cabin air is exchanged entirely every 2-3 minutes. Thus cabin air is exchanged approximately 20-30 times per hour. Compare that with the average household, which exchanges its volume only about five times per hour.

Clearly a very large volume of air enters and exits the cabin in a very short time. Without very precise modifications, passengers would experience severe drafts. Engineering

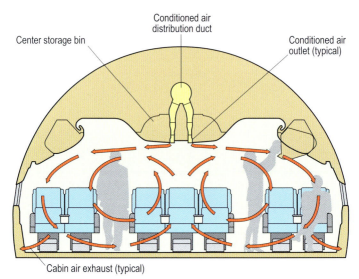

Fig. 4.2 **Cabin picture demonstrating air flow.**

modifications have reduced this "wind tunnel effect" by using laminar flow. Cabin air enters from air ducts running the length of the cabin overhead. Air supplied then exits at approximately the same row, thereby reducing airflow in fore and aft directions. This effectively limits the spread of passenger-generated contaminants (**Fig. 4.2**).

Contamination

While the laminar flow serves to minimize spread of passenger-generated contaminants, the major barrier to particulate matter on all modern aircraft is the high-efficiency particulate air (HEPA) filter. This is the standard filter used in most hospital intensive care units, operating rooms, and industrial clean rooms. A rating is given on efficiency based on the ability of the filter to remove particles greater than 0.3 microns. For reference, bacteria and fungi are on the order of greater than 1 micron in size. Viruses, however, may range on the order of 0.003-0.05 microns. Less data exist on these organisms, but it is known that clumping of virus particles facilitates their removal via HEPA filters.

Studies have been done collecting air samples from various locations and assaying for microorganisms. Locations included municipal buses, shopping malls, sidewalks, downtown streets, and airport departure lounges. It was found that microbial aerosols in the aircraft cabin were much less than in other public locations. While there does exist a risk of disease transmission simply based on the number of passengers and the close proximity, it does not appear to be any greater aboard aircraft than that for any of the other modes of public transportation. Interestingly, aircraft cabin microbial aerosols were reported lower during night flights when presumably there was less passenger activity and were higher during daytime flights when passengers were more likely to get out of their seats to walk up and down the airplane aisle.

In addition to pathogenic organisms, the concern over other contaminants exists as well, including carbon dioxide, carbon monoxide, and ozone. Carbon dioxide levels have been equated with poor air quality in buildings and other public spaces. However, data collected on 92 different US flights found carbon dioxide, carbon monoxide, and ozone levels well below maximum Federal Aviation Administration (FAA) and Occupational Safety and Health Administration standards. Thus passenger symptoms of fatigue, headache, nausea, and upper respiratory tract irritation are likely to stem from other factors, including flight duration, noise levels, dehydration, and circadian dysrhythmia. The American Society of Heating Refrigeration and Air Conditioning Engineers has recently proposed Standard 161P, which makes recommendations for cabin air quality for all commercial passenger aircraft carrying 20 or more passengers.

Humidity and Temperature
In addition to the previously discussed factors that affect cabin air quality, no discussion would be complete without mentioning humidity and temperature. The cabin milieu is much like that of a desert environment (12-21% humidity). Relative humidity can be between 5 and 35% on most aircraft. The low humidity is caused by the frequent renewal of cabin air with outside air. With outside air temperatures being well below 0°F (−18°C), little appreciable moisture or heat is brought into the cabin. Air bled off the engines must be circulated and warmed to bring it to a comfortable range. Exposure to this environment for prolonged periods is known to cause dehydration due to insensible water loss as well as to exacerbate respiratory conditions. It is of interest to note, however, that the low humidity can actually inhibit bacterial and fungal growth.

TRANSMISSION OF COMMUNICABLE DISEASES ON AIRCRAFT
Seasonal viral influenza, measles, chickenpox, meningococcal meningitis, and the common cold are examples of communicable diseases that can be transmitted from person to person in close proximity within enclosed spaces such as the aircraft cabin. Transmission is usually through aerosols of infected respiratory secretions resulting from coughing and sneezing by infected individuals or by direct contact items and furnishings contaminated with infectious secretions. In response to heightened public health concerns over global transmission and spread of emerging agents such as pandemic flu virus strains (avian influenza H5N1, H7N9), severe acute respiratory syndrome (SARS), Middle East respiratory syndrome (MERS-CoV), multidrug-resistant tuberculosis, and hemorrhagic fever viruses such as Lassa, Ebola, and others, the International Air Transport Association (IATA) and the International Civil Aviation Organization work closely with the World Health Organization (WHO) and national public health authorities such as the Centers for Disease Control and Prevention (CDC) to develop and implement guidelines to minimize the spread of disease through air travel and transport.

Despite the policy of most major airlines to reduce exposure to infectious diseases during air travel through denial of boarding to individuals perceived to be ill, exposure does nonetheless occur. Some individuals are contagious before overt symptoms are manifested and recognized. (See further considerations in the section below entitled "The Air Carrier Access Act 1986.")

When a contagious source passenger is identified, usually days after the flight has been completed, public health authorities and the airline carrier must work together to notify and screen all passengers who traveled with the source passenger and have been assessed to be at risk of exposure. It is important to document the level of infectiousness of the source passenger. In the case of *Mycobacterium tuberculosis*, factors such as anatomic involvement, positive acid-fast bacilli smears, history of transmission, and prior treatment of the source case must be considered. Further, the proximity to the source case and duration of exposure all figure into the post-exposure notification algorithm. Literature clearly reflects that proximity to the source case is one of the most important variables in the transmission of infectious disease. Thus, a passenger traveling in first class need not necessarily be notified of a source case seated in the rear of the aircraft in the coach section. Similarly, those whose exposure was limited to less than 8 hours are very unlikely to need notification.

Exceptions to this rule clearly exist, however. Consider the case of a jet delayed on the ground for 3 hours due to engine problems with 54 passengers on board. The ventilation system on board the aircraft was apparently inoperative. Of those on board, 72% became infected with influenza. The attack rate varied linearly with time spent on board the aircraft. This would demonstrate that any alteration from standard boarding, taxi, and takeoff protocols might be significant in determining infectivity of a source case and the need to notify other passengers.

The worldwide spread of SARS in 2003 illustrated to public health authorities the need to develop reliable methods to quickly locate and notify passengers who may have been exposed in-flight to communicable diseases. Because of passenger data privacy concerns, airlines have traditionally performed passenger notifications when alerted by public health authorities to do so. However, US public health agencies led by the CDC have taken a more active role and now may require airlines to release electronic passenger data by issuing a Directive Order in the event of a confirmed possible exposure in-flight. In addition, there is now a requirement for the commander of an aircraft destined for a US airport to report immediately to the nearest CDC Quarantine Station any death or illness among passengers or crew, *prior to* arrival. Reportable illnesses include high or persistent fevers, particularly if accompanied by a rash or jaundice, as well as moderately severe diarrhea.

Avian flu H5N1 virus causes outbreaks of serious disease in poultry and wild birds in countries around the world. Although it is not easily transmitted to humans, more than 500 human cases have been reported since 2003 in parts of Asia, Africa, Eastern Europe, and the Middle East, with a case mortality rate of about 60%. Transmission of avian flu H5N1 to humans usually involves direct contact with infected birds, but if the virus mutates and becomes more easily spread from human to human (e.g., airborne by the respiratory route), this could start an influenza pandemic or worldwide outbreak of disease. Avian influenza H7N9 virus continues to cause severe outbreaks of disease on poultry farms in China, in other Asian countries, and in the US. So far, human cases reported from Asia have not led to sustained human-to-human transmission. Considering the possibility of an avian flu pandemic in the future, IATA in cooperation with the CDC developed guidelines for airline personnel meeting passengers arriving from known outbreak areas, as well as for airline cleaning and maintenance crews who may potentially be exposed. All guidelines emphasize basic hygiene practices to prevent becoming ill, such as hand washing with soap and water or an alcohol-based hand gel, separation of any ill passengers and providing them with a surgical mask or tissues to cover the mouth and nose, use of disposable gloves when handling blood or body fluids, and prompt reporting of the illness to public health authorities. Specialized personal protective equipment such as respirators or gowns is not recommended except in direct patient-care situations, although the use of surgical masks when around symptomatic individuals in public areas may be considered. Specialized passenger screening techniques such as thermal screening to identify febrile passengers when pre-boarding that were utilized during the SARS epidemic in some international locations are not being recommended at this time.

Following the 2014 Ebola virus disease (EVD) outbreak in West Africa, a new "Traveler Public Health Declaration Form" (www.iata.org) was developed for use by public health officials to pre-screen travelers departing from the outbreak areas. The WHO published "Travel and Transport Risk Assessment: Interim Guidance for Public Health Authorities and the Transport Sector" in September 2014 with regard to EVD control. This document may be accessed online at www.who.int.

SUPPLEMENTAL OXYGEN DURING AIR TRAVEL

For the travel advisor encountering with a patient requiring oxygen during air travel, it is essential that the following be considered. Oxygen is considered by the FAA to be hazardous cargo. Oxygen, as well as any other oxidizing agents, can pose serious hazards to the safety of the aircraft and passengers. Consider the downing of an airliner when oxygen-generating cylinders were inappropriately stored in the cargo hold, killing all on board. Due to the inherent dangers of transporting oxygen, strict regulations surrounding its transport exist.

For the passengers who will require supplemental oxygen during air travel, it is imperative to be acquainted with each carrier's policy regarding supplemental oxygen. While passengers cannot bring their own oxygen on board, most air carriers can provide oxygen with adjustable or non-adjustable flow meters to passengers who require it. There is a fee for this service, and advance notice is required, 24-48 hours or longer. Further, a physician's statement is necessary attesting to the ability of the patient to be medically cleared to an altitude of 8000 ft with supplemental oxygen. The statement must include flow rates, continuous or intermittent usage, and type of delivery system (mask vs. nasal cannula). Additionally, the need for oxygen supplies on the ground during layovers or transfers must be considered. Typically such service is not available from the airline and must be arranged in advance through a local supplier in the layover city or through the home oxygen service.

In the late 2000s, the FAA began allowing passengers who require supplemental oxygen in-flight to use a portable oxygen concentrators (POCs). Only specified models of POCs have received FAA approval (www.faa.gov/about/initiatives/cabin_safety/portable_oxygen). In addition, specific requirements must be met, including possessing an adequate supply of batteries, pre-notification given to the airline, proper storage during take-off and landing, and the possession of a written doctor's statement detailing the passenger's oxygen requirements. Individual airlines should be consulted about specific requirements. See also Chapter 16 for additional details on travel with respiratory conditions.

THE AIR CARRIER ACCESS ACT OF 1986: DENIAL OF BOARDING/PASSENGER ACCEPTANCE

While the airline may make certain regulations to assure the safety of the traveling public, it may in no way limit the ability of those with disabilities to board the aircraft, with rare exception. The Air Carrier Access Act of 1986 was established to ensure that persons with disabilities, as per the Americans with Disabilities Act definition, are treated without discrimination in any way, consistent with safe carriage of all passengers. This act, known as the "FAA final rule," required the Department of Transportation to publish air carrier access guidelines adopted in March 1990 (14 CFR Part 382). This regulation, which applies only to US-based carriers, states that a carrier may not refuse carriage of a passenger solely based on disability. Nor can it limit the number of disabled individuals on a flight. Further, a carrier may not limit transportation of an individual simply because his or her appearance or behavior is disturbing. Some take this to mean that any "sick" passenger must be accepted.

Exceptions to the "FAA final rule" do exist, however. A carrier may refuse to transport an individual if the carrier deems transportation of the passenger to be a risk to health or safety of the public or to be a clear violation of FAA rules. One such example of when an air carrier might justifiably refuse boarding to a disabled individual would include the inability to perform exit row functions when there is no other seat availability. Also, a carrier may refuse boarding to a passenger known to harbor communicable disease or a passenger who requires respiratory equipment not compatible with the aircraft.

The large responsibility to accept all disabled or ill passengers who do not pose a risk to the traveling public has made necessary the creation of the Complaint Resolution Official (CRO). This position is specifically mandated by Air Carrier Access Rules to resolve complaints or disagreements regarding the transportation of individuals with disabilities. This official or department is usually located in a central location and may involve discussion with an in-house consultant or physician. The physician may request information regarding the clinical scenario prior to making a decision on acceptance or denial of passenger boarding. The CRO may also be called on to make a decision regarding diversion of a flight during which the safety of a passenger or crew member might be jeopardized if it were to continue. Clearly, the issue of traveling with a disability or medical need can best be accomplished through early communication with the air carrier and its special assistance coordinator. Further advice and information for physicians who must advise passengers on travel or medical certifications is available though the Aerospace Medical Association (www.asma.org). (See also Chapter 16, "Traveling with Chronic Medical Conditions.")

DEEP VENOUS THROMBOSIS AND AIR TRAVEL

Sitting inactive for long periods of time predisposes even young, healthy individuals to developing deep vein thrombosis (DVT) in the lower extremities, but, as noted below, some travelers with certain health conditions face an even higher risk during long-distance travel. When a blood clot breaks away from the vein and travels to arteries serving the lungs, it is called a pulmonary embolism (PE), a life-threatening event with a mortality rate of more than 50% in some surveys. DVT and PE are often called venous thromboembolism (VTE).

The development of DVT in travelers during or shortly after long-distance air travel was given the popular name "economy class syndrome" because many travelers wanted to blame the ever-diminishing space of economy class seats on aircraft as the cause of the ailment. However, causal links have not been demonstrated. Limited data show the risk of air travel-associated DVT is similar among passengers in first class and economy class sections, and the etiology of air travel-associated DVT is probably multifactorial. A published study reported a lower incidence of symptomless DVT in a group of long-distance air travelers who used elastic compression stockings compared with those who did not and supports the concept that long periods of sitting and inactivity are plausible risk factors contributing to DVT. Cases of DVT have been reported following long train and automobile trips. In addition, other studies suggest that activation of coagulation induced by hypobaric hypoxia during air travel is another separate and important trigger of thrombosis. Dehydration developing during long flights could also contribute to increased blood coagulability. Personal health issues contributing to increased risk for air travel-associated DVT are shown in **Table 4.2**.

DVT of the lower extremities can be symptomless or symptoms may appear during or shortly after the flight. Although prolonged sitting commonly may cause some swelling of both lower legs, asymmetrical swelling and/or a cramp or tenderness in one lower leg, or swelling and bruising behind the knee of one leg, are symptoms of a blood clot. Chest symptoms usually appear 2-4 days or more after the initial clot in the calf, and signal PE. There may be shortness of breath, rapid breathing or panting, painful breathing, fever, coughing up blood, and/or fainting (often the first sign, especially in older people). Immediate medical evaluation is mandatory if chest or other systemic symptoms develop, because prompt diagnosis of and treatment for pulmonary embolism could be life saving.

All long-distance air travelers, but especially those whose trips are 8 hours or more, should consider the following DVT prevention guidelines in **Table 4.3**.

TURBULENCE-RELATED INJURIES

There are few published studies on the incidence of passenger injuries due to trauma during air travel. Episodes of turbulence can contribute to in-flight trauma by causing overhead luggage bins to open up, spilling contents onto passengers seated below, and by causing

---

TABLE 4.2   Risk Factors for Air Travel-Associated DVT

Sitting motionless for long periods (8 hours or more)

Adulthood, especially advanced age

Prior injuries to blood vessels (e.g., leg trauma, surgery, radiation therapy)

Estrogen use (oral contraceptives or hormone replacement therapy)

Pregnancy

Severe obesity

Infections

Inflammatory diseases (e.g., rheumatoid arthritis, Crohn disease, systemic lupus erythematosus)

Inherited clotting disorders (e.g., factor V Leiden, prothrombin gene mutation). *Note:* Uncommon in Asian, African, and Native American populations

Cancer (some cancers release prothrombotic substances)

Smoking

TABLE 4.3   DVT Prevention Guidelines

Sit in an aisle seat if possible to allow ease of getting up and around.

Get up and walk up and down the airplane aisle periodically when it's safe to do so.

Do calf muscle exercises once an hour while seated to promote muscular pumping action of venous blood back into the central circulation.

Drink plenty of water (about 1 glass per hour) and stay well hydrated—an added benefit is that trips to the lavatory will compel one to get up and move around.

Avoid excess consumption of coffee and alcohol, which have a diuretic effect and may contribute to dehydration.

Avoid drugs that promote sleepiness and long periods of immobility.

Below-knee graduated compression stockings providing 15-30 mmHg of pressure at the ankle during travel are recommended for air travelers with one or more of the health conditions associated with increased risk of DVT (Table 4.2).

Aspirin or anticoagulants to prevent VTE are not routinely recommended for long-distance travelers, but pharmacologic thromboprophylaxis may be prescribed on an individual basis for some travelers considered to be at particularly high risk, according to evidence-based clinical practice guidelines from the American College of Chest Physicians.

DVT, Deep vein thrombosis; *VTE,* venous thromboembolism.

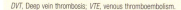

traumatic injuries in unrestrained and ambulatory persons. In one limited report, 462 injuries caused by objects falling from overhead bins were reported in a 3-year period; >90% were head injuries to passengers seated in aisle seats. In a 10-year retrospective study of turbulence-related injuries among airline cabin crew, about one-half involved serious injuries, with the most frequent type being lower extremity fractures, especially the ankle. The conundrum is that sitting in an aisle seat and ambulating in the airplane aisle are recommended for prevention of VTE in passengers, but the risk of turbulence-related injuries could be lowered by sitting in a window seat and being restrained by a seat belt as much as possible.

IN-FLIGHT MEDICAL EMERGENCIES

With the aging of the population and the increase in commercial air travel now involving several billion passengers a year, it only follows that an increase in the number of in-flight medical emergencies would also occur. However, the incidence of these events is hard to estimate. Although medical events during flight are reported, the information was not collected in a standardized format, and it is difficult to compare data across carriers and regions. Two recently published retrospective studies of in-flight medical emergencies show that most cases were related to syncope, respiratory symptoms, or gastrointestinal symptoms, but potential cardiac symptoms such as chest pain were most often associated with diversion of the flight.

In 2004 the FAA implemented FAR 121.803, which specifies that all US-based commercial airlines must carry a defibrillator and an enhanced emergency medical kit. Airplanes that weigh more than 7500 lb and that have at least one flight attendant are subject to this rule. The items in the enhanced medical kit are listed in **Table 4.4**. Many airlines carry additional items in their onboard medical kits; however, it should be noted that IATA does not regulate the contents of emergency medical kits of international airlines, some of which may be inadequate to provide an effective emergency response.

Medical personnel are frequently onboard and can assist fellow passengers during a medical emergency. Due to the perceived reluctance for physicians or other medical personnel to render aid for fear of legal repercussions, a "Good Samaritan" provision was included in the Aviation Medical Assistance Act of 1998, which limits air carrier and non-employee passenger liability unless the assistance is grossly negligent or willful misconduct is evident. It has been suggested that volunteer physicians or other medically qualified volunteers

TABLE 4.4 Contents of Enhanced Medical Kit
Sphygmomanometer
Stethoscope
Three sizes of oral airways
Syringes
Needles
50% dextrose injection
Epinephrine
Diphenhydramine
Nitroglycerin tabs
Basic instructions
Non-sterile gloves
Oral antihistamine[a]
Non-narcotic analgesic[a]
Aspirin[a]
Atropine[a]
Bronchodilator inhaler[a]
Lidocaine and saline[a]
Intravenous (IV) fluid administration kit[a]
Bag valve mask (BVM) with self-reinflating bag (brand name AMBU bag)[a]
Cardiopulmonary Resuscitation (CPR) masks[a]

[a]Required under FAR 121.803.

(e.g., emergency department nurse, advanced nurse practitioner, or advanced paramedic) responding to an in-flight medical incident stay within the scope of their training and practice, request access to the on-board emergency medical kit, and coordinate their efforts with the flight crew and remote response/call center physician (if available).

Automatic External Defibrillators

The role of the AED is expanding in public access areas. As per figures published by the American Heart Association, sudden cardiac death occurs in about 1000 people per day in the United States. The chance of survival in such an event is less than 1 in 10. As in the teaching for all basic and advanced rescue personnel, the adage "shock first and shock fast" is of paramount importance. With ventricular fibrillation being the most common and the most treatable rhythm disturbance found at time of cardiac death, the importance of AEDs cannot be understated.

The implementation by the FAA of FAR 121.803 has seen the installation of AEDs in all major commercial passenger aircraft maintained by US airlines. All flight crew members including pilots receive training in the location, function, and intended use of AEDs, and flight attendants receive initial and recurring training in cardiopulmonary resuscitation and the use of AEDs every 2 years. This far-reaching regulation has gone a long way in making air travel safer for the thousands of passengers who fly with medical conditions both known and undiagnosed.

BEHAVIORAL PROBLEMS DURING AIR TRAVEL

Passengers behaving badly contribute to the increasing discomfort of air travel, and their behavior most often can be ascribed to a lack of courtesy and common sense. The behavior of the flying public reflects on the informality, self-indulgence, and permissiveness of modern society. Passengers engaging in personal grooming and hygiene tasks, including changing baby diapers in the close quarters of the economy class seat row, demonstrate gross bad manners. Crying babies and unruly children may cause nearby passengers to feel irritated and miserable. Alcohol intoxication, side effects of recreational and even prescribed drugs, sleep deprivation, jet lag, and/or mental stress may create acute psychological problems in certain passengers during air travel that could possibly result in injury to others who try to intercede. While airlines continue to work on ways to prevent, manage, and control passengers behaving badly, individual travelers who are affected should exit their seats if possible and quietly ask for assistance from a flight attendant, rather than directly confronting the person or persons creating the disturbance. Chapter 16, "Travel with Chronic Medical Conditions," and Chapter 17, "Mental Health and Travel," also contain advice on neuropsychiatric conditions and travel.

ACKNOWLEDGMENTS

Sincere thanks and appreciation to Thomas N. Bettes, M.D., M.P.H., who wrote the original chapter on "Air Carrier Issues in Travel Medicine" for the third and fourth editions of this book. This chapter has been adapted from his excellent foundation chapter.

FURTHER READING

Bettes, T.N., McKenas, D.K., 1999. Medical advice for commercial air travelers. Am. Fam. Physician 60, 801–810.
A concise, clinically oriented review for primary care providers advising traveling patients.

Centers for Disease Control and Prevention (CDC), 2014. Infection Control Guidelines for Cabin Crew Members on Commercial Aircraft. Available at <www.cdc.gov/quarantine/air/index> (accessed April 25, 2015).
This is a useful link for access to general health and infection control guidelines pertaining to commercial aircraft, as well as guidelines for specific outbreak situations (e.g., seasonal influenza, avian influenza, MERS-CoV, Ebola).

Chandra, A., Conry, S., 2013. In-flight medical emergencies. West. J. Emerg. Med. 14, 499–504.
Retrospective review of studies and high-quality topic summaries related to in-flight medical emergencies published between 1980 and 2010. Excellent discussion of approach to patient and clinical practice guidelines in the unique cabin environment.

Cummins, R.O., Schubach, J.A., 1989. Frequency and types of medical emergencies among commercial air travelers. JAMA 264, 1295.
This early study of medical emergencies associated with air travel showed that cardiovascular incidents occurred on the ground prior to boarding and after disembarking as well as on board the aircraft, suggesting that a reduction of stress factors associated with travel might be prudent for patients with cardiovascular disease.

Kahn, S.R., Lim, W., Dunn, A.S., et al., 2012. Prevention of VTE in nonsurgical patients: Antithrombotic Therapy and Prevention of Thrombosis, 9th ed: American College of Chest Physicians Evidence-Based Clinical Practice Guidelines. Chest 141 (Suppl. 2), e217–18S.
Evidence-based clinical practice guidelines contain recommendations on prevention of VTE for long-distance travelers.

Kenyon, T.A., Vaway, S.E., Ihle, W.W., et al., 1996. Transmission of multidrug-resistant *Mycobacterium tuberculosis* during a long airplane flight. N. Engl. J. Med. 334, 933–938.
A detailed analysis of the transmission of multidrug-resistant tuberculosis during long-haul air travel that demonstrates variables of seating and passenger activity in relation to the source case among passengers who had PPD skin test conversion on post-travel follow-up.

Peterson, D.C., Martin-Gill, C., Guyette, F.X., et al., 2013. Outcomes of medical emergencies on commercial airline flights. N. Engl. J. Med. 368, 2075–2083.
Retrospective review of 11,920 in-flight emergency calls from five domestic and international airlines to a physician-directed medical communications center during 2008-2010. Diagnoses, treatment plans, and outcomes are discussed in detail.

Wick, R.L., Jr., Irvine, L.A., 1995. The microbiological composition of airliner cabin air. Aviat. Space Environ. Med. 66, 220–224.

This study is interesting because it compares bacterial counts and mold counts in samples of airplane cabin air with air samples from city buses, shopping malls, and city street corners.

World Health Organization (WHO), 1998. Tuberculosis and Air Travel: Guidelines for Prevention and Control, third ed. WHO, Geneva. Available at <www.who.int/tb> (accessed April 21, 2015).

An essential reference containing guidelines and an algorithm for evaluating infectiousness in a source case of airplane tuberculosis and the need to notify other passengers after the flight.

World Health Organization (WHO), 2014. WHO Travel and Transport Risk Assessment: Interim Guidance for Public Health Authorities and the Transport Sector. WHO, Geneva. Available at <www.who.int/evd> (accessed April 21, 2015).

Interim guidance to address transmission and control of Ebola virus disease, to be used as a reference for developing national responses.

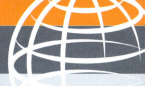

CHAPTER 5

Immunizations for Travelers

Elaine C. Jong

 Access evidence synopsis online at ExpertConsult.com.

Recommendations for travel immunizations are based on a risk assessment of each traveler's general health, trip itinerary, and knowledge of current health conditions at a given destination. Most travelers seek protection against vaccine-preventable diseases, yet their acceptance of the vaccines recommended for travel may depend largely on other concerns, such as number of doses and vaccine schedules, route of administration (oral vs. injection), and cost. Many first-time international travelers are surprised by the number of vaccines that may be advised for a given itinerary. On the other hand, experienced repeat travelers may be pleased by the availability of new vaccines that may be better tolerated, provide greater efficacy, and have a longer duration of protection compared with older products.

Travelers planning adventure or expedition travel, extended stays abroad, or whose work may necessitate multiple trips abroad with very short notice should be encouraged to seek advice for travel immunizations well in advance (up to 6 months) of anticipated departure. This allows time for optimal scheduling of vaccine doses and procurement of vaccines that may be in short supply or difficult to obtain. For travelers with little advance notice, accelerated schedules may be used for some travel vaccines, and multiple vaccine doses may be given at different sites on the same day, limited only by the recipient's anticipated tolerance for multiple injections and associated minor adverse side effects. Up to six live virus vaccines may be given on the same day without interfering with immune efficacy. **Table 5.1** lists some conditions that may cause vaccine interactions or interfere with the expected immune protection. In general, attenuated live virus vaccines and bacterial vaccines are contraindicated during pregnancy and in persons with altered immune competence (see Chapters 14-16). This chapter will cover the approach to adult travel immunizations. Pediatric travel immunizations are covered in Chapter 12.

ROUTINE IMMUNIZATIONS

Immunizations may be organized into three categories termed the "3 Rs": routine, required, and recommended. Routine vaccines are those vaccines usually given as part of national public health childhood immunization programs. Although most travelers seek pre-travel care for "travel" immunizations, documenting completion of the routine vaccines (or immunity to the given vaccine-preventable disease) and identifying recommended booster doses are just as important as the travel vaccines. Many low-resource countries are still working toward implementation of childhood immunization programs that cover 90% of the pediatric population, a public health goal identified by the World Health Organization (WHO) Expanded Program on Immunizations. Thus, during international travel, adult travelers may be exposed to vaccine-preventable communicable diseases that are no longer commonly transmitted in industrialized countries, such as measles, polio, and chickenpox. Dosage schedules for adult routine immunizations are given in **Table 5.2**.

TABLE 5.1   Vaccine Interactions

Vaccine	Interaction	Precaution
Immune globulin	Measles/mumps/rubella (MMR), varicella, polio, and hepatitis A vaccines	Give these vaccines at least 2 weeks before immune globulin (IG) or 3-11 months after IG, depending on IG product, indication, and dose received.
Oral typhoid vaccine	Antibiotic therapy	Do not administer oral typhoid vaccine concurrently with antibiotics.
Oral typhoid vaccine	Proguanil malaria chemoprophylaxis	Schedule an interval of at least 10 days between final dose of oral typhoid vaccine and proguanil (Malarone = atovaquone + proguanil).
Virus vaccines, live (MMR, oral polio, varicella, yellow fever)	Other live virus vaccines	Give live virus vaccines on same day, or separate doses by at least 1 month.
Virus vaccines, live (MMR, oral polio, varicella, yellow fever)	Tuberculin skin test (PPD)	Do skin test on same day as receipt of a live virus vaccine, or 4-6 weeks after, because live virus vaccines can impair the response to PPD skin test.

Updated from Jong, E.C., 1993. Immunizations for international travelers. In: The Travel Medicine Advisor. American Health Consultants, Atlanta.

The American Committee on Immunization Practices (ACIP) at the Centers for Disease Control and Prevention (CDC) is the federal agency that develops official guidelines for immunizations in the United States. Current recommendations for childhood immunizations include the following vaccines: combined diphtheria, tetanus, and (acellular) pertussis (Dtap), *Haemophilus influenzae* type b conjugate, hepatitis A, hepatitis B, influenza, measles/mumps/rubella, pneumococcal conjugate, poliovirus, rotavirus, and varicella. The standard immunizations recommended by the ACIP for administration to pre-adolescent children at 11-12 years of age include tetanus, diphtheria, and (acellular) pertussis (Tdap), meningococcal conjugate, and human papillomavirus (HPV) vaccines, as well as the second dose of measles, mumps, rubella (MMR) and varicella (chickenpox) vaccines if these had not yet been given (Chapter 12).

When individuals seek travel immunizations, this provides a natural opportunity for them to catch up on any missed doses of their routine immunizations. Adult travelers may be due for booster doses of vaccines for tetanus/diphtheria, polio (for travel to polio outbreak areas), and/or measles (if a second dose after infancy was not received). As varicella is a disease of young adults rather than children in many tropical countries, persons lacking a definite history of previous varicella infection or of having received two doses of varicella vaccine may benefit from primary immunization or should complete their immunization by receiving a second dose of varicella vaccine prior to travel.

Hepatitis A Vaccine as a Routine Immunization
Hepatitis A is the most common vaccine-preventable disease associated with travel and should be a high priority for those over the age of 1 year who have not previously received it or had the natural disease. In 1999, the ACIP recommended that hepatitis A vaccine be administered to all 2-year-olds living in 11 Western states in the United States, where heightened transmission of hepatitis A virus infections was occurring. In 2006, the ACIP issued a new recommendation for hepatitis A immunization of all children at 1 year of age. Thus, hepatitis A vaccine is now a standard immunization for children but should be considered a travel vaccine for older children and adults.

TABLE 5.2 Dosage Schedules for Adult Routine Immunizations

Vaccine	Primary Series	Booster Interval
Influenza virus, inactivated	One dose[a] IM or SC	Annual immunization with current vaccine
Influenza virus, live attenuated	One application by nasal inhalation	Annual immunization with current vaccine
Measles/mumps/rubella[b] (for children >15 months and adults)	One dose[a] SC	Boost measles vaccine at 12-18 years old; if a second dose was not received after childhood, boost measles vaccine once in adult life before international travel for people born after 1957 and before 1980
Pneumococcus conjugate (13 valent)	One dose SC	Give one dose at 65 years of age or older, preferably 6-12 months before the pneumococcus polysaccharide (23 valent) vaccine. (See text for alternate schedules)
Pneumococcus polysaccharide (Pneumovax) (23-valent)	One dose[a] SC	One booster 5 years after the first dose if the primary dose was received at <65 years of age
Poliomyelitis, enhanced inactivated killed vaccine, safe for all ages)	Give doses[a] one and two SC or IM 4-8 weeks apart; give dose three 6-12 months after dose two	Give a booster dose once to people before travel in areas at risk if 5 or more years since the last dose of vaccine
Tetanus and diphtheria toxoids adsorbed (Td) (for children >7 years of age and for adults)	Three doses[a] SC or IM: give doses one and two 4-8 weeks apart, give dose three 6-12 months later	Routine booster dose every 10 years
Combined tetanus, diphtheria, and acellular) pertussis (Tdap) (Adacel)	One dose at 11-12 years of age to boost childhood combined diphtheria, tetanus and (acellular) pertussis (Dtap) immunization	Give a single dose to boost childhood immunity; may substitute Tdap once for one of the adult Td booster doses
Varicella[b] (Varivax) (for children >13 years of age and for adults)	Two doses[a] SC given 4-8 weeks apart	None; give a second dose of vaccine if only one dose was received in childhood.

[a]See manufacturer's package insert for recommendations on dosage.

[b]May be contraindicated in patients with any of the following conditions: pregnancy, leukemia, lymphoma, generalized malignancy, immunosuppression from HIV infection or treatment with corticosteroids, alkylating drugs, antimetabolites, or radiation therapy.

IM, Intramuscularly; SC, subcutaneously.

Adapted from Jong, E.C., 1993. Immunizations for international travelers. In: The Travel Medicine Advisor. American Health Consultants, Atlanta.

Hepatitis B Vaccine as a Routine Immunization

Hepatitis B vaccine was incorporated into the recommended childhood immunization schedule in 1990. Adults born before 1990 may require the full three-dose hepatitis B vaccine primary series as a catch-up vaccine for protection against inadvertent exposures associated with travel.

Influenza Vaccine

Annual immunization against viral influenza is recommended by the ACIP for all persons 6 months of age or older who do not have medical contraindications to the vaccine. The influenza viruses undergo minor mutations of surface antigens from season to season in a process termed "antigenic drift"; thus the influenza vaccine is re-formulated each year in between flu seasons, according to WHO guidelines, to provide protection against strains of the influenza virus predicted to be in circulation during the season ahead. The newly formulated influenza vaccines are usually released in the early fall.

Both inactivated influenza vaccine (IIV) and live attenuated influenza vaccine (LAIV) products are available. The inactivated influenza vaccines are given by intramuscular (IM) or intradermal (ID) injection. The LAIV is approved for use in persons 2-49 years old and is administered by intranasal application. Both IIV and LAIV are effective in adults. If the flu season has already started in the community, susceptible persons should be immunized with either flu vaccine type that is immediately available. (See Chapter 12 for details on pediatric recommendations.) An IIV administered by ID injection is approved for use in persons 18-64 years. The elderly >65 years old may have a decreased response to IIV; a high-dose IIV formulated for this age group should be used.

Despite the recommendation for universal immunization against viral influenza, flu vaccine coverage rates in the general population remain suboptimal. Flu vaccine should be recommended to all international travelers because prolonged air travel, fatigue, and exposure to crowds in various closed environments may predispose them to air-borne infections. The CDC identified a particular risk for viral influenza infections among travelers during the summer sailing season of Alaska cruise ship tours. The risk is thought to be associated with exposure of susceptible travelers to influenza-infected persons among the other travelers and tourist industry staff, particularly those from the Southern Hemisphere where the seasonal climate patterns are opposite to those in the Northern Hemisphere.

If flu vaccine is unavailable for travelers during their travel season, the inclusion in the traveler's medical kit of one of the antiviral drugs active against influenza virus, either oseltamivir (Tamiflu®, chemoprophylaxis or early treatment) or zanamivir (Relenza®, early treatment), should be discussed with the travelers who will be at potential risk.

Pneumococcal Vaccine

Immunization of adults ≥65 years of age against invasive pneumococcal disease is routinely recommended by the ACIP. The current recommendation is for the 13-valent pneumococcal conjugate vaccine (PCV13) to be given first in a series, with the 23-valent pneumococcal polysaccharide vaccine (PPSV23) administered 6-12 months after. However, since this recommendation is relatively recent (2014), the following regimens are also acceptable: if PPSV23 was received first, administer PCV13 after an interval of at least 1 year or more; if the first dose of PPSV23 was received prior to 65 years of age, give the first dose of PCV13 at ≥65 years of age (at least 1 year after the first PPSV23), and then give a second dose of PPSV23 at 6-12 months after the PCV13.

REQUIRED TRAVEL IMMUNIZATIONS

The immunizations for international travel identified as "required" usually refer to those covered by the WHO International Health Regulations (IHR). Historically, yellow fever, cholera, and smallpox vaccines were subject to WHO regulations. However, the requirements for cholera and smallpox vaccines for international travel were dropped several decades ago. At the present time, yellow fever vaccine is the only vaccine that may be required for entry into member countries, according to current WHO regulations. In addition, Saudi Arabia requires evidence of immunization with meningococcal vaccine to be submitted with visa applications of inbound travelers for travel during the time of the annual Hajj.

In response to the international spread of wild polio virus (WPV) from certain countries in Africa, the WHO declared a public health emergency of international concern in May 2014 and issued temporary polio vaccine recommendations under the authority of IHR (2005) for long-term travelers and residents departing from countries with WPV in circulation. Proof of polio vaccine received between 4 weeks and 12 months before the date of departure from the polio-affected country might be *required* of such travelers. Updates on country vaccine requirements are posted on the WHO website (www.who.int) and the CDC Travelers' Health website (www.cdc.gov/travel).

The international traveler should have all current immunizations recorded in the "International Certificate of Vaccination or Prophylaxis," a document in folded booklet form printed on yellow paper and approved by the WHO. The booklet has a special page for official validation of the yellow fever vaccine and is recognized as an official document all over the world. The WHO officially removed cholera vaccination from the IHR in 1973. If given, the cholera vaccination can be recorded in the space provided for "Other Vaccinations." *Likewise, a traveler's receipt of meningococcal ACWY vaccine and/or polio vaccine should also be documented in the International Certificate of Vaccination or Prophylaxis.*

Yellow Fever Vaccine

Yellow fever is a viral infection transmitted by *Aedes aegypti* mosquitoes in equatorial South America and Africa. The endemic zones are shown in **Figure 5.1**. Immunization is required for entry into some countries within the endemic zones or may be recommended to travelers going to rural tropical areas within the endemic zones or to both rural and urban areas during yellow fever outbreaks.

Yellow Fever (YF) Vaccine

YF vaccine is a live attenuated viral vaccine prepared from the 17D strain of YF virus (YF Vax™, Sanofi). The WHO controls the production of YF vaccine, sets requirements, and approves certain laboratories for its manufacture. The vaccine leads to seroconversion rates of 95% or higher, a protection rate of over 99% in immunocompetent recipients, and a duration of immunity after one dose, which appears to be lifelong. The YF vaccine is given as a single dose for primary immunization, and the recommended booster interval is 10 years (**Table 5.3**).

YF Vaccine Booster Doses

In 2015, the ACIP recommended that routine booster doses of YF vaccine are not necessary for travelers to endemic areas because of studies showing that the primary YF vaccination elicits sustained immunity and probable lifelong protection in healthy recipients. The ACIP recommendation is in agreement with an earlier 2013 recommendation from the WHO Strategic Advisory Group of Experts on Immunization. However, since the 10-year booster dose requirement is scheduled to be removed from WHO IHR by June 2016, in the interim some travelers may find that a YF vaccine booster is still necessary for entry into certain countries. Travelers and travel health advisors can find updated country-by-country YF vaccine requirements at the WHO and CDC websites.

YF Vaccine Precautions and Contraindications

The vaccine virus is cultured in eggs and is not recommended for persons with a history of severe allergy (anaphylaxis) to eggs. A review of reports submitted to the US Vaccine Adverse Events Reporting System from 1990 through 1997 found a rate of 1/131,000 for anaphylaxis after immunization with yellow fever vaccine. The package insert contains instructions for skin-testing persons with an uncertain history of allergy to eggs. YF vaccine is contraindicated in infants <6 months of age because of the significant but rare risk of vaccine-associated neurotropic disease in such young infants after immunization (estimated rate 1 per 8 million doses). If possible, YF immunization should be delayed until the infant is ≥9 months of age (Chapter 12). YF vaccine is generally not recommended during pregnancy except when travel to a highly endemic area cannot be avoided or postponed by the pregnant traveler, and the risk of the actual disease is thought to be greater than the theoretical risk of adverse effects from the vaccine.

Additional contraindications to receiving the YF vaccine include immune suppression caused by underlying disease (e.g., malignancy, HIV infection, congenital immune deficiency) or by medical therapy (e.g., treatment with daily corticosteroids, cancer chemotherapy, radiation therapy, organ transplant therapy). Most travel experts would consider administering YF vaccine to travelers at risk if the CD4 cell count is >400 μL in an HIV-infected person or if the corticosteroid dosage is <20 mg prednisone/day.

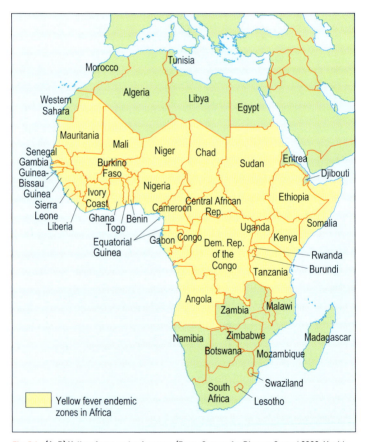

Fig. 5.1 **(A, B) Yellow fever endemic zones.** (From: Centers for Disease Control 2008. Health Information for International Travel, 2007–2008. US Government Printing Office, Washington, DC. Available at <http://wwwn.cdc.gov/travel/yellowBookCh4-YellowFever.aspx#668>.)

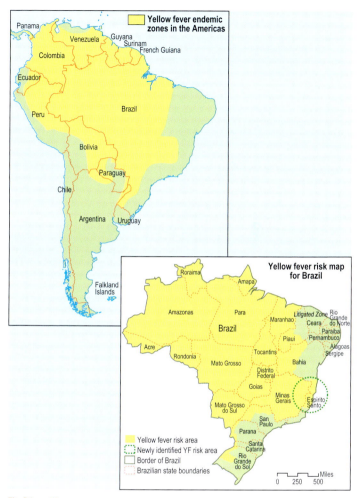

Fig. 5.1, cont'd

YF Vaccine-Associated Viscerotropic Disease (YEL-AVD)

YEL-AVD is likely related to the transient viremia that normally occurs after receipt of this live attenuated virus vaccine. In cases reported to the WHO and CDC, YEL-AVD occurred 2-5 days after receiving YF vaccine and is a febrile illness leading to multiple organ system failure as manifested by fever, myalgia, arthralgia, hepatitis, thrombocytopenia, disseminated intravascular coagulation, lymphopenia, rhabdomyolysis, hypotension, and oliguria. Review of the reported cases shows that the risk of YEL-AVD is very rare (13 cases reported per >100 million vaccine doses) and that the risk involved *first-time* vaccine recipients. The risk increases with age, with a rate of 3.5/100,000 vaccine recipients reported for persons 65-74 years of age, and an almost three-fold increase in rate to 9.1/100,000 among vaccine recipients aged >75 years old. Thus, careful review of the proposed itinerary with regard to risks

TABLE 5.3   Dosage Schedules for Adult Travel Immunizations

Vaccine	Primary Series	Booster Interval
Cholera, oral inactivated whole cell recombinant B subunit (WC/rBS) (Dukoral)	Two doses[a] PO 10-14 days apart according to package directions	Booster for continued risk of exposure to cholera at approximately 6-month intervals, more frequently when the vaccine is used for protection against traveler's diarrhea due to ETEC heat-labile toxin.
Hepatitis A (Havrix)	Two doses[a] IM at 0 and 6-12 months	Protective immunity following receipt of first dose; second dose promotes long-lasting immunity.
Hepatitis A (VAQTA)	Two doses[a] IM at 0 and 6-18 months	Protective immunity following receipt of first dose; second dose promotes long-lasting immunity.
Hepatitis B (Engerix B) (standard schedule)	Three doses[a] IM at 0, 1, and 6 months	Need for booster not determined.
Hepatitis B (Recombivax) (standard schedule)	Three doses[a] IM at 0, 1, and 6 months	Need for booster not determined.
Hepatitis B (Engerix B) (accelerated schedule)	Three doses[a] IM at 0, 1, and 2 months	A 4th dose is recommended 12 months after the first dose to assure long-lasting immunity.
Hepatitis A/B (Twinrix) (standard schedule)	Three doses[a] IM at 0, 1, and 6 months	Need for booster not determined; persistence of anti-HAV and anti-HBsAg antibodies in adults for at least 10 years after primary immunization.
Hepatitis A/B (Twinrix) (accelerated schedule)	Three doses[a] IM on days 0, 7, and 21-30	A 4th dose is recommended 12 months after the first dose to assure long-lasting immunity.
Immune globulin (IG) (hepatitis A protection)	One dose[a] IM in gluteus muscle (2-mL dose for 3 months' protection; 5-mL divided dose for 5 months' protection)	Boost at 3- to 5-month intervals depending on initial dose received for continued risk of exposure.
Japanese encephalitis-purified inactivated virus (Ixiaro)	Two doses IM on days 0 and 28	Booster dose may be given 12 months after the first dose for continued risk of exposure.
Meningococcal (A/C/Y/W-135) diphtheria toxin conjugate vaccine (MCV4/MenACWY-D) (Menactra)	One dose IM	Not determined; estimated protective immunity 7 years or more.
Meningococcal (A/C/Y/W-135) CRM197 conjugate vaccine (MenACWY-CRM) (Menveo)	One dose IM	Not determined.
Meningococcus (A/C/Y/W-135) polysaccharide vaccine (MPSV4) (Menimmune)	One dose[a] SC	Estimated protective immunity 3-5 years; may boost with MenACWY-D or MenACWY-CRM vaccine.
Meningococcal B-4C (Bexsero)	Two doses at 1 month apart	Not determined.
Meningococcal B-FHbp (TruMemba)	Three doses at 0, 2, and 6 months	Not determined.

TABLE 5.3   Dosage Schedules for Adult Travel Immunizations—cont'd

Vaccine	Primary Series	Booster Interval
Rabies (HDCV) (Imovax) or Rabies (PCEC) (RabAvert)	Three doses[a] (1 mL IM in the deltoid area) on days 0, 7, and 21 or 28	Boost after 2 years for continued risk of exposure, or test serum for antibody level.
Tick-borne encephalitis (Encepur) (standard or conventional schedule)	Three doses SC on days 0, 28, and 300)	Boost 3 years after the last dose.
Tick-borne encephalitis (Encepur) (rapid schedule)	Three doses[a] SC on days 0, 7, 21	First booster dose at 15 months after the first vaccine dose; 2nd booster at 36 months after the first booster.
Tick-borne encephalitis (FSME-Immuno) (standard or conventional schedule)	Three doses[a] SC at months 0, 1-3, and 9-12 months after dose two	Boost 3 years after the last dose.
Tick-borne encephalitis (FSME-Immuno) (rapid schedule)	Three doses[a] SC on 0, 7, and 21 days	First booster dose at 15 months after the first vaccine dose; second booster at 36 months after the first booster.
Tuberculosis (BCG vaccine)[b]	One dose[a] percutaneously with multiple-puncture disk	Re-vaccinate after 2-3 months those who remain tuberculin negative to 5 TU skin test.
Typhoid, Vi capsular polysaccharide (Typhim Vi)	One dose[a] SC	Boost after 2 years for continued risk of exposure.
Typhoid, oral (Vivotif) (for persons >6 years of age)	One capsule[a] PO every 2 days for four doses	5 years; use full four-dose series for booster.
Yellow fever[b]	One dose[a] SC	10 years[c].

[a]See manufacturer's package insert for recommendations on dosage.
[b]Caution: may be contraindicated in patients with any of the following conditions: pregnancy, leukemia, lymphoma, generalized malignancy, immunosuppression from HIV infection or treatment with corticosteroids, alkylating drugs, antimetabolites, or radiation therapy.
[c]Recommendation for a booster dose is undergoing revision at the time of writing. Check the CDC Travelers' Health website for updates (http://www.cdc.gov/travel).
BCG, Bacillus Calmette-Guérin; ETEC, enterotoxic Escherichia coli; HAV, hepatitis A virus; HBsAg, Hepatitis B surface antigen; IM, intramuscularly; PO, by mouth; SC, subcutaneously.
Adapted from Jong, E.C., 1993. Immunizations for international travelers. In: The Travel Medicine Advisor. American Health Consultants, Atlanta, GA.

and benefits of YF vaccine is particularly important in advising senior travelers. However, the protection offered by the vaccine probably outweighs the risks in those who are traveling to regions endemic for yellow fever, regardless of age.

YF Vaccine Letter of Waiver

If a person for whom the vaccine is contraindicated must travel to a country where yellow fever vaccine is required for entry, a signed statement on letterhead stationery that states that the yellow fever vaccine could not be administered to the traveler because of medical contraindications will be accepted in lieu of the vaccination statement, according to WHO regulations. Alternately, the medical provider can complete the "Medical Contraindication to Vaccination" section of the International Certificate of Vaccination or Prophylaxis.

Meningococcal ACWY Vaccines

Due to outbreaks of meningococcal disease among Hajj pilgrims with secondary spread of meningococcal infections to family and friends after the pilgrims returned home, in 2003 Saudi Arabia implemented a *requirement* for meningococcal vaccine for all persons seeking to travel in Saudi Arabia during the annual Hajj. Either the quadrivalent meningococcal vaccine containing capsular polysaccharides from *Neisseria meningitidis* serogroups A, C, W, Y (MCPSV4) or one of the quadrivalent meningococcal conjugate vaccines containing the same capsular polysaccharides conjugated to a protein carrier (MCV4/MenACWY-D or MenACWY-CRM) will meet the requirement. In some countries, bivalent meningococcal polysaccharide or conjugate vaccines eliciting immunity against serogroups A and C may be commonly available; however, the A/C vaccine does not protect travelers in outbreaks involving serogroup Y or W-135 disease, such as has been the case in some of the Hajj outbreaks (**Fig. 5.2**). Meningococcal vaccine is also *recommended* for travelers going to live and work in certain areas of Africa (sub-Saharan), South America (Brazil), or other parts of the world where meningococcal disease is hyperendemic or epidemic among the residents.

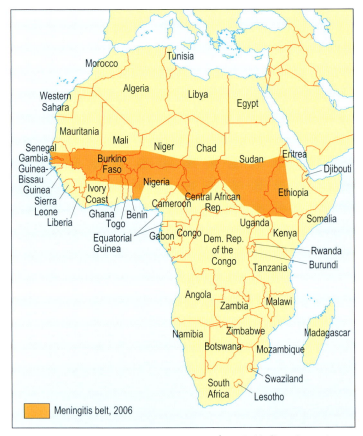

Fig. 5.2 **Areas with frequent epidemics of meningococcal meningitis.** (From: Centers for Disease Control 2008. Health Information for International Travel, 2007–2008. US Government Printing Office, Washington, DC. Available at <http://wwwn.cdc.gov/travel/yellowBookCh4-Menin.aspx#651>.)

The ACIP recommends *routine* immunization against meningococcal disease with ACWY quadrivalent vaccine for young people 11-18 years old and for incoming college freshmen who will live in large residence halls on campus (some institutions *require* immunization for matriculation because of the increased risk of meningococcal transmission in such student populations). Meningococcal vaccination is also recommended for persons at increased risk of disease, such as microbiologists who may be routinely exposed to strains of *N. meningitidis*, military recruits, persons with complement component deficiencies, and persons with anatomic or functional asplenia. Meningococcal B vaccine is discussed under "Recommended Travel Vaccines" below.

The meningococcal conjugate vaccines promote eradication of the nasopharyngeal carrier state due to the high levels of mucosal antibodies elicited, and there is a strong antibody response to subsequent booster doses of the vaccine. Use of a meningococcal conjugate vaccine is preferred for those persons who need imminent as well as possible future protection against meningococcal disease because immunity can be effectively boosted by additional conjugate vaccine doses, although the meningococcal polysaccharide vaccine is sufficiently protective for use in travelers and others anticipating limited exposure to meningococcal disease.

The duration of immunity following immunization with a conjugate vaccine is estimated to be 7 years, although no formal booster interval has been recommended at this time. Persons who received the MPSV4 vaccine in the past and who remain at risk of exposure to meningococcal disease may be boosted with a conjugate vaccine.

Meningococcal ACWY-Diphtheria Toxin Protein Conjugate (MenACWY-D) Vaccine

MenACWY-D vaccine (Menactra®, Sanofi) is a quadrivalent vaccine derived from serogroups A/C/W-135/Y capsular polysaccharides conjugated to diphtheria toxin protein, which enables enhanced immunogenicity through activation of a strong T-cell immune response in vaccine recipients. The vaccine is licensed for use among persons 9 months through 55 years of age and given as a single dose administered by IM injection.

Meningococcal ACWY-CRM Conjugate (MenACWY-CRM) Vaccine

MenACWY-CRM vaccine (Menveo®, Novartis) is a quadrivalent vaccine derived from serogroups A/C/W-135/Y capsular polysaccharides conjugated to diphtheria toxin mutant CRM197. The vaccine is licensed for use among persons 2 months through 55 years of age and given as a single dose administered by IM injection.

Meningococcal Polysaccharide A/C/Y/W-135 Vaccine (MPSV4)

MPSV4 vaccine (Menimmune®, Sanofi) is a quadrivalent capsular polysaccharide vaccine inducing immunity against serogroups A/C/Y/W-135. A single dose administered by subcutaneous (SC) injection provides immunity for approximately 3-5 years among healthy recipients, although vaccine efficacy is variable in young children. A second dose of vaccine after 2 or 3 years is recommended for children living in high-risk areas who received the first vaccine dose at <4 years of age.

Polio Vaccine

Polio vaccine is given as part of the routine immunization series to infants and children in the United States. A four-dose series of inactivated poliovirus vaccine (IPV) administered by IM or SC injection is given at 2, 4, and 6-18 months of age, and at 4-6 years old (Chapter 12). IPV (Ipol®, Sanofi) is the only polio vaccine used in the United States since 2000, when a policy decision to discontinue the use of oral polio vaccine was made in order to avoid the rare occurrence of vaccine-associated paralytic poliomyelitis from the attenuated live virus vaccine. Oral polio vaccine is still in use in countries outside the United States.

A single lifetime IPV booster dose is recommended for adult travelers 18 years and older who are traveling to countries with recognized circulation of WPV or to countries that border countries that have areas with WPV in circulation. WPV circulation has been reported in Afghanistan, Pakistan, Middle Eastern countries, Egypt, Nigeria, and other countries located in a belt across sub-Saharan Africa. Outbound long-term (≥4 weeks) travelers and residents of WPV-affected countries may be *required* to show proof of polio vaccination between 4 weeks and 12 months before departure under WHO IHR in order to prevent importation of polio into polio-free countries by infected travelers. The CDC regularly updates its website regarding which countries have ongoing transmission of polio and which countries may require proof of polio vaccination from exiting travelers.

Cholera Vaccine

There is no WHO regulation requiring cholera vaccine for entry into any country. Currently available cholera vaccines are discussed under "Recommended Travel Vaccines" below.

Smallpox Vaccine

The smallpox vaccine (vaccinia virus vaccine) is no longer available commercially. Limited supplies are released on a case-by-case basis from the CDC based on individual review. Research scientists and healthcare workers who work with the smallpox virus and closely related viruses are candidates for immunization. The last case of smallpox acquired through natural transmission was reported in 1977, and the requirement for smallpox vaccine for international travel was removed from the WHO regulations in 1982.

RECOMMENDED TRAVEL VACCINES

Recommended travel vaccines are those that are given to travelers based on the anticipated level of risk of exposure. Vaccines in this category may include hepatitis A, immune globulin (for hepatitis A), hepatitis B, typhoid fever, cholera, meningococcal disease, rabies, Japanese encephalitis, and tick-borne encephalitis vaccines. Immunization against tuberculosis or a tuberculosis skin test may also be recommended for some travelers. Brief descriptions of each vaccine are given below. Table 5.3 lists dosage schedules for adult travel immunizations.

Hepatitis A Vaccine

Hepatitis A is a serious viral infection with an oral-fecal transmission pattern similar to polio, cholera, typhoid, hepatitis E, and traveler's diarrhea. Hepatitis A infections are reported to be the leading cause of vaccine-preventable illness occurring among non-immune international travelers, where the incidence rate can be as high as 20 cases/1000 travelers per month among travelers during rural or adventure travel in developing countries. A lower rate, 3-6 cases/1000 travelers per month, has been observed among travelers going to tourist areas or hotels and resorts in developing countries.

The hepatitis A case fatality rate associated with acute infections is <0.1% in childhood from <1 to 14 years of age. There is an age-related rise in the disease mortality rate: 0.4% from 15 to 39 years of age, 1.1% in persons >40 years of age, and 2.7% in persons >50 years of age. Although up to 60% of adults >40 years of age from industrialized countries may have immunity to hepatitis A through clinical or subclinical infection, most travelers <40 years old are susceptible. If time allows, a serum test for hepatitis A antibody could be performed in people who are of foreign birth, resided overseas, travel frequently in non-industrialized countries, have a history of a previous illness with jaundice, or were born before 1945; unnecessary immunization may be avoided if a person has protective antibodies from hepatitis A infection in the past.

Hepatitis A Virus (HAV) Vaccine

Several safe and highly efficacious inactivated HAV vaccines have become available commercially since the 1994 release of Havrix® (GlaxoSmithKline). Havrix is an inactivated HAV vaccine derived from the HM-175 viral strain and given by injection. The others include VAQTA® (Merck), an inactivated parenteral HAV vaccine derived from the CR-326F strain; Avaxim® (Sanofi), an inactivated parenteral HAV vaccine derived from the

GBM viral strain; and Epaxal® (Crucell), an inactivated parenteral virosomal HAV vaccine derived from the RG-SB viral strain. Havrix and VAQTA are available worldwide. The other inactivated HAV vaccines are distributed mostly in Western Europe, and a live-attenuated hepatitis A vaccine Biovac-A (Pukang) approved by the WHO is available in Asia and South America. The immunization schedules for the inactivated HAV vaccines listed above consist of a single primary dose given by IM injection into the deltoid muscle, resulting in protective antibody titers within 2-4 weeks (98-100% seropositivity rate). The first vaccine dose is followed by a booster dose 6-12 months later, producing levels of antibody predicted to give protection for ≥10 years. After the primary series of two doses, additional boosters are not currently advised.

Delayed Hepatitis A Vaccine Booster Dose

In some cases, travelers return for their booster dose of inactivated hepatitis A vaccine later than the recommended time of 6-12 months after the primary dose. Based on the results of clinical studies, delaying the booster dose up to 66 months after primary vaccination did not seem to influence the anamnestic immune response to the booster dose. These findings suggest that a booster dose given later than the recommended 6-12 months will still be highly effective.

Hepatitis A Vaccine Interchangeability

Using one of the inactivated hepatitis A vaccines for the primary dose and then using a hepatitis A vaccine made by a different manufacturer for the booster dose is not a recommended or officially approved practice. However, it appears from the preliminary results of clinical studies that Havrix and VAQTA may be used interchangeably without significant loss of protective antibody levels elicited (data from Merck Vaccine Division).

Immune Globulin (IG)

Immune globulin (purified human immune globulin) may be used to provide temporary protection against hepatitis A virus infection through the passive transfer of pre-formed antibodies against hepatitis A present in the IG (at least 100 IU/mL) and is given to travelers who are unable to receive hepatitis A vaccine. Duration of protection is dependent on dose, with a dose of 0.06 mL/kg (10 mg IgG/kg) administered as a deep IM injection into the gluteus maximus muscle providing up to 3-4 months' protection (**Table 5.3**).

Concurrent Administration of Hepatitis A Vaccine with Immune Globulin

Updated recommendations no longer call for concurrent administration of IG when hepatitis A vaccine is given <2 weeks before trip departure. The vaccine induces a vigorous antibody response in normal hosts that may not totally protect the recipient against infection but will most likely protect the recipient from developing severe disease, in the case the vaccine recipient is exposed to hepatitis A virus before the vaccine-induced antibodies are at a level (>20 mIU/mL) sufficient to prevent infection. Using this rationale, hepatitis A vaccine has been successfully used for post-exposure immunization of susceptible persons during hepatitis A outbreaks.

Hepatitis B Virus (HBV) Vaccine

In many parts of Asia and Africa, up to 15% of the general population may be asymptomatic carriers of hepatitis B virus. Travelers going to Asia and Africa who will live and work among the residents, such as missionaries, healthcare personnel, volunteer relief workers, teachers, students, adventure travelers, and other travelers who might have intimate or sexual contact with the residents, should consider immunization against hepatitis B. In addition, inadvertent exposures to hepatitis B among travelers can occur during medical procedures (emergency or elective) and personal grooming/esthetic activities (shaving, manicures/pedicures, tattoos, piercings, etc.). Although hepatitis B vaccine has been recommended for routine immunization of children in the United States since the early 1990s, many adult travelers at potential risk of infection would not have received hepatitis B vaccine as a routine immunization.

Two recombinant hepatitis B virus vaccines are available: Recombivax HB® (Merck) and Engerix-B® (GlaxoSmithKline). The standard dosage schedule for both vaccines consists of doses administered by IM injection into the deltoid muscle at 0, 1, and 6 months.

Hepatitis B Vaccine Low-Responders or Nonresponders

Among travelers who are at high risk of hepatitis B exposure, such as healthcare workers, volunteer relief workers, missionaries, long-term travelers and expatriates, the possibility of vaccine recipients who do not seroconvert with protective levels of antibody after immunization should be considered. Known risk factors are increasing age (>30 years old), chronic medical conditions, obesity, smoking, male gender, and vaccine administration into the buttock.

Immune protection against Hepatitis B virus is measured by serum levels of antibodies to Hepatitis B surface antigen (Anti-HBs). Anti-HBs testing should be performed 1-6 months after the last dose of vaccine. If there is no seroconversion (≥10 mIU/mL), one additional dose of HBV should be given, and the anti-HBs titer re-checked 4-12 weeks later. If there is still no measurable antibody response, the second series is completed with two additional doses given at monthly intervals after that. Limited data from clinical studies have shown that anti-HBs titers and protection do not always correlate closely, such that even those with low or undetectable titers may still be protected after immunization due to cellular immunity, with an amnestic antibody response following a subsequent exposure to hepatitis B virus or the hepatitis B vaccine years afterward.

Accelerated Hepatitis B Vaccine Schedules

Engerix B vaccine has a Food and Drug Administration (FDA)-approved accelerated dosage schedule of 0, 1, and 2 months. This may allow full immunization of a traveler with limited time before departure; however, a booster dose at 12 months is recommended to assure long-lasting immunity. Another accelerated schedule approved for adolescents and adults calls for the first two doses of either hepatitis B vaccine to be given 1 or 2 months apart, and for the third dose to be given at least 4 months after the first dose; in this case, a booster dose at 12 months is not required.

Hepatitis A/B Combination Vaccine

A hepatitis A/B combination vaccine (Twinrix®, GlaxoSmithKline Biologicals) was released in 2001 in the United States and is approved for use in persons 18 years of age or older. The vaccine contains 720 ELISA (enzyme-linked immunosorbent assay) units of hepatitis A antigen and 20 μg of hepatitis B antigen, and the standard immunization series consists of three doses given at 0, 1, and 6 months. Clinical studies have shown that the combination hepatitis A/B vaccine is highly efficacious and safe, with long-term protection demonstrated up to 10 years after primary immunization. The use of this combination vaccine will be convenient for travelers and other persons who need protection against both diseases, and decreases the total number of vaccine injections required (3 vs. 5). A pediatric formulation of the hepatitis A/B vaccine is not licensed in the United States but is available in other countries.

Accelerated Hepatitis A/B Vaccine Schedule

Hepatitis A/B vaccine (Twinrix) given on 0, 7, and 21-30 days elicits a high level of protective antibody against both hepatitis A and hepatitis B, 1 month following the third dose. A fourth dose at 12 months is recommended to boost the longevity of the immune response to the accelerated schedule. The accelerated hepatitis A/B Twinrix schedule was FDA approved in the United States in 2006. The accelerated hepatitis A/B vaccine schedule should be considered for last-minute travelers at risk whose departure date is 21-30 days from the date of the travel clinic appointment. If the departure date is <21 days from the clinic encounter, the traveler should be immunized with one dose of monovalent hepatitis A vaccine, concurrently with monovalent hepatitis B vaccine on a standard schedule, or consideration should be given to an accelerated hepatitis B vaccine schedule.

Typhoid Vaccine

The incidence of typhoid fever among US travelers is relatively low (58-174 cases per 1 million travelers), but among reported cases in the United States, 62% were acquired during international travel. Mexico, Peru, India, Pakistan, and Chile are countries where the risk of transmission appears particularly high. Sub-Saharan Africa and Southeast Asia are also regarded as areas of increased risk for typhoid fever. The risk of typhoid fever infections to the traveler is further heightened by the multidrug-resistance patterns emerging in *Salmonella typhi* strains around the world to antibiotics commonly used in the treatment of gastrointestinal infections, including the widely used fluoroquinolones.

Avoidance of potentially contaminated food and drink during travel is important, even if the typhoid vaccine is received. The protection against typhoid fever afforded by immunization may be overwhelmed by ingestion of highly contaminated food: protection rates of 43-96% were reported in field trials with the oral live-attenuated typhoid vaccine among residents of endemic areas. However, only limited data are available to predict actual protection rates in people who travel from non-endemic areas to endemic areas for typhoid. There are two typhoid vaccines available in the United States: the oral Ty21A typhoid vaccine and the parenteral Vi capsular polysaccharide typhoid vaccine. Neither typhoid vaccine will give protection against paratyphoid fever, caused by strains of *Salmonella paratyphi*.

Ty21A Oral Typhoid Vaccine

The oral typhoid vaccine (Vivotif®, Crucell) contains a live attenuated strain of *Salmonella typhi* bacteria (Ty21A). The vaccine is in capsule form and is recommended for people 6 years of age and older. A primary (or booster) series consists of four capsules, one taken every other day on an empty stomach over the course of 1 week. The booster interval is 5 years, and another four-capsule regimen is used to renew immunity. A liquid suspension form of this vaccine is available in Europe, and this facilitates administration of the vaccine to children and others who have difficulty in swallowing capsules. Persons who were previously immunized with one of the parenteral typhoid vaccines and who now desire immunization with the oral vaccine should receive the full four-capsule series. Safety of the live oral Ty21a typhoid vaccine in immune-compromised persons has not yet been demonstrated, and this vaccine should not be administered to these persons. The vaccine is not recommended for pregnant women because of lack of data regarding its safety (Category C).

Ty21A Typhoid Vaccine and Concomitant Drugs

Any conditions interfering with multiplication of the vaccine strain bacteria in vivo may result in an insufficient bacterial antigen stimulus to induce a protective response. The live oral typhoid vaccine should not be administered during an acute gastrointestinal illness nor if the individual is receiving treatment with sulfonamides, doxycycline, or other antibiotics. The antimalarial drugs chloroquine and mefloquine may be administered concomitantly with the oral typhoid vaccine without decreasing the immune response rate. However, proguanil, one component of the atovaquone/proguanil (Malarone) fixed-dose combination drug used for prevention and treatment of chloroquine-resistant malaria, does significantly decrease the immune response to oral typhoid vaccine. Therefore, proguanil and atovaquone/proguanil should be administered ≥10 days after the final dose of the vaccine.

Ty21A Oral Typhoid Vaccine and Other Vaccines

Concomitant administration of oral polio vaccine, oral cholera vaccine, or yellow fever vaccine does not appear to suppress the immune response of the oral typhoid vaccine.

Vi Capsular Polysaccharide (ViCPS) Typhoid Vaccine

A highly purified Vi capsular polysaccharide typhoid vaccine (Typhim Vi®, Sanofi) elicits immunity 10 days following receipt of a single primary dose by IM injection. The ViCPS typhoid vaccine is usually very well tolerated, has a low rate of adverse effects, and is safe for use in children >2 years old, pregnant women, and travelers with a compromised immune system. The protection elicited by the Vi polysaccharide typhoid vaccine is similar to that seen following immunization with the live oral Ty21A typhoid vaccine. The booster interval for the ViCPS typhoid vaccine is 2 years.

ViCPS Typhoid Vaccine Combined with Hepatitis A Vaccine

Typhoid fever and hepatitis A viral infections are both transmitted through oral-fecal contamination of food and beverages, thus protection against both diseases is indicated for many international travelers. Several studies have shown that simultaneous administration of the Vi polysaccharide typhoid vaccine (Typhim Vi™) and hepatitis A vaccine (Havrix or VAQTA) at different injection sites results in no significant increase in adverse side effects nor in impaired efficacy of either vaccine.

Cholera Vaccine

Travelers going to cholera-endemic or cholera-epidemic areas are encouraged to follow food and water precautions as recommended for prevention of all forms of travel-associated diarrhea (see Chapter 8). Travelers going to such areas who have underlying gastric conditions, such as achlorhydria or partial gastric resection, or who take medications that block gastric acid production (e.g., H2 blockers, proton pump inhibitors) may have increased susceptibility to cholera infection and should be considered as priority candidates for cholera immunization. Other prime candidates for cholera vaccine are healthcare workers who plan work in areas of high endemicity for cholera, for example, India or sub-Saharan Africa, or in refugee camps and/or communities during a known outbreak of cholera. There are two oral cholera vaccines (OCV) that are WHO-prequalified for use in areas at risk for cholera. Both are whole-cell killed vaccines of *Vibrio cholerae* O1.

Killed Whole-Cell B Subunit Oral Cholera Vaccine (WC/rBS OCV)

WC/rBS oral cholera vaccine (Dukoral®, Crucell) is approved for use in persons 2 years of age and older. In addition to stimulating immunoprotection against cholera, the vaccine has been shown to offer some protection against traveler's diarrhea due to antibodies elicited against the recombinant cholera B subunit toxin component cross-reacting with the heat-labile toxin secreted by enterotoxic *Escherichia coli* (ETEC) (see Chapter 8). Two doses are taken orally at least 1 week apart (up to 6 weeks), and the vaccine provides protection against cholera for 2 years and short-term (3 months) protection against traveler's diarrhea caused by ETEC. Children 2-6 years old should take 3 doses 1 week apart. Protection starts 1 week after the last dose of the vaccine is taken, with a protective efficacy range of 50-86%. Adverse side effects consist of gastrointestinal symptoms rarely reported. Dukoral is not licensed in the United States but is available in Canada and some countries in Western Europe, South America, and Asia. In Canada Dukoral is available without prescription for prevention of traveler's diarrhea, but a prescription is required for the vaccine to be used for prevention of cholera.

Killed Whole-Cell Bivalent (O1 and O139 Serogroups) Oral Cholera Vaccine (BivWC OCV)

BivWC OCV (Shanchol™, Shantha Biotechnics-Sanofi Company) is not currently available in the United States but has been used in vaccine programs to prevent cholera in endemic areas, mainly in Asia, and BivWC OCV also was used to control disease spread during the cholera outbreak in Haiti in 2010 after the earthquake. The vaccine can be used in persons 1 year of age and up; two doses are given orally 2 weeks apart. Onset of protection is from 7 to 10 days after the second dose, and the vaccine is estimated to provide 65% protection lasting at least 5 years.

Meningococcal Serogroup B Vaccine

Quadrivalent meningococcal vaccines against serogroups A, C, Y, and W-135 are discussed above in "Required Travel Vaccines." At the time of writing, there is no WHO IHR for meningococcal serogroup B (MenB) vaccine, although sporadic and sustained outbreaks of serogroup B disease have been reported throughout the world. The ACIP *recommends* MenB vaccine for certain high-risk groups, including persons with complement deficiency or functional asplenia (status post-splenectomy, sickle cell anemia), microbiologists with routine exposure to *N. meningitidis* isolates, and persons identified at increased risk because of ongoing serogroup B meningococcal outbreaks in the community. International travelers such as healthcare providers, teachers, students, and missionaries going to live and work in areas with ongoing serogroup B meningococcal outbreaks may also wish to avail themselves of MenB vaccine protection; they need to plan ahead to allow completion of the given vaccine series before departure. There is currently no ACIP recommendation for universal MenB immunization of incoming US college freshman who will live in campus housing; however, in 2015, ACIP did vote to follow the recommendation of ACIP's meningococcal working group, which stated that the serogroup B meningococcal vaccine series "may be administered to adolescents and young adults 16 through 23 years of age," further specifying that 16-18 years is the preferred age for vaccination.

Two meningococcal B (MenB) vaccines are FDA licensed and available in the United States at the time of writing, both approved for use in persons 10-25 years old. Once started, the MenB vaccine series should be completed with the same product.

Meningococcal B-4C Vaccine (MenB-4C)

MenB-4C vaccine (Bexsero, Novartis Vaccines) contains three recombinant proteins: *Neisseria* adhesin A, factor H binding protein (FHbp) fusion protein, and *Neisseria* heparin binding antigen, plus outer membrane protein PorA serosubtype P1.4. It is administered by injection of two doses at least 1 month apart.

Meningococcal B-FHbp Vaccine (MenB-FHbp)

MenB-FHbp vaccine (TruMemba, Wyeth Pharmaceuticals) consists of two purified recombinant FHbp antigens and is licensed to be given as a series of three doses, with the second dose at 2 months and the third dose at 6 months after the first.

Rabies Vaccine

Animal bites, especially dog bites, present a potential rabies hazard to international travelers who travel to rural areas in Central and South America, the Middle East, Africa, and Asia. Pre-exposure rabies immunization is recommended for rural travelers, especially adventure travelers who go to remote areas, and for expatriate workers, missionaries, and their families living in countries where rabies is a recognized risk. Veterinarians, animal handlers, cavers, field biologists, and laboratory workers are also considered at high risk of rabies exposure.

Pre-exposure rabies immunization with the three-dose primary vaccine series simplifies the post-bite medical care of a person following an animal bite. Without pre-exposure immunization, the bitten person needs treatment with both rabies immune globulin (RIG) and a series of four doses of a modern tissue culture-derived vaccine administered as soon as possible after the incident. Both RIG and high-quality rabies vaccine doses may be difficult for the international traveler to access in the areas of greatest rabies risk. More detailed recommendations for post-bite treatment are discussed below.

Pre-Exposure Rabies Vaccines

There are two inactivated rabies virus vaccines available, both derived from viruses grown in tissue culture cells: human diploid cell vaccine (HDCV, Imovax™, Sanofi) and purified chick embryo cell vaccine (PCEC, Rabavert™, Novartis). These vaccine products may be used interchangeably in the pre-exposure rabies immunization: a total of three doses (1.0 mL each) of rabies vaccine are administered by IM injection on days 0, 7, and 21 or 28. Mild local reactions to rabies vaccine are common and consist of erythema, pain, and swelling at the injection site. Mild systemic symptoms including headache, dizziness, nausea, abdominal pain, and myalgias may develop in some recipients. In approximately 5% of people receiving booster doses of HDCV for pre-exposure prophylaxis and in a few receiving post-exposure immunization, a serum sickness-like illness characterized by urticaria, fever, malaise, arthralgias, arthritis, nausea, and vomiting may develop 2-21 days after a vaccine dose is received.

Rabies Vaccine Booster Doses

Whether or not a traveler requires boosters of rabies vaccine depends on that traveler's risk of exposure to rabies. For low-risk itineraries, no booster is recommended. For those with "frequent" risk (e.g., spelunkers, veterinarians, and staff in rabies-epizootic areas) serologic testing is advised every 2 years, with booster vaccination if the antibody titer is below protection levels. For those with "continuous" exposure (e.g., rabies research lab workers), serological testing is advised every 6 months with booster vaccination if the antibody titer is below a protective level.

Rabies Post-Exposure Vaccine and Rabies Immune Globulin (RIG)

Receipt of pre-exposure rabies immunization simplifies the care of a person if a high-risk bite is sustained. In addition to immediate wound care (vigorous cleansing, debridement, loose approximation of skin edges, and antibiotics to prevent wound infection), two additional 1-mL IM doses of rabies vaccine on days 0 and 3 are recommended for optimal protection.

If a person who has not received pre-exposure rabies vaccine is bitten while in a rabies-endemic area, post-exposure care for the bite includes a dose (20 IU/kg) of RIG, with one-half the dose infiltrated at the wound site if possible and the remainder given by IM injection. In addition, four doses (1 mL) of rabies vaccine should be given by IM injection on days 0, 3, 7, and 14. A fifth dose of rabies vaccine on day 28 after the bite injury is recommended for patients with immune compromise.

Human-derived RIG and tissue culture-derived rabies vaccine are difficult to obtain in many rabies-endemic areas. The supply of RIG in developing countries is likely to be derived from horse serum, and administration of horse-derived RIG is accompanied by a significant risk of serum sickness. The rabies vaccines available in developing countries could be Semple-type vaccines, derived from infected brain tissue of laboratory animals. Such preparations have a potential for serious adverse side effects and decreased protective efficacy compared with the modern tissue culture-derived rabies vaccines.

Japanese Encephalitis Virus Vaccine

Japanese encephalitis (JE) is a viral infection primarily transmitted by *Culex* mosquitoes in Asia, Southeast Asia, and the western Pacific (**Fig. 5.3**). Transmission is year round in the tropical and subtropical zones and during the late spring, summer, and early fall in the temperate climate zones. Pigs and some species of aquatic birds are natural reservoirs of the virus, while the mosquito vectors breed extensively in flooded rice fields and irrigation projects. JE virus infections may cause an asymptomatic infection or a nonspecific febrile illness that is not recognized or diagnosed. Residents living in JE transmission areas appear to acquire immunity through natural infections over the years, thus reported cases of symptomatic disease and serious neurologic sequelae are seen most often in children younger than 15 years of age and in the elderly. There is no specific treatment, and care is supportive: up to one-third of diagnosed cases survive with permanent cognitive and neurologic impairments, and approximately one-third of patients die.

JE virus is considered the most common cause of vaccine-preventable encephalitis in Asia. Approximately 68,000 cases are reported annually among residents in the countries and areas at risk. The incidence of JE cases is decreasing in endemic countries and areas where immunization against JE has been incorporated into standard childhood vaccine programs or where targeted community vaccine programs against JE have been implemented. However, factors such as climate change, land use patterns, and human migration within the endemic areas are contributing to the emergence of JE in new geographic areas and among new populations, thus resulting in negligible net change in JE incidence statistics in some countries despite vaccine prevention efforts.

JE is not usually considered a risk for short-term travelers visiting only well-developed urban destinations and resorts within JE endemic areas. However, even in countries with long-standing JE vaccine programs and no reported human infections, the JE virus continues

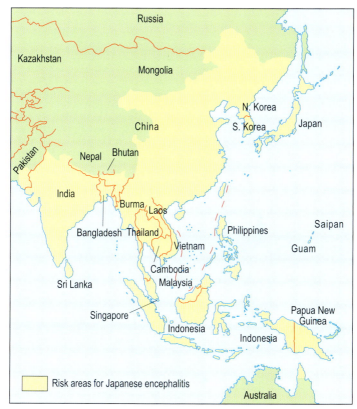

Fig. 5.3 **Geographic distribution of Japanese encephalitis.** (From: Centers for Disease Control 2008. Health Information for International Travel, 2007–2008. US Government Printing Office, Washington, DC. Available at <http://wwwn.cdc.gov/travel/yellowBookCh4-Japaneseencephalitis .aspx#638>.)

to be present in the environment and can be detected in sentinel animals and in birds. Thus, JE transmission from natural reservoirs to non-immune humans is an ever-present risk to travelers in countries where JE transmission appears to be "under control" based on numbers of reported cases.

Since JE has been acquired by short-term travelers as well as long-stay travelers, all travelers going on trips of any length to endemic areas during JE transmission season (when biting mosquitoes are present), especially to rural agricultural areas where pig farming is present, should be educated about the risk of JE and the availability of a safe, effective vaccine to prevent the disease. Furthermore, since urban development encroaching on agricultural lands is typical in many parts of Asia and can bring infected mosquitoes into the proximity of susceptible urban dwellers, and backyard piggeries may serve as local JE reservoirs, even travelers planning strictly urban stays in Asia and Southeast Asia should be educated about the risk of JE transmission. Personal protective measures to prevent mosquito bites such as wearing protective clothing, using insect repellents, and sleeping under permethrin-treated bed nets (see Chapter 1) are also important toward decreasing the traveler's risk of JE infection and other mosquito-borne infections (e.g., malaria, dengue fever).

Japanese Encephalitis Purified Inactivated Virus Vaccine (JE-PIV)

The JE-PIV vaccine Ixiaro™ (Valneva) derived from the SA 14-14-2 JE virus strain cultured in Vero cell tissue cultures was licensed by the FDA in 2009 for use in adults 17 years of age and older, and in 2013 for use in children 2 months through 16 years. Two doses of JE-PIV vaccine administered 28 days apart by IM injection will elicit protective levels of antibodies for up to 12 months after the first vaccine dose. The dose is 0.5 mL for adults and children 3 years of age and up. For children 2 months through 2 years, the vaccine dose is 0.25 mL (one-half the adult dose). A booster dose is recommended 1 year after primary immunization for continued risk of exposure in adults; there are limited data about booster doses in children. Local pain and tenderness at the injection site are the most commonly reported adverse side effects, with up to 10% of adult vaccine recipients reporting headache, myalgia, fatigue, and an influenza-like illness. In children, fever was the most commonly reported systemic symptom following a vaccine dose. Clinical studies suggest that a single dose of JE-PIV may effectively boost protective antibodies in persons who were immunized in the past with the previously available mouse brain-derived JE vaccine. A recently published randomized controlled trial showed that strong short-term immunity could be elicited in healthy adults by administering JE-PIV vaccine on an accelerated regimen with the two-dose primary series administered 1 week apart (off-label at the time of writing).

Tick-Borne Encephalitis Vaccine

Tick-borne encephalitis (TBE) is caused by infection with either of two closely related viruses: Central European encephalitis virus (CEEV) in Europe (Austria, Czechoslovakia, Germany, Hungary, Poland, Switzerland, Northern Yugoslavia) and Russian Spring Summer encephalitis virus (RSSEV) in the Commonwealth of Independent States (the former Soviet Union) during the months of April through August. There is overlap of the areas of transmission in Eastern Europe (**Fig. 5.4**). TBE is transmitted to humans by bites from infected *Ixodes ricinus* ticks usually found in forested areas of endemic regions (**Fig. 5.5**). However, systemic infection after ingestion of unpasteurized dairy products from infected cows, goats, or sheep can also occur.

Disease caused by this infection can lead to serious neurological sequelae or even fatal outcomes. Medical care consists of symptomatic treatment, as there is no specific cure. Immunization against TBE is the primary mode of prevention for populations living in endemic areas and travelers to those areas. The availability of TBE vaccines in mostly endemic areas and the multiple-dose immunization schedule mean that most travelers from North America who anticipate a need for protection against TBE will not be able to obtain pre-travel immunization. Travelers planning outdoor activities (hiking, biking, camping) in areas where TBE is a risk need to rely on personal protection measures to prevent tick bites. Travelers to such areas should be also advised to avoid ingestion of unpasteurized dairy products.

FSME-Immuno TBE Vaccine

Vaccination against TBE is currently not available in the United States. FSME-Immuno TBE vaccine (Immuno, Vienna) is available in Canada and Europe. The vaccine is produced in chick embryo cell cultures, and primary immunization consists of three doses given by SC injection. Another TBE vaccine called Encepur TBE Vaccine is manufactured by Chiron (Behring) and is distributed in European and Asian countries. Clinical studies have shown that the two vaccines are interchangeable and that administration using the rapid schedule of 0, 7, and 21 days with a booster dose of vaccine given at 15 months after the last vaccine dose yields rapid onset of protection and sustained high antibody titers over a 300-day observation period.

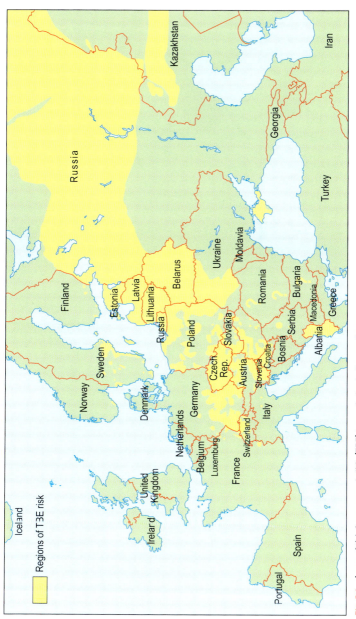

Fig. 5.4 **Areas of tick-borne encephalitis (TBE) transmission in Eastern Europe.**

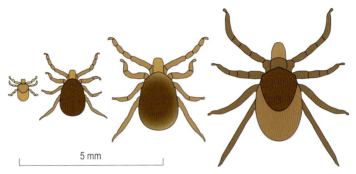

5 mm

Fig. 5.5 Tick vector (transmitter) of tick-borne encephalitis. *Ixodes ricinus*, from left to right: larva, nymph, adult female, adult male. (Courtesy of Fedor Gassner, Wageningen University.)

Tuberculosis (BCG) Vaccine

People going on short trips for tourism or business to countries where tuberculosis (TB) is much more common among the general population than in the United States are not considered to be at great risk of contracting TB. Travelers who will live among foreign residents or who will work in foreign orphanages, schools, hospitals, or other facilities may be at significant risk of exposure to infection with TB, which is commonly spread from person to person by inhalation of infected respiratory droplets in closed environments. Such travelers should be skin tested with tuberculin purified protein derivative (PPD) and control antigens (such as *Candida* and *Trichophyton*) or an interferon-gamma release assay (IGRA), such as QuantiFERON-TB Gold In-Tube test (QFT-GIT) or SPOT TB test (T-Spot), before and after the trip. Persons who convert to a skin test–positive status or from a negative to a positive IGRA following international travel need further evaluation and are candidates for consideration of prophylactic treatment with isoniazid or other drugs to prevent TB disease.

Occasionally, children in families going abroad for extended residence are requested by the receiving country to provide proof of bacillus Calmette-Guérin (BCG) vaccine receipt to qualify for a visa. A BCG vaccine is commercially available in the United States and is approved by the American Academy of Pediatrics Committee on the Control of Infectious Diseases for use in children going to live in areas where TB is prevalent or where there is a likelihood of exposure to adults with active or recently arrested TB. The BCG vaccine also might be considered appropriate in the case of uninfected (PPD skin test–negative) healthcare workers who are going to work in areas where there is a high endemic prevalence of tuberculosis in the population and who will have limited access to medical diagnosis and treatment.

Bacillus Calmette-Guérin Vaccine (BCG)

BCG vaccine is widely used all over the world for childhood immunization against TB, although this has never been a public health policy in the United States. There is no consensus on the protective efficacy of BCG vaccines, and estimates of protection have varied from study to study. Epidemiologic data suggest that the vaccine may be more useful in protecting children from disseminated extrapulmonary complications of tuberculosis, including TB meningitis, than in protecting adults from primary pulmonary infection.

Persons immunized with BCG vaccine become PPD skin test–positive for several years afterward, regardless of the degree of protection conferred by the vaccine. As a general rule, the longer the duration since BCG administration and the larger the PPD skin reaction, the more likely it is that the PPD skin reaction represents a true positive. In those who have received BCG vaccine, the IGRA is preferred over a PPD for diagnosis of latent TB infection.

Like other live attenuated vaccines, BCG vaccine is contraindicated in people with immunosuppression caused by congenital conditions, chemotherapy, radiation therapy, HIV infection, or another condition resulting in impaired immune responses. Pregnancy also is considered a relative contraindication.

CONCLUSION

Despite the availability of safe, highly efficacious vaccines against many of the diseases that are health risks to international travelers, there are several factors that influence travelers' acceptance of immunization recommendations. Practical concerns include the time available before trip departure, past history of allergies to or intolerance of specific vaccines, avoidance of multiple vaccine doses administered by injection, and the traveler's overall budget for pre-travel health preparations. Other factors influencing the traveler's choice of travel immunizations include his or her cultural perceptions of the health risks presented by a given itinerary, whether or not adventure travel away from normal tourist routes is planned, and anticipated access to organized medical care and/or medical evacuation in case of medical illness while traveling abroad.

FURTHER READING

Beran, J., Douda, P., Gniel, D., et al., 2004. Long-term immunity after vaccination against tick-borne encephalitis with Encepur using the rapid vaccination schedule. Int. J. Med. Microbiol. 293 (Suppl. 37), 130–133.
The rapid vaccination schedule makes it feasible for some travelers going to TBE transmission areas to obtain protection before exposure to this vaccine-preventable disease.

Centers for Disease Control and Prevention, 2015. Vaccination coverage among adults, excluding influenza vaccination—United States, 2013. MMWR Morb. Mortal. Wkly Rep. 64, 95–103.
This report shows that despite continuing efforts to improve vaccine awareness among US healthcare providers, pharmacists, and the public, adult vaccination coverage remains low for most routinely recommended vaccines. This highlights the importance of using the travel clinic visit as an opportunity to review the traveler's status with regard to routine immunizations and to advise on the required and recommended travel vaccines.

Centers for Disease Control and Prevention, 2016. Health Information for International Travel. DHHS (Department of Health and Human Services), Atlanta, GA. Available at <http://wwwnc.cdc.gov/travel/page/yellowbook-home> (accessed July 26, 2015).
Essential comprehensive reference for travel health providers and travelers. Provides official US public health guidelines and policies on international health issues, harmonizes recommendations from US health professional academies and societies, and references WHO recommendations. Available in printed form and a variety of electronic formats.

Charles, R.C., Hilaire, I.J., Mayo-Smith, L.M., et al., 2014. Immunogenicity of a killed bivalent (O1 and O139) whole cell oral cholera vaccine, Shanchol, in Haiti. PLOS Negl. Trop. Dis., May 2014 81, e2828, 1-8,
Field studies on the use of a killed whole cell bivalent oral cholera vaccine in a cholera outbreak in Haiti, outside the historical cholera endemic areas in Asia where residents may have had prior exposures to cholera that influence the magnitude of their cholera vaccine response. This article reports efficacy of a two-dose regimen in eliciting a protective immune response in children and adults.

Connor, B.A., Blatter, M.M., Beran, J., et al., 2007. Rapid and sustained immune response against hepatitis A and B achieved with combined vaccine using an accelerated administration schedule. J. Travel Med. 14, 9–15.
Clinical study demonstrating efficacy and benefits of an accelerated administration schedule for hepatitis A and B combination vaccine. The accelerated schedule is useful for "last minute" travelers and health care personnel who need vaccine protection against hepatitis A and B "in a hurry."

Gershman, M.D., Staples, J.E., 2013. World Health Organization reports that 10-year yellow fever vaccine booster is not necessary. CID: 57 (October 1) Available at <http://cid.oxfordjournals.org> (accessed February 1, 2014).

Report on a new recommendation from the WHO Strategic Advisory Group of Experts that a single dose of yellow fever vaccine is sufficient to confer sustained immunity and lifelong protection.

Jellinek, T., Burchard, G.D., Dieckmann, S., et al., 2015. Short-term immunogenicity and safety of an accelerated pre-exposure prophylaxis regimen with Japanese encephalitis vaccine in combination with a rabies vaccine: a phase III, multicenter, observer-blind study. J. Travel Med. 22, 225–231.

Clinical trial demonstrating that the immunogenicity of an accelerated 1-week JE vaccine regimen was non-inferior to that of the standard JE vaccine regimen and had no impact on concomitant rabies vaccination. This accelerated regimen would be useful for travelers departing for JE-endemic areas on short notice but is not licensed at the time of writing.

World Health Organization, 2010. Cholera vaccines WHO position paper. Wkly Epidemiol Rec. No13 85, 117–128. Available at <http://www.who.int/wer/2010/wer8513.pdf> (accessed July 14, 2015).

World Health Organization, 2014. Use of oral cholera vaccine in humanitarian emergencies. Available at <http://www.who.int/cholera/vaccines/OCV_in_humanitarian_emergencies-_15Jan2014_pdf> (accessed July 14, 2015).

These two documents from the WHO provide detailed information on cholera vaccines, manufacturers, supplies, and use in cholera outbreaks and provide essential information for relief workers, disaster response teams, and program planners involved in cholera outbreak areas.

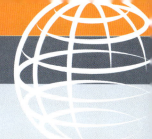

CHAPTER 6

Malaria Prevention

Hans D. Nothdurft and Kevin C. Kain

 Access evidence synopsis online at ExpertConsult.com.

Malaria is the most important parasitic disease in the world. Human malaria is a blood-borne protozoal infection caused by five species of the genus *Plasmodium*: *P. falciparum, P. vivax, P. ovale, P. malariae,* and *P. knowlesi.* The infection is transmitted through the bite of infected female *Anopheles* mosquitoes. Less commonly, malaria may be transmitted by blood transfusion, with shared needle use, or congenitally, from mother to fetus. Ecologic change and economic and political instability, combined with escalating malaria drug resistance, have led to a worldwide resurgence of this parasitic disease. The 2014 World Malaria Report (World Health Organization [WHO] and United Nations Children's Fund [UNICEF]) estimated there were more than 220 million cases and more than 600,000 deaths annually resulting from malaria.

Malaria is not just a problem in the developing world, however. The combination of increases in international travel and increasing drug resistance has resulted in a growing number of travelers at risk of contracting malaria. It is estimated that as many as 30,000 travelers from industrialized countries contract malaria each year. However, this incidence is likely to be an underestimate because of the failure to take into account those who are diagnosed and treated abroad and the prevalence of underreporting. The majority of *P. falciparum* cases imported into North America and Europe are acquired in Africa (85%), and travel to the African continent is still on the rise.

The overall case fatality rate of imported *P. falciparum* malaria varies from 0.6 to 3.8% but may be much higher in the elderly. The fatality rate of severe malaria may be ≥20% even when managed in modern intensive care units; however, cases of imported malaria and associated fatalities remain largely preventable, provided high-risk travelers use appropriate chemoprophylaxis and measures to reduce insect bites, and physicians promptly recognize infections and initiate appropriate treatment.

APPROACH TO MALARIA PREVENTION

This chapter highlights the important principles of malaria prevention. The interested reader is referred to **Table 6.1** and the references for additional sources of information and country-specific malaria risk. There are four principles—adapted from the WHO's ABCD of malaria protection—of which all travelers to malarious areas should be informed:

A Be **A**ware of the risk and the symptoms and understand that malaria is a serious infection.

B Avoid mosquito **B**ites.

C Take **C**hemoprophylaxis when appropriate.

D Seek immediate **D**iagnosis and treatment if fever develops during or after travel.

These principles, which are key issues to be considered when advising travelers on protection against malaria, are discussed in further detail below and summarized as a checklist in **Table 6.2**.

Protection against malaria can be summarized into the following four principles.

TABLE 6.1   Internet Resources for Travel Health Information and Country-Specific Malaria Risk

http://www.cdc.gov/travel/ US Centers for Disease Control and Prevention (Travelers' Health Section)	On-line references include full text of Health Information for International Travel 2016, with full adult and pediatric recommendations, including malaria risks and recommendations.
http://www.who.int/ith/en WHO (International Travel and Health Information Resource Page)	Includes updates on country-specific malaria risk.
www.TravelHealth.gc.ca Health Canada (Travel Medicine Resource Page)	See Information for Travel Medicine Professionals. Contains CATMAT guidelines, travel bulletins, and updates for preventing and treating malaria in travelers.

CATMAT, Committee to Advise on Tropical Medicine and Travel.

1. Assessing Individual Risk

Estimating a traveler's risk is based on a detailed travel itinerary and specific risk behaviors of the traveler (examples in parentheses represent increasing risk). The risk of acquiring malaria varies according to the geographic area visited (e.g., Southeast Asia vs. Africa), the travel destination within different geographic areas (urban vs. rural travel), type of accommodations (well screened or air conditioned vs. camping), duration of stay (1-week business travel vs. 3-month overland trek), season of travel (low vs. high malaria transmission season), and elevation of destination (malaria transmission is rare above 2000 m). In addition to the location, travelers can influence their own risk by how well they comply with preventive measures, such as treated bed nets and chemoprophylactic drugs, and the efficacy of these measures.

Additional information can be obtained from studies using malaria surveillance data that estimate risk of malaria in travelers. For example, relative risk assessments show that travelers are 207 times more likely to acquire malaria in sub-Saharan Africa compared with low-risk areas, and the relative risk decreases with other destinations studied such as South Asia (53.8), Central America (37.8), Southeast Asia (11.5), and South America (8.3). Risk of infection if no chemoprophylaxis is used varies from >20% per month in regions of Papua (formerly Irian Jaya) to 1.7-2.4% per month in West Africa to 0.01% per month in Central America. Of note, the estimated risk of malaria for travelers to Thailand in one study was 1:12,254, which may be less than the risk of a serious adverse event secondary to malaria chemoprophylaxis. Such data can also help provide an estimate of the cost/benefit ratio for the use of various chemoprophylactic drugs in different geographic areas. Good sources of updated malaria information and country-specific risk are available online from the WHO, Centers for Disease Control and Prevention (CDC), and Health Canada (Table 6.1).

2. Preventing Mosquito Bites (Personal Protection Measures)

All travelers to malaria-endemic areas need to be instructed in how best to avoid bites from *Anopheles* mosquitoes that transmit malaria. Any measure that reduces exposure to the evening and nighttime feeding female *Anopheles* mosquito will reduce the risk of acquiring malaria. Different brands of effective insect repellents are available, but some should not be used on babies and small children. Insecticide-impregnated bed nets (with permethrin or other chemicals) are safe for children and pregnant women and are—together with use of repellents—an effective prevention strategy that is underused by travelers. Additional details are provided in Chapter 1.

TABLE 6.2   Checklist for Travelers to Malarious Areas

The following is a checklist of key issues to be considered in advising travelers.

1. Risk of malaria

   Travelers should be informed about their individual risk of malaria infection and the presence of drug-resistant *P. falciparum* malaria in their areas of destination. Pregnant women and adults taking young children should question the necessity of the trip.

2. Anti-mosquito measures

   Travelers should be instructed how to protect themselves against mosquito bites.

3. Chemoprophylaxis (when appropriate)

   Travelers should be:

   a. Advised to start chemoprophylaxis before travel and to use prophylaxis continuously while in malaria-endemic areas and for 1 or 4 weeks after leaving such areas (depending on the drug used).

   b. Questioned about drug allergies and other contraindications for drug use.

   c. Informed that antimalarial drugs can cause side effects; if these side effects are serious, medical help should be sought promptly and use of the drug discontinued. Mild nausea, occasional vomiting, or loose stools should not prompt discontinuation of chemoprophylaxis, but medical advice should be sought if symptoms persist.

   d. Warned that they may acquire malaria even if they use malaria chemoprophylaxis.

   e. Warned that they may receive conflicting information regarding antimalarial drugs overseas but that they should continue their prescribed medication unless they are experiencing moderate to severe adverse effects.

4. In case of illness, travelers should be:

   a. Informed that symptoms of malaria may be mild and that they should suspect malaria if they experience a fever or flu-like illness (unexplained fever).

   b. Informed that malaria may be fatal if treatment is delayed. Medical help should be sought promptly if malaria is suspected, and a blood sample should be taken and examined for malaria parasites on one or more occasions (if possible, blood smears should be brought home for review).

   c. Reminded that self-treatment (if prescribed) should be taken only if prompt medical care is not available within 24 hours and that medical advice should still be sought as soon as possible after self-treatment.

   d. Reminded to continue to take chemoprophylaxis in cases of suspect or proven malaria.

5. Special categories:

   Pregnant women and young children require special attention because of the potential effects of malaria illness and inability to use some drugs (e.g., doxycycline).

Adapted from World Health Organization, 2012, International Travel and Health.

3. Use of Chemoprophylactic Drugs Where Appropriate

The use of antimalarial drugs and their potential adverse effects must be weighed against the risk of acquiring malaria (as described previously). The following questions should be addressed before prescribing any antimalarial drug:

a. Will the traveler be exposed to malaria?

b. Will the traveler be in a drug-resistant *P. falciparum* zone?

c. Will the traveler have prompt access to medical care (including blood smears prepared with sterile equipment and then properly interpreted) if symptoms of malaria were to occur?

d. Are there any contraindications to the use of a particular antimalarial drug?

An overview of antimalarial drug regimens based on drug-resistance zones is provided in **Figure 6.1** and **Table 6.3**. It is important to note that a number of travelers to low-risk areas, such as urban areas and tourist resorts of Southeast Asia, continue to be inappropriately

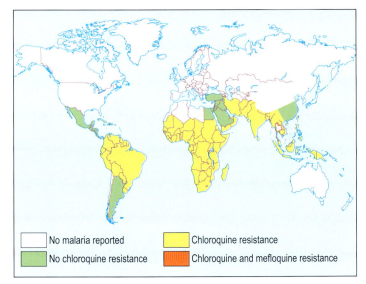

Fig. 6.1 **Map of malaria-endemic areas and zones of drug-resistance. See Fig. 6.2 for detail.** *Note*: This is meant as a *visual aid only*. The reader is referred to additional important details of malaria drugs and country-specific malaria risk available online (see Table 6.1) or in references. (From Health Canada. 2004. Canadian recommendations for the prevention and treatment of malaria among international travelers. CCDR 30S1.)

prescribed antimalarial drugs that result in unnecessary adverse events but offer little protection. Improved traveler adherence with antimalarial drugs is more likely when travel medicine practitioners make a concerted effort to identify and carefully counsel the high-risk traveler and avoid unnecessary drugs in the low-risk individual.

4. Seeking Early Diagnosis and Treatment If Fever Develops during or after Travel

Travelers should be informed that although personal protection measures and antimalarial drugs can markedly decrease the risk of contracting malaria, these interventions do not guarantee complete protection. Symptoms resulting from malaria may occur as early as 1 week after first exposure and as late as several years after leaving a malaria zone, whether or not chemoprophylaxis has been used. Most travelers who acquire falciparum malaria will develop symptoms within 2 months of exposure. Falciparum malaria can be effectively treated early in its course, but delays in therapy may result in a serious and even fatal outcome. The most important factors that determine outcome are early diagnosis and appropriate therapy. Travelers and healthcare providers alike must consider and urgently rule out malaria in any febrile illness that occurs during or after travel to a malaria-endemic area (see Chapters 20 and 21).

CURRENT CHEMOPROPHYLACTIC DRUG REGIMENS

Antimalarial drugs are selected based on individual risk assessment (as discussed previously) and drug-resistance patterns (**Figs. 6.1**, **6.2**, and **Tables 6.1**, **6.3**, and **6.4**). Chloroquine-resistant *P. falciparum* (CRPF) is now widespread in all malaria-endemic areas of the world, except for Mexico, the Caribbean, Central America, Argentina, and parts of the Middle

TABLE 6.3   Malaria Chemoprophylactic Regimens for At-Risk Individuals According to Zones of Drug-Resistance[a]

Zone	Drug(s) of Choice[b]	Alternatives
No chloroquine resistance	Chloroquine	Doxycycline or atovaquone-proguanil
Chloroquine resistance	Atovaquone-proguanil or doxycycline or mefloquine[c]	Primaquine[d]
Chloroquine and mefloquine resistance	Atovaquone-proguanil or doxycycline	
Adult doses		
Atovaquone-proguanil	One tablet daily	
Chloroquine phosphate	300 mg (base) weekly	
Doxycycline	100 mg daily	
Mefloquine	One tablet weekly (250 mg salt in the United States; base elsewhere)	
Primaquine	30 mg (base) daily[d]	

Note: Protection from mosquito bites (insecticide-treated bed nets, *N,N*-diethyl-meta-toluamide [DEET]-based insect repellents, etc.) is the first line of defense against malaria for all travelers. In the Americas and Southeast Asia, chemoprophylaxis is recommended only for travelers who will be exposed outdoors during evening or night time in rural areas.
[a]See detailed information in Table 6.4.
[b]Chloroquine and mefloquine are to be taken 1-3 weeks before entering malarial areas, continued during the stay in malarial areas, and taken for 4 weeks after leaving malarial areas. Doxycycline may be started 1 day before entering malarial areas but must be continued for 4 weeks after departure. Atovaquone-proguanil and primaquine are started 1 day before entering the malarial area and may be discontinued 7 days after leaving the malaria-endemic area.
[c]Adhere to boxed warning about contraindications before prescription.
[d]Contraindicated in glucose-6-phosphate dehydrogenase (G6PD) deficiency and during pregnancy. Not presently licensed for this use. Must perform the G6PD level test before prescribing.

East and China. *P. falciparum* malaria resistant to chloroquine and mefloquine is still rare except on the borders of Thailand with Cambodia and Myanmar (Burma). Resistance to sulfadoxine-pyrimethamine is now common in the Amazon basin and Southeast Asia and is increasing in many regions of Africa. Chloroquine-resistant *P. vivax* is also becoming an important problem, particularly in Papua New Guinea, Papua (formerly Irian Java), Vanuatu, Myanmar, and Guyana. More recently *P. knowlesi* has been indentified in Southeast Asia as causing clinical malaria resembling falciparum malaria.

Chloroquine-Sensitive Zones

Chloroquine is the drug of choice for travel to areas where chloroquine resistance has not been described. Chloroquine is active against the erythrocytic forms (**Fig. 6.3**) of sensitive strains of all species of malaria, and it is also gametocidal against *P. vivax*, *P. malariae*, and *P. ovale*. Except for its bitter taste, chloroquine is usually well tolerated and has a low incidence of serious adverse events. Dark-skinned persons may experience generalized pruritus that is not indicative of drug allergy. Retinal toxicity that may occur with long-term high doses of chloroquine used in the treatment of other diseases is extremely unlikely with chloroquine given as a weekly malaria chemosuppressive agent. Chloroquine use is suitable for people of all ages and for pregnant women. Because insufficient drug is excreted in breast milk to protect the infant, nursing infants should be given chloroquine. Contraindications include people who are glucose 6-phosphate dehydrogenase (G6PD) deficient or hypersensitive to 4-aminoquinoline compounds. Administration of the oral live typhoid vaccine and live cholera vaccine should be completed 3 days before chloroquine use, and chloroquine may suppress the antibody response to primary pre-exposure rabies vaccine.

Continued text to page 80

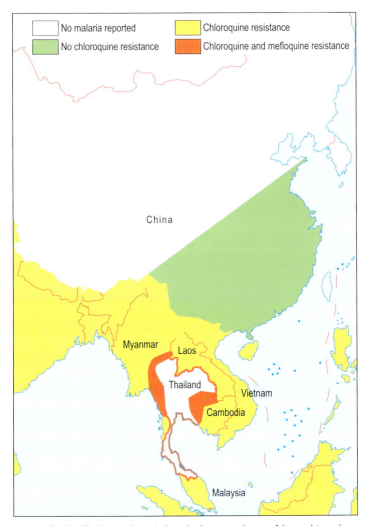

Fig. 6.2 Detail of Fig. 6.1 showing malaria-endemic areas and zones of drug resistance in Southeast Asia. *Note*: This is meant as a visual aid only. The reader is referred to additional important details of malaria drugs and country-specific malaria risk available online (see Table 6.1) or in references. (From Health Canada. 2004. Canadian recommendations for the prevention and treatment of malaria among international travelers. CCDR 3051.)

TABLE 6.4 Antimalarial Drugs, Doses,[a] and Adverse Effects (Listed Alphabetically)

Generic Name	Packaging	Adult Dose	Pediatric Dose	Adverse Effects
Artemether/Lumefantrin	20 mg Artemether and 120 mg Lumefantrine in 1 tablet	Prevention: not indicated Treatment: 80 mg/480 mg (=4 Tbl.) initially, after 8 hours: 4 Tbl., then twice daily 4 Tbl. On day 2 and 3 (total = 24 Tbl.)	Prevention: not indicated Treatment: Licensed from 5 kg body weight. Total treatment: 6 doses (initially, then after 8, 24, 36, 48, and 60 hours) 5– <15 kg: 1 tablet/dose 15– <25 kg: 2 tablets/dose 25– < 35 kg: 3 tablets/dose ≥ 35 kg and >12 years: 4 tablets/dose	Frequent: GI symptoms, headache, dizziness Rare: QTs prolongation, cardiac arrhythmia, hemolysis
Atovaquone-proguanil	250 mg atovaquone and 100 mg proguanil (adult tablet)	Prevention: 1 tablet daily Treatment: 1000 mg atovaquone and 400 mg proguanil (4 tablets) once daily ×3 days	Prevention: 11–20 kg 1/4 tablet; 21–30 kg 1/2 tablet; 31–40 kg 3/4 tablet; >40 kg 1 tablet; (see Chapter 12 for AP pediatric tablet dosing schedule) Treatment: 20 mg/kg atovaquone and 8 mg/kg proguanil once daily ×3 days	Frequent: nausea, vomiting, abdominal pain, diarrhea, increased transaminases Rare: seizures, rash

Continued

TABLE 6.4 Antimalarial Drugs, Doses,[a] and Adverse Effects (Listed Alphabetically)—cont'd

Generic Name	Packaging	Adult Dose	Pediatric Dose	Adverse Effects
Chloroquine[b] phosphate	150 mg base	Prevention: 300 mg base once weekly Treatment: 1.5 g base ×3 days[c]	Prevention: 5 mg base once weekly 5-6 kg or <4 months: 25 mg base 7-10 kg or 4-11 months:[c] 50 mg base 11-14 kg or 1-2 years: 75 mg base 15-18 kg or 3-4 years: 100 mg base 19-24 kg or 5-7 years: 125 mg base 25-35 kg or 8-10 years: 200 mg base 36-50 kg or 11-13 years: 250 mg base 50 kg or 14 years: 300 mg base Treatment: 25 mg salt/kg total over 3 days	Frequent: pruritus in black-skinned individuals, nausea, headache Occasional: skin eruptions, reversible corneal opacity Rare: nail and mucous membrane discoloration, nerve deafness, photophobia, myopathy, retinopathy with daily use, blood dyscrasias, psychosis and seizures, alopecia
Doxycycline[d]	100 mg	Prevention: 100 mg once daily Treatment: 1 tablet twice daily for 7 days (plus quinine) (see Chapter 20)	Prevention: 1.5 mg salt/kg once daily (max. 100 mg daily) <25 kg or <8 years: contraindicated 25-35 kg or 8-10 years: 50 mg 36-50 kg or 11-13 years: 75 mg ≥50 kg or ≥14 years: 100 mg Treatment: 1.5 mg salt/kg twice daily (max. 200 mg daily) <25 kg or <8 years: contraindicated 25-35 kg or 8-10 years: 50 mg twice daily 36-50 kg or 11-13 years: 75 mg twice daily 50 kg or ≥14 years: 100 mg twice daily (plus quinine) (see Chapter 20)	Frequent: GI upset, vaginal candidiasis, photosensitivity Rare: allergic reactions, blood dyscrasias, azotemia in renal diseases, hepatitis

Mefloquine	250 mg base	Prevention:	Prevention:	Common:
		250 mg base once weekly	<5 kg: no data	transient dizziness diarrhea, nausea,
		Treatment:	5-9 kg: 1/8 tablet	vivid dreams, nightmares,
		see text	10-19 kg: 1/4 tablet	irritability, mood alterations,
			20-30 kg: 1/2 tablet	headache, insomnia
			30-45 kg: 3/4 tablet	Rare:
			>45 kg: 1 tablet once weekly	seizures, psychosis, prolonged
			Treatment:	dizziness
			see text	
Quinine	330 mg salt	Prevention:	Prevention:	Common:
		not indicated	not indicated	cinchonism
		Treatment:	Treatment:	
		see text	see text	
Primaquine	15 mg base	Prevention:	Prevention:	Occasional:
(Note: Must		prophylaxis: 30 mg base	0.5 mg base/kg daily	GI upset, hemolysis in G6PD
perform G6PD		daily (see text)	Terminal prophylaxis or radical cure: 0.5 mg	deficiency, methemoglobinemia
testing before		Terminal prophylaxis or	base/kg per day ×14 days[f]	
use)		radical cure: 30 mg		
		base/day for 14 days[e]		

G6PD, Glucose 6-phosphate dehydrogenase; GI, gastrointestinal.

[a] Dose for chemoprophylaxis, unless specified for "Treatment."

[b] Chloroquine sulfate (Nivaquine) is not available in the United States and Canada but is available in most malaria-endemic countries in both tablet and syrup form.

[c] Generally, 2 tablets twice per day on days 1 and 2, then 2 tablets on day 3 (total of 10 tablets).

[d] For treatment only in combination with other antimalarials.

[e] Doses increased to 30 mg base/day due to primaquine-resistant/tolerant P. vivax.

[f] Doses increased to 0.5 mg base/kg/day due to primaquine-resistant/tolerant P. vivax.

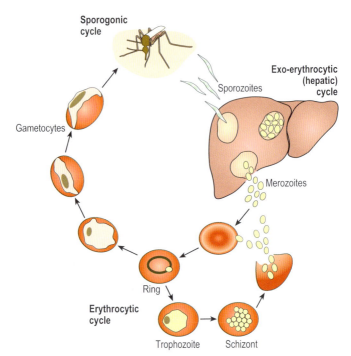

Fig. 6.3 **Life cycle of the malaria parasite in humans.** (Courtesy of Dr. Lena Serghides. Adapted from Serghides L., et al. 2005. CD36 and malaria: friend or foes? Trends Parasitol. 19(10):461–469.)

Chloroquine-Resistant Zones

For many travelers to these areas, a choice between atovaquone-proguanil (AP) (e.g., Malarone™), doxycycline (e.g., Vibramycin™), or mefloquine (e.g., Lariam™), will have to be made. Less commonly primaquine may be used. Deciding which agent is best requires an individual assessment of risk of malaria and the specific advantages and disadvantages of each regimen (**Table 6.5**). For drugs such as mefloquine and doxycycline to be optimally effective, they need to be taken for 4 weeks after leaving a malaria-endemic area, although traveler adherence with this component has been traditionally poor. Agents such as AP and primaquine are called causal prophylactics because they kill malaria early in its life cycle in the liver, and therefore may be discontinued 1 week after leaving an endemic area (**Fig. 6.3**). This advantage makes these drugs attractive for high-risk but short-duration travel. It is important to note that none of these agents is ideal, and all carry a risk of adverse events that are distressing enough to travelers that 1-7% will discontinue their prescribed chemo- prophylactic regimen.

Atovaquone Plus Proguanil (Malarone)

Malarone is a fixed-dose combination of atovaquone and proguanil hydrochloride. AP works against the erythrocytic stages of all the *Plasmodium* parasites and the liver-stage (causal prophylaxis) of *P. falciparum*. The AP combination is effective against *P. falciparum* malaria strains that are resistant to a variety of other antimalarial drugs.

TABLE 6.5   Clinical Utility Score for Current Malaria Chemoprophylactic Regimens

Drug	Efficacy[a]	Tolerance[b]	Convenience[c]	Causal[d]	Cost[e]	Total
Atovaquone-proguanil	3	3	2	2	1	11
Doxycycline	3	2	2	0	3	10
Mefloquine	3	1	3	0	2	9
Primaquine	2	2	1[f]	2	3	10

Note: Scores and weighting are arbitrary and can be modified/individualized to specific travelers and itineraries.
[a]Efficacy: 1, <75%; 2, 75-89%; 3, ≥90%.
[b]Tolerance: 1, occasional disabling side effects; 2, rare disabling side effects; 3, rare minor side effects.
[c]Convenience: 1, daily and weekly dosing required; 2, daily dosing required; 3, weekly dosing required.
[d]Causal: 0, no causal activity; 2, causal prophylactic (may be discontinued within a few days of leaving risk area).
[e]Cost: 1, >US$100/month; 2, US$50-100/month; 3, <US$50/month.
[f]Requires a pre-travel G6PD measurement, resulting in a lower convenience score.

Atovaquone inhibits parasite mitochondrial electron transport at the level of the cytochrome bc1 complex and collapses mitochondrial membrane potential. The plasmodial electron transport system is 1000-fold more sensitive to atovaquone than the mammalian electron transport system, which likely explains the selective action and limited side effects of this drug. Proguanil is metabolized to cycloguanil, which inhibits dihydrofolate reductase and impedes the synthesis of folate cofactors required for parasite DNA synthesis. AP works synergistically since proguanil, which alone has no effect on mitochondrial membrane potential or electron transport, significantly enhances the ability of atovaquone to collapse mitochondrial membrane potential; however, this is not mediated through the cycloguanil metabolite. This might explain why proguanil enhances atovaquone activity even in the presence of documented cycloguanil resistance or in patients deficient in the cytochrome P450 enzymes required for the conversion of proguanil to cycloguanil.

In randomized, controlled trials, AP was highly efficacious in preventing *P. falciparum* malaria in both adults and children. Four published trials have examined the protective efficacy of AP in semi-immune adults and children living in malaria-endemic areas. The overall efficacy of AP in the prevention of *P. falciparum* malaria in these trials was 98% (95% CI 91.9-99.9%). The protective efficacy of AP for prevention of *P. falciparum* malaria in non-immune adults and children has been examined in five clinical trials, four of which were randomized, and three blind. Collectively, the protective efficacy of AP was 96-100% (95% CI 48-100%). Only one randomized, double-blind, placebo-controlled trial has evaluated the protective efficacy of AP against *P. vivax*. The protective efficacy of AP was 84% (95% CI 45-95%) for *P. vivax* and 96% (95% CI 71-99%) for *P. falciparum*. As AP does not appear to eradicate *P. vivax* hypnozoites, it is suggested that travelers to areas where the transmission rates of *P. vivax* are high should receive consideration for presumptive antirelapse therapy with primaquine.

Controlled trials indicate that AP at prophylactic doses is well tolerated by adults and children with drug discontinuation rates of 0-2%. The most commonly reported adverse events are headache and abdominal pain (which can often be reduced by taking AP with food); however, in placebo-controlled trials, these occurred at similar rates as in placebo recipients. In two large randomized, double-blind clinical trials in non-immune subjects traveling to a malaria-endemic area, chemoprophylactic drugs were well tolerated, but AP was significantly better tolerated than either mefloquine or chloroquine/proguanil (CP) in these studies. Participants receiving AP reported significantly lower rates of neuropsychiatric adverse events (14% vs. 29%) compared with mefloquine, significantly lower gastrointestinal adverse events (12% vs. 20%) compared with CP, and lower drug discontinuation rates compared with both. In another randomized trial in travelers, AP was the best-tolerated chemoprophylactic with discontinuation rates of 1.8% versus 3.9% for mefloquine and doxycycline and 5.2% for CP. Additionally, efficacy and tolerability have been examined in pediatric travelers using a randomized comparative trial of AP versus CP. There were no prophylactic failures, but AP was better tolerated with no premature discontinuation of AP due to an adverse event, compared with a 2% discontinuation rate with CP.

AP is currently indicated for the prophylaxis and treatment of *P. falciparum* malaria including areas where chloroquine and/or mefloquine resistance has been reported. Travelers who have experienced intense exposure to *P. vivax* and *P. ovale* should be considered for radical treatment with primaquine on leaving the malaria-endemic area. Because of its causal activity, AP is taken 1 day prior to travel in a malarious zone, daily while exposed, and for 7 days on leaving.

AP is contraindicated in those with severe renal impairment and in those with a history of hypersensitivity to any of the drug components. AP is currently approved for the prevention of malaria in children >5 kg and adults in the United States, Australia, and Europe. A lack of data exists for the use of AP during pregnancy or breast feeding, and it is not currently recommended for chemoprophylaxis. Although a recent but small study suggests that AP is safe and well tolerated in pregnancy, additional data are needed. AP should not be given with other proguanil-containing medications, or with tetracycline, rifampin, rifabutin, and metoclopramide, which significantly reduce the plasma concentration of atovaquone.

Doxycycline

Doxycycline is a relatively slow-acting schizonticidal agent and, while not appropriate on its own for treatment, is efficacious as a solo chemoprophylactic agent against drug-resistant *P. vivax* and *P. falciparum* malaria.

A number of randomized trials have examined the efficacy of doxycycline as a chemoprophylactic in non-immune and semi-immune populations. The reported protective efficacy in these trials was excellent, ranging from 92 to 100% against *P. falciparum* and *P. vivax*. In comparative trials in areas with chloroquine-resistant *P. falciparum* malaria, doxycycline has been shown to be equivalent to mefloquine and AP and superior to azithromycin and chloroquine-proguanil. Parasite resistance to doxycycline has not been reported to be an operational problem in any malaria-endemic area thus far. Poor adherence to daily use rather than true drug resistance is the major reason for doxycycline failures.

Overall, a number of comparative studies have shown that doxycycline is well tolerated as a chemoprophylactic agent and has relatively few reported side effects. In clinical trials, doxycycline was tolerated as well as or better than placebo or the comparator drug, with few serious adverse events reported. The most commonly reported adverse events related to doxycycline use are nausea, vomiting, abdominal pain, and diarrhea. Esophageal ulceration is a rare but well-described adverse event associated with doxycycline use. Taking doxycycline with food and plentiful fluids and remaining in an upright position for ≥1 hour can reduce adverse gastrointestinal effects. Dermatologic reactions, including photosensitivity, are also adverse events frequently associated with doxycycline use. Although doxycycline has a lesser effect on normal bacterial flora than other tetracyclines, it still increases the risk of oral and vaginal candidiasis in predisposed individuals.

Doxycycline is currently indicated as an agent of choice for prevention of mefloquine-resistant *P. falciparum* malaria or an alternative to AP or mefloquine for the prevention of CRPF malaria. Doxycycline should be taken once daily, beginning 1-2 days before entering a malarious area, and should be continued while there. Because of its poor causal effect, it must be continued for 4 weeks after leaving the risk area. Doxycycline is contraindicated during pregnancy, in breast-feeding women, and in children <8 years old, and should not be taken within 1-3 hours of administering Bismuth subsalicylate, an oral antacid, or iron. Long-term safety (>3 months) of daily doxycycline use has not been established among travelers, but chronic use of related tetracyclines by young healthy adults in acne treatment protocols is a common clinical practice.

Mefloquine

Mefloquine is a potent, long-acting blood schizontocide (**Fig. 6.3**) and has >90% protective efficacy against all malarial species including *P. falciparum* resistant to chloroquine and pyrimethamine-sulfonamide combinations. The CDC and WHO list mefloquine as one of the drugs of choice for high-risk travelers to chloroquine-resistant regions such as sub-Saharan Africa and New Guinea. Mefloquine is effective in the prevention of CRPF malaria, except for rural Thai border regions with Myanmar and Cambodia, where parasites display multidrug resistance, including to mefloquine. Although there is general agreement about the drug's efficacy, the drug tolerance has been called into question. Approximately 25-50% of mefloquine users report side effects, the majority of which are mild and self-limited. The most frequent adverse events reported by mefloquine users are nausea, strange dreams, dizziness, mood changes, insomnia, headache, and diarrhea. Severe neuropsychiatric reactions (psychosis, convulsions) are infrequent with prophylactic doses and are reported to occur in approximately 1/6000 to 1/13,000 individuals. Less severe but nonetheless troublesome neuropsychologic adverse events (e.g., anxiety, depression, nightmares) disabling enough to result in drug discontinuation are reported in 0.2-3.9% of users. There is no evidence that the long-term use of mefloquine (>1 year) is associated with additional adverse effects.

Data from well-designed prospective and randomized trials show that, for the most part, mefloquine is well tolerated. Overall mefloquine withdrawal rates in comparative trials were estimated to be 1-5%, indicating high acceptance rates comparable to other chemoprophylactic regimens and suggesting that <5% of individuals would need to switch to an alternative drug regimen. In randomized controlled trials comparing mefloquine with AP or doxycycline in non-immune travelers, all agents were effective and well tolerated, but AP and doxycycline were significantly better tolerated.

Contraindications to the use of mefloquine include a history of psychiatric illness including anxiety and depression, seizure disorder, and a history of hypersensitivity to mefloquine or related substances including quinine. Precautions include its use in children weighing <10 pounds, cardiac conduction disturbances or arrhythmia, and the concurrent use of quinine-like drugs (e.g., halofantrine and mefloquine should not be used together). In 2013 the Food and Drug Administration (FDA) and European Medicines Agency (EMA) issued a boxed warning on contraindications before the prescription of mefloquine and made it mandatory that a mefloquine user should carry a wallet pass.

The manufacturers of mefloquine also caution about its use by drivers, pilots, and machine operators because of concerns that it may affect spatial orientation and motor coordination. There are no data on mefloquine use by scuba divers; however, caution is advised because of the risk of neurologic symptoms developing at depth and because signs and symptoms of decompression illness (dizziness, headache, nausea, fatigue) may be attributed to the drug, thus potentially delaying recognition and appropriate treatment for the decompression problem. Mefloquine is metabolized through the liver, so should be avoided in travelers with chronic hepatic dysfunction, and can also cause an asymptomatic increase in the liver function tests during therapy. Travelers on drugs such as warfarin or cyclosporin A should start mefloquine 3-4 weeks in advance of departure, so that prothrombin times or cyclosporine A levels can be monitored and adjusted as needed.

For a traveler to a CRPF destination who plans to engage in special physical activities, such as those mentioned previously, and who cannot take AP or doxycycline (see later discussion), a practical approach would be to start the traveler on mefloquine approximately 3 weeks before departure and monitor for adverse events. It has been suggested by many travelers that if the drug is taken in the evening, side effects are mostly relegated to the hours of sleep and effects on physical performance the next day are potentially lessened.

Travelers who will be at immediate high risk of drug-resistant falciparum malaria may be given a loading dose of mefloquine. Data from several trials indicate that mefloquine taken once a day for 3 days before travel followed by standard weekly doses is an effective way to rapidly achieve therapeutic blood levels (in 4 days compared with 7-9 weeks with standard weekly dosing of mefloquine). Approximately 2-3% of loading-dose recipients discontinued mefloquine (most commonly for gastrointestinal upset and dizziness), and most of these did so during the first week. Alternatively, mefloquine can be initiated 2-3 weeks before travel to achieve higher blood levels before entering malaria-endemic areas. Either strategy permits an assessment of drug tolerance before travel and allows a change to a suitable alternative if required.

Primaquine

Primaquine is an 8-aminoquinoline that has antimalarial activity against both blood and tissue stages and can be used as a chemoprophylactic agent as well as for "terminal" prophylaxis. Recent randomized controlled field trials have convincingly demonstrated the prophylactic potential of primaquine, showing a protective efficacy of 85-95% against both *P. falciparum* and *P. vivax* infections.

Primaquine has been shown to be tolerated as well as or better than other standard regimens but may cause nausea and abdominal pain that can be decreased by taking the drug with food. Of importance, primaquine may cause oxidant-induced hemolytic anemia with methemoglobinemia, particularly in individuals with a deficiency of G6PD. It is contraindicated in patients with G6PD deficiency and also during pregnancy. If not already documented, a traveler's G6PD status should be determined with a G6PD blood test before primaquine is prescribed. The use of primaquine as a malaria chemoprophylaxis regimen during travel is off-label (FDA, April, 2015). However, in the absence of contraindications, primaquine may be a useful alternative prophylactic agent to consider for selected travelers, and because of its causal acitvity may be discontinued 1 week after leaving an endemic area.

If the risk of *P. vivax* infection is thought to be particularly high (e.g., in long-term expatriates and soldiers) a 14-day course of primaquine phosphate ("radical" or "terminal" prophylaxis, also called presumptive antirelapse therapy) may be given at the conclusion of the standard post-travel chemoprophylaxis regimen to eliminate latent hepatic parasites (as indicated by the FDA label). See section below, Primaquine for Relapse Prevention.

Chloroquine and Mefloquine-Resistant Zones

For evening and overnight exposure in rural regions along the Thai-Myanmar and Thai-Cambodian border, doxycycline or AP are the drugs of choice.

Contrasts in Prophylaxis Recommendations among Health Organizations

As mentioned above, the major health organizations including the CDC, Health Canada, the UK Foreign and Commonwealth Office (FCO), and the WHO all have detailed information available on their websites about malaria chemoprophylaxis and areas of drug resistance, by country (**Table 6.1**). It should be noted that these sites are constantly being updated and need to be updated and checked frequently. Areas of controversy between different advisory groups include the Indian subcontinent, Latin America, and parts of southern Africa, including South Africa, Namibia, and Botswana, where despite studies showing significant chloroquine resistance, some groups still continue to recommend chloroquine or chloroquine combinations.

Frequent Short-Term Travel to High-Risk Areas

If travelers are expecting to take several short trips over a period of months to areas of high malarial transmission, the use of causal antimalarials such as AP and primaquine should be strongly considered. Since standard chemoprophylactic drugs such as doxycycline and mefloquine require use for 4 weeks after malaria exposure, travelers in this situation would be constantly on antimalarials for many months. Causal drugs, due to their activity on the parasite liver stages, need to be taken only for a short time (1 week) after leaving the malaria-endemic area and are more user-friendly for this type of travel. Examples might include living in Bangkok (no malaria risk) but with frequent travel to rural areas of Laos or Cambodia for a few days each month. A similar situation exists in Nairobi, Kenya (one of few malaria-free areas in East Africa), where travel outside the city places individuals at risk of chloroquine-resistant *P. falciparum* malaria.

Summary

In summary, the use of antimalarials for chemoprophylaxis should be carefully directed at high-risk travelers where their benefit most clearly outweighs the risk of adverse events. None of the available regimens is ideal for all travelers, and the travel medicine practitioner should attempt to match the individual's risk of exposure to malaria to the appropriate regimen based on drug efficacy, tolerance, and safety. As a guide to facilitate decision making, we have generated a Clinical Utility Score, in which different attributes of each drug regimen, such as efficacy, tolerance, convenience, and cost, are weighted based on clinical trials and experience with these drugs (**Table 6.5**). The scores assigned are arbitrary, and other groups and users may weight each variable somewhat differently depending on the specific needs and risk of drug-resistant malaria. For example, a traveler to rural Papua may weigh efficacy more heavily than cost or convenience.

Dosing regimens may affect the traveler's acceptance of and compliance with the regimen prescribed. Chloroquine and mefloquine are taken once weekly beginning 1-3 weeks before travel, during travel, and for 4 weeks after leaving the endemic area. Doxycycline is taken once a day beginning 1-2 days before travel, during travel, and for 4 weeks after leaving an endemic area. The fixed dose combination drug AP (atovaquone plus proguanil) is taken once a day beginning 1-2 days before travel and every day during travel; because AP is active against liver stages of malaria, it can be discontinued 1 week after leaving an endemic area.

OTHER DRUGS

Drug Regimens to Avoid for Chemoprophylaxis

Amodiaquine

Amodiaquine, a drug that is structurally similar to chloroquine, is not recommended for use as a chemoprophylactic agent, although it is still used for therapy in parts of sub-Saharan Africa. Potential severe adverse events include agranulocytosis and hepatitis.

Artemisinin Derivatives, Alone or in Combination with Other Antimalarials

Artemisinin derivatives, including Artesunate, either alone or in combination with other malaria drugs such as lumefantrine, are a class of extremely effective therapeutic agents; however, there is currently no role for these drugs in malaria chemoprophylaxis.

Chloroquine plus Proguanil

An older alternative for travelers with contraindications or intolerance to mefloquine, AP, or doxycycline is the combination of weekly chloroquine plus daily proguanil. This combination is no longer recommended in the United States, Canada, and many countries of Europe to prevent malaria due to high levels of resistance in many malaria-endemic areas. Proguanil is not available in the United States but is available in Canada, Europe, and many malaria-endemic countries. The combination of proguanil and chloroquine is considered safe during pregnancy. Reported side effects of proguanil include mouth ulcerations, gastrointestinal upset, and hair loss. The gastrointestinal side effects may be lessened by taking the drugs with meals. Chloroquine plus proguanil is more efficacious in sub-Saharan Africa than chloroquine alone, but it is considerably less efficacious than doxycycline, mefloquine, or AP. Many failures have been reported in travelers taking this combination, and users must be informed that they are taking a less efficacious regimen.

Halofantrine

Halofantrine continues to be used in some countries as a therapeutic agent for malaria; however, it is not recommended for the prevention or treatment of malaria due to its potential to cause potentially fatal cardiac arrhythmias and prolongation of the QTc intervals, which can be accentuated when used in combination with other antimalarials that can affect cardiac conduction such as mefloquine.

Pyrimethamine plus Sulfadoxine (Fansidar)

This drug combination interferes with folic acid metabolism in the parasite: pyrimethamine inhibits dihydrofolate reductase, and sulfadoxine inhibits dihydropteroate synthetase. Fansidar was used as a weekly chemoprophylactic regimen against CRPF malaria in the 1980s, but an unacceptable rate of serious and sometimes fatal hypersensitivity reactions that developed during therapy with the weekly dose resulted in withdrawal of the recommendation for its use in prophylaxis. At present, Fansidar is still used for treatment in Africa.

Pyrimethamine plus Dapsone

This drug combination is marketed as Maloprim in many malaria-endemic areas outside the United States and, like Fansidar, interferes with folic acid metabolism in the parasite. This drug combination is not as efficacious as mefloquine, AP, or doxycycline in preventing malaria. However, the tablets containing the fixed-dose combination are relatively inexpensive and often sold over the counter in foreign countries; thus travelers have been known to start taking this drug during travel in lieu of more efficacious antimalarial drugs, on the advice of other travelers or local pharmacies. Travelers should be told to avoid Maloprim and should be educated about the possible and potentially serious dose-related toxicity (bone marrow suppression) of this drug combination.

Quinine

While quinine remains a first-line therapeutic agent for CRPF malaria, it is not used as a prophylactic drug due to its short half-life and its frequent treatment-associated adverse effects, including nausea, vomiting, headache, tinnitus, cardiovascular toxicity, and risk of blackwater fever with prolonged use.

STANDBY EMERGENCY MALARIA THERAPY (SBET)

Most travelers will be able to obtain prompt medical attention when malaria is suspected and therefore will not require a self-treatment regimen. Under unusual circumstances individuals at risk of malaria may be unable to seek medical care within 24 hours and may require self-treatment for presumptive malaria. However, because of the nonspecific symptoms of malaria, the potentially serious risk of incorrectly treating another disease, and the potential toxicity of malaria therapy, self-treatment should never be undertaken lightly; consultation with a tropical medicine expert is recommended before individuals are placed on self-treatment protocols. Travelers should be advised that the clinical presentation of malaria is variable and may mimic other diseases. An alternate diagnosis that requires treatment may be present, particularly in travelers who have been compliant with chemoprophylaxis. The most frequent symptoms of malaria are fever, headache, and generalized aches and pains. Fever, which may or may not be cyclical, is almost always present. Malaria can be misdiagnosed as "influenza" or another febrile illness, so that an early and accurate diagnosis is essential. Travelers for whom self-treatment has been recommended should be told that self-treatment is not considered definitive treatment but is a temporary, life-saving measure until they can receive medical attention. Self-treatment for malaria should be used only if travelers develop fever and professional medical care is not available within 24 hours. After self-treatment, medical attention should still be sought as soon as possible.

Rapid detection of malaria using immunochromatographic or dipstick tests may be available to some travelers. The sensitivity and specificity of these tests in research labs appears promising (>90%). However, the accuracy of these tests is not known in the hands of inexperienced operators and with ambient temperatures in the tropics. A summary of self-treatment regimens is presented in **Table 6.6**. Below is summarized important information about SBET regimens and those to avoid. Note that individuals who are on chemosuppression should never attempt treatment with the same drug, as there is the potential for additive toxicity and reduced efficacy.

TABLE 6.6   Self-Treatment Regimens[a]

A. For individuals in chloroquine-sensitive regions and not on chloroquine prophylaxis: self-treatment with chloroquine should be taken (Table 6.4). Seek medical help as soon as possible. Chloroquine prophylaxis should be started.

B. For individuals in chloroquine-sensitive regions and already on chloroquine prophylaxis: self-treatment with atovaquone-proguanil should be taken (Table 6.4). Seek medical help as soon as possible. Chloroquine prophylaxis should be resumed.

C. In chloroquine or chloroquine- and mefloquine-resistant *P. falciparum* regions, treatment recommendations for uncomplicated *P. falciparum* include the following (Table 6.4): begin oral atovaquone-proguanil (Table 6.4). Seek medical help as soon as possible. Appropriate prophylaxis should be resumed.

OR

Begin oral Artemether/Lumefantrine (Table 6.4). Seek medical help as soon as possible. Appropriate prophylaxis should be resumed.

[a]*Note*: To be used only if fever develops and medical care is not available within 24 hours. Self-treatment is not routine and in the United States and Canada is considered only for certain travelers and certain circumstances. If vomiting occurs within 30-60 minutes of dose, repeat full dose. If vomiting occurs 1-2 hours after dose, repeat one-half dose.

Atovaquone plus Proguanil (Malarone™)

Atovaquone-proguanil (AP; see the previous discussion) is an attractive agent for emergency self-treatment, provided the traveler is not taking this agent for prophylaxis. Apart from occasional gastrointestinal intolerance (reduced by taking the drug with food), treatment doses of AP are well tolerated (adult dose, 4 tablets/day for 3 days). It is safe for children (>10 pounds), but its safety in pregnancy and during breast feeding are unknown, and until additional data are available it should be avoided in these situations (see Chapter 14).

Artemether/Lumefantrin (Coartem™, Riamet™)

Coartemether (Riamet™ in Europe, Coartem in Africa and the United States) is a combination of artemether and lumefantrine. Coartemether is licensed in most European countries, Australia, and the United States for the treatment of uncomplicated malaria in adults and children >10 pounds and is becoming widely distributed in Africa. A six-dose regimen of artemether-lumefantrine appears more effective than antimalarial regimens not containing artemisinin derivatives.

Coartemether is generally well tolerated. Reported adverse effects are mostly gastrointestinal upset, headache, and dizziness. Coartemether is contraindicated for patients with a family history of sudden heart death or prolongation of the QTc interval. Also contraindicated is the concomitant use of drugs that might prolong the QTc interval and induce CYP3A4 (e.g., erythromycin, ketoconazole, rifampicine, carbamazepine, phenytoin, and St. John's wort).

The safety of artemisinin derivatives in pregnancy has not been established.

SPECIAL THERAPEUTIC CONSIDERATIONS

The Pregnant Traveler

Falciparum malaria in a pregnant woman poses significant risks for the mother, fetus, and the neonate. *P. falciparum* infection during pregnancy increases the risk of spontaneous abortion and stillbirth, intrauterine growth retardation, premature delivery, and maternal mortality. Travel by pregnant women or women who might become pregnant to destinations where CRPF malaria is transmitted should be avoided or deferred when possible. This advice is based on the fact that most effective antimalarial regimens against CRPF are neither recommended nor adequately studied during pregnancy, especially in the first trimester.

If a pregnant woman must travel to a CRPF malaria-endemic area, the use of insect repellents and treated bed nets (see Chapter 1) should be strongly encouraged. If the travel is to an area where there is intense transmission of CRPF with high-grade chloroquine resistance and travel cannot be deferred, mefloquine may be considered for chemoprophylaxis. For areas with less intense transmission, some experts recommend that chloroquine and proguanil chemoprophylaxis can be considered, although its efficacy is certainly limited. Some sources recommend dietary supplementation with folic acid for pregnant women taking proguanil.

At present there are insufficient data available on the use of AP in pregnancy or breast feeding, and therefore it is not recommended unless the potential benefit outweighs the potential risk to the fetus. Doxycycline is contraindicated in pregnancy and breast feeding. Conception should be delayed until 1 week after completion of doxycycline. Primaquine is contraindicated in pregnancy though is considered safe in breast feeding provided that the infant and mother are both screened for G6PD deficiency. There is currently no safe and effective chemoprophylaxis regimen for pregnant women at risk of mefloquine-resistant *P. falciparum* malaria.

The Infant Traveler

Malaria chemoprophylaxis in the very young infant is difficult to achieve. Although most antimalarial drugs taken by the mother will be present in breast milk, drug concentrations are not considered high enough to provide an adequate protective dose to the nursing infant. Thus malaria prevention in the nursing infant must be addressed separately from what is recommended to the mother.

For pediatric travelers to malarious areas where chloroquine is still effective, the chloroquine dose can be adjusted based on weight (**Table 6.4**). Chloroquine phosphate pediatric suspension is available in some destination countries, but not in the United States or Canada. If the suspension is not available, chloroquine phosphate tablets (250 mg salt = 150 mg chloroquine base) can be ground up by the pharmacist, and the weight-adjusted dose plus a filler can be put into capsules. Once a week, the capsule can be opened and the chloroquine powder mixed into a syrup to be given to a child. Chocolate syrup is recommended over fruit syrups and jams, as chocolate can effectively mask the extremely bitter taste of the chloroquine and make the mixture palatable to a child.

AP (Malarone) (available in a one-quarter-strength pediatric tablet) and mefloquine dosage for children can be adjusted based on weight for those weighing more than 10 pounds. Doxycycline is contraindicated in children <8 years old. In addition to chemoprophylaxis, the use of insect repellents formulated for pediatric use and insecticide-impregnated bed nets is recommended (see Chapters 1 and 12).

The Immunocompromised Traveler

P. falciparum malaria has been shown to increase HIV-1 replication and increase proviral loads and may cause faster progression of HIV-1 disease. HIV-1 infection also appears to make malaria worse and is associated with higher parasitemia infections and an increase in clinical malaria.

Another concern is antimalarial and antiretroviral drug interactions. Both mefloquine and protease inhibitors are metabolized by cytochrome P450. Inducers or inhibitors of cytochrome P450 might be expected to alter drug levels of these agents. Mefloquine has been shown to decrease the drug levels of ritonavir, but ritonavir had little effect on mefloquine. There is reported to be less interaction between mefloquine and other protease inhibitors such as nelfinavir or indinavir. There are few available data on the interaction of other antiretrovirals with mefloquine. Atovaquone increases the level of some nucleoside reverse transcriptase inhibitors, but whether this increases the risk of adverse drug events is unknown. There are also few data available regarding the potential interaction of proguanil and antiretroviral agents.

Doxycycline may cause photosensitivity, similar to antiretrovirals such as abacavir, and predispose to candidiasis, potential problems for HIV-infected individuals.

Because of potential or unknown interactions between antiretroviral and antimalarial drugs, it may be advantageous to start an antimalarial drug in advance of the recommended start date in order to monitor for any adverse effects.

As in other travelers, a CRPF malaria infection could result in a serious and life-threatening illness, so insect precautions and malaria chemoprophylaxis appropriate to the itinerary should be strongly encouraged. Travel advice for the HIV-infected traveler is discussed more fully in Chapter 15.

The Traveler without a Spleen

Overwhelming infection from encapsulated bacteria, such as *Haemophilus influenzae*, *Streptococcus pneumoniae*, and *Neisseria meningitidis* (meningococcus) is a recognized risk in persons who have undergone splenectomy. Medical advisors have postulated that malaria also would be more difficult to control in the splenectomized host, since the spleen serves as a major site for removal of parasitized red cells from the circulation. A review of the clinical course and treatment of malaria in a group of splenectomized patients, although based on a limited number of observations, suggested that splenectomized patients were significantly more likely to have *P. falciparum* parasitemia and febrile symptoms than controls. Parasite densities reached significantly higher levels, and mature parasite stages were more often seen in the peripheral blood, in asplenic individuals.

Long-Term Travelers

Few data are available on efficacy and tolerability of long-term malaria chemoprophylaxis. The long-term traveler requires expert advice on malaria risk and seasonality and practical guidance regarding long-term use of medications, especially since adherence is an issue over long periods of travel or deployment. Mefloquine has been used successfully for up to 2.5 years and was shown to be well tolerated and effective in preventing falciparum malaria. Toxic accumulation does not occur during long-term intake. AP can be used for long-term travelers, and US and Canadian guidelines do not limit the period of prophylaxis, although there is a 28-day limit in some countries. Few data exist on the long-term (>6-month) use of doxycycline in malaria chemoprophylaxis. Insect protection measures such as insecticide-treated bed nets and effective insect repellents are an essential component of malaria protection for long-term travelers.

PRIMAQUINE FOR RELAPSE PREVENTION

Terminal chemoprophylaxis, "the radical cure," or presumptive antirelapse therapy, refers to treatment with primaquine phosphate, an antimalarial compound that can eradicate latent malaria (*P. vivax* or *P. ovale*) incubating in the liver. Currently, the standard adult regimen consists of primaquine phosphate at a dose of 30 mg base daily with food for 2 weeks. An alternative regimen consists of three tablets (45 mg base) once a week for 8 weeks (**Table 6.4**). Common side effects are nausea and malaise.

The risk of latent hepatic malaria infections causing attacks of relapsing malaria beyond the standard 4-week period of post-travel malaria chemoprophylaxis increases with the degree of exposure to mosquito bites in the malarious area. Although post-travel primaquine therapy is not routinely advised, travelers who spent prolonged periods in rural areas of malarious countries or who report an inordinate number of mosquito bites may be candidates for primaquine therapy.

Treatment with primaquine is usually initiated at the time of the last dose of post-travel chemoprophylaxis or the last dose of treatment for a malaria attack caused by *P. vivax* or *P. ovale*. Primaquine can cause severe hemolytic anemia in persons with red cells low in G6PD, which is more common in persons of African, Asian, or Mediterranean origin. G6PD testing should be used before initiation of primaquine therapy.

Primaquine-Resistant or Tolerant *P. vivax*

P. vivax strains that do not respond to the formerly used dosage regimen of primaquine (adults, 15 mg base/day) for terminal prophylaxis have been reported from Papua, Papua

New Guinea, India, South America, and Somalia. Since primaquine tolerance is widespread, most experts now recommend using 30 mg base/day for adults for all cases of *P. vivax* malaria (0.5 mg/kg in children), provided the individual has a normal G6PD level. Primaquine is associated with nausea and vomiting, which can be reduced by giving the drug with food.

FURTHER READING

Canadian Government, 2014. Guidelines for Malaria. Available at: <http://www.phac-aspc.gc.ca/site/eng/463465/publication.html>.

Centers for Disease Control and Prevention, 2014. Health information for international travel. Available at <http://wwwnc.cdc.gov/travel/page/yellowbook-home-2014>.

Grynberg, S., Lachish, T., Kopel, E., et al., 2015. Artemether-lumefantrine compared to atovaquone-proguanil as a treatment for uncomplicated *Plasmodium falciparum* malaria in travelers. Am. J. Trop. Med. Hyg. 92, 13–17.

Hatz, C., Soto, J., Nothdurft, H.D., et al., 2008. Treatment of acute uncomplicated *falciparum* malaria with artemether-lumefantrine in nonimmune populations: a safety, efficacy, and pharmacokinetic study. Am. J. Trop. Med. Hyg. 78, 241–247.

Health Canada (CATMAT), 2014. Canadian recommendations for the prevention and treatment of malaria. Available at <http://www.phac-aspc.gc.ca/tmp-pmv/prof-eng.php>.

Høgh, B., Clarke, P.D., Camus, D., et al., 2000. Atovaquone-proguanil versus chloroquine-proguanil for malaria prophylaxis in non-immune travellers: a randomised, double-blind study. Malarone International Study Team. Lancet 356, 1888–1894.

International Association of Medical Assistance to Travelers (IAMAT), 2015. World Malaria Risk Chart. IAMAT, Guelph, Ontario, Canada. Available at <https://www.iamat.org/assets/files/World%20Malaria%20Risk%20Chart%202015.pdf>.

Leder, K., Black, J., O'Brien, D., et al., 2004. Malaria in travelers: a review of the GeoSentinel surveillance network. Clin. Infect. Dis. 39, 1104–1112.

Lell, B., Luckner, D., Ndjavé, M., et al., 1998. Randomised placebo-controlled study of atovaquone plus proguanil for malaria prophylaxis in children. Lancet 351, 709–713.

Maltha, J., Gillet, P., Jacobs, J., 2013. Malaria rapid diagnostic tests in travel medicine. Clin. Microbiol. Infect. 19, 408–415.

Nosten, F., van Vugt, M., 1999. Neuropsychiatric adverse effects of mefloquine—what do we know and what should we do? CNS Drugs 11, 1–8.

Overbosch, D., Schilthuis, H., Bienzle, U., et al., 2001. Atovaquone-proguanil versus mefloquine for malaria prophylaxis in nonimmune travelers: results from a randomized, double-blind study. Clin. Infect. Dis. 33, 1015–1021.

Public Health England, 2014. Guidelines for malaria prevention in travellers from the UK. Available at <https://www.gov.uk/government/publications/malaria-prevention-guidelines-for-travellers-from-the-uk>.

Ryan, E.T., Kain, K.C., 2000. Health advice and immunizations for travelers. N. Engl. J. Med. 342, 1716–1725.

Schlagenhauf, P., Petersen, E., 2012. Standby emergency treatment of malaria in travelers: experience to date and new developments. Expert Rev. Anti Infect. Ther. 10, 537–546.

Schlagenhauf, P., Tschopp, A., Johnson, R., et al., 2003. Tolerability of malaria chemoprophylaxis in nonimmune travelers to sub-Saharan Africa: multicenter, randomised, double-blind, four-arm study. BMJ 329, 1078.

Shanks, G.D., Gordon, D.M., Klotz, F.W., et al., 1998. Efficacy and safety of atovaquone/proguanil for suppressive prophylaxis against *Plasmodium falciparum* malaria. Clin. Infect. Dis. 27, 494–499.

World Health Organization (WHO), 2014, International Travel and Health. Available at <http://www.who.int/ith/en/>.

World Health Organization (WHO), 2014. World Malaria Report. Available at <http://www.who.int/malaria/publications/world_malaria_report_2014/en/>.

CHAPTER 7

Water Disinfection

Howard D. Backer

RISK OF WATER-BORNE INFECTION

Water disinfection is an essential component of the prevention strategy for enteric infections. In developing countries, surface water may be highly contaminated with human waste. The World Health Organization (WHO) reports that 780 million people still lack access to an improved drinking water supply, and 2.4 billion people lack access to improved sanitation. This lack of safe drinking water, sanitation, and hygiene accounts for an estimated 2 million deaths in children under 5 years of age, nearly 90% of diarrhea in all ages, and as much as 4% of all deaths globally. Urban tap water may become contaminated from aged, overwhelmed sanitation plants and deteriorating water distribution systems. Bottled water is a convenient solution, but in some places, it may not be superior to the tap water. Moreover, the plastic bottles create a huge ecological problem, since most developing countries do not recycle plastic bottles. Even in developed countries with low rates of diarrhea illness, wilderness travelers who rely on surface water for drinking and residents in areas affected by a disaster should take steps to ensure microbiologic quality. In the United States, there have been water-borne outbreaks of *Giardia*, *Shigella*, *Campylobacter*, *Escherichia coli* O157:H7, norovirus, and *Cryptosporidium*, some from untreated surface water and others from community water systems.

The list of potential water-borne pathogens is extensive and includes bacteria, viruses, protozoa, and parasitic helminths. More than 120 different enteric viruses alone can be transmitted by fecal-contaminated water. Most of the organisms that can cause traveler's diarrhea can be water-borne; however, the majority of travelers' intestinal infections are probably transmitted by food. Cholera and *Salmonella typhosa* are well known to cause extensive water-borne outbreaks. Water is considered the main route of transmission for hepatitis E and is one of the potential routes for hepatitis A and salmonellosis.

Risk of illness depends on the number of organisms ingested, which in turn depends on the degree of water contamination from human and animal waste, immune status and individual susceptibility, and virulence of the organism (**Table 7.1**). Microorganisms with small infectious dose can even cause illness through recreational water exposure such as swimming as a result of inadvertent water ingestion. Organisms that have been implicated recently in outbreaks resulting from recreational water exposure (including several in the United States) include *Giardia*, *Cryptosporidium*, *Shigella*, *E. coli* O157:H7, norovirus, and gastroenteritis from other unidentified enteric viruses.

Persistence of microorganisms in water facilitates the potential for transmission; cold water greatly prolongs survival (**Table 7.2**). Some enteric bacteria can also survive and even multiply in organic-rich tropical waters. There is a common misconception that streams "purify" themselves over a short distance. Natural die-off of organisms and the disinfection effects of ultraviolet light decrease the number of viable microorganisms, but these are not reliable enough to ensure potable water in a stream. Microorganisms also clump to particles and settle to the bottom in still water but are easily stirred up and redistributed. This does suggest that when taking surface water from a lake, one should try to obtain the water from

TABLE 7.1   Minimal Infectious Dose

Organism	Minimal Infectious Dose
Salmonella	10^5
Vibrio cholerae	10^3
Cryptosporidium	30
Giardia	10
Enteric viruses	1-10

TABLE 7.2   Survival of Microorganisms in Water

Organism	Survival
Vibrio cholerae	4-5 weeks in cold water
Giardia lamblia	2-3 months at 5-10° C
	10-28 days at 15° C
Cryptosporidium	12 months in cold water
Enteric viruses	6-10 days at 15-25° C
	30 days at 4° C
Norovirus	61 days in ground water at 25° C
Hepatitis A	12 weeks in temperate water
	6-12 months in cold water
Salmonella, Shigella	Half-life 16-24 h in temperate stream

underneath the surface, where particles float from surface tension, while not disturbing bottom sediment.

Many organisms, such as *Giardia*, *Salmonella*, and *Cryptosporidium*, can be zoonotic and have animal reservoirs, but most surface water contamination probably comes from human fecal contamination. It is important to properly dispose of personal waste. Wilderness hikers and backpackers should bury feces 6-10 inches in the soil, at least 100 feet from any water source and any natural drainage.

Accurate information concerning water quality is difficult to obtain in any country. Where sanitation systems are lacking, which is still the case in many rural areas of developing countries, all surface water should be considered highly contaminated, and tap water should be highly suspect. Any water that receives partially treated wastes, including in North America, is likely to contain pathogenic microorganisms, especially protozoa. Unfortunately, natural metals such as arsenic or chemical and nuclear wastes from industrial dumping and agricultural and mining run-off may be unrecognized or unacknowledged pollutants of water supplies. Expatriates and long-term travelers staying in a given area should try to obtain information from the Consulate or other expatriates about the safety of the local municipal water supplies.

FIELD TECHNIQUES FOR WATER TREATMENT

Fortunately, there are reliable field methods for ensuring the microbiologic safety of drinking water. A large body of recent research confirms the beneficial effect of all standard techniques at the household or individual point of use level to improve water quality and reduce diarrheal illness (**Table 7.3**). The main methods to eliminate microorganisms from water are heat, filtration, chemical disinfection, and ultraviolet treatment. Other techniques may be needed to improve the esthetic quality of the water or to remove chemical contamination. Each technique is discussed along with its respective advantages and disadvantages. Understanding the principles of water disinfection helps in choosing a method appropriate for the risk, location, and size of the group.

TABLE 7.3   Efficacy and Effectiveness of Point-of-Use Technologies for Household Use in the Developing World Households

Treatment Process	Pathogen	Optimal Log Reduction[a]	Expected Log Reduction[b]	Diarrheal Disease Reduction[c]
Ceramic filters	Bacteria	6	2	63% (51-72%) for candle filters 46% (29-59%) for bowl filters
	Viruses	4	0.5	
	Protozoa	6	4	
Free chlorine	Bacteria	6	3	37% (25-48%)
	Viruses	6	3	
	Protozoa	5	3	
Coagulation/ chlorination	Bacteria	9	7	31% (18-42%)
	Viruses	6	2-4.5	
	Protozoa	5	3	
Biosand filtration	Bacteria	3	1	47% (21-64%)
	Viruses	3	0.5	
	Protozoa	4	2	
SODIS	Bacteria	5.5	3	31% (26-37%)
	Viruses	4	2	
	Protozoa	3	1	

[a]Skilled operators using optimal conditions and practices (efficacy); log reduction: pretreatment minus post-treatment concentration of organisms (e.g., 6 log = 99.999% removal).
[b]Actual field practice by unskilled persons (effectiveness). Depends on water quality, quality and age of filter or materials, following proper procedure, and other factors.
[c]Summary estimates from published data. Depends on consistency and correct use of technique, integrity of techniques (e.g., cracked filter), and other household sanitation measures.
SODIS, Solar disinfection.
Data from multiple studies analyzed and summarized by Sobsey 2008; with data from Bielefeldt 2009; Sobsey 2002; WHO 2011(table 7.8).

Definitions

Disinfection, the desired result of field water treatment, means the removal or destruction of harmful microorganisms. Technically, it refers only to chemical means such as halogens, but the term can be applied to heat and filtration.

Pasteurization is similar to disinfection but specifically refers to the use of heat, usually at temperatures below 212°F (100°C), to kill most enteric pathogenic organisms. Disinfection and pasteurization should not be confused with *sterilization,* which is the destruction or removal of all life forms. The goal of disinfection is to achieve *potable* water, indicating that a water source, on average over a period of time, contains a "minimal microbial hazard," so the statistical likelihood of illness is minimized.

Purification is the removal of organic or inorganic chemicals and particulate matter to remove offensive color, taste, and odor. It is frequently used interchangeably with disinfection (e.g., Environmental Protection Agency [EPA] classification of water purifier), but purification, as used here, may not remove or kill enough microorganisms to ensure microbiologic safety.

Heat

The advantages of heat for water disinfection are the following:
- It is widely available.
- It imparts no additional taste to the water.
- It inactivates all enteric pathogens.
- Efficacy of heat treatment is not compromised by contaminants or particles in the water, as in the case of halogenation and filtration.

The major disadvantages of heat are the following:

- Heat does not improve the taste, smell, or appearance of poor-quality water.
- In many areas natural fuel is scarce or unavailable; 1 kg of wood is required to boil 1 L of water.
- Liquid fuels are expensive for developing countries and heavy to carry for the wilderness traveler.

Heat inactivation of microorganisms is exponential and follows first-order kinetics. Thermal death point is reached in a shorter time at higher temperatures, whereas temperatures as low as 140° F (60° C) are effective with a longer contact time. Pasteurization uses this principle to kill food-borne enteric food pathogens and spoiling organisms at temperatures between 140 and 158° F (60-70° C), well below boiling.

Heat resistance varies with different microorganisms, but common enteric pathogens are readily inactivated by heat (**Table 7.4**). Bacterial spores (e.g., *Clostridium* spp.) are the most resistant; some can survive 212° F (100° C) for long periods. *Clostridium* spores are wound pathogens that are ubiquitous in soil, lake sediment, tropical water sources, and the stool of animals and humans. Water sterilization is not necessary for drinking, since these most resistant organisms are not water-borne enteric human pathogens.

Protozoan cysts, including *Giardia*, *Entamoeba histolytica*, and *Cryptosporidium* are sensitive to heat, killed rapidly at 131-140° F (55-60° C). Parasitic helminth eggs and larvae, and cercariae of schistosomiasis, are equally susceptible to heat.

Vegetative bacteria and most enteric viruses are killed rapidly at temperatures above 140° F (60° C) and within seconds by boiling water. Typical pasteurization processes include heating to 145-149° F (63-65° C) for up to 30 min or flash pasteurization using high temperature-short time at 160-162° F (71-72° C) for 15-30 seconds. Recent data confirm

---

TABLE 7.4   Data on Heat Inactivation of Microorganisms[a]

Organism	Lethal Temperature/Time
Giardia	131° F (55° C) for 5 min
	212° F (100° C) immediately
Entamoeba histolytica	Similar to *Giardia*
Nematode cysts Helminth eggs, larvae, cercariae	122-131° F (50-55° C) (time not specified but should be similar to *Cryptosporidium*)
Cryptosporidium	113-131° F (45-55° C) for 20 min
	148° F (64.2° C) for 2 min
	162° F (72° C) heated up over 1 min
Escherichia coli	131° F (55° C) for 30 min
	140-144° F (60-62° C) for 10 min
Salmonella and *Shigella*	149° F (65° C) for <1 min
Vibrio cholerae	212° F (100° C) for 30 s
Enteric viruses	131-140° F (55-60° C) for 20-40 min
	158° F (70° C) for <1 min
	167° F (75° C) for <0.5 min
Hepatitis A	185° F (85° C) for 1 min
	140° F (60° C) for 10 min
Hepatitis E	140° F (60° C) for 30 min
Bacterial spores	>212° F (100° C)

[a]Endpoint in most studies is death of 100% of organisms. Some studies use 99.9% inactivation, but longer time in contact with heat will rapidly result in inactivation of all micro-organisms.

TABLE 7.5 Boiling Temperature and Altitude	
Elevation	Boiling Point of Water
10,000 ft (3048 m)	194°F (90°C)
14,000 ft (4267 m)	187°F (86°C)
19,000 ft (5791 m)	178°F (81°C)

that common water-borne enteric viruses, including hepatitis A virus (HAV), are readily inactivated at these temperatures.

In recognition of the difference between pasteurizing water for drinking purposes and sterilizing for surgical purposes, most sources now agree that boiling for 10 min is not necessary. Heating water on a stove or fire takes time, which counts toward disinfection while the temperature rises from 131°F (55°C) to the boiling temperature. Although attaining boiling temperature is not necessary, it is the only easily recognizable endpoint without using a thermometer. Therefore, any water brought to a boil should be adequately disinfected. For an extra margin of safety, the water should be brought to a boil, the stove turned off, and the pot covered for a few minutes before using the water. The WHO concurs with this conclusion, but the Centers for Disease Control and Prevention (CDC) and the EPA still recommend boiling for 1 min to allow for an extra margin of safety. The boiling point decreases with increasing altitude, but this is not significant with regard to the time and temperature required for thermal death (**Table 7.5**).

The use of hot tap water, "too hot to touch," has been suggested to prevent traveler's diarrhea in developing countries. However, testing shows considerable variation in the temperature of hot tap water (most between 131 and 140°F (55-60°C), but some lower) and in maximum tolerated temperature-to-touch (below 131°F (55°C) for some people). If no other means of water treatment is available, using hot tap water that has been kept hot in a tank for some time is a reasonable alternative. Travelers staying in hotels or other accommodations with electricity can conveniently bring water to a boil with a small electric heating coil or with a lightweight electric beverage warmer brought from home.

In hot, sunny climates, temperatures adequate for pasteurization can be achieved by solar heating using a solar oven or simple reflectors.

Filtration

Many commercial products are available for individuals and groups to filter water in the field. Advantages of filtration include:

- Filters are simple to operate.
- Filters add no unpleasant taste, and many will improve the taste and appearance of water.
- Most filters require no holding time, and water can be consumed as it comes out of the filter.
- It may be rationally combined with halogens if the filter is not rated for viral removal.

Disadvantages of filtration include:

- It is expensive compared with halogen treatment.
- Filters can be heavy and bulky, which may be significant if carrying the gear oneself.
- Many filters will not remove viruses sufficiently and may require a second step with halogens to assure viral inactivation.
- A cracked filter element or a leaking seal can allow channeling of water around the filter and will let contaminated water pass through the device.
- Filters clog quickly if the water is dirty or has a lot of suspended particles and eventually will clog from filtering even "clear" surface water. Most micropore filters include a prefilter for larger particulates. Laboratory paper filters with a pore size of about 20-30 μm or even coffee filters can be used to prefilter the larger particulate debris from dirty water and may also retain parasitic eggs and larvae (see the section on Clarification below for other methods). The user should know how to clean or replace the filter elements to re-establish flow.

TABLE 7.6a   Levels of Filtration

Filtration Level	Minimal Pore Size (μm)	Particles Removed
Microfiltration	0.1	Protozoa, bacteria, algae, particles, sediment
Ultrafiltration	0.001	Viruses, colloids, some dissolved solids
Nanofiltration	0.0001	All microorganisms, dissolved substances, salts, endotoxins
Reverse osmosis	0.00001	All of above plus monovalent ions and nearly all organic molecules

TABLE 7.6b   Susceptibility of Microorganisms to Filtration

Organism	Approximate Size (μm)	Maximum Filter Pore Size (μm)
Nematode eggs	30 × 60	20
Giardia	6-10 × 8-15	3-5
Entamoeba histolytica	5-30 (average 10)	3-5
Cyclospora	8-9	3-5
Cryptosporidium oocysts	2-6	1
Enteric bacteria	0.5 × 3-8	0.2-0.4
Viruses	0.03	0.01

The effectiveness of filters depends on pore size (**Tables 7.6a and 7.6b**), but other variables influence filter efficiency, including the characteristics of the filter media and the water, as well as flow rate. Microfilters are effective for removing protozoa and bacteria, algae, most particles, and sediment but allow dissolved material, small colloids, and some viruses to pass through. Ultrafiltration membranes are required for complete removal of viruses, colloids, and some dissolved solids. Nanofilters can remove other dissolved substances, including salts (sodium chloride) and endotoxins from water. Reverse osmosis removes monovalent ions (desalination) and nearly all organic molecules.

Filtration is usually a two-step process: physical (separation of particles from liquid) and chemical (attachment of microorganisms to the medium), which may allow increased efficacy of virus removal. Most field filters are not membranes but rather depth filters, with maze-like passageways that trap particles and organisms smaller than the average passage diameter.

Most field devices are microfilters that are adequate for cysts and bacteria but may not sufficiently remove viruses, which are a major concern in water with high levels of fecal contamination. It is important for point-of-use filters to achieve the EPA standard of 4-log reduction (99.99%) of viruses, given the small infectious dose. Most viruses adhere to larger particles or clump together into aggregates that may be removed by the filter, in addition to any electrochemical adherence to the filter media. Reverse osmosis filters that desalinate will also remove viruses; however, these are currently too expensive and slow for use in a hand pump for land travel. Iodine resin filters will kill bacteria and viruses by contact with the iodine, not by mechanical filtration. Several portable filters have test results that meet the EPA standards for removal of viruses: General Ecology First-Need mechanical microfilter claims electrochemical removal of viruses; Sawyer Water Purifier, Lifestraw, MSR and other products that use hollow fiber membrane filtration remove viruses with ultrafiltration capability.

Some filters can be readily and inexpensively built in developing areas. One is a ceramic filter shaped like a flower pot or rounded cone made from local substances like porous fired clay (diatomaceous earth). The other is a biosand filter that uses successive layers of progressively more coarse sand and gravel. The uppermost layer of fine sand further builds a biologic layer that contributes to the filtration effectiveness.

If the water supply is suspected of being heavily contaminated with biologic wastes and additional assurance is needed, then a second step with chemical treatment of the water before or after filtration can kill viruses. Many filters contain a charcoal stage that will remove the halogen, if applied prior to filtration. Alternately, prior filtration allows lower halogen doses to be used for the chemical inactivation step.

Filters for international and wilderness travelers are listed in **Table 7.7**.

CLARIFICATION

The appearance of cloudy water can be improved by several other means. Large particles will settle out over a period of several hours by *sedimentation*. The supernatant can then be filtered and/or chemically treated. Smaller suspended particles can be removed by *coagulation-flocculation*. A pinch of alum, an aluminum salt, is added to a gallon of water, mixed well, and then stirred occasionally for 30-60 min. The quantity added does not need to be precise, and more can be used as needed. The small particles clump (flocculate) and then settle out over minutes to hours. The supernatant is then decanted, or the mixture is poured through a paper filter before proceeding with microfiltration and/or chemical treatment. Coagulation-flocculation removes many microorganisms as well as other impurities from the water, greatly improving taste, smell, and microbiologic safety of cloudy water. However, coagulation-flocculation should not be used as a sole step for disinfection; it should be followed by chemical treatment, filtration, or ultraviolet treatment.

Granular Activated Charcoal

Granular activated charcoal (GAC) improves water quality by removing organic pollutants and chemicals by adsorption. GAC can remove objectionable color, taste, and smell from water. Although some microorganisms will adhere to GAC or become trapped in charcoal filters, GAC does *not* remove all microorganisms; thus, it does not disinfect. In fact, charcoal beds become colonized rapidly with nonpathogenic bacteria. One rational use of GAC is to remove the color and taste of iodine or chlorine after disinfection. If used to remove halogen, one must wait until *after* the required contact time before running water through charcoal or adding charcoal to the water. Granular activated charcoal is commonly incorporated into point-of-use water filters (**Table 7.7**).

CHEMICALS

Chemical means of disinfection include the halogens, chiefly chlorine and iodine, and their chemical species that form in aqueous solution, e.g., hypochlorite. Chlorine dioxide is also considered in this section.

Halogens (chlorine and iodine) have the following advantages:

- They are excellent disinfectants for bacteria, viruses, *Giardia*, and amebic cysts.
- Iodine and chlorine are widely available in several forms.
- They are inexpensive.
- They can be applied with equal ease to large and small quantities of water, and dosing is flexible.
- Taste can be removed.

Disadvantages include:

- They can potentially be toxic (mainly iodine).
- Taste can be unpleasant at concentrations of 4-5 mg/L and above.
- The potency of some products (tablets and crystals) is affected by prolonged exposure to moisture, heat, and air.
- Liquids are corrosive and stain clothing.
- Iodine and chlorine do not kill *Cryptosporidium* when used in usual field doses.

TABLE 7.7 Portable Field Water Filters and Purification Devices

Manufacturer, Product/ Manufacturer's Website[a]	Microbial Claims[b]	Operation	Primary Filter, Additional Elements, Stages, Comments[c]	Capacity	Retail Price (US$)[d]
Aquamira www.mcnett.com Water filter bottle and Frontier	P, B, V	In line, drink-through in sport bottle, water bag, or gravity drip	Prefilter, porous plastic microfilter, new Redline filter for virus removal, carbon shell. May be used in conjunction with Aquamira water treatment—chlorine dioxide stabilized solution	1-2 people	20-50
Aquarain www.aquarain.com					
Aquarain 200 and 400	P, B	Gravity drip	Stacked bucket filter with one to four candle filters with ceramic elements. Carbon core, stainless steel housing	Small group	240-320
British Berkfeld www.jamesfilter.com					
Big Berkey and multiple other models	P, B	Gravity drip	Bucket filter, one to four ceramic elements with carbon matrix or candle filters of compressed carbon. Available in stainless steel or Lexan housing with 1.5-6 gallon lower reservoir.	Household or moderate-sized group	240 (100-320)
General ecology www.generalecology.com			Claims for viral removal are based on electrostatic attraction in structured matrix compressed carbon block filter. Variety of sizes and configurations also available for in-line use and electric-powered units		
First Need XLE	P, B, V	Hand pump	Compressed charcoal	Small group	120
Base camp	P, B, V	Hand pump or electric	Compressed charcoal element similar to First Need. High flow, high capacity. Stainless steel housing. Prefilter. Electric models also available	Large group	700
Trav-L-Pure	P, B	Hand pump	Same compressed charcoal filter element as First Need in plastic housing	Small group	230

Hydro-photon www.hydro-photon.com		Hand-held purifier		Ultraviolet purifier uses batteries with timer. Active end of unit is held in bottle or other small container of water.	1-2 people	
Multiple Steripen models: Classic Opti Adventurer Ultra Freedom Aqua	P, B, V			Units differ in size, battery (AA, CR 123, rechargeable), LED display, and other features.		50-100
Katadyn www.katadyn.com				Unless otherwise specified, filter elements are 0.2 μm ceramic depth filter.		
My Bottle	P, B, V	Sport bottle		Iodine resin with filter for protozoan cysts, and granular activated charcoal	1-2 people	40-60
Hiker and Hiker Pro	P	Hand pump		Pleated glass-fiber 0.3-μm filter with granular activated charcoal core and prefilter; for high-quality source water, removes "most" bacteria	1-2 people	60-85
Gravity Camp and Basecamp	P, B	Gravity drip		Pleated glass fiber 0.3 μm with activated carbon; reservoir bag with in-line filter	Small group	60
Mini	P, B	Hand pump		Ceramic filter with prefilter	1-2 people	90
Pocket	P, B	Hand pump		Ceramic filter with prefilter	Small group	300
Ceradyn and Gravidyn	P, B	Gravity drip		Bucket filter, three ceramic candles; optional activated carbon core filters with Gravidyn	Small-large group	160-190
Combi	P, B	Hand pump		Ceramic filter and activated carbon cartridge; can be converted for in-line faucet use	Small group	180
Expedition	P, B	Hand pump		Ceramic filter with intake pre-filter; stainless steel housing	Large group	1250
Survivor 06 Survivor 35 (power units also available)	P, B, V	Hand pump		Reverse osmosis filter; desalinates as well as disinfects; for ocean survival; very low flow rate; power units available	1-2 people	1000-2200

Continued

TABLE 7.7 Portable Field Water Filters and Purification Devices—cont'd

Manufacturer, Product/ Manufacturer's Website[a]	Microbial Claims[b]	Operation	Primary Filter, Additional Elements, Stages, Comments[c]	Capacity	Retail Price (US$)[d]
Cascade Designs www.cascadedesigns.com					
MSR Sweetwater microfilter	P, B	Hand pump	0.2-μm depth filter with granular activated carbon and pre-filter; purifier solution (chlorine) as pre-treatment to kill viruses	Small group	90
Miniworks EX	P, B	Hand pump	Ceramic filter with activated carbon core and pre-filter	Small group	90
HyperFlow and AutoFlow	P, B	Pump or gravity drip	Microfilter (0.2 μm) with hollow-fiber technology	Small group	100-120
Guardian	P,B,V	Hand pump	Hollow fiber technology with 0.02 micron pore size to remove viruses.	Small group	350
Sawyer www.sawyerproducts.com					
Water filter Point One Biologic (available in wide array of packaged products)	P, B	Multiple applications including sport bottle and in-line cartridge, gravity drip, bucket filter, or faucet attachment	Hollow-fiber technology, 0.1 μm in versatile filter cartridge	1-2 people or small group	40-90
Water purifier Zero Point Two (available in wide array of packaged products)	P, B, V	Multiple applications, same as Point One filter	Hollow-fiber technology, 0.02 μm, in versatile filter cartridge	1-2 people or small group	130-220

[a]This is not a comprehensive list. Models change frequently. A manufacturer's website is provided if it contains product information; otherwise, search manufacturer and brand with any major search engine to find large retail sites that provide detailed product information.

[b]B, Bacteria; P, protozoa; V, viruses.

[c]Consider additional features, such as flow rate, filter capacity, size, and filter weight.

[d]Prices vary.

- There is some degree of imprecision because the actual residual concentration (after halogen demand is met) is not known.
- Some understanding of the process is helpful to achieve reliable results and reasonable taste.

Vegetative bacteria are markedly sensitive to halogens. Viruses and *Giardia* are sensitive but require higher concentrations or longer contact times. *Cryptosporidium* cysts are highly resistant to halogens. Little is known about *Cyclospora*, but it is assumed to be similar to *Cryptosporidium*. Certain parasitic eggs, such as *Ascaris*, are also resistant, but these are not commonly spread by water. (All these resistant cysts and eggs are susceptible to heat or filtration.)

Primary factors determining the rate and proportion of microorganisms killed are the concentration of halogen (measured in mg/L) or the equivalent, parts per million (ppm), and the length of time organisms are exposed to the halogen (contact time, measured in minutes) (**Table 7.8**). An increase in either halogen concentration or contact time allows a decrease in the other. Theoretically, for given conditions of temperature and pH, doubling contact time allows half the concentration of halogen to achieve the same results. In clear water, this principle can be used to decrease the taste of halogen. Due to many unknown factors in the field, extending contact time even longer adds a margin of safety.

Secondary factors are temperature of the water, organic contaminants in the water, and pH. Cold slows reaction time, so in cold water, the contact time should be increased. Alternatively, the dose could be increased in cold water. Some halogen is absorbed by organic impurities in the water, so an increased dose is required if water is cloudy (high turbidity); longer contact time may not be effective. The better solution is clarification prior to use of halogen. Although clear surface water probably requires minimal halogen, some impurities (at least 1 mg/L) must be assumed, so it is prudent to use 4 mg/L as a target halogen concentration for clear water and to allow extra contact time, especially if the water is cold. Water pH usually becomes a factor only in highly alkaline waters but not for usual surface water, which is neutral to slightly acidic.

TABLE 7.8   Experimental Data for 99.9% Kill with Halogens at pH 6-8

Organism	Halogen	Concentration (mg/L)	Time (min)	TEMPERATURE	
				(°C)	(°F)
Giardia	Chlorine	4.0	60	3-5	37-41
		8.0	30	3-5	37-41
		3.0	10	15	59
		1.5	10	25	77
	Iodine	1.5	10	25	77
		3.0	15	20	68
		7.0	30	3	37
Enteric viruses	Chlorine	0.5	40	2	36
		0.3	30	25	77
	Iodine	0.3	30	25	77
Norovirus	Free chlorine	1	10	5	10
		5	20 seconds	5	2.7
Poliovirus	Iodine	20	1.5	25	77
Escherichia coli	Chlorine	0.03	5	2-5	36-41
	Iodine	1.0	1	2-5	36-41
Cryptosporidum	Chlorine	80	90		

Recommendations for chlorine and iodine disinfection of water with regard to concentration, temperature, and contact times are given in **Table 7.9**. Both chlorine and iodine are available in liquid and tablet form. **Table 7.10** describes some commercially available halogen products.

Choice of Halogen

Iodine has some advantage over chlorine for field disinfection. Dilute iodine solutions are less affected by nitrogenous wastes or pH, and most people prefer the taste at treatment levels. However, there is concern over physiologic activity. Some alteration in thyroid

TABLE 7.9 Halogen Disinfection of Water

Iodine Products	Amount to Release 4 ppm in 1 L	Amount to Release 8 ppm in 1 L[a]
Iodine tabs	½ tab	1 tab
Tetraglycine hydroperiodide	*or*	
EDWGT	1 tab in 2 L	
Potable aqua		
Globaline		
2% Iodine solution (tincture) (do not use decolorized iodine)	0.2 mL; 5 gtt	0.4 mL; 10 gtt
10% Povidone-iodine solution	0.35 mL; 8 gtt	0.70 mL; 16 gtt
Saturated iodine crystals in water (Polar Pure)	13 mL	26 mL

Chlorine Products[b]	Amount for 5 ppm in 1 L	Amount for 10 ppm in 1 L
Household bleach (5% sodium hypochlorite)	0.1 mL	0.2 mL
	2 gtt	4 gtt
Household bleach (8.25%)	1 gtt	2 gtt
Chlorination–flocculation	1 tablet in 2 L	1 tablet (8 ppm)
Chlor-Floc		
AquaCure		

Contact time in minutes at various water temperatures[c]

Concentration of Halogen	5°C	15°C	30°C
2 ppm	240	180	60
4 ppm	180	60	45
8 ppm	60	30	15

[a]For cloudy water, it is preferable to clarify water prior to using halogens to reduce the need for high levels of halogen, improving the taste. For cold water, use the lower dose and increase the contact time.
[b]Formula for calculation of chlorine dose to achieve specific halogen concentration in large volumes of water (from Lantagne 2014):

$$\text{Dose (mg}_{Cl}/\text{L}_{water}) = \left(\text{bleach concentration (\%)} \times \frac{10{,}000\ \text{mg}_{Cl}/\text{L}_{Cl}}{1\%} \times \text{bleach added (mL}_{Cl}) \times \frac{1\text{L}_{Cl}}{1000\ \text{mL}_{Cl}} \right) \Big/$$
$$(\text{volume of water (L}_{water}))$$

[c]Recent data indicate that very cold water requires prolonged contact time with iodine or chlorine to kill *Giardia* cysts. These contact times in cold water have been extended from the usual recommendations to account for this and for the uncertainty of residual concentration.
EDWGT: Emergency Drinking Water Germicidal Tablets.

TABLE 7.10   Commercial Halogen Products[a]

Saturated solution of iodine in water

Polar Pure

Iodine crystals, 8 g in 3-oz bottle; bottle cap is used to measure; directions and color dot thermometer on bottle (temperature affects iodine concentration in bottle); capacity: 2000 quarts; weight: 5 oz; yields 4 ppm iodine when recommended dose is added to 1 quart of clean water. Warm water to 20° C (68° F) before adding iodine to shorten contact time. Since it is not feasible to warm all water, extend contact time to 1-2 h for very cold water.

Saturated aqueous solution of crystalline iodine is an excellent and stable source of iodine.

Iodine Solutions

Iodine solutions for topical disinfection can be used for water; however, these solutions also contain iodide, which has physiologic activity but no disinfection activity:

Tincture of iodine: 2% iodine, 2.4% iodide

Lugol's solution: 5% iodine, 10% iodide

Strong iodine: 2% iodine, 9.0% iodide

Decolorized iodine: 0% iodine

Betadine solution contains 9-12% iodine bound to a large neutral molecule that serves as a sustained-release reservoir of free iodine, resulting in 2-10 ppm free iodine in aqueous solution.

Iodine tablets

Potable Aqua (Wisconsin Pharmacal, Jackson, WI)

Emergency Drinking Water Germicidal Tablets (Coghlan's, Winnipeg, MB, Canada, www.coghlans.com)

Iodine-containing tablets (tetraglycine hydroperiodide) release approximately 7-8 mg iodine when added to water. One tablet is added to 1 quart of water. In cloudy or cold water, add two tabs. Contact time is only 10-15 min in clear, warm water, much more in cold, cloudy water. Neutralizing tablets contain ascorbic acid.

This method was developed by the military for troops in the field. Advantages are unit dose and short contact time, but these concentrations create strong tastes that are not acceptable to many users. Options to improve taste include adding one tablet to 2 quarts of clear water to yield about 4 mg/L (and extend contact time), or using the neutralizer tablets. Clarify cloudy water first.

Flocculation plus chlorination

Chlor-Floc (Deatrick & Associates, Alexandria, VA)

PUR, Purifier of Water (Proctor and Gamble, Cincinnati, OH, http://www.pghsi.com/safewater/development.html)

Aqua Cure (distributed by Safesport Manufacturing, Denver, CO)

Tablets or powder that contain a flocculating agent and source of chlorine to clarify and disinfect water. The process was developed and tested by the military and is still used by some services for individual troops in the field. Chlor-Floc and Aqua Cure are similar products containing sodium dichloro-isocyanurate (NaDCC) with proprietary flocculating agents and a buffering system. A cloth filter is provided. One tablet provides 8 ppm available chlorine. Proctor and Gamble recently developed packets of powder for humanitarian use in developing countries or disaster situations that contains ferric sulfate as a coagulant and calcium hypochlorite.

Household bleach (sodium hypochlorite)

The Centers for Disease Control and Prevention (CDC) and World Health Organization (WHO) advocate chlorination for point-of-use household water disinfection, using a 1% hypochlorite solution to provide a dosage of 1.875 or 3.75 mg/L of sodium hypochlorite with a contact time of 30 min.

Continued

TABLE 7.10   Commercial Halogen Products—cont'd

NaDCC (chlorine)

Aquaclear (Gal Pharm, Ireland, imported by BCB Survival Equipment)

Aquatabs (Global Hydration Water Treatment Systems, Kakabeka Falls, Ontario, Canada)

NaDCC is a stable, nontoxic chlorine compound that forms a mildly acidic solution, which is optimal for hypochlorous acid, the most active disinfectant of the free chlorine compounds. Free chlorine is in equilibrium with available chlorine that remains in compound, providing greater biocidal capacity. NaDCC is more stable and provides more free, active chlorine than other available chlorine products for water disinfection. Available as individually wrapped effervescent tablets for small quantities or in bulk quantities and higher concentrations in screw-cap tubs for disinfection of large quantities of water or for shock chlorination of tanks and other storage systems.

Calcium hypochlorite (dry chlorine)

Calcium hypochlorite is a stable, concentrated, dry source of hypochlorite that is commonly used for chlorination of swimming pools. It is widely available in tablets or tubs of granules through chemical supply or swimming pool supply stores.

Redi-Chlor (Continental Technologies, Little River, KS) distributes calcium hypochlorite tablets in blister packs that come in different strengths and can be broken in half or fourths to treat various quantities of water. Recommended dose results in 2-5 mg/L residual chlorine. This is a convenient source of hypochlorite, which can also be used for superchlorination.

Silver

Micropur (www.katadyn.com)

Silver in tablet, liquid, or crystal form. Unit dosages available for small volumes of water or for big storage tanks. Most common formulation: silver-containing tablets in individual bubble packing; add one tab to 1 quart of water. Mix thoroughly and allow 2 h contact time.

Claims: "For the disinfection and storage of clear water." "Reliably kill bacterial agents of enteric diseases but *not* worm eggs, ameba, viruses." "Neutral to taste, simple to use and innocuous." Treatment of water will ensure protection against reinfection for 1-6 months.

Silver is approved by the EPA to be marketed in the USA as a "water preservative" that can maintain bacteria-free water for up to 6 months. Although there are proven antibacterial effects, silver tablets are not licensed as a water purifier in the United States. Note there are no claims for viruses and protozoa, because concentrations may not be adequate to kill these organisms.

Silver and chlorine

Micropur Forte (Katadyn Corporation, Wallisellen, Switzerland, www.katadyn.com)

This product combines silver and chlorine in tablet or liquid form. Chlorine ensures destruction of viruses and bacteria in clear, untreated surface water. Silver maintains microbiologic purity of water for up to 6 months. If water is consumed right away, there is no reason to use this product, because the silver adds little advantage to chlorine alone.

Chlorine dioxide

Aquamira (McNett Outdoor, Bellingham, WA)

Pristine (Advanced Chemicals, Vancouver, British Columbia)

MicroPur MP-1 (Katadyn Corporation)

Various products in tablet, liquid, or powder form containing "stabilized" chlorine dioxide that generates active disinfectant through mixing two ingredients or through dissolution of the tablets in water. Advantages of chlorine dioxide are greater effectiveness than chlorine at equivalent doses and the ability to inactivate *Cryptosporidium* oocysts with reasonable doses and contact times. Chlorine dioxide does not have extended persistence in water, so should not be used to maintain microbiologic purity of stored water. Testing suggests tablets may be more effective than solutions.

---

^aExtensive data exist for the effectiveness of iodine and chlorine (see text and Table 7.9)

function can be measured when iodine is used for water disinfection, and goiters have been associated with excessive iodine levels in water. There is the potential for hypersensitivity reactions (although these have not been described for iodinated water) and for exacerbation of pre-existing thyroid problems.

Therefore iodine use is *not* recommended in the following circumstances:

- Unstable thyroid disease
- Known iodine allergy
- During pregnancy for periods longer than several weeks (because of the risk of neonatal goiter).

Despite studies documenting use of iodine for prolonged periods without problems, WHO recommends limiting iodine water disinfection to emergency use of a few weeks. The military developed iodine tablets and still uses them in some situations, but the disadvantages of unpleasant taste and color and alteration of thyroid function have led them to substitute chlorine tablets combined with a flocculent for many small group field applications.

Taste of halogens may be improved by the following:

- Using GAC *after* contact time (included as a final stage in many filters)
- Reducing the halogen concentration and increasing the contact time in clean water
- Removing taste by chemical means. A tiny pinch or several granules of ascorbic acid (vitamin C, available in powder or crystal form) or sodium thiosulfate (nontoxic, available at chemical supply stores) will reduce iodine to iodide or chlorine to chloride, which has no taste or color; these must be added *after* the required contact time. Many flavored drink mixes contain ascorbic acid. Note that iodide still has physiologic activity. Hydrogen peroxide will also reduce chlorine to chloride (see the section on Superchlorination-Dechlorination below).

Superchlorination-Dechlorination

The above principle of chemical reduction is used in this process. Chlorine (hypochlorite) can be used in very high doses of 100-200 mg/L for reliable disinfection, then dechlorinated (reducing hypochlorite to chloride), effectively removing taste and smell with no toxicity. This is an extremely effective way to maintain potability of water stored for prolonged periods, dechlorinating batches as needed. It is also a very good technique for disinfecting large quantities of water. There are currently no commercial products using this technique; however, ingredients can be purchased from chemical supply (30% peroxide) and swimming pool supply (calcium hypochlorite granules) stores.

About $\frac{1}{4}-\frac{1}{2}$ tsp/L of calcium hypochlorite (65% available chlorine) is added to water to achieve very high concentrations of chlorine for disinfection, tested only by strong smell. After a reasonable contact time of 30-60 min, add about 6 drops 30% hydrogen peroxide (usual wound care strength is 3%) and stir or agitate, which causes formation of soluble nontoxic calcium chloride. Excess peroxide bubbles off as oxygen, but hydrogen peroxide is also a disinfectant. If titrated correctly, treated water has no chlorine taste. Ingredients should be kept in separate 3-4 oz plastic bottles and are highly stable if kept in a cool, dry place. Measurements do not need to be exact, but it takes some experimentation and experience to balance the two and achieve optimal results. Hydrogen peroxide 30% is extremely corrosive and burns skin, so handle cautiously.

Iodine Resins

Iodine resins are considered a contact disinfectant: iodine binds to microorganisms that come into contact with the resin aided by electrostatic forces, but leaves only small amounts of iodine dissolved in the water. Organisms are effectively exposed to high iodine concentrations when passing through the resin, allowing reduced contact time; however, some contact time is necessary. *Cryptosporidium* oocysts may become trapped in the resin, but of those passing through, half are viable at 30 min.

The resins have been incorporated into many different filter designs available for field use. Most contain a 1-µm cyst filter, which should effectively remove *Cryptosporidium* as well as *Giardia* and any other halogen-resistant parasitic eggs or larva. Their operation assumes that resins kill bacteria and viruses rapidly and the filter membrane removes cysts, so minimal contact time is required for most water. A carbon stage removes residual dissolved iodine to prevent excessive iodine ingestion in long-term users. The effectiveness of an individual resin matrix depends on ensuring contact of every microorganism with iodine resin (no channeling of water). Cloudy or sediment-laden water may clog the resin, as it would with any filter, or coat the resin, inhibiting iodine transfer. Due to variable test results and amounts of ingested iodine, most models are no longer marketed in the United States; however, some products are still available for international use.

Chlorine Dioxide

Chlorine dioxide (ClO_2), a potent biocide, has been used for many years to disinfect municipal water and in numerous other large-scale applications. Until recently, chlorine dioxide could be used only in large-scale water treatment applications, but several new chemical methods for generating chlorine dioxide on-site can now be applied in the field for small quantity water treatment, allowing this technique to gain wider use for disinfection of both community and point-of-use drinking water supplies in developed countries. Chlorine dioxide is capable of inactivating most water-borne pathogens, including *Cryptosporidium parvum* oocysts, at practical doses and contact times. It is at least as effective a bactericide as chlorine and in many cases superior. It is far superior as a virucide. Chlorine dioxide is not stable in solution and does not produce a lasting residual (**Table 7.10**).

OTHER CHEMICAL DISINFECTANTS

Mixed Species Disinfection (Electrolysis)

Passing a current through a simple brine salt solution generates free available chlorine and other "mixed species" disinfectants that have been demonstrated effective against bacteria, viruses, and bacterial spores. The process can be used on both large and small scales. The resulting solution has greater disinfectant ability than a simple solution of sodium hypochlorite and has even been demonstrated to inactivate *Cryptosporidium*, suggesting that chlorine dioxide (see below) is among the chemicals generated. Testing and large-scale products are available on the Miox website (http://www.miox.com/). The pocket-sized device (Miox Purifier) is no longer marketed, but an individual user product for point of use in developing areas is in production (SE 200 Electrochlorinator) by Cascade Designs (Seattle, WA; http://sites.path.org/water/community-water/products/technology-se200/).

Potassium Permanganate

Potassium permanganate is a strong oxidizing agent with some disinfectant properties. It was used extensively before hypochlorites as a drinking water disinfectant. In some parts of the world, it is still used on a small scale for this purpose and also for washing fruits and vegetables. It is most commonly used as a 1-5% solution for disinfection and often sold as packets of 1 g to be added to 1 L of water. At these concentrations, the solutions are deep pink to purple and can stain surfaces. Although bacterial inactivation can be achieved with moderate concentrations and contact times, it cannot be recommended for field use, since quantitative data are not available for viruses or protozoan cysts.

Hydrogen Peroxide

Hydrogen peroxide (H_2O_2) is a strong oxidizing agent but considered a weak disinfectant for water disinfection use. Small doses (1 mL of 3% H_2O_2 in 1 L water) are effective for inactivating bacteria within minutes to hours, depending on the level of contamination. Viruses require high doses and longer contact times. Lack of data for protozoan cysts and quantitative data for dilute solutions prevents it from being useful by itself as a field water disinfectant. In higher concentrations, it can be used to sterilize industrial and food processing equipment. It is considered safe enough for use in foods, yielding oxygen and water as innocuous end products.

Silver

Silver is widely used as a disinfectant, although the literature on antimicrobial effects of silver is confusing. Silver ion has bactericidal effects in low doses, but disinfection requires several hours at the recommended concentration of 50 ppb. An advantage is absence of taste, odor, and color. One factor limiting its use is that it readily adsorbs to container surfaces, making it difficult to control the concentration. However, this characteristic is also used beneficially, coating surfaces with silver to release small amounts. Another caution is that silver has physiologic activity, but doses used for water treatment are unlikely to cause side effects such as agyria, a permanent discoloration of the skin and mucous membranes. The use of silver as a drinking water disinfectant has been much more popular in Europe, but in the United States, it is approved only for maintaining bacteriological quality of stored water.

Citrus

Citrus juice contains limonene, which has biocidal properties. Lemon or lime juice has been shown to destroy *Vibrio cholerae* at a concentration of 2% (equivalent of 2 tbs/L of water) with a contact time of 30 min. Lime juice also killed 99.9% of *V. cholerae* on cabbage and lettuce leaves and inhibited growth of *V. cholerae* in rice foods, suggesting that adding sufficient lime juice to water, beverages, and other foods can reduce disease risks. Commercial products using citrus cannot yet be recommended as primary means of water disinfection, rather than an ancillary or emergency measure.

Ultraviolet Light

In sufficient doses, all water-borne enteric pathogens are inactivated by ultraviolet (UV) radiation. Bacteria and protozoan parasites require lower doses than enteric viruses and bacterial spores. *Giardia* and *Cryptosporidium* are susceptible to practical doses of UV light and may be more sensitive because of their relatively large size. The germicidal effect of UV light depends on light intensity and exposure time. Advantages of UV treatment include:

- UV irradiation is effective against all microorganisms.
- Treatment does not require chemicals and does not affect the taste of the water.
- It works rapidly, and extra dosing to the water presents no danger; in fact, it is a safety factor.
- Available from sunlight (see section on SODIS below)

Disadvantages include the following:

- UV irradiation with lamps requires a power source and is costly.
- No residual disinfection power; so water may become re-contaminated or re-growth of bacteria may occur.
- Particulate matter can shield microorganisms from UV rays.

UV lamp disinfection systems are widely used to disinfect drinking water at the community and household level. Steri-Pen, a portable, battery-operated UV water disinfection system for individual use has recently been developed (Hydro-Photon, Blue Hill, ME; http://www.hydrophoton.com/). The use of this portable technology is currently limited to small volumes of clear water, but its simplicity is very appealing (**Table 7.7**).

Solar Irradiation (SODIS)

UV irradiation by sunlight in the UV-A range can substantially improve the microbiologic quality of water and thereby reduce diarrheal illness in communities employing this technique in developing countries. Recent work has confirmed the efficacy and optimal procedures of the solar disinfection (SODIS) technique. Transparent bottles (e.g., clear plastic beverage bottles), preferably lying on a dark surface, are exposed to sunlight for a minimum of 4 h; some investigations demonstrate improved benefit from several sequential days. Oxygenation induces greater reductions of bacteria, so agitation is recommended before solar treatment in bottles.

UV and thermal inactivation are synergistic for solar disinfection of drinking water in transparent plastic bottles. Above 55°C (131°F), thermal inactivation is of primary importance. Use of a simple reflector or solar cooker can achieve temperatures of 65°C (149°F), which will pasteurize the water (see section on Heat disinfection).

Where strong sunshine is available, solar disinfection of drinking water is an effective, low-cost method for improving water quality and may be of particular use in refugee camps and disaster areas.

Nanoparticles: Solar Photocatalytic Disinfection

Several nanomaterials have been shown to have strong antimicrobial properties and are being evaluated for use in water disinfection and purification. They are already being used widely in industrial purification, but they show great potential for point-of-use applications as well. The metals, including silver, titanium dioxide (TiO_2), and zinc oxide, are of particular interest for water disinfection applications because they can be activated by UV light to produce potent oxidizers. In addition to being an excellent disinfectant for various microorganisms, this process is unique in its ability to break down complex organic contaminants and most heavy metals into carbon dioxide, water, and inorganics. For field water disinfection, nanoparticles coated with TiO_2 can be integrated into a plastic bag and remain active for hundreds of uses

SUMMARY OF PREFERRED TECHNIQUES

Considerations for choosing a specific field disinfection technique are listed in **Tables 7.11** and **7.12**. The optimal technique for an individual or group depends on the number of

TABLE 7.11	Method(s) of Choice for Various Source Water Conditions			
	"Pristine" Wilderness Water with Little Human or Domestic Animal Activity	Tap Water in Developing Country	DEVELOPED OR DEVELOPING COUNTRY	
			Clear Surface Water Near Human and Animal Activity[a]	Cloudy Water
Primary concern	Usually high quality; isolated contamination	Bacteria, *Giardia*, small numbers of viruses	All enteric pathogens, including *Cryptosporidium*	All enteric pathogens and other contaminants that inhibit treatment
Effective methods	Any single-step method[b]	Any single-step method[b]	• Heat or • Filtration plus halogen (can be done in either order) or • Chlorine dioxide or • Ultra Violet (commercial product) or • Filtration with hollow fiber filter rated for viruses	CF followed by second step (heat, filtration, or halogen treatment)

[a]Includes agricultural run-off with cattle grazing, or sewage treatment effluent from upstream villages or towns.
[b]Includes heat, filtration, halogens, chlorine dioxide, or ultraviolet treatment.
CF, Coagulation–flocculation.

TABLE 7.12 Summary of Advantages and Disadvantages of Disinfection Techniques

	Heat	Filtration	Halogens	Chlorine Dioxide	Two-Step Process	UV Treatment
Availability	Wood can be scarce	Many commercial choices	Many products	Several new products generate ClO_2	Filtration plus halogen or clarification plus second stage	Portable commercial devises available
Cost	Fuel and stove costs	Moderate expense, but low per unit of water treated	Cheap	Generally inexpensive (depends on method)	Depends on choice of stages	Commercial devices relatively expensive
Effectiveness	Can sterilize or pasteurize	Most filters not reliable for viruses	*Cryptosporidium* and some parasitic eggs are resistant	All pathogenic organisms	Highly effective, should cover all pathogenic organisms	All pathogenic organisms
Optimal application	Clear water	Clear or slightly cloudy; turbid water clogs filters rapidly	Clear; need increased dose if cloudy	Clear water, but ClO_2 less affected by nitrogenous compounds	May be adapted to any source water	Requires clear water, small volumes
Taste	Does not change taste	Can improve taste, especially with charcoal stage	Tastes worse unless the halogen is removed or "neutralized"	Unchanged, may leave some chlorine taste	Depends on sequence and choice of stages; generally improves	Unchanged
Time	Boiling time (min)	Filtration time (min)	Contact time (min–h)	Prolonged to ensure *Cryptosporidium* disinfection	Combination of time for each stage	Min
Other considerations	Fuel is heavy and bulky	Adds weight and space; requires maintenance to keep adequate flow	Works well for large quantities and for water storage. Some understanding of principles is optimal. Damaging if spilled or if container breaks.	More experience and testing would be reassuring. Likely to replace iodine for field use.	More rational to use halogens first if filter has charcoal stage. CF is best means of cleaning very turbid water, then followed by halogen, filtration, or heat.	Sunlight for emergency situations when no other method is available; commercial product for high-quality source water and small groups

CF, Coagulation–flocculation; *UV*, ultraviolet.

persons to be served, space and weight considerations, quality of source water, personal taste preferences, and availability of fuel. Unfortunately, optimal protection for all situations may require a two-step process of (1) filtration or coagulation-flocculation and (2) halogenation, because halogens do not kill *Cryptosporidium* and most filters miss some viruses. In recognition of the need for two-stage treatment of microbiologically contaminated water, many microfilters are packaged with a chlorine solution. Generally the halogen is added first, with filtration as the second step. Heat is effective as a one-step process but will not improve esthetics if the water is cloudy or poor tasting. In addition, fuel supplies may limit the use of heat. Newer techniques generating chlorine dioxide or using ultraviolet light (in clear water) or titanium dioxide nanoparticles are also one-step processes.

When the water will be stored for a period of time, such as on a boat, in a motor home, or as collected rainwater, halogens should be used to prevent the water from becoming contaminated. This can be supplemented before or after storage by filtration. Superchlorination-dechlorination is especially useful in this situation, because high levels of chlorination can be maintained for long periods, and when ready for use, the water can be poured into a smaller container and dechlorinated. If another means of chlorination is used, a minimum residual of 3-5 mg/L should be maintained in the stored water. Iodine will work for short but not for prolonged storage, since it is a poor algaecide. After initial disinfection, silver also can be used to maintain microbiologic quality.

On long-distance, ocean-going boats where water must be desalinated during the voyage, only reverse osmosis membrane filters are adequate.

FURTHER READING

Arnold, B.F., Colford, J.M. Jr., 2007. Treating water with chlorine at point-of-use to improve water quality and reduce child diarrhea in developing countries: a systematic review and meta-analysis. Am. J. Trop. Med. Hyg. 76 (2), 354–364.

Backer, H.D., 2011. Field water disinfection. In: Auerbach, P.S. (Ed.), Wilderness Medicine, sixth ed. Elsevier, Philadelphia (Chapter 67), pp. 1324–1359.

Backer, H., Hollowell, J., 2000. Use of iodine for water disinfection: iodine toxicity and maximum recommended dose. Environ. Health Perspect. 108, 679–684.

Bielefeldt, A.R., 2011. Appropriate and sustainable water disinfection methods for developing communities. In: Buchanan, K. (Ed.), Water Disinfection. Nova Science Publishers, New York City, NY, pp. 45–75.

Brunkard, J.M., Ailes, E., Roberts, V.A., et al., 2011. Surveillance for waterborne disease outbreaks associated with drinking water—United States, 2007-2008. MMWR Surveill. Summ. 60 (12), 38–68.

Cairncross, S., Baker, S., Brown, J, et al., 2011. Department for International Development Evidence Paper: Water, Sanitation and Hygiene. London School of Hygiene and Tropical Medicine, London.

CDC, Effect of chlorine in inactivating selected microorganisms. 2012 [Accessed 2/12/16]. Available at <http://www.cdc.gov/safewater/effectiveness-on-pathogens.html>.

Centers for Disease Control and Prevention (CDC), 2001. Safe Water Systems for the Developing World: A Handbook for Implementing Household-Based Water Treatment and Safe Storage Projects. Centers for Disease Control and Prevention, Atlanta, GA. Available at <http://www.cdc.gov/safewater/manual/sws_manual.pdf>.

Clasen, T., Schmidt, W.P., Rabie, T., et al., 2007. Interventions to improve water quality for preventing diarrhoea: systematic review and meta-analysis. BMJ 334 (7597), 782.

Fewtrell, L., Kaufmann, R.B., Kay, D., et al., 2005. Water, sanitation, and hygiene interventions to reduce diarrhoea in less developed countries: a systematic review and meta-analysis. Lancet Infect. Dis. 5 (1), 42–52.

Hlavsa, M.C., Roberts, V.A., Anderson, A.R., et al., 2011. Surveillance for waterborne disease outbreaks and other health events associated with recreational water—United States, 2007-2008. MMWR Surveill. Summ. 60 (12), 1–32.

Lantagne, D., 2008. Sodium hypochlorite dosage for household and emergency water treatment. J. Am. Water Works Assoc. 100, 106–119.

Lantagne, D., Person, B., Smith, N., et al., 2014. Emergency water treatment with bleach in the United States: the need to revise EPA recommendations. Environ. Sci. Technol. 48 (9), 5093–5100.

LeChevallier, M., Kwok-Keung, A., 2004. Water Treatment and Pathogen Control: Process Efficiency in Achieving Safe Drinking Water. IWA Publishing, on behalf of the World Health Organization (WHO), Geneva, Switzerland. Available at <http://www.who.int/water_sanitation_health/dwq/9241562552/en/>.

Li, Q., Mahendra, S., Lyon, D.Y., et al., 2008. Antimicrobial nanomaterials for water disinfection and microbial control: potential applications and implications. Water Res. 42 (18), 4591–4602.

McDonnell, G.E., 2007. Antisepsis, Disinfection, and Sterilization. ASM Press, Washington, DC.

McGuigan, K.G., Conroy, R.M., Mosler, H.J., et al., 2012. Solar water disinfection (SODIS): a review from bench-top to roof-top. J. Hazard. Mater. 235–236, 29–46.

Meierhofer, R., Wegelin, M., 2002. Solar Water Disinfection: A Guide for the Application of SODIS. SANDEC Report No. 06/02. Swiss Federal Institute of Environmental Science and Technology (EAWAG) and Department of Water and Sanitation in Developing Countries (SANDEC), St. Gallen, Switzerland.

Ngwenya, N., Ncube, E.J., Parsons, J., 2013. Recent advances in drinking water disinfection: successes and challenges. Rev. Environ. Contam. Toxicol. 222, 111–170.

Powers, E.M., 1993. Efficacy of flocculating and other emergency water purification tablets. Technical Report Natick/TR-93/033. United States Army Natick Research, Development and Engineering Center, Natick, MA.

Sobsey, M., 2003. Managing Water in the Home: Accelerated Health Gains from Improved Water Supply. World Health Organization, Geneva, WHO/SDE/WSH/02.07. Available at <http://www.who.int/water_sanitation_health/dwq/wsh0207/en/index.html> (accessed February 6, 2007).

Sobsey, M.D., Stauber, C.E., Casanova, L.M., et al., 2008. Point of use household drinking water filtration: a practical, effective solution for providing sustained access to safe drinking water in the developing world. Environ. Sci. Technol. 42 (12), 4261–4267.

US Army, 2005. Sanitary Control and Surveillance of Field Water Supplies. Department of Army Technical Bulletin (TB Med 577). Departments of the Army, Navy, and Air Force, Washington, DC. December 15.

WHO and UNICEF, 2013. Progress on Sanitation and Drinking Water: 2013 Update. WHO and UNICEF, France. Available at <http://apps.who.int/iris/bitstream/10665/81245/1/9789241505390_eng.pdf>.

World Health Organization, 2007. Combating Waterborne Disease at the Household Level. Geneva, Switzerland. Available at <http://www.who.int/household_water/advocacy/combating_disease.pdf?ua=1>.

World Health Organization, 2011. Guidelines for Drinking Water Quality. WHO. Available at: <https://www.google.com/url?sa=t&rct=j&q=&esrc=s&source=web&cd=1&cad=rja&uact=8&ved=0ahUKEwijzq2R9PXKAhVD82MKHeMGAhsQFggcMAA&url=http%3A%2F%2Fwww.who.int%2Fwater_sanitation_health%2Fpublications%2F2011%2Fdwq_guidelines%2Fen%2F&usg=AFQjCNFpnY4Yd6GRKVRhfbdkUVudQ3QV8A&sig2=eR_qfqsJstWnPp4RxfOGSQ> (Accessed 2/12/2016).

World Health Organization, 2015. Technical Brief: Boil Water, WHO/FWC/WSH/15.02; Accessed 2/12/16. Available at <http://www.who.int/water_sanitation_health/dwq/Boiling_water_01_15.pdf?ua=1>.

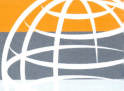

CHAPTER 8

Traveler's Diarrhea: Prevention and Self-Treatment

Charles D. Ericsson

Access evidence synopsis online at ExpertConsult.com.

Traveler's diarrhea is a common malady affecting up to 60% of international travelers during a 2-week trip. Areas of the world can be divided into high, intermediate, and low risk for acquiring traveler's diarrhea (**Fig. 8.1**). Lowering risk from high to intermediate speaks to excellent efforts by many countries to improve their food and beverage hygiene. However, in the preparation of travelers for self-treatment or prophylaxis of traveler's diarrhea, intermediate risk is managed practically as if the risk were high. Traveler's diarrhea is usually a self-limited illness consisting of 4-6 days of loose stools, sometimes accompanied by low-grade fever, nausea, abdominal cramping, headache, and/or general malaise. Up to 25% of sufferers will alter their activities, 15% will be confined to bed, and 1% will be hospitalized.

Classic traveler's diarrhea occurs when immunologically naïve persons move from industrialized nations to developing areas of the world. Travelers moving in the opposite direction experience far less illness. While travelers might experience gastrointestinal (GI) upset after exposure to new foods and spices, classic traveler's diarrhea is caused by microorganisms contaminating food and, to a much lesser extent, beverages. Other risk factors have been elucidated, but most are either inherent to the chosen itinerary or are host factors that are not amenable to modification (**Table 8.1**).

Enteropathogens associated with traveler's diarrhea include bacteria, viruses, and parasites. A majority of cases of the syndrome are caused by bacteria, which explains the success of antibiotics in treatment and prevention. Pre-travel vaccinations against enteropathogens can protect against typhoid (a rare cause of traveler's diarrhea), cholera (rare among tourists and business travelers), and hepatitis A (not classically included as a cause of traveler's diarrhea, since it does not always cause loose stools). A degree of cross protection against common enterotoxigenic *Escherichia coli* can be achieved with oral cholera vaccine; however, protection is modest, requires two doses completed prior to travel, and does not provide enough protection against other causes of traveler's diarrhea to obviate preparing the traveler for self-treatment and prophylaxis. The immune protection afforded by vaccination and natural protective mechanisms of the GI tract (mainly gastric acidity) can be overwhelmed by the ingestion of heavily contaminated food or water. Some pathogens such as *Shigella* can cause disease after ingestion of a relatively low infectious inoculum.

Common-sense food and water precautions during travel should guard against contracting traveler's diarrhea. However, contamination is ubiquitous in developing countries, and many travelers simply do not exercise the stringent precautions required to prevent disease. Despite efforts in travel medicine clinics to educate clientele about food and water hygiene, risk remains high among most travelers to high-risk areas of the world. For this reason a primary goal during a pre-travel clinic visit is to prepare the traveler for self-treatment and sometimes to prescribe chemoprophylaxis.

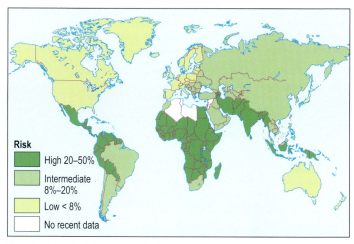

Fig. 8.1 **Worldwide risks for traveler's diarrhea.** (With permission of Steffen, R., Hill, D.R., DuPont, H.L., 2015. Traveler's diarrhea: a clinical review. JAMA 313, 71–80.)

TABLE 8.1 Risk Factors for Traveler's Diarrhea

Risk Factor	Comments
Age	Highest in infants and young adults
Source of food and water	Quality may depend on type of travel, adherence to dietary precautions
Type of travel	Adventurous travelers, prolonged stays
Decreased gastric acidity	Acid-reducing medications, achlorhydria, hypochlorhydria, gastrectomy
Immune deficiency	HIV infection with low CD4 count; IgA deficiency
Blood group O	Increased risk of severe disease with *Vibrio cholerae* El Tor

HIV, Human immunodeficiency disease; *IgA*, immunoglobulin A.

ETIOLOGY

Bacteria are responsible for the majority of cases of traveler's diarrhea, with viruses and parasites accounting for significantly lower numbers; however, the ratios depend somewhat on the geographic region, time of year, and presence of local outbreaks (e.g., norovirus and diarrhea aboard a cruise ship). In many cases of traveler's diarrhea, no etiologic agent can be identified unless a research laboratory is engaged. While clinical presentation does not usually predict the pathogen that will be isolated, occasionally, bloody or mucoid stools and high fever signal dysentery caused by one of the invasive pathogens.

Enterotoxigenic strains of *E. coli* (ETEC) bacteria are the most common identifiable cause of acute diarrhea in travelers visiting developing and tropical countries, with the exception of Southeast Asia, where *Campylobacter* is the most prevalent organism, followed closely by ETEC. The heat labile toxin of ETEC is similar to cholera toxin; it causes prolonged secretion of isotonic fluid containing high amounts of bicarbonate and potassium throughout all segments of the small bowel via stimulation of adenylate cyclase. Oral cholera vaccine elicits antibodies to the B subunit of cholera toxin that cross-react with the heat-labile toxin of ETEC, and this is the basis for the vaccine's partial protection against traveler's diarrhea.

The heat-stable toxin alters fluid transport via stimulation of guanylate cyclase in the jejunum and ileum only. Many ETEC strains produce both toxins.

Campylobacter species, mostly *C. jejuni*, are common etiologic agents of traveler's diarrhea, especially in Southeast Asia, but are less frequently isolated in many other regions of the world. Seasonal variance occurs in rates of *Campylobacter* infections: peak incidence in the United States or United Kingdom occurs in the summer or spring, whereas in North Africa it peaks during the drier winter months.

Other bacterial enteric pathogens less frequently isolated in cases of traveler's diarrhea include species of *Salmonella*, *Shigella*, *Aeromonas*, *Plesiomonas shigelloides*, *Vibrio cholerae*, *V. parahaemolyticus*, *V. vulnificus*, and *Yersinia enterocolitica*.

Norovirus, implicated in outbreaks of food-borne gastroenteritis, is a common cause of gastroenteritis in adults and accounts for as high as 10-15% of the cases of traveler's diarrhea in some studies. Rotavirus is less common among adult travelers. Infections with hepatitis A virus or hepatitis E virus can account for some cases of traveler's diarrhea.

The parasites causing acute diarrhea in travelers are usually protozoans, including *Giardia lamblia*, *Cryptosporidium* sp., *Cyclospora cayetanensis*, *Entamoeba histolytica*, *Isospora belli*, and *Dientamoeba fragilis*. Although less common, helminthic infections can also account for diarrhea in travelers.

Food, fish, and shellfish poisoning (Chapters 33 and 34) can also be included among occasional to rare causes of acute diarrhea in travelers.

PREVENTION OF TRAVELER'S DIARRHEA
Potential preventive strategies for traveler's diarrhea include dietary precautions, appropriate immunizations, and chemoprophylactic agents.

Dietary Precautions
Adherence to advice on food and water precautions should logically reduce the risk from all forms of traveler's diarrhea (**Table 8.2**). Most travelers to urban destinations and tourist attractions do not need to learn techniques for water purification (Chapter 7); clean, bottled water is readily available for most travelers around the world. However, adherence to principles of food and beverage hygiene is difficult to sustain for most, particularly longer-term or adventurous, travelers. Families with small infants should consider keeping young infants off the ground and maintaining breast feeding during the trip.

Immunizations
Oral cholera vaccines are only modestly effective against ETEC strains and are not readily available worldwide. Vaccines against hepatitis A and typhoid are effective, but these

TABLE 8.2   Ten Tips for Selection of Safe Food and Water
1. Drink purified, bottled water or carbonated beverages.
2. Eat foods that are thoroughly cooked and served piping hot.
3. Eat fruits that have thick skins (they should be peeled at the table by the traveler).
4. Avoid salads made with raw vegetables, especially leafy green vegetables.
5. Do not use ice cubes, even in beverages containing alcohol.
6. Eat and drink dairy products made only from pasteurized milk.
7. Avoid shellfish and raw or undercooked seafood, even if "preserved" or pickled with vinegar or the juice of lemon or lime.
8. Do not buy and eat food sold by street vendors.
9. If canned beverages are cooled by submersion of the can in a bucket of ice water or in a stream, dry off the outside of the container before drinking the contents.
10. Use purified water for brushing teeth and for taking medications.

TABLE 8.3   Drug Regimens for Prevention of Traveler's Diarrhea

Drug[a]	Adult Dosage	Comments
Bismuth subsalicylate (Pepto-Bismol)	2 tablets, or 60 mL liquid suspension, orally, four times a day	Less effective than antibiotic prophylaxis; contraindicated in people allergic to aspirin, taking other salicylate-containing drugs, or who are pregnant. Not recommended for children.
Fluoroquinolone[b] Ciprofloxacin 500 mg Norfloxacin 400 mg Ofloxacin 200 mg Levofloxacin 500 mg	1 tablet once daily	Contraindicated in pregnancy and in people allergic to quinolones; beware of drug interaction with theophylline and caffeine.
Rifaximin 200 mg	1-2 tablets daily	Only 0.4% absorbed. Should be safe in pregnancy (not studied). Where *Campylobacter* is prevalent, 2 tablets daily is preferred owing to high MICs of the organism (not studied)

[a]Both trimethoprim-sulfamethoxazole and doxycycline showed benefit in prophylaxis in old studies; rising resistance among enteropathogens around the world has now rendered these drugs passé.
[b]All fluoroquinolones should work equally well.
MIC, Minimum inhibitory concentration.

pathogens account for very few cases of traveler's diarrhea. No vaccines are currently available to prevent the many remaining causes of traveler's diarrhea.

Chemoprophylaxis

Medications that can be used to prevent traveler's diarrhea are shown in **Table 8.3**.

Bismuth Subsalicylate

A daily regimen of bismuth subsalicylate (Pepto-Bismol®), taken as two tablets chewed four times a day for up to 3 weeks, affords about 65% protection against traveler's diarrhea. As a prophylactic agent it is relatively expensive and is not available worldwide.

Mechanisms of action of bismuth subsalicylate include antibacterial, antisecretory, and toxin-adsorptive effects. Adverse effects can include black-colored tongue and stools, constipation, and tinnitus. While bismuth subsalicylate has relatively low toxicity, it should be used with caution in those who are already taking salicylate and in patients with salicylate sensitivity, bleeding disorders, impaired renal function, or peptic ulcer disease. Bismuth subsalicylate is not recommended for children owing to the risk of Reye syndrome.

Antibiotic Prophylaxis

Most prophylactic antibiotic regimens involve taking a single daily dose throughout the trip. Taking an antibiotic for prevention of traveler's diarrhea is controversial. Fully informed travelers might prefer chemoprophylaxis after they weigh the risks and benefits of taking preventative antibiotics compared with waiting until the onset of symptoms and initiating a course of effective self-treatment. Certain travelers (business travelers, politicians, athletes, or honeymooners) taking short, critically important trips (where even a single day of illness might seriously ruin the purpose of the trip) might be offered antibiotic prophylaxis. Defining criticality of a trip is probably best left to the informed traveler. In addition, prophylactic antibiotics may be prudent in travelers with inflammatory bowel disease, brittle diabetes, acquired immune deficiency syndrome, or chronic renal impairment.

Effectiveness of antibiotic prophylaxis depends on the spectrum of activity of the antibiotic used relative to the antibiotic-resistance patterns among the local bacterial enteropathogens. Daily doses of doxycycline, trimethoprim-sulfamethoxazole (TMP/SMX), fluoroquinolones (norfloxacin, ciprofloxacin, and ofloxacin), and rifaximin have been shown to be successful in diarrhea prevention studies. However, in most of the developing world widespread resistance to doxycycline and TMP/SMX exists among enteric pathogens, so these agents can no longer be recommended. Fluoroquinolone resistance is increasingly reported, especially for *Campylobacter* spp. and *Shigella* spp. in Southeast Asian countries such as Thailand, and limits the utility of fluoroquinolones as preventive agents.

The non-absorbed agent rifaximin prevents diarrhea. The agent is well tolerated, has uses in multiple enteric diseases, and has a strong safety record when used chronically in the prevention of hepatic encephalopathy. While it performs poorly in the treatment of invasive pathogens, it can prevent disease by invasive pathogens. It is arguably best positioned as a preventative agent. Azithromycin is commonly recommended for empiric treatment in areas with high levels of fluoroquinolone resistance, but it is not recommended for prophylaxis. The doses of drugs that can be recommended for prevention of diarrhea are shown in **Table 8.4**.

Arguments against the use of antibiotic prophylaxis include altering normal enteric flora and possibly rendering the host more susceptible to infection. Risk of allergic reactions is also a consideration. For instance, fluoroquinolone antibiotics can cause GI upset, rash, and drug interactions and might predispose to *Clostridium difficile* overgrowth. For most travelers, carrying an antibiotic for self-treatment of traveler's diarrhea is the primary approach to management, and antibiotic prophylaxis is a secondary approach.

Probiotics

Several studies have examined the use of probiotics in the prevention of acute diarrhea. A meta-analysis of the available data from 34 masked, randomized, placebo-controlled trials suggests that probiotics reduced the risk of traveler's diarrhea by a meager 8% (95% CI–6-21%). The protective effect did not vary significantly among probiotic strains used alone or in combinations of two or more strains. Probiotics are popular among some travelers, and they are safe, but they cannot be recommended as a substitute for antibiotics in the prevention of traveler's diarrhea.

EMPIRIC SELF-TREATMENT

The majority of travelers will do well if they are instructed to follow the guidelines for safe food and water selection and if they carry a supply of appropriate medications for empiric self-treatment. Treatment of traveler's diarrhea consists of (1) oral rehydration, (2) symptomatic treatment, and (3) empiric antibiotic treatment. As a rule the traveler developing diarrhea within days of return from a developing country can be advised simply to take the medications already prescribed for self-treatment. A trip to the doctor or a costly laboratory work-up can usually be avoided.

Oral Rehydration

Dehydration due to abnormal losses of body fluids through watery diarrhea can accentuate the general feeling of misery. A wide variety of liquids can be used for oral rehydration, including mineral water, canned juices, carbonated caffeine-free beverages, bouillon, Gatorade®, etc. In the event of severe dehydrating diarrhea, many commonly available liquids contain excess sugar and insufficient electrolytes for optimal replacement. Commercially formulated preparations for oral rehydration solution (ORS) can be purchased premixed and in powdered form convenient for mixing in clean water. For the vast majority of travelers, concocting their own ORS is logistically impossible. Furthermore, most traveler's diarrhea, even presenting with severe symptoms, is simply not dehydrating if treated early with an antibiotic plus loperamide regimen (see below). Loperamide has both antimotility and antisecretory properties. The pathogen of leading concern for the possibility of developing dehydration is ETEC, owing to its secretory toxin production. However, unlike cholera toxin, ETEC toxin is not bound irreversibly to the gut, so once an antibiotic kills the organism the secretory effect of the toxin abates in a matter of hours.

TABLE 8.4   Drugs for Self-Treatment of Traveler's Diarrhea in Adults

Drug	Adult Dosage	Comments[a]
Symptomatic medications		
Bismuth subsalicylate (Pepto-Bismol)	30 mL (or 2 tabs) q30 min × 8 doses	The maximum recommended dose is 240 mL/day (16 tablets).
Loperamide (Imodium®)	Take 2 caplets (2 mg each) for first dose; then 1 after each loose stool; do not exceed 8 caplets (16 mg) in 24 h	Antiperistaltic drug; use with caution in dysentery; sold over the counter.
Antibiotics		
Trimethoprim/ sulfamethoxazole (Bactrim®, Septra®)[b]	160-mg/800-mg tab (1 double-strength tab) every 12 hours for 3 days	Do not use in sulfa-allergic patients; less effective against traveler's diarrhea in many areas of the world due to drug-resistance; drug of choice for *Cyclospora* (treat for 7 days).
Norfloxacin (Noroxin®)	400-mg tablet every 12 hours for 3 days	Do not use in pregnancy or in children <18 years old.
Ciprofloxacin (Cipro®)	500-mg tablet every 12 hours for 3 days, or 750-mg tablet once[c]	Do not use in pregnancy or in children <18 years old.
Levofloxacin (Levaquin®)	500-mg tablet once or every 24 hours for 3 days	Do not use in pregnancy or in children <18 years old. Continue therapy for 3 days if inadequate response after first dose or if fever or bloody stool is present.
Azithromycin (Zithromax®)	1 g as a single oral dose or 500 mg once daily for 3 days[b]; 500 mg or 1 g as a single dose[c]	Drug of choice for quinolone-resistant *Campylobacter* strains; use for traveler's diarrhea in persons unable to use fluoroquinolones.
Rifaximin (Xifaxan®)	200-mg tablet three times a day for 3 days	Effective drug treatment for ETEC or pathogen-negative TD; poorly absorbed following an oral dose. Do not use for invasive pathogens.

[a]See Chapter 12 for pediatric guidelines for treatment of diarrhea.
[b]This drug has been studied at both doses for treatment of *Campylobacter*.
[c]Doses for traveler's diarrhea when *Campylobacter* is not prevalent.

Symptomatic Treatment

Regardless of specific etiology, most people will feel better if symptomatic relief from frequent stools and abdominal cramps can be obtained.

Bismuth subsalicylate taken in treatment doses (**Table 8.4**) can reduce the number of stools and is a reasonable choice for initial treatment of mild diarrhea in adults. However, travelers must be warned that they should not take doses of antibiotics (e.g., doxycycline and fluoroquinolones) and bismuth subsalicylate or any product containing bivalent cations at the same time, because of decreased absorption of the antibiotic. If diarrhea develops while using bismuth subsalicylate prophylaxis or if a treatment dose of bismuth subsalicylate was taken but is not giving adequate relief, an oral dose of antibiotic should be delayed by several hours.

Loperamide (Imodium®) is useful for obtaining rapid symptomatic relief from frequent bowel movements and abdominal cramps. Loperamide has an antiperistaltic effect on the intestines, which slows intestinal transit and delays excretion, as well as an antisecretory effect. Studies have shown beneficial results using loperamide and antibiotics in combination for traveler's diarrhea, including dysentery. Using loperamide alone in nondysenteric disease was effective in the majority of patients, but 17% opted to take an antibiotic for better relief. Antimotility agents, including loperamide, should not be given without a concurrent antibiotic in patients with dysentery. Loperamide is not usually recommended in young children due to the risk of side effects such as respiratory depression, drowsiness, and ileus, although in those observations the agent had often been given in too high doses or was continued well beyond the recommended duration of use. Because Lomotil® (the combination of diphenoxylate HCl and atropine sulfate) is habit forming and is no more effective than safer loperamide, it is no longer recommended.

The clay-based products such as attapulgite or kaolin (Kaopectate®) bind water in the colon. In studies these products caused a slightly firmer stool but did not impact the frequency of diarrhea.

Empiric Antibiotic Treatment

Several studies have shown that if self-treatment with loperamide plus one of the antibiotics is started shortly after the onset of nondysenteric traveler's diarrhea, relief can be obtained by many patients within 24 hours. The benefits of antibiotic plus loperamide cannot be predicted by the severity of the onset of diarrhea. A proportion of those treated will benefit from the loperamide regardless of the severity of presentation. Choice of an antibiotic will be dictated by several factors, including the resistance profile of the enteric pathogens likely to be encountered at the destination, age of the traveler, and any underlying medical illnesses.

Any illness that is characterized by high fever (>102° F), severe abdominal pain, or the passage of grossly bloody stools (dysentery) mandates treatment with an antibiotic, and oral rehydration might also be indicated. While loperamide actually benefited patients with dysenteric shigellosis when combined with ciprofloxacin, many experts prefer not to use loperamide when treating overt dysentery. Seeking medical attention at the onset of severe disease in many locations of the developing world will too often result in unnecessary hospitalization and administration of intravenous fluids. Starting an antibiotic (with or without loperamide) early in the course of severe disease often suffices to afford adequate relief and an excellent outcome. If relief of severe disease is not realized within a day or two or if dehydration develops despite self-treatment, medical help should be sought.

If diarrhea is caused by a virus, loperamide will be beneficial, but a course of antibiotic self-therapy is unlikely to influence the outcome. If diarrhea is caused by a resistant bacterial agent or by a parasite, illness might persist beyond the empiric treatment regimen, and the traveler should seek medical consultation.

Fluoroquinolone Antibiotics

The fluoroquinolone antibiotics (e.g., norfloxacin, ofloxacin, levofloxacin, and ciprofloxacin) are active against the majority of bacteria commonly implicated in traveler's diarrhea in many parts of the world. Although the fluoroquinolones are generally accepted as one of the antibiotics of choice for empiric treatment of traveler's diarrhea in adults, growing resistance to this class of antibiotics among *Campylobacter* spp. in some Southeast Asian countries poses a significant challenge to its usefulness for empiric treatment of traveler's diarrhea. In Thailand, for instance, the rate of fluoroquinolone resistance of *Campylobacter jejuni* is extremely high.

Azithromycin

Azithromycin is highly efficacious as a treatment for traveler's diarrhea, including in areas where *Campylobacter* spp. have developed fluoroquinolone resistance. In a study comparing azithromycin (500 mg) or ciprofloxacin (500 mg) daily for 3 days for the treatment of acute diarrhea among US military personnel in Thailand, azithromycin was superior to ciprofloxacin in decreasing the excretion of *Campylobacter* and as effective as ciprofloxacin in shortening the duration of illness. In another study in Thailand, treatment with a single 1-g dose of azithromycin was significantly more efficacious (96% cure rate) compared with a 3-day regimen of azithromycin at 500 mg daily (85% cure rate) and a 3-day regimen of levofloxacin at 500 mg daily (71% cure rate). In a study conducted among adult travelers in Mexico (where ETEC is prevalent and *Campylobacter* is uncommon), azithromycin given as a single oral dose (1 g) was comparable with levofloxacin (500 mg) for the treatment of traveler's diarrhea, with >90% cure rates in both regimens. When *Campylobacter* is not a concern, azithromycin, in combination with loperamide, can be given as a single 500-mg dose with beneficial results comparable to the use of higher doses.

Rifaximin

Rifaximin, a semisynthetic derivative of rifamycin, is a poorly absorbed antibiotic that is approved for the treatment of traveler's diarrhea in persons 12 years of age and older at a dose of 200 mg three times a day for 3 days. Rifaximin is not recommended for treatment of diarrhea accompanied by fever or blood in the stool, as it shows inadequate efficacy in the treatment of diarrhea due to invasive enteropathogens. In a recent study comparing treatment of traveler's diarrhea (where ETEC was the prevalent pathogen) with rifaximin alone (200 mg three times daily for 3 days), loperamide alone (4 mg initially followed by 2 mg after each unformed stool), or a combination of both drugs using the same dosing regimen, rifaximin-loperamide therapy provided rapid symptomatic improvement compared with either agent alone. The problem with recommending rifaximin plus loperamide as preferred initial empiric therapy is that travelers might need to be armed additionally with an agent predictably active against invasive pathogens in the event rifaximin fails to afford adequate relief.

SPECIAL CONSIDERATIONS

People stricken with diarrhea who are unable to tolerate oral rehydration owing to severe nausea and vomiting may need medical attention and intravenous fluids in a hospital. In particular, this may be the case in hot climates, where insensible water loss is greater and where heat stroke may be a danger.

People taking diuretics need to be especially cautious in the face of severe, watery diarrhea and probably should stop the diuretic during the acute diarrheal illness. In the event of severe diarrhea lasting >1 or 2 days, such people should seek medical attention for a blood pressure check, an examination of the heart and lungs, and a serum potassium check.

In the case of many pathogens, the likelihood of developing diarrhea is inoculum dependent. People with decreased gastric acidity due to achlorhydria, gastric resection, frequent antacids, or medication with H_2 blocking agents or proton pump inhibitors may be more susceptible to illness and therefore may be in special need of pre-travel medical counseling on preventive measures for traveler's diarrhea.

FURTHER READING

Adachi, J.A., Ericsson, C.D., Jiang, Z.D., et al., 2003. Azithromycin found to be comparable to levofloxacin for the treatment of US travelers with acute diarrhea acquired in Mexico. Clin. Infect. Dis. 37, 1165–1171.
Clinical trial showing comparable efficacy of azithromycin in treatment of traveler's diarrhea.

Connor, B.A., Riddle, M.S., 2013. Post-infectious sequelae of travelers' diarrhea. J. Travel Med. 20 (5), 303–312.
Discussion of a common clinical scenario in returned travelers and underscores importance of traveler's diarrhea prevention when possible.

DuPont, H.L., Haake, R., Taylor, D.N., et al., 2007. Rifaximin treatment of pathogen-negative travelers' diarrhea. J. Travel Med. 14, 16–19.
Empiric rifaximin plus loperamide treatment resulted in symptomatic improvement among travelers with traveler's diarrhea in an ETEC region.

DuPont, H.L., Ericsson, C.D., Farthing, M.J.G., et al., 2009. Expert review of the evidence base for prevention of travelers' diarrhea. J. Travel Med. 16, 149–160.
Expert review.

DuPont, H.L., Ericsson, C.D., Farthing, M.J.G., et al., 2009. Expert review of the evidence base for self-therapy of travelers' diarrhea. J. Travel Med. 16, 161–171.
Expert review.

Ericsson, C.D., DuPont, H.L., Okhuysen, P.C., et al., 2007. Loperamide plus azithromycin more effectively treats travelers' diarrhea in Mexico than azithromycin alone. J. Travel Med. 14, 312–319.
Clinical trial showing benefit of adding antiperistaltic agent (loperamide) to an antibiotic regimen for traveler's diarrhea.

Sazawal, S., Hiremath, G., Dhingra, U., et al., 2006. Efficacy of probiotics in prevention of acute diarrhea: a meta-analysis of masked, randomized, placebo-controlled trials. Lancet Infect. Dis. 6, 374–382.
Probiotics had only a modest beneficial effect in prevention of traveler's diarrhea.

Steffen, R., Hill, D.R., DuPont, H.L., 2015. Traveler's diarrhea: a clinical review. JAMA 313, 71–80.
State-of-the-art review of traveler's diarrhea by recognized travel medicine experts.

Tribble, D.R., Sanders, J.W., Pang, L.W., et al., 2007. Traveler's diarrhea in Thailand: randomized, double-blind trial comparing single-dose and 3-day azithromycin-based regimens with a 3-day levofloxacin regimen. Clin. Infect. Dis. 44, 338–346.
Clinical trial showing effectiveness of azithromycin in treatment of traveler's diarrhea in areas of fluoroquinolone-resistant pathogens.

CHAPTER 9

Disequilibrium: Jet Lag, Motion Sickness, Cold Exposure, and Heat Illness

Stephen A. Bezruchka

 Access evidence synopsis online at ExpertConsult.com.

When travelers cross several time zones, go to hot or cold climates, or are subject to novel motion stimuli, they may face problems adapting to new environmental situations. This chapter presents some common states of disequilibrium likely to be encountered by the traveler and suggests practical approaches to the problems. Socioeconomic position, class, or economic status can affect individuals with these conditions profoundly, but like most afflictions, studies ignore these factors. Increasingly, we can expect more displaced people that present with travel-related conditions to be poor. Evidence from which to base prevention, advice, and treatment in these circumstances is limited at best, so experience and clinical judgment, tailored to the specific situation the traveler faces, are paramount.

JET LAG

When many time zones are crossed quickly, the traveler's normal sleep–wake cycle is disrupted and is put into conflict with the body's underlying physiologic circadian rhythms. The traveler experiences disturbed sleep, loss of mental efficiency, and fatigue during the day—symptoms commonly known as "jet lag," which when combined with the fast-paced, security-conscious stress of travel today can make the traveler feel even more uncomfortable. "Surface travel lag" is almost unheard of, but there are stresses inherent in any travel away from home that, combined with the increasing sleep deprivation that has become a part of so-called normal everyday life, can result in similar symptoms.

Jet lag symptoms increase with the number of time zones crossed and generally begin when there is a 2-hour difference. The incidence of jet lag in travelers is almost universal, and symptoms can persist for 1 week or more. Circadian rhythms may take up to 2 weeks to adjust. Specific complaints include insomnia, daytime sleepiness and fatigue, poor concentration, slowed reflexes, indigestion, hunger at odd hours, irritability, depression, exacerbation of major psychiatric disorders, increased vulnerability to infections, headache, myalgias, and dysphoria. Sleep disturbances persist longer than the other symptoms. The lower oxygen content aboard jet planes may exacerbate the symptoms.

Older people tend to have more difficulties, although experienced travelers and those with more convenient travel arrangements report fewer symptoms. "Morning types"—individuals who tend to go to bed earlier and awaken earlier in the day—may be more susceptible than "evening types." There is little data on the impact of co-existing morbidity on jet lag, although those with pre-existing sleep disorders are expected to have worse symptoms. Travelers may have affective disorders from jet lag desynchronization. Chronic jet lag has been associated with neuro-anatomic changes, persistent cognitive deficits, and other health problems.

Performance errors in pilots, reduced functioning among athletes, and decreased mental performance among diplomats are ascribed to jet lag. Those crossing many time zones quickly should be advised to avoid potentially hazardous activities on arrival until symptoms

121

improve. Operating dangerous machinery including motor vehicles, undertaking risky recreational activities, and making critical decisions are to be avoided. Competing athletes are advised to schedule sufficient arrival days before events. Melatonin and nonbenzodiazepine benzodiazepine-receptor agonists (NBRAs; see below) are not banned by the World Anti-Doping Agency, so athletes could consider their use.

While the role of socioeconomic status, class, or other contextual markers has not been studied in the severity of jet lag symptoms, individuals under both acute and chronic stress can be expected to fare worse than those who have more control over their lives. Wealthy travelers are likely to have increased access to preferred travel schedules, choice airline seats, comfortable layovers, purchased food and refreshments, pharmaceuticals, luggage-handling services, massages, traveling nannies, etc., in contrast to the harried, resource-poor family on a once-in-a-lifetime journey.

Prevention and Treatment

Minimizing the effects of jet lag is best accomplished by a multifactorial approach. Few controlled studies have examined the various means of preventing jet lag, and none has compared different available modalities. Current approaches are reviewed in order of ease of use for travelers.

Melatonin

A nonvisual, photoreceptive, monosynaptic retinohypothalamic tract directly mediates the synchronization of the sleep–wake cycle with the light–dark cycle. Melatonin from the pineal gland modulates this link, as does the light–dark cycle. Melatonin is produced only during nighttime darkness in sighted individuals and is affected only by exposure to bright light. Melatonin resets the phase shift curve marking the circadian phase position. Ingestion of an appropriately timed physiologic dose (0.5 mg) of exogenous melatonin can shift the phase response curve the required number of hours of time zone change. Several studies demonstrate benefits on subjective rating of jet lag. Melatonin delays circadian rhythm when taken in the morning and advances it when taken later in the day. **Table 9.1** shows one possible schedule for timing melatonin ingestion for eastward and westward travel beginning the day before departure and continuing for 3 days after arrival. This is time zone traverse-specific.

Times for exposure to bright light are also given there, since light exposure is synergistic with melatonin. The suggested physiologic melatonin dose can produce drowsiness before departure, so the dose can be adjusted downward to that which does not cause unacceptable drowsiness and repeated every 2 hours to a total of 0.5 mg. Over-the-counter preparations available in the United States in health food stores are not standardized nor can potencies be guaranteed. Liquid preparations allow titration of an appropriate dose for an individual. Melatonin is not available in some countries and in others only by prescription. There are no data on long-term safety of exogenous melatonin ingestion nor any reports of safety during pregnancy. A Cochrane review by Herxheimer found reports of short-term adverse effects of melatonin to include confusion, ataxia, headache, convulsant effects, and blood-clotting issues (prothrombin increased or decreased, suspected interaction with warfarin), as well as cardiovascular symptoms including chest pain and dyspnea. People with epilepsy and those taking warfarin or other anticoagulants should not use melatonin without an informed medical discussion.

An alternative dosing schedule is to take melatonin at bedtime on arrival at the destination. Most trials have used large doses, 5-8 mg, continued for 3-7 days after arrival. A commonly reported side effect on this regimen is drowsiness after ingestion.

Nonbenzodiazepine Benzodiazepine-Receptor Agonists (NBRAs)

Short-term pharmacologic manipulation of the sleep–wake cycle with hypnotic drugs to induce sleep is a convenient way to manage jet lag in healthy travelers. There may not be much improvement in performance, and hypnotics do not appear to adjust circadian rhythms in humans. The short-acting drugs known as nonbenzodiazepine benzodiazepine-receptor

TABLE 9.1 Jet-Lag Treatment with Melatonin

Time Zone Change	1-6 h	7-9 h	≥10 h
	Time to take melatonin the day before and the day of departure		
Travel from east to west	When you awake	When you awake	When you awake
Travel from west to east	About 15:00 h (3 pm)	About 15:00 h (3 pm)	When you awake
Time to take melatonin on arrival			
Travel from east to west	Day 1: when you awake	Day 1: when you awake	Day 1: when it is the same time at departure as when you took it yesterday
	Days 2 and 3: 1-2 h later than the day before	Days 2 and 3: 1-2 h later than the day before	Days 2 and 3: 1-2 h later than the day before
Travel from west to east	Day 1: when it is the same time at departure as when you took it yesterday	Day 1: when it is the same time at departure as when you took it yesterday	Day 1: when it is the same time at departure as when you took it yesterday
	Days 2 and 3: 1-2 h earlier than the day before	Days 2 and 3: 1-2 h earlier than the day before	Days 2 and 3: 1-2 h earlier than the day before
	Time periods to be in or to avoid bright light		
Travel from east to west	Get bright light later in the day	Get bright light in the middle of the day, avoid bright light later in the day	Get bright light in the morning and avoid it the rest of the day
Travel from west to east	Get bright light in the morning	Get bright light in the middle of the day, avoid bright light earlier in the day	Get bright light in the middle of the day, avoid bright light later in the day

Adapted from Bezruchka, S.A., 1999. The Pocket Doctor. The Mountaineers, Seattle, pp. 54-56.

agonists (NBRAs) have become very popular sleep agents, as typified by zolpidem. Others include zopiclone or the enantiomer eszopiclone, and the even shorter-acting zaleplon. They may be used to treat early awakening, while using melatonin, although studies are lacking and more adverse effects may be expected. Zolpidem, like some short-acting benzodiazepines such as triazolam, has been shown to have idiosyncratic side effects including amnesia, dysphoria, excitability, and somnambulism. Consider a home-based trial before departure to gauge the side effects. Some travelers use these agents during flights, taking them at the destination's sleep time.

The usual adult dose of hypnotics should be halved for first-time users and for geriatric patients, and travelers on NBRAs should be warned not to drink alcoholic beverages or to use other medications that cause drowsiness (e.g., antihistamines) concurrently. Triazolam has been banned or allowed only limited use in several European countries due to reported adverse side effects (psychosis). Other benzodiazepines are longer acting and less suitable for use. Use of these drugs has been associated with increased mortality.

Ramelteon

Ramelteon is a melatonin receptor agonist approved for insomnia and is said to not cause rebound insomnia like the NBRAs and benzodiazepines. It appears to have phase-shifting

TABLE 9.2 Pharmaceuticals to Consider for Jet Lag

Drug	Adult Dose[a]	Elimination Half-Life
Hypnotics		
Zolpidem (Ambien®)	5-10 mg p.o. hsb	3-5 h
Zaleplon (Sonata®, Starnoc®Andante®)	5-10 mg p.o. hsb	1-2 h
Eszopiclone (Lunesta®)	1 mg p.o. hsb	6 h
Zopiclone (Imovane®)	7.5 mg p.o. hsb	6 h
Oxazepam (Serax®)	10-15 mg p.o. hsb	8-10 h
Circadian rhythm agents		
Ramelteon (Rozerem®)	1-8 mg p.o. hsb	1-2 h
Melatonin	See text and Table 9.1	
Wakefulness promoters		
Armodafinil	150 mg p.o. am. on arrival	

[a]Use half the dose for elderly patients or first-time users. b, bedtime.

effects for treating jet lag. One study found that doses of 1 mg at bedtime for four nights in the new destination decreased sleep latency, but light exposure may be more beneficial. Drug interactions and hepatotoxicity may limit extensive use in those with co-morbidities. Ramelteon could also be used like the NBRAs above.

Table 9.2 lists pharmaceuticals to consider for jet lag.

Armodafinil
One study has found that armodafinil, a wakefulness-promoting drug, increased wakefulness after eastward travel in a dose of 150 mg in the morning on arrival. Side effects such as headache, nausea, and diarrhea may limit its use. Modafinil may also be useful but neither drug is FDA-approved for this use.

Agomelatine
Older people who adapt less well to jet lag could be treated with agomelatine, a melatonergic antidepressant, although studies of its efficacy are lacking, and it is not available in the United States.

Sleep Schedule Adjustment
Traditional advice has been to adjust the sleep schedule, beginning 3 days before departure, gradually moving bedtime closer to the customary time at the destination. For instance, if traveling eastward, a traveler would try to go to bed 1 hour earlier each succeeding night in the 3-day period before departure. Smartphone applications are available to help calculate sleep times. If traveling westward, the traveler would try to stay up 1 hour later each night in the pre-travel period. Because it is easier to stay up later than to retire earlier, westward flights across a few meridians result in faster adaptation than eastward ones. Naps should be avoided on eastbound trips. It is useful to exercise before, during, and after the flight and to maintain good hydration.

If traveling across multiple time zones and returning after a day or two, it is better not to try to adjust to the proximate destination but to maintain the home sleep schedule. If traversing more than three time zones, scheduling a stop-over of a day or more in the travel itinerary may help with readjustment of the sleep–wake cycle. Resetting the watch early on each flight to the new local time at destination is advisable for orientation. On arrival at the destination, activities should be scheduled that are appropriate for the new local time. For the first few days after arrival at a destination, major decisions should be avoided if possible, and important meetings should be scheduled at the individual's most alert time of

TABLE 9.3	Resetting the Circadian Clock with Bright Light			
Direction of Travel	External Clock	Behavioral Change	Circadian Clock	Light Exposure
West to east	Turn watch forward	Earlier bedtime, earlier awakening	Turn back circadian clock	Bright light in early morning at destination
East to west	Turn watch backward	Later bedtime, later awakening	Advance circadian clock	Bright light in afternoon at destination

the day at home. Vigorous physical exercise on arrival—mid-morning for travel east and late afternoon for going west—helps.

Bright Light Exposure

The circadian clock can be shifted by exposure to bright light. Such techniques are of no value for the blind. To use principles of phototherapy to reset the circadian clock, the traveler should expose him- or herself to intense bright light (7000-12,000 lux, comparable to that of natural sunlight at sunrise). An exposure time of approximately 5-9 hours is needed. Light episodes before 0400 (at the originating time zone) retard the circadian clock, whereas those after 0400 (at the originating time zone) advance the clock. Thus travelers going eastward should expose themselves to bright light for a few hours early every morning after arrival at the destination. Those traveling westward should expose themselves to bright light in the late afternoon. Three to four days of such light exposure will entrain the original clock and allow it to be reset for sleeping at the destination time zone bedtime (**Table 9.3**).

The required light level can be measured with a digital camera (operating in manual mode). When set for ISO50, a camera meter reading of f:5.6 at 1/60 s indicates the brightness comparable to 11,000 lux. Short wavelength light exposure (blue, green), even if less intense, may be more effective than white light.

Wearing an eye shield on the plane or sitting by an unshaded window at the appropriate times can contribute toward circadian clock resetting during the journey. Enhancing destination time–appropriate sleep with ear plugs or playing soothing sounds on an audio device may help. On arrival, sunglasses are best not worn when it is necessary to get exposed to bright light, and it is advisable to be outdoors when possible. Wear a visor and/or sunglasses when outdoors in bright light that is not at an appropriate time. When indoors, the window curtains should be open and bright room lights should be kept on during the period of phototherapy. Indoor light is much dimmer than required, but it can shift the circadian clock.

Often travel schedules and conditions may prevent a traveler from using scheduled exposures to bright light to facilitate an adaptation to the new time zone.

Jet Lag Diet and Other Remedies

The Argonne National Laboratory Jet Lag Diet tries to reset the circadian rhythm by alternative feasting and fasting, beginning 3 days before departure, and by timing the consumption of high-protein breakfasts and lunches, high-carbohydrate dinners, and caffeine. There is one study using it to advantage in US soldiers traversing nine time zones. Websites calculate this timed diet, and there are apps for smartphones to help adjust to the new time zone. Slow-release caffeine in a dose of 300 mg taken in the morning on arrival appears to have benefits to increase wakefulness. This may be more beneficial than 2 cups of espresso coffee. Other remedies, such as "anti-jet lag" pills sold over the counter or plant products, are of questionable efficacy.

In summary, jet lag is unavoidable; there are substantial individual variations in symptoms; and there are many ways of minimizing its effects.

MOTION SICKNESS

Motion sickness is not a true disease but a normal response to a stimulating situation. It can be induced in anyone with a normally functioning vestibular system, given the right stimulation, but it is not produced by voluntary movement. People who lack vestibular function are immune. Vertigo, by contrast, is a sensation of movement without the stimulation of activity or sequelae of motion.

Motion sickness as a generic term includes sea sickness, motor vehicle sickness, air sickness, and other disorders such as ski sickness. One study collected data from 20,029 passengers on ferries on sea routes across the English Channel, Irish Sea, and North Sea and found that more than one-third of passengers reported some symptoms of motion sickness, and 7% vomited. The incidence of illness was greater in females than males, and there was a slight decline in incidence with age. Those who traveled frequently reported less motion sickness; this was presumed due to either habituation or self-selection.

Overpacked buses on winding mountain roads are common sites where adventure travelers experience motion sickness symptoms directly, while others may find it induced by a camel ride. Ski sickness is a special form of motion sickness produced by unusual and contradictory sensory information among the visual, vestibular, and somatosensory systems and develops while performing winding turns on uneven ground, with insufficient visual control, especially on foggy or white-out days with reduced visibility.

Women may be twice as susceptible to motion sickness as men, and more so toward the end of menstruation. Pregnant women are at an increased risk of motion sickness. Those with a history of migraine may be more at risk. A past history of motion sickness is strongly predictive of future problems. Children experience more symptoms and tend to outgrow them. Youth who engage in proprioceptive physical and sporting activities at an early age may be less susceptible. Retention of adaptation to motion sickness stimuli is retained for at least 1 month.

Nausea is a common presentation of motion sickness and may be preceded by pallor and cold sweats; eventually, vomiting occurs. Sufferers may express a desire for cool, fresh air, although ambient air temperature is not found to influence susceptibility. Hypersalivation, yawning, hyperventilation, and frontal headache are reported. Drowsiness, lethargy, inhibition of gastric motility, and loss of performance proficiency are the secondary symptoms of motion sickness. Diminished gastric motility reduces the absorption of oral drugs. Lethargy may take longer to resolve once the stimulus is gone. Altitude sickness should be included in the differential diagnosis.

Prevention

Studies on motion sickness use self-reports or laboratory experiments simulating space sickness or extreme sea conditions. Advice is based on such limited information and anecdotal reports. General advice includes resting before the anticipated motion and beginning with an empty stomach. Generally, high-sodium foods, as well as those that are calorie dense or high in protein or fat, including cheese and milk products, may be more associated with symptoms, as is an increased frequency of eating. One study suggested a pleasant taste of food was more important than composition, although liquid high-protein, low-carbohydrate consumption produced less cardiac vagal tone. An ear plug in the nondominant side has been reported to help minimize symptoms.

Seeking a place in the vehicle where motion is least, sitting in a semi-reclining position, and minimizing head motion, as well as looking at the horizon, help. In a car, sit in the front seat and look out the front window at distant scenery. On an airplane, consider a window seat over the wings, and look out of the windows. For the susceptible on a ship, choose a cabin on a middle deck near the waterline. If lacking other modalities for an individual highly susceptible to seasickness, consider advising the use of a blindfold when inside a room on a ship. Symptoms of motion sickness may decrease with prolonged exposure to changing vestibular and optokinetic stimuli, for example, developing one's "sea legs."

TABLE 9.4   Medication for Motion Sickness

Drug	Adult Dose	Side Effects
Granisetron (Kytril®)	2 mg p.o. single dose	
Ondansetron (Zofran®)	8 mg p.o. single dose	
Phenytoin (Dilantin®)	200 mg p.o. single dose	
Cyclizine (Marezine®)	50 mg p.o. q4-6 h	Minimal sedation
Dimenhydrinate (Dramamine®)	50 mg p.o. q4-6 h	Sedation
Meclizine (Bonine®, Antivert®)	25-50 mg p.o. q6-12 h	Mild sedation
Promethazine (Phenergan®)	25 mg p.o., p.r. q8-12 h	Moderate sedation
Scopolamine patch (Transderm Scop®)	¼–1 patch applied to bare skin q72 h	Dry mouth, blurry vision
Scopolamine hydrobromide	0.4 mg p.o. q6 h	Dry mouth, blurry vision
Ephedrine sulfate	25 mg p.o. q6-12 h	Cardiovascular (counteracts sedation)
Pseudoephedrine	30-60 mg p.o. q6-12 h	Cardiovascular (counteracts sedation)
Dextroamphetamine (Dexedrine®)	5 mg p.o. q a.m.	Cardiovascular (counteracts sedation)

Those who are particularly susceptible to motion sickness could undergo desensitization through exercise procedures. Search the Web for "motion sickness desensitization" to find resources. Physical therapists specializing in vestibular disorders could be consulted. However, behavior modification techniques, including cognitive therapy, biofeedback, and desensitization therapy, require frequent exposure to motion over a considerable time to be effective.

Antihistamines

Several pharmaceuticals are useful to alleviate the symptoms of motion sickness, especially if they are started prophylactically before severe symptoms are manifest (**Table 9.4**). H1 receptor antihistamines useful for motion sickness include cyclizine, dimenhydrinate, and meclizine. Cyclizine is thought to affect gastric dysrhythmias; dimenhydrinate may work as a sedative; and meclizine affects the vestibular system. Common side effects include sedation and a dry mouth. These antihistamines are available without a prescription in the United States, but availability elsewhere should be determined. Caution is advised for use by the elderly, as these drugs may cause confusion and hallucinations, and caution is advised for use in pregnant women, although the common antihistamines are considered category B.

Scopolamine Patch

Scopolamine (an anticholinergic), when administered in the form of a transcutaneous drug patch, is widely used for prevention of motion sickness. The 0.5-mg patch is placed behind the ear, where skin permeability is highest, providing therapeutic levels of scopolamine for up to 3 days. The patch should be applied 4-8 hours before exposure to motion and must be worn for as long as the stimulus is present. Initial enthusiasm for this drug has waned because side effects are unpleasant, efficacy is disputed, and there is concern that the patch may decrease adaptation to motion sickness. Side effects include dry mouth (50%), blurred vision (25%), and occasional anisocoria. Lower doses (cutting the patch into halves or quarters) is not approved according to the package insert but may provide adequate protection and lessened side effects in some people. Scopolamine should not be used in those with conditions such as prostatic hypertrophy and glaucoma.

Scopolamine may cause drowsiness, impaired short-term memory, toxic psychosis (hallucinations, confusion, disorientation, confabulation), acute angle-closure glaucoma, or urinary retention in susceptible people, especially the elderly. Side effects can become more severe after a long period of use. Anticholinergic intoxication can result after ≥16 days, especially if an allergic skin reaction develops where the adhesive patch is applied, thus allowing greater absorption of the drug. Withdrawal symptoms, including hypersalivation and increased gastrointestinal motility, are possible with prolonged use. Physiologic chemical dependency has been reported. Consider advising use of the patch for long journeys (≥3 days) in those who have a history of severe motion sickness. Oral scopolamine (0.4 mg) can be used for faster onset and shorter duration of drug activity.

Sympathomimetics

Sympathomimetics can potentiate the prophylactic effects of scopolamine and antihistamines and tend to counteract the sedation caused by these drugs. Ephedrine and dextroamphetamine are effective, useful additions for prophylaxis of motion sickness when either scopolamine or an antihistamine does not work well enough (**Table 9.4**) or there is an intense stimulus for <6 hours. Pseudoephedrine could be used in this case as well. The combination of promethazine plus dextroamphetamine has been found to have limited impact on psychomotor performance and to not increase sleeplessness. Sympathomimetics should not be prescribed for patients with cardiovascular risk factors or disease because the drugs are associated with palpitations, tachycardia, and elevation of blood pressure. Patients also need to be warned about possible central nervous system (e.g., restlessness, dizziness, tremor) and gastrointestinal (e.g., anorexia, dry mouth, change in bowel habits) side effects.

Phenytoin

Phenytoin and other anticonvulsants prevent motion sickness but are not widely used. One study found that a therapeutic dose of phenytoin was four times more efficacious than any other single pharmacologic agent in delaying onset of artificially induced motion sickness; it was twice as effective as a scopolamine/dextroamphetamine combination. The dosage used was 15 mg/kg per day given in divided doses at 4-hour intervals over a 20-hour period before the experiment. A blood level of 9 µg/mL appears to be protective. This regimen could have useful clinical applications, as phenytoin in this study did not produce sedation or any decrease in performance.

Other Drugs

Promethazine (a phenothiazine derivative) is used orally to prevent motion sickness. Drugs used to protect against radiation-induced nausea and vomiting, such as granisetron and ondansetron, have been used by pilots flying jet planes where psychomotor performance was maintained, although laboratory studies dispute their ability to influence motion sickness symptoms. Other drugs that have been proposed on the basis of anecdotal or small study reports include nifedipine (calcium channel blocker), triptan serotonin agonists (rizatriptan) in those with a history of migraine headaches, and selegiline (phenethylamine derivative). Ginger has been reported as a remedy for seasickness; however, studies have yielded conflicting results, perhaps owing to variation in the type of preparation used and the experimental design.

Anecdotal reports and small studies support the use of acupressure at the "P6 point" with a commercial device (Accu-Band, ReliefBand, Traveleeze, or Sea-Band) to prevent motion sickness.

Treatment

There are no controlled studies of different drugs to treat large patient populations experiencing the symptoms of motion sickness. Most reports use a variety of experimental situations to induce motion sickness in the subjects. Generally, intramuscular doses of prochlorperazine or trimethobenzamide are effective in treating nausea and vomiting. Rectal suppositories of prochlorperazine or trimethobenzamide may be effective, but onset of action is slower because of unpredictable absorption through the rectal mucosa. In one study of motion sickness in weightless conditions simulating outer space, 50 mg of promethazine or

0.5 mg of intramuscular (i.m.) scopolamine were reported to be effective, but 25 mg of promethazine or 50 mg of dimenhydrinate were not. Caution is necessary in using these agents for treatment if they have already been administered for prophylaxis.

For treatment of the secondary symptoms, IM ephedrine (25 mg) or dimenhydrinate (50 mg) are effective for dizziness, and parenteral metoclopramide (5 mg) aids in gastric emptying.

Nonpharmaceutical treatment of motion sickness may be attempted by putting the afflicted into the driver's seat, the cockpit pilot's chair, or other appropriate active-engaging positions. Keep the head and chest balanced over the hips. Controlled breathing and other behavioral measures may help. Do not read. Debilitated seasick persons need a safety harness if there is a risk they may be washed overboard. Those at bed rest should be supine, face up, head still, eyes closed, and secure in a well-ventilated area.

COLD EXPOSURE

Exposure to cold conditions is more common in travelers and residents due to increasing numbers pursuing recreation in cold environments and from disasters occurring to residents in such places.

Temperature homeostasis is problematic in the cold because humans lose heat easier than they retain it. Humans are relatively incapable of increasing metabolic rate when the temperature drops. The heat balance equation sums conductive, convective, radiative, and evaporative heat exchange. Body fat and skin thickness may protect from cold injury because of low thermal conductivity. About 40% of heat loss from a naked human is mediated by convection at an ambient temperature of 29° C (84° F) and a wind velocity of 0.9 m/s (2 mph). Radiant heat loss under the same conditions accounts for 45% of the total. Evaporative heat loss is the remainder, with half of that coming from the respiratory tract.

Peripheral thermal sensors to cold are found immediately beneath the epidermis, whereas warm receptors are deeper in the dermis and are 10 times more sensitive when there is rapid temperature change. They are not uniformly distributed, and there are many more cold receptors. The forehead, for example, has many more cold sensors than the lower leg. The upper torso has the greatest cold receptor density and sensitivity, with the lower torso, arms, and legs having similar numbers but with much lower sensitivity to cold. Measuring the core temperature assesses the overall status of the regulatory system, but this can be difficult to do in the environmental situations where problems occur. Carry low-reading thermometers in situations where cold conditions prevail. Electronic devices may be easier to read quickly by a stressed, cold operator. The debate on which site to monitor temperature is academic.

The major involuntary response to cold is to vasoconstrict the peripheral circulation and to contract muscles in shivering. Active exercise will increase body temperature, which will plateau 30-40 min after initiation, with higher levels resulting in higher core temperature increases. But even when exercising at 50% of maximal aerobic capacity, the increase is only 1° C. Aging results in a weakening of the vasoconstrictor response to cold, and older individuals do not shiver as much. (Sweating in response to passive heating is also lessened with aging.) Cyclical hormonal changes in women impact these responses. During pregnancy, the thermoregulatory system is very sensitive to heat produced by exercise, with steady-state core temperature during exercise dropping, possibly lessening thermal stress on the fetus.

Thermoregulation is affected by chronic exposure to very cold environments and by chronic exercise in both warm and cold situations, so an acclimated individual can work with less increase in core temperature. Ethnic groups who traditionally lived in warm environments may be more at risk of cold injury, as they appear to have less heat output or cold-induced vasodilation.

There may be some acclimatization to cold, with a cold-induced vasodilatation, or "hunting response," in some individuals. However, for most people, wearing appropriate clothing, wearing mittens rather than gloves, having chemical hand warmers, avoiding extreme conditions, keeping the feet and hands dry, avoiding direct finger contact with cold surfaces, eating plenty, and maintaining sufficient hydration are important steps to prevent cold injury. Drinking cold water from a stream is more efficient than eating snow. Getting out of the wind can decrease convective exchange, as can putting on dry clothes. Moist or wet skin increases heat loss. To keep the skin dry and limit heat loss, Arctic explorers did not wash. Dressing in multiple layers gives better insulation through greater air trapping. Wearing a base layer of clothing made of materials with wicking properties helps keep the skin dry. A helpful mnemonic referring to clothing is "**COLD**": **C**lean, **O**pen with exercise to limit sweating, **L**oose layers to retain heat, and **D**ry to limit conductive heat loss.

Donning an extra layer, exercising, or getting into a warm shelter require conscious decisions that may be impaired by alcohol and other drugs as well as by mental illness. Alcohol offers no protection and increases heat loss. Some drugs inhibit shivering. Underlying conditions that predispose to cold injury include malnutrition, poverty, stress, and exertion. Individuals with peripheral neuropathy may lack nociception and not vasoconstrict appropriately.

The type and duration of cold contact determines the extent of injury and is compounded by wind chill. Exposed head and neck areas can suffer high heat loss, as these areas do not vasoconstrict effectively. Fatigue and apathy increase the risk of cold injury. A dissociative state resulting from cold can limit self-help. In cold injury situations those who maintain cognitive abilities must help those who have become limited.

Nonfreezing Cold Injuries

Nonfreezing cold injuries include pernio and trench foot (immersion foot). Frostbite represents localized freezing, while systemic injury is termed "hypothermia."

Pernio

Pernio, a prolonged chilblain, can result from water and winter activities following consecutive days of wearing wet boot liners and socks and having continually wet feet. Cold and moisture produce swelling and tenderness, but after prolonged exposure, usually 12 hours or more, deep pain and disabling tissue sensitivity as well as eschar formation can result. These changes follow sympathetic nerve instability and vascular hypersensitivity to cold that produces a vasculitis. Prevention depends on maintaining awareness, keeping the feet dry, changing socks, and checking the feet daily. Treatment includes drying and massage as well as active gentle warming and elevation. Chronic sequelae can occur.

Trench Foot

Trench foot has its origins in the military where troops stood for days in water-filled trenches. Today it can be seen in adventure travelers who become cold, wet, exhausted, and dehydrated and are unable to care for themselves, who go to bed with wet feet, or who continue to put on wet socks and tight boots day after day, leading to peripheral vasoconstriction and tissue ischemia. It can happen in warm water as well as cold and is seen in homeless populations. There is a pre-hyperemic phase followed by a hyperemic period lasting weeks with considerable pain and deep aching during which time victims cannot tolerate even light pressure on their feet. Vascular injury produces very reactive blood vessels, so the limb can easily blanch on elevation and become deep purple-red when lowered, manifesting a peripheral vasoneuropathy. Initial management is the same as for pernio, but pain relief is often problematic.

Freezing Injuries

Freezing injuries when mild are termed "frostnip," and when severe, "frostbite." They are relatively common in very cold environments as well as in major cities during the winter, including cities in the United States and Canada. With dogged persistence in cold, high, and hazardous environments, severe freezing injuries are a predictable risk among adventure travelers. Often the victims lack proper equipment but persist in the circumstances rather than retreat. Urban freezing injuries can result from poverty and the inability to protect oneself from the environment, which can occur because of equipment breakdown or from a lack of community responses.

When onset of frostbite is considered, giving a dose of aspirin or ibuprofen to enhance circulation has been suggested. Or the foot or hand may be placed in a companion's armpit or groin for 10 minutes. At altitude give oxygen if available. Prevent hypothermia. Treatment for frostbite can be delayed until the victim has been evacuated and will no longer need the affected extremity for rescue efforts. Once a foot has become frozen, using it until it can be actively rewarmed is preferable to the possibility of warming attempts followed by refreezing. Fingers are more problematic, as they become useless with frostbite. Rapid thawing for all frostbite injuries is by immersion in water between 40 and 42° C. The actual temperature is crucial for maximal tissue survival. Aggressive pain control is required. Topical treatment to blisters is with aloe vera, but whether or not to debride is controversial. Subsequent treatment strategies over the last 40 years have focused on expectant observation as viable tissue becomes demarcated. Recent strategies have attempted to use systemic and topical agents, as in burn care, and contemporary methods such as intravenous radioisotope scanning, angiography, duplex imaging, or digital plethysmography to assess tissue viability before various medical interventions such as thrombolysis or amputation are considered.

Hypothermia

Hypothermia results when there is decreased heat production, increased heat loss, or impaired thermoregulation. Thermogenesis is decreased in the very young and the elderly. Older individuals tend to have impaired heat conservation. Ataxia or subtle signs in early stages of hypothermia may be missed by companions.

Diagnosis of hypothermia may be difficult in the environmental conditions encountered during travel because of survival exigencies. Hypothermia reflects body heat loss with a core body temperature of <35° C. Moderate hypothermia occurs below 32° C and is severe below 28° C. Shivering is lost in moderate hypothermia, which is accompanied by hypoventilation, hypotension, bradycardia, and hemoconcentration. Moderate hypothermia requires active external and non-invasive rewarming.

Severe hypothermia presents with pulseless apnea. The victim may appear lifeless, but the advanced cardiac life support adage that "you are not dead until you are warm and dead" applies, unless it can be determined that death occurred before cooling, such as by asphyxia or lethal injury. Gentle handling of the comatose victim is required because of sensitivity to the development of cardiac arrhythmias. The task is to rescue, examine, insulate, and transport, using whatever skills and facilities are available. There is no standard approach. No predictive scale, such as the Glasgow Coma Scale, has been validated, and no controlled studies exist. Positive predictors of survival include rapid cooling rate, presence of ventricular fibrillation during cardiac arrest, and narcotic or ethanol intoxication. The greatest risks to survival may be asphyxia, slow rate of cooling, invasive rewarming, asystole, and development of acute respiratory distress syndrome.

Guiding principles for initial treatment of hypothermia in the field include gently removing clothing and drying the patient, while keeping him or her horizontal to minimize orthostatic hypotension from autonomic dysfunction. Avoid exertion, which could result in a further decline in core temperature (afterdrop), and do not massage the extremities, which suppresses shivering and increases skin vasodilatation, which also can enhance core temperature afterdrop. Mildly hypothermic conscious victims can be given warm sweet fluids to drink. Stabilize injuries, administer warmed intravenous fluids if possible, attempt active rewarming with heated inhalation, and promote truncal warming via hot water bottles applied to the axillae and groin. Oxygenation is critical. Insulate with whatever can be improvised. Conditions in remote circumstances may require prolonged rescue efforts where little actual rewarming may take place, but further heat loss should be thwarted.

Once in a clinical setting, external rewarming with radiant heat, hot water bottles, heating pads and blankets, forced hot air, and warm water immersion can be used. Core rewarming with heated inhaled gases, heated IV infusions, and lavage of internal cavities with warm fluids can be considered, as can the use of extracorporeal circulation. Active methods can be used in the elderly in whom mild hypothermia does not respond to passive efforts. The rate of active rewarming is debatable, but hourly rates exceeding 0.5° C do not seem to increase mortality. Efforts to treat cardiac arrest may not be successful until considerable rewarming has occurred. Rapid cooling of young victims, such as in sudden cold drowning, can be followed by full recovery without long-term sequelae.

HEAT ILLNESS

The human body is only about 25% efficient, meaning most of our metabolic energy production is added to the body as heat. Despite being better able to tolerate heat than cold, humans continue to die in considerable numbers during heat waves around the world. In the adult, basal heat production is about 60-70 kcal/h; excitement, fear, certain drugs, catecholamines, and thyroid hormones can increase heat production moderately, and physical work can produce up to 1000 kcal/h of thermal energy.

To diffuse excess heat, skin vasodilates and blood shifts from the splanchnic circulation to the skin. Sweat forms, then skin cools as the sweat vaporizes, thus keeping a temperature gradient between heated blood and the skin and promoting heat loss. If evaporation cannot occur because the air surrounding the skin is already saturated, sweat continues to form, but heat loss is curtailed. In these situations, extreme heat production (i.e., work) must be limited.

Children are more at risk of developing heat illness than adults because they are less efficient thermoregulators: they have a lower rate of sweating and a higher set point at which sweating starts. Children produce more metabolic heat per unit weight for a given workload and have a comparatively lower cardiac output than adults. Their larger surface area in proportion to body weight can result in greater heat absorption from the environment. Furthermore, they acclimatize more slowly than adults, and so need to reduce the intensity of activities in a hot environment for a longer period.

Serious heat illness is preventable. Chronic stress, fear, and low socioeconomic status can predispose to heat illness, as was well demonstrated in the 1995 heat wave in Chicago, with the greatest risk among African-American inhabitants residing in city slums, who lacked access to transportation and were socially isolated. Hypertension was the commonest co-morbidity in a study of survivors who suffered substantial mortality within a year. Hispanics were less affected because of their social cohesion. During the 1980 heat wave in St. Louis and Kansas City, the rates of those affected were six times higher in the lowest socioeconomic status compared with the highest socioeconomic status. Poorer people can be expected to have more complications from the stress of heat illness, including more opportunistic infections and prolonged recovery. Climate change is likely to increase exposure to heat illness, especially for the poor.

Organizers of events taking place in hot weather have a responsibility to prevent heat illness. Plenty of hydration stations, with trained spotters for potential victims, must be provided. A response system to deal with potential problems must be set up. It is appropriate to cancel events when there is a significant risk of serious heat illness from environmental factors, such as when the wet-bulb globe temperature (WBGT) is above 25° C. Runners with a fast finishing pace are especially at risk. There are numerous anecdotes of world-class athletes, as well as high school football players, who have died as a result of heat illness.

Communities will need to mobilize for the coming heat waves that are predicted as a part of global warming. The challenge is to recognize increased risk for those living in the relative poverty and social isolation conditions that often co-exist. Often those who died did not seek help or were incapable of following advice that was offered. During the heat wave in France in 2003, the highest mortality risk was in cities, especially in Paris among isolated elderly living in top-story single rooms. That air conditioners are not commonly used in France added to the impact of this tragedy. During heat waves, consider promoting visits to air-conditioned malls for the isolated, relatively poor individuals at highest risk. Providing air-conditioned shelters and lowering energy costs during hot periods are other measures to consider as public health efforts. The Occupational Health and Safety Admin-istration has a Heat Safety Tool app for smartphones to monitor risk levels.

Acclimatization

Acclimatization is the process whereby the body adapts to a hot environment. With repeated exposures to heat stress, for any given work load, the cardiac output increases; there is expansion of circulating blood volume; and metabolic adaptations occur in skeletal muscle. Sweat production increases, and to conserve blood volume, the sodium concentration in sweat decreases. As a result, there is less heat production for a given amount of work, but increased sweating increases the tendency to dehydration. Each liter of water lost through sweating raises rectal temperature 0.3° C, speeds heart rate 8 beats/min, and decreases cardiac output 1 L/min.

Acclimatization does not occur without work or exercise that elevates body temperature; the cardiovascular system must be capable of responding to these increased demands. A gradual increase in the time and intensity of physical exertion over 8-10 days is advised for those who will be active in the heat. It takes 2 weeks or more for maximal acclimatization.

Those in excellent physical condition are better able to tolerate the heat. The obese are at an increased risk of heat illness. Those with a febrile or gastrointestinal illness are at greater risk. The drugs described under heat stroke predispose to heat illness. Motor vehicle driver vigilance and other measures of performance are diminished under heat stress.

The best indication of the heat-acclimatized state is the capability to sweat profusely during heat stress. Prudent advice is to wear clothing that is lightweight and loose fitting, with only one layer of absorbent material. As much skin as possible should be exposed to facilitate sweat evaporation.

Water consumption should increase, since hypohydration is a major contributor to dif-ficulty adapting to heat stress. Voluntary drinking replaces about two-thirds of the body water lost as sweat. Individuals commonly dehydrate 2–6% of their body weight during hot-weather exercise, even when fluids are available. Drinking on schedule makes better sense: 1 L 2 hours before, a $\frac{1}{2}$ L 15 minutes before, and 250 mL every 15 minutes during the practice or game. Weight and urine should be monitored; urine should be copious, clear, and pale. Sports drinks containing electrolytes and carbohydrates offer no advantage over cold water in maintaining plasma volume or electrolyte concentrations during exercise. Carbohydrate solutions may offer an advantage in endurance activities. Alcohol and caffeine dehydrate.

Acclimatization to heat will be less efficient in those with lower socioeconomic position, so such people and communities will be more vulnerable to heat illness, as has been well demonstrated in the United States. There is a moral hazard in not looking out for the common good, as was evidenced in heat waves and other disasters.

Environmental Heat Illness

Heat illness is a continuum from subtle impairment in performance or heat stress to lethal heat stroke. Specific entities are described in this section.

Heat Syncope

Heat syncope includes orthostatic symptoms or fainting occurring in a person who has not undergone heat acclimatization and who is exposed to a high environmental temperature. It results because not enough salt and water have been retained and is more common in those with heart disease and those taking diuretics. The risk of heat syncope disappears as acclimatization occurs.

Heat Edema

Heat edema is seen during acclimatization and is caused by salt and water retention resulting from aldosterone production. It is seen more often in women; salt supplementation can be a precipitating factor. Heat edema vanishes as one is fully acclimatized.

Heat Tetany

Heat tetany results from hyperventilation on exposure to hot air, leading to respiratory alkalosis, paresthesias, and occasionally frank tetany.

Heat Cramps

Heat cramps are painful muscle contractions occurring in workers or athletes; they are associated with hyponatremia caused by fluid replacement of profuse sweat with free water but not salt. Typically, the victims are acclimatized, exercising, and requiring copious sweat production to control temperature. The muscles involved are those being exercised, and symptoms tend to occur toward the end of the activity. Cramps last a few minutes and disappear spontaneously. A hot environment for the exercise is not mandatory. Salt replacement is important at the first sign of premonitory muscle twitching.

Heat Exhaustion

Heat exhaustion results from body water loss and electrolyte depletion. It is common during exercise and work during heat waves but can occur as a result of heavy sweating while undergoing intense exercise in temperate climates. Typically, postural hypotension develops immediately on termination of exercise in the heat by unacclimatized persons. Although there is a continuum, patients tend to suffer from one of two categories: water depletion or salt depletion.

Early warning signs include a flushed face, hyperventilation, headache, dizziness, nausea, arm tingling, piloerection, paradoxical chilliness, incoordination, and confusion. Pain may not be present and there may be euphoria.

The water-depletion variety can occur in the very young or very old who experience dehydration but cannot act on their thirst to replenish their water losses. Soldiers, laborers in the desert, boiler-room workers, and athletes who ingest salt without adequate water are also commonly afflicted. Symptoms include thirst, fatigue, dysphoria, and impaired judgment. Examination shows dehydration and an elevated body temperature. Left untreated, heat stroke can result as the body temperature rises.

The salt-depletion variety is seen in those who replace fluid losses with water without salt; they do not experience thirst as a predominant symptom. Unlike heat cramps, salt depletion heat exhaustion tends to occur in unacclimatized individuals who exhibit systemic symptoms. Symptoms can include myalgias, nausea, vomiting, and diarrhea, as well as weakness, fatigue, and headache. Hypotension and tachycardia are seen; the body temperature is not elevated unless dehydration results from the vomiting. Replacement of sodium chloride results in rapid improvement.

Confusion is an early sign of heat injury. Delirium has been reported. Commonly, individuals with heat exhaustion suffer from both water and salt depletion; they exhibit a variety of symptoms and are often misdiagnosed as having a viral syndrome. Giving aspirin to exercising patients who develop heat exhaustion can paradoxically increase body temperature.

Treatment of Heat Exhaustion

When treating heat exhaustion, if hypernatremia and scant concentrated urine are present, one should assume water deficiency, calculate the water deficit, and treat. Water should be given orally if the patient is conscious and not vomiting. If shock is present, the patient should first be treated with plasma-expanding fluids; otherwise, replace volume with 5% dextrose intravenously (IV) until the serum sodium has fallen to near normal, and then add hypotonic saline to the infusion. Half the water deficit should be replaced over 3-6 hours. In children, give half normal saline initially until urine output is established, then decrease to quarter normal saline along with 5% dextrose. Hydration and electrolyte balance should be corrected to normal over at least 48 hours in children to avoid seizures. Severe prolonged central nervous system (CNS) symptoms may take days to resolve. Those presenting with primary salt depletion respond quickly to salty oral fluids or normal saline IV if they cannot drink.

Heat Stroke

Heat stroke results from a failure of the thermoregulatory mechanisms to meet heat stress; extreme elevations of body temperature occur, as well as end-organ dysfunction and damage. Risk factors in healthy individuals include environmental extremes (e.g., Hajj in Saudi Arabia, where up to 1000 cases per day may occur with a mortality rate around 50%), salt and water depletion, infection, fever after immunization, lack of acclimatization, obesity, fatigue, and consumption of drugs that suppress sweating (e.g., anticholinergics, drugs for Parkinson disease, phenothiazines, and antihistamines). Other drugs known to predispose to heat stroke include diuretics, which cause salt and water depletion; tricyclics, which increase heat production; butyrophenones, which disturb hypothalamic regulation of temperature and the ability to recognize thirst; and sympathomimetics, which increase psychomotor activity.

Health conditions that are risk factors for the development of heat stroke include those compromising cardiovascular function, diabetes mellitus, hyperthyroidism, potassium deficiency, and alcoholism. Other conditions that result in impaired sweat production are also associated with heat stroke and include prickly heat (miliaria), healed extensive thermal burns, scleroderma, and congestive heart failure.

Relative poverty, advanced age, and lacking an air conditioner or the resources to run it have been found to be major risk factors in US cities during heat waves.

Classic Heat Stroke

Classic heat stroke occurs in sedentary individuals exposed to several days of environmental heat stress in whom thermoregulatory mechanisms stop functioning. It can occur at lower temperatures if the relative humidity is high. The skin is hot, dry, and flushed. Hyperthermia is invariably present, with a body temperature above 40.6° C (105° F), with some CNS disturbance present. Confusion may be the earliest sign, with an inability of victims to recognize their own illness. Eventually, coma may ensue. A respiratory alkalosis is usually present. Pre-existing organic disease increases mortality.

Exertional Heat Stroke

Exertional heat stroke is found in males performing heavy muscular exercise on warm, humid days. In the United States, it is seen in competitive long-distance runners, football players (>75 fatalities per year in the United States among amateurs), and military recruits. Victims are volume depleted and exhibit neurologic symptoms such as strange behavior, confusion, or even coma. Relative bradycardia may be seen in highly conditioned athletes with this disorder. Sweating persists in more than half the cases. These individuals present with a relatively cool, clammy skin, but with an extremely elevated core temperature (up to 44.5° C). However, by the time the individual is seen, his temperature may have dropped to the more typical febrile range but with all the other complications present as a result of widespread organ damage: rhabdomyolysis disseminated intravascular coagulation, lactic acidosis, hyperuricemia, and hypokalemia. A moderate to severe metabolic acidosis is seen. Few cases are seen in women. Patients who recover from heat stroke are more susceptible to recurrent attacks.

Differential Diagnosis of Heat Stroke in Travelers

Be sure to check temperatures of potential heat illness victims when they are first evaluated in the field. Infections, including cerebral falciparum malaria, can occur in environments similar to those where heat stroke occurs. Encephalitis, meningitis, and typhoid fever can present with a picture similar to heat stroke. Shaking chills suggest that fever is due to an infectious etiology. Drug-induced heat illness, especially anticholinergic poisoning, may be difficult to diagnose. Cocaine, methamphetamine, and other sympathomimetic agents may be involved. Sweating suggests that anticholinergic poisoning is not present. Over half of heat stroke patients have constricted, pinpoint pupils, which also militate against anticholinergic poisoning.

Treatment of Heat Stroke

Treatment of heat stroke is a medical emergency, and delay in cooling is the single most important factor leading to death. Begin cooling at the site of collapse by disrobing, fanning, and bathing the skin with cool water. Monitor rectal temperature every 5-10 min during resuscitation. The duration of hyperthermia is the most important factor affecting survival. Reasons for delay include failure to make the diagnosis and lack of facilities to rapidly cool. Mortality is still high, at close to 10%.

Cool the Patient

The victim should be removed from the hot environment, and aggressive cooling techniques improvised depending on what is available. The classic treatment is to immerse the patient in a tub of ice water and massage the skin briskly. Although cold-induced vasoconstriction can theoretically impair heat loss, this method has been used successfully. No other technique yet proposed claims better results. Tepid or tap water may be as good as ice water for cooling and may be more comfortable. Alternatively, the patient can be wetted down with water and rubbed briskly with ice bags, keeping a large fan blowing on the patient, which may be better tolerated than ice-water immersion in confused individuals. If the ice supply is limited, it should be applied to the head, neck, abdomen, axillae, and groin. Special beds (physiologic body-cooling unit or the King Saud University cooling bed) have been constructed to allow the spraying of pressurized water at 15° C on the nude body; they were designed for use in countries where heat stroke occurs to many on pilgrimage. In evacuation, consider an open vehicle and mist sprays. No pharmacologic agent has been shown to help, including dantrolene, although antipyretic agents have not been evaluated.

Support the Vital Signs

A heat stroke patient should be transported to a medical facility with rapid correction of fluid and electrolyte abnormalities; hypoglycemia, if present, should be treated. Diazepam (IV) should be given for seizures, severe cramping, or shivering, which impair cooling. Consider gastric, rectal, thoracic, bladder, or peritoneal lavage cooling. Central venous monitoring can guide fluid therapy and avoid fluid overload. If the victim is comatose, endotracheal intubation is recommended.

Prevention of Heat Stroke

Heat stroke can be prevented by encouraging people to drink enough fluids (especially important for children, elderly people, and those with debilitating conditions), adjusting dosages of drugs affecting fluid balance and thermoregulation in travelers to warm climates, and limiting activity during heat extremes. Exercise in the heat should be commensurate with fitness level, with the hottest hours of the day avoided and rest periods taken. Those engaged in strenuous activity during hot weather need to drink more frequently and copiously than thirst dictates. Consuming 400-500 mL of water before exertion, and then a cup or more (300 mL) of water for every 20 min of exercise in the heat should be encouraged. Splashing or spraying the skin with water intermittently can promote evaporative cooling, and access to air-conditioned spaces is essential. Salt tablet consumption is not routinely recommended.

If someone feels ill or "overstressed" during exercise, he or she should stop and seek a cool area. This is especially important for driven individuals in peer-group situations. After a febrile illness, individuals should be especially cautious of further heat exposure.

FURTHER READING

Jet lag: an app for light exposure time to help with jet lag: <http://entrain.math.lsa.umich.edu>

Heat illness: OHSA website on heat illness in outdoor workers where you can download a Heat Safety Tool app: <https://www.osha.gov/SLTC/heatillness/index.html>

Motion sickness: motion sickness site with much useful information: <http://www.dizziness-and-balance.com/disorders/central/motion.htm>

Auerbach, P.S. (Ed.), 2012. Wilderness Medicine. Elsevier/Mosby, Philadelphia, PA.
Comprehensive chapters on cold and heat disorders for the clinician.

Keystone, J.S., Kozarsky, P.E., Freedman, D.O., et al. (Eds.), 2013. Travel Medicine. Saunders, Oxford.
Comprehensive chapters on jet lag and motion sickness for the clinician.

Herxheimer, A., Petrie, K.J., 2009. Melatonin for the prevention and treatment of jet lag. Cochrane Database Syst. Rev. (2).
Sack, R.L., 2010. Jet lag. NEJM 362 (5), 440–447.
A readable useful review.

Srinivasan, V., Singh, J., Brzezinski, A., et al., 2014. Jet lag: use of melatonin and melatonergic drugs. In: Srinivasan, V., Brzezinski, A., Oter, S., et al. (Eds.), Melatonin and Melatonergic Drugs in Clinical Practice. Springer, New Delhi, pp. 367–378.
Detailed review of studies of these agents.

Weich, S., Pearce, H.L., Croft, P., et al., 2014. Effect of anxiolytic and hypnotic drug prescriptions on mortality hazards: retrospective cohort study. BMJ 348, g1996.
Sobering material on possible mortality hazards from use of these commonly prescribed agents.

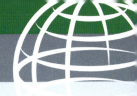

CHAPTER 10

High-Altitude Travel

Andrew M. Luks

Increasing numbers of people are traveling to high altitude for work or pleasure. While the rewards of such travel are often great and include opportunities to see places of great beauty or historical and cultural significance, to accomplish lifelong objectives, or to simply have an enjoyable vacation, there are risks associated with such travel. Unacclimatized lowlanders are at risk for one of several forms of acute altitude illness within the first several days of ascent, while individuals with underlying medical problems may be at risk for worsening control of those problems or other complications.

This chapter provides information for counseling individuals seeking advice about how to prevent such problems. After defining the term "high altitude" and describing features of the high-altitude environment and the physiologic responses to hypobaric hypoxia, the chapter describes a general approach to three types of patients who may present for evaluation: the traveler who has never been to high altitudes before and seeks advice on ensuring a safe trip, the returning traveler who had a problem on a prior trip and seeks advice on how to avoid repeating such problems in the future, and the potentially at-risk traveler with underlying medical problems that may be exacerbated by hypobaric hypoxia or may predispose to acute altitude illness.

WHAT CONSTITUTES "HIGH ALTITUDE"?

Although there are no firm definitions, the term "high altitude" generally refers to regions located above 1500 m (~5000 ft) in elevation. While some physiologic responses to hypoxia begin just above this threshold, acute altitude illness does not generally occur until an individual ascends above 2340 m (~8000 ft). For most healthy individuals, it is only when traveling above this latter threshold that the altitude should be taken into account with trip planning. For individuals with underlying medical conditions, however, the effect of the altitude may need to be considered at lower elevations. Regardless of underlying health status, the further an individual travels above these thresholds, the greater the potential for altitude-related problems.

The majority of high-altitude travelers will not ascend above 5500-6500 m, a range that includes common trekking destinations such as Mt. Kilimanjaro (5895 m) and Everest base camp (5350 m). Select individuals, typically those engaged in mountaineering expeditions, do ascend above this range and are exposed to extreme degrees of hypoxia that pose significant physiologic challenges and markedly increase the risk of acute altitude illness if proper acclimatization measures are not undertaken.

THE ENVIRONMENT AT HIGH ALTITUDE

The defining environmental feature at high altitude is the nonlinear decrease in barometric pressure with increasing elevation. This change, which is more pronounced at higher latitudes and during the winter months, leads to decreased ambient partial pressure of oxygen

(PO₂) that, in turn, lowers the PO_2 throughout the body and triggers several important physiologic responses (described later).

Other important environmental changes include lower air density, increased ultraviolet (UV) light exposure, decreased humidity, and decreased ambient temperature. The lower air density is likely too small to be of clinical significance, while the increased UV exposure decreases the time necessary to develop sunburn and ultraviolet keratitis ("snow blindness"), particularly with travel on snow-covered terrain. The decrease in humidity increases insensible water losses through the respiratory tract and the risk of dehydration, particularly when individuals engage in physical exertion, while the decrease in temperature may increase the risk of hypothermia and frostbite depending on the full range of environmental conditions at the time of travel.

Air quality often improves in the mountains, but this is not always the case. Greater solar radiation increases smog potential, while extensive valley systems can trap pollutants during temperature inversions, particularly when near urban centers. Finally, wood and yak-dung stoves are common heat sources in rural areas of the Himalaya and elsewhere, leading to poor air quality when these stoves are in high use.

PHYSIOLOGIC RESPONSES TO HYPOBARIC HYPOXIA

The decrease in PO_2 at all points along the oxygen transport cascade from inspired air to the alveolar space, arterial blood, and tissues causes physiologic responses across multiple organ systems, which facilitates adaptation to the hypobaric hypoxia (**Table 10.1**). Some of the responses, such as the increase in minute ventilation, start within minutes of exposure, while other responses, such as erythropoiesis, take several weeks before their full effect is realized. The magnitude of these responses varies considerably between individuals, and this

TABLE 10.1   Physiologic Responses to Hypobaric Hypoxia

System	Responses
Pulmonary responses	Arterial hypoxemia triggers increased peripheral chemoreceptor output, leading to an increase in minute ventilation and a respiratory alkalosis.
	The respiratory alkalosis blunts the initial ventilatory responses.
	With continued time at high altitude, minute ventilation rises further due to renal compensation for the respiratory alkalosis and increased sensitivity of the peripheral chemoreceptors.
	Alveolar hypoxia triggers hypoxic pulmonary vasoconstriction, leading to an increase in pulmonary vascular resistance and pulmonary artery pressure.
Cardiac responses	Cardiac output increases, largely due to an increase in heart rate.
	Stroke volume declines due to a decrease in plasma volume.
	Myocardial contractility is preserved.
	Systemic blood pressure increases to a variable extent.
Renal responses	Variable increase in diuresis and natriuresis following ascent leads to a decrease in circulating plasma volume.
	Arterial hypoxemia triggers increased secretion of erythropoietin (EPO) within 24-48 hours of ascent.
	There is an increase in bicarbonate excretion, as compensation for the acute respiratory alkalosis.
Hematologic responses	There is an initial increase in hemoglobin concentration and hematocrit due to reduction in plasma volume.
	Over days to weeks, there are further increases in red blood cell mass, hemoglobin concentration, and hematocrit due to increased EPO concentrations.

variability plays a large role in determining tolerance of hypobaric hypoxia and susceptibility to acute altitude illness.

Because of these environmental changes and physiologic responses to hypobaric hypoxia, high-altitude travelers are at risk for a range of problems they might not experience at lower elevations and may present for evaluation with one of several possible concerns:

- **The altitude-naïve traveler** who has never ascended to high altitude before and seeks advice on how to ensure a safe trip
- **The returning traveler** who had problems on a prior high-altitude trip and seeks information about what happened and how to prevent such problems in the future
- **The potentially at-risk traveler** who has underlying medical problems that may worsen at high altitude or predispose to acute altitude illness.

The remainder of this chapter describes an approach to each of these situations.

THE ALTITUDE-NAÏVE TRAVELER

Many travelers have never been to high altitude and seek advice about what to expect in this environment and how to prevent problems. Alternatively, individuals who have traveled to high altitude before without difficulty may be going to significantly higher elevations and are now concerned about similar issues. Effective counseling of such travelers encompasses a range of topics described in detail below.

Normal Responses to High Altitude

Even if they avoid acute altitude illness, individuals feel different at high altitude than at lower elevations as a result of the environmental changes and physiologic responses to hypobaric hypoxia. These differences (**Table 10.2**) should be reviewed as part of pre-trip counseling, as this can prevent misinterpretation of normal responses as evidence of illness and facilitate identification of those individuals who are truly becoming ill.

High-altitude travelers who are otherwise well commonly report poor sleep quality, insomnia, vivid dreams, and frequent awakenings. A major contributor to these problems is periodic breathing, in which periods of crescendo-decrescendo breathing movements are punctuated by apneas lasting from 5 to 20 seconds. While overall sleep quality tends to improve over time, periodic breathing can persist or worsen during long stays at high altitude.

Exercise is also challenging at high altitude. At any given level of work, heart rate and minute ventilation are higher than at sea level, and, unlike at sea level, arterial oxygen saturation decreases with progressive exercise. Even following extensive pre-trip physical training, individuals experience more intense breathlessness during exertion, particularly during the first few days at altitude. Importantly, however, on stopping to rest, dyspnea typically resolves within a short time (~1-2 min).

Recognition of Acute Altitude Illness

All high-altitude travelers should be able to recognize the three main forms of acute altitude illness: acute mountain sickness (AMS), high-altitude cerebral edema (HACE), and

TABLE 10.2 How Travelers Feel Different at High Altitude Compared with the Altitude of Residence
• Heart rate at rest and with any level of exertion higher than at altitude of residence
• Increased respiratory rate and tidal volume
• More frequent sighs
• Increased frequency of urination
• Dyspnea on exertion that resolves quickly with rest
• Difficulty sleeping, including frequent arousals, insomnia, vivid dreams
• Transient lightheadedness on rising to a standing position

high-altitude pulmonary edema (HAPE). The clinical features of these diseases are described in **Table 10.3**, while information about their underlying pathophysiology is described in several excellent reviews listed at the end of this chapter. Of these entities, AMS is by far the most common and the most likely to be encountered during high-altitude travel. HACE and HAPE are uncommon but potentially fatal if not recognized promptly and warrant attention in pre-travel counseling.

For individuals ascending to and remaining at a given elevation, the risk for these problems lasts up to 5 days following ascent. Individuals ascending to steadily higher elevations, as on a climbing expedition, remain at risk until they begin to descend from their maximum elevation, at which point the risk of illness decreases significantly and eventually disappears entirely as descent continues.

A challenge in recognizing AMS is the nonspecific nature of the symptoms, as headache can be seen as a result of dehydration, carbon monoxide intoxication from cooking in a poorly ventilated tent, and other causes. Similarly, symptoms of HAPE can be present in other respiratory disorders such as pneumonia and pulmonary embolism. However, while it is always important to consider a broad differential diagnosis, compatible symptoms and signs arising following ascent should be considered altitude illness until proven otherwise.

Risk Factors for Acute Altitude Illness

The primary reason individuals develop acute altitude illness is they ascend too high, too fast, where "fast" refers to the number of meters ascended per day rather than the walking pace itself. For example, an individual ascending to 5000 m over 3 days and remaining at that elevation is more likely to get sick than an individual completing the same ascent over 7 days.

There is an important interaction between the altitude attained and the time spent at that altitude that affects risk; individuals who ascend rapidly but descend quickly after reaching the summit may avoid altitude illness, whereas individuals who complete the same ascent at the same rate but remain on the summit for many hours face a higher risk of problems.

There is considerable inter-individual variability in susceptibility to acute altitude illness, such that some individuals acclimatize well and tolerate seemingly fast ascents while others develop problems even with appropriate ascent profiles. While susceptibility to altitude illness is likely a multigenetic trait, the specific genetic polymorphisms have not been identified, and we lack a simple, reliable means of predicting which travelers face risk following ascent.

A common misperception is that being in good physical condition protects against acute altitude illness. To the contrary, highly fit endurance athletes are just as susceptible to AMS, HACE, and HAPE as unconditioned individuals and must adhere to the same principles of altitude illness prevention.

Prevention of Acute Altitude Illness

Effective prevention relies on a combination of both nonpharmacologic and pharmacologic measures.

Nonpharmacologic Measures

Because the primary risk factor for acute altitude illness is an overly rapid ascent, the single best preventive measure is to undertake an adequately slow ascent to the target elevation. In particular, once above 3000 m, individuals should not increase their sleeping elevation by more than 300-500 m per night and, every 3-4 nights, should take a rest day and remain at the same elevation for a second night. While simple in its prescription, this rule of thumb can be hard to follow, as the logical stopping points on most major trekking or climbing routes are not spaced at 500 m intervals. In such situations, rather than focusing on the elevation gain for each day of the trip, one can focus on the overall rate of gain for the entire trip. If excessive gains in elevation are necessary on particular days, rest days can be added to the itinerary to decrease the overall ascent rate. As individuals gain experience traveling at high altitude they can deviate from these guidelines based on their personal

TABLE 10.3 Clinical Features and Management of Acute High-Altitude Illnesses

Acute Altitude Illness	Timing and Altitude of Onset	Clinical Features	Prevention	Treatment
Acute mountain sickness (AMS)	Seen at altitudes ≥2340 m Altitude of onset varies significantly between individuals Subacute onset of symptoms within 6-10 hr of ascent to a given elevation	Headache plus one or more of the following: nausea, vomiting, lethargy, sustained light-headedness Normal neurologic exam and normal mental status	Slow ascent (above 2500 m, limit increases in sleeping elevation to 500 m/day) Avoid overexertion Acetazolamide or dexamethasone with moderate- to high-risk ascent profiles	Stop ascending Acetaminophen or NSAIDs for headache Antiemetics Mild to moderate illness: acetazolamide Severe cases: dexamethasone Descend if symptoms do not improve in 1-2 days or worsen on appropriate treatment Further ascent possible if symptoms resolve
High-altitude cerebral edema (HACE)	Seen at altitudes ≥3000 m, with increasing incidence at higher elevations Subacute onset of symptoms. Sudden onset of symptoms should prompt search for alternative causes	Preexisting AMS or concurrent HAPE symptoms (not universally present) Ataxia, altered mental status Severe lassitude, somnolence, coma Focal neurologic deficits uncommon and should prompt consideration of other diagnoses Potentially fatal if not recognized and treated promptly	Slow ascent Avoid overexertion Acetazolamide or dexamethasone with moderate- to high-risk ascent profiles	Descend until symptoms resolve If descent not possible, supplemental oxygen or a portable hyperbaric chamber Dexamethasone
High-altitude pulmonary edema (HAPE)	Seen at altitudes ≥2500 m, with cases documented at lower elevations in patients with history of pulmonary vascular diseases Subacute onset within 2-5 days of ascent	Mild: dyspnea and arterial O₂ desaturation out of proportion to that seen in normal individuals with similar ascent rates at a given elevation; decreased exertional tolerance, dry cough Severe: dyspnea with mild exertion or at rest; cough with pink, frothy sputum; cyanosis May see concurrent signs or symptoms of AMS or HACE but not universally present Potentially fatal if not recognized promptly	Slow ascent Avoid overexertion Nifedipine for individuals with prior history of HAPE (alternative: phosphodiesterase inhibitors)	Descend until symptoms resolve Avoid heavy exertion on descent If descent not possible, supplemental oxygen or a portable hyperbaric chamber Nifedipine or phosphodiesterase inhibitor (may not be necessary if supplemental oxygen available) Avoid concurrent use of nifedipine and phosphodiesterase inhibitor

NSAIDs, Nonsteroidal anti-inflammatory drugs.

tolerances of hypobaric hypoxia, but for the altitude-naïve traveler, they represent the appropriate initial approach.

Travelers should also avoid overexertion, heavy alcohol consumption, and opiate pain medications. Forced hydration is often recommended as a tool for decreasing the risk of altitude illness but has never been shown to be of benefit. Constant vigilance to adequate fluid intake does, however, prevent dehydration, whose symptoms mimic those of AMS.

Pharmacologic Measures

Information about the medications used to prevent AMS, HACE, and HAPE are provided in **Tables 10.3** and **10.4**. Because AMS and HACE may have a common pathophysiology, medications used to prevent AMS should prevent HACE. Several options are available for HAPE prevention, but these are reserved for individuals with a history of HAPE and are not used in the altitude-naïve traveler. Despite recent attention in the literature, ibuprofen has not replaced acetazolamide or dexamethasone as the preferred option for pharmacologic prophylaxis.

Not all travelers require pharmacologic prophylaxis. Instead, the decision to use medications should be based on an assessment of the risk associated with a planned ascent profile (**Table 10.5**). Pharmacologic prophylaxis is not necessary with low-risk ascent profiles but should be strongly considered with moderate- to high-risk itineraries.

Treatment of Acute Altitude Illness

As with prevention, the therapeutic approach to altitude illness is based on a combination of nonpharmacologic and pharmacologic measures. The most important treatment principle is to stop ascending and, in some cases, to descend to lower elevation. Patients with mild to moderate AMS may remain at the same elevation while undergoing treatment, while those with incapacitating AMS, HACE, or HAPE should descend. Descent raises the barometric pressure and the PO_2 at each step of the oxygen transport cascade, thereby terminating the pathophysiologic processes contributing to these diseases. Five hundred to 1000 m of descent is usually sufficient in most cases, although more severely ill patients should be evacuated as to as low an altitude (and as quickly) as possible. When descent is not feasible due to weather or logistical factors, supplemental oxygen or portable hyperbaric chambers are suitable alternatives, if available.

A general treatment approach for each disease, including pharmacologic measures, is described in **Table 10.3**, while the appropriate doses for the medications used in treatment are provided in **Table 10.4**. Clinical experience suggests that dexamethasone is more effective than the acetazolamide for treating moderate to severe AMS. The use of medications in HAPE varies based on the clinical setting; travelers who access health facilities may only require supplemental oxygen, while those in more remote settings should receive either the nifedipine, tadalafil, or sildenafil. No further ascent should be undertaken until the individual is asymptomatic while off medications. Strong consideration should be given to adding pharmacologic prophylaxis with continued ascent following an episode of altitude illness.

THE RETURNING TRAVELER

Travelers returning from trips to high altitude often present for evaluation of problems that developed during their sojourn. The range of problems for which they may seek evaluation is broad and includes the acute altitude illnesses described above and a host of other problems that may or may not be related to the altitude, such as vision changes due to retinal hemorrhages or prior refractive surgery, neurologic disorders such as seizures or transient focal neurologic deficits, respiratory problems such as persistent cough or pneumonia, and chest pain on exertion. Depending on the problem, the common concerns in such evaluations are determining what happened, whether the individual can return to high altitude in the future, and what preventive measures would be useful on such trips.

TABLE 10.4 Doses and Other Considerations for Medications Used in the Prevention and Treatment of Acute Altitude Illness

Medication	Dose for Prevention	Dose for Treatment	Other Considerations
Acetazolamide	125 or 250 mg every 12 h	250 mg every 12 h	Contraindicated in patients with cirrhosis Avoid in patients with severe ventilatory limitation (FEV_1 <25% predicted) Avoid in patients on chronically high doses of aspirin Caution in patients with documented sulfa allergy
Dexamethasone	2 mg every 6 h or 4 mg every 12 h	AMS: 4 mg every 6 hr HACE: 8 mg once then 4 mg every 6 h	May increase blood glucose values in diabetic patients Avoid in patients at risk for peptic ulcer disease Caution in patients at risk for strongyloidiasis
Nifedipine	30 mg sustained-release version every 12 h	30 mg sustained-release version every 12 h	Caution in patients using medications metabolized by CytP450 system Caution with concurrent use with other antihypertensive medications
Sildenafil	50 mg every 8 h[a]	50 mg every 8 h[a]	Avoid concurrent use of nitrates and alpha-blockers Caution in patients taking medications metabolized by CytP450 system
Tadalafil	10 mg every 12 h	10 mg every 12 h[b]	Avoid concurrent use of nitrates and alpha-blockers Caution in patients taking medications metabolized by CytP450 system
Salmeterol	125 μg every 12 h[c]	Not used for treatment	Potential for adverse effects in patients with coronary artery disease prone to arrhythmia

[a]Clinical utility for prevention or treatment not demonstrated.
[b]Clinical studies have shown benefit only in HAPE prevention.
[c]Not used as monotherapy for HAPE prevention. Recommended only as adjunct to pulmonary vasodilator therapy.
AMS, Acute mountain sickness; *FEV₁*, forced expiratory volume in the first second; *HACE*, high-altitude cerebral edema; *HAPE*, high-altitude pulmonary edema.

Determining What Happened

A major challenge in these assessments is the fact the symptoms and signs have typically resolved by the time the patient presents for evaluation. If the traveler accessed medical care at the time of the problem, he or she may have medical records, including chest radiographs and laboratory studies, that can be used as part of the assessment. In many cases, however, individuals descend to lower elevation and return home without any formal evaluation at the time of their problem. All that is available in such situations is the individual's oral description of the events and perhaps an oxygen saturation value if someone on their trip

TABLE 10.5 Risk Categories for Acute Altitude Illness in Unacclimatized Individuals Ascending to High Altitude[a]

Risk Category	Description
Low	• Individuals with no prior history of altitude illness and ascending to ≤2800 m • Individuals taking ≥2 days to arrive at 2500-3000 m with subsequent increases in sleeping elevation <500 m/day and an extra day for acclimatization every 1000 m
Moderate	• Individuals with prior history of AMS and ascending to 2500-2800 m in 1 day • No history of AMS and ascending to >2800 m in 1 day • All individuals ascending >500 m/day (increase in sleeping elevation) at altitudes above 3000 m but with an extra day for acclimatization every 1000 m
High	• Individuals with a history of AMS and ascending to >2800 m in 1 day • All individuals with a prior history of HACE and HAPE • All individuals ascending to >3500 m in 1 day • All individuals ascending >500 m/day (increase in sleeping elevation) above >3000 m without extra days for acclimatization • Very rapid ascents (e.g., <7-day ascents of Mt. Kilimanjaro)

[a]Altitudes listed refer to the altitude at which the person sleeps. Ascent is assumed to start from elevations <1200 m.
AMS, Acute mountain sickness; *HACE,* high-altitude cerebral edema; *HAPE,* high-altitude pulmonary edema.
Adapted from Luks, A.M., McIntosh, S.E., Grissom, C.K., et al., 2014. Wilderness Medical Society Practice Guidelines for the Prevention and Treatment of Acute Altitude Illness: 2014 update. Wilderness Environ. Med. 25, S4–S14.

was carrying a pulse oximeter. The absence of corroborating data in such cases places a high premium on thorough history taking.

A key question is whether the problem was directly related to the hypobaric hypoxia at high altitude. A general rule of thumb is that symptoms and signs developing after ascent and resolving with descent are typically attributable to high altitude. There are exceptions to this rule, however, as vision deficits from symptomatic high-altitude retinal hemorrhages can persist for weeks following descent, while seizures associated with high altitude may terminate before descent. The timing of onset relative to the ascent can also be useful. AMS, HACE, and HAPE typically develop within 1-5 days of ascent to a given elevation, and, as a result, problems developing after that time period at a given altitude are more likely attributable to another issue. When available, pulse oximetry can aid in evaluating patients with respiratory issues. Patients with HAPE, for example, develop severe hypoxemia, and it is hard to ascribe respiratory problems at high altitude to HAPE if the individual had oxygen saturation values similar to those of healthy members of their trip.

Further Evaluation

For problems other than the acute altitude illnesses, the need for further evaluation depends on the particular problem. While individuals who developed chest pain on exertion at high altitude or those with symptomatic retinal hemorrhages, for example, warrant further evaluation by the appropriate specialist, other problems, such as persistent cough, may not warrant immediate assessment.

For individuals who developed acute altitude illness, a general principle is that prior performance at high altitude is a good but not perfect predictor of outcomes on subsequent trips. For example, an individual who developed AMS following a single-day ascent to 3000 m is likely but not guaranteed to develop AMS on a similar ascent in the future. Similarly, studies have shown that HAPE-susceptible individuals have about a 60% chance of recurrence on subsequent trips to the same elevation.

Individuals with AMS and HACE do not warrant any further testing to determine future risk, as there are no widely accessible means for this assessment. Because HAPE-susceptible individuals have a characteristic phenotype marked by excessive rises in pulmonary artery pressure in response to resting hypoxia and normoxic and hypoxic exercise, consideration can be given to evaluating for such responses in individuals with a concerning history. Such testing is not widely available, however, and, as a result, in individuals with a clear history of the diagnosis, it may be acceptable to forego such testing and just use pharmacologic prophylaxis on future trips.

Risk Mitigation for Future Trips

Individuals with a history of AMS, HACE, or HAPE can return to high altitude in the future. While those with AMS may not require pharmacologic prophylaxis with future ascents if they are going to lower elevations or using a slower ascent rate, individuals with HACE or HAPE should use pharmacologic prophylaxis, as the consequences of these illnesses are potentially great (**Tables 10.3** and **10.4**). Individuals should be counseled to ascend at a slower rate than on their prior trips.

When there is uncertainty about the likelihood of a problem recurring on future trips, consideration can be given to doing graded exposures to high altitude in more controlled settings. For example, prior to a committing trek into a distant, remote area, the individual can do a series of test trips to areas from which they can readily descend or access medical facilities in the event of problems.

THE POTENTIALLY AT-RISK TRAVELER

While many high-altitude travelers have no prior medical history, it is highly likely that some individuals who present for pre-travel counseling will have underlying medical conditions. Many of these travelers will have mild, well-controlled problems that pose little risk at high altitude, while others may have severe or difficult-to-control issues that could predispose to problems during the planned trip. Regardless of the severity of the condition, individuals with underlying medical issues warrant assessment to determine whether those issues will worsen at high altitude or affect the risk of acute altitude illness.

A Framework for Assessing Risk

A challenge of these evaluations is that, with the exception of several common conditions such as asthma, coronary artery disease, hypertension, and sleep apnea, the evidence base for pre-travel assessment of the full spectrum of problems with which patients may present is limited, and providers may find few, if any, studies that address risk for their patient's specific condition. In such situations, the assessment can be framed around four general questions.

Question 1: Is the Individual at Risk for Severe Hypoxemia or Impaired Tissue Oxygen Delivery?

While all individuals develop hypoxemia to varying degrees at high altitude based on how high they ascend, certain categories of patients, including those with moderate to severe chronic obstructive pulmonary disease, interstitial lung diseases, severe cystic fibrosis, and cyanotic congenital heart disease, will develop more severe hypoxemia than normal, particularly during exertion. This not only may lead to increased dyspnea and poor exertional tolerance but, in some studies, has been associated with an increased risk of AMS. With anemia, the arterial PO_2 will be the same at rest as in normal individuals, but oxygen carrying capacity and oxygen delivery are decreased, which may also lead to severe dyspnea and exercise limitation.

Question 2: Is the Individual at Risk for Impaired Ventilatory Responses to Hypoxia?

As described in **Table 10.2**, arterial hypoxemia normally triggers an increase in minute ventilation, whose role is to maintain the alveolar and arterial PO_2 at adequate levels. Individuals with severely impaired respiratory mechanics, as in severe chronic obstructive pulmonary disease, obesity hypoventilation syndrome, and many neuromuscular disorders, or those with impaired respiratory drives may not be able to mount the expected ventilatory responses. This, in turn, will cause greater degrees of hypoxemia and, as a result, increased dyspnea, impaired exertional tolerance, and, possibly, an increased risk of AMS.

Question 3: Is the Individual at Risk Due to the Expected Pulmonary Vascular Responses to Hypobaric Hypoxia?

As noted in **Table 10.2**, decreases in the alveolar PO_2 at high altitude lead to an increase in pulmonary vascular resistance, which raises pulmonary artery pressure. This change is well tolerated in most individuals but could pose problems for patients with pulmonary hypertension or right heart disease, as the literature contains several reports documenting the development of HAPE or worsening right heart function in patients with underlying pulmonary hypertension exposed to ambient hypoxia during either travel to high altitude or commercial flight. How severe the underlying pulmonary hypertension or right heart dysfunction must be to predispose to problems remains unclear, as the patients in these reports had varying degrees of pulmonary hypertension, but the presence of this issue should raise concern in the pre-travel evaluation.

Question 4: Will Environmental Features of High Altitude or the Expected Physiologic Responses to Hypobaric Worsen the Underlying Medical Condition?

Certain features of the environment at high altitude or the expected physiologic responses to hypoxia can affect some medical conditions. For example, cold, dry air may adversely affect airway function in asthmatic individuals, particularly those with exercise-induced symptoms, while increased sympathetic nervous system activity can worsen blood pressure in hypertensive individuals. The expected hypoxemia at high altitude can trigger vaso-occlusive crises in sickle cell disease patients or potentially provoke myocardial ischemia in patients with inadequately controlled coronary artery disease. A complete discussion of how various diseases are affected by high altitude is beyond the scope of this chapter. The expected outcomes for several common diseases are described in **Table 10.6**, while more extensive reviews on this topic are listed at the end of the chapter.

If the answer to all of these questions is "no," the individual is likely safe to travel to high altitude without further evaluation or risk-mitigation strategies beyond the general prevention measures described above. Individuals with nonreassuring answers, however, may require further evaluation and one of several possible risk reduction measures.

Further Evaluation

For individuals deemed to be at risk based on nonreassuring answers to the first three questions noted above, the best way to evaluate potential outcomes at high altitude is to expose these individuals to hypoxia and monitor their responses. Because access to hypobaric chambers is limited, the most feasible approach is the hypoxia altitude simulation test, in which an individual breathes a hypoxic gas mixture while symptoms and physiologic responses such as heart rate, oxygen saturation, and blood pressure are monitored. The test can be supplemented with echocardiography to assess the pulmonary vascular responses to hypoxia. The test has advantages over published prediction rules designed to estimate the degree of hypoxemia experienced by lung disease patients at high altitude, as it allows direct measurement of oxygen saturation while breathing the gas mixture, but its utility is limited in several respects; it is hard to simulate the full duration of time and the full range of ambient hypoxia an individual may experience on his or her trip. An individual might not develop symptoms during the short duration of this test but could develop problems after several days at high altitude. For individuals planning trips to distant places such as the Himalaya or Andes Mountains, another option would be test trips under more controlled conditions prior to the intended trip by, for example, taking shorter trips to the Alps or Rocky Mountains, where symptoms and pulse oximetry can be monitored and the individual can easily descend or access health facilities in the event of problems. For nonreassuring answers to the fourth question above, the approach varies based on the clinical

TABLE 10.6 Common Medical Conditions and High-Altitude Travel

Disease or Condition	Key Issues for High-Altitude Travel
Asthma	Well-controlled patients can travel as high as 6000 m and possibly higher.
	Avoid travel with worsening asthma control or following an acute exacerbation.
	Continue inhaler regimen at high altitude and travel with an adequate supply of rescue medications.
Chronic obstructive pulmonary disease	Avoid high-altitude travel in patients with FEV_1 <1 L, CO_2 retention, pulmonary hypertension, or recent exacerbation.
	Assess the need for supplemental oxygen in patients with FEV 1.0-1.5 L.
	Monitor pulse oximetry following ascent.
	Continue inhaler regimen at high altitude and travel with an adequate supply of rescue medications.
Congestive heart failure	Avoid high-altitude travel with poorly compensated disease or following a recent exacerbation.
	Okay to ascend with well-compensated disease to altitudes <3000 m.
	Monitor weight and blood pressure following ascent and adjust medications according to pre-arranged plan.
Coronary artery disease	Avoid high-altitude travel with unstable angina, ischemia at low levels of exertion, or recent acute coronary syndrome (<3-6 months, no revascularization).
	Consider risk stratification with exercise treadmill test prior to planned travel.
	Reduce level of exertion to slightly lower than that done at sea level. No de novo exercise at altitude if not exercising at sea level.
	Continue existing medications at high altitude.
Diabetes mellitus	Increase frequency of blood glucose monitoring.
	Avoid overly strict glucose control early in the trip due to concerns about glucometer accuracy at high altitude.
	Evaluate for co-morbid conditions (e.g., coronary artery disease) that could worsen at high altitude.
	Avoid vigorous exercise at high altitude if not experienced with high-level exercise at sea level.
Hypertension	Mild or well-controlled disease: no indication for medication adjustments or routine blood pressure monitoring.
	Poorly controlled or labile hypertension: monitor blood pressure following ascent and adjust medications for severely elevated blood pressures (>180/120 with symptoms or >220/140 without symptoms).
Obstructive sleep apnea	Patients with moderate to severe disease should travel with CPAP machine if access to power can be assured.
	Consider adding acetazolamide to decrease the incidence of central sleep apnea.
Pregnancy	Evaluate pre-travel to ensure the pregnancy remains low risk.
	Avoid high-altitude travel with complicated or high-risk pregnancies (e.g., impaired placental function, chronic hypertension, intrauterine growth retardation, anemia).
	Exercise at levels lower than at home; avoid dehydration.
	Avoid travel into remote areas in the third trimester.

TABLE 10.6 Common Medical Conditions and High-Altitude Travel—cont'd	
Disease or Condition	**Key Issues for High-Altitude Travel**
Pulmonary hypertension	Avoid high-altitude travel without supplemental oxygen with moderate to severe disease (mean PA pressure >35 mmHg or systolic PA pressure >60 mmHg). In less severe disease, consider adding pulmonary vasodilator therapy or supplemental oxygen.
Sickle cell diseases	Sickle cell anemia: avoid high-altitude travel due to increased risk of sickling and vaso-occlusive and splenic crises. Sickle cell trait: high-altitude travel likely okay, but patients should avoid heavy exertion and seek medical attention for left upper quadrant pain (possible splenic crisis).

CPAP, Continuous positive airway pressure; *FEV,* forced expiratory volume.

circumstances. Patients with coronary artery disease may require stress testing, for example, while patients with recent exacerbations of heart failure, asthma, chronic obstructive pulmonary disease, or recent stroke or myocardial infarction within the past 6 months may simply need to forego their planned trip.

Risk Mitigation Strategies

The most important principle of risk mitigation is to ensure the underlying medical problem is under good control at the time of the planned trip. Patients with evidence of worsening asthma, for example, should not embark on high-altitude travel, particularly into remote areas away from medical care. A second important principle is to ensure that patients remain on their baseline medications or therapies during their trip. Some individuals, such as those with diabetes, heart failure, or poorly controlled hypertension, should consider monitoring aspects of their disease more carefully during the trip and adjusting medications according to a pre-specified plan. Individuals at risk for disease exacerbations, such as those with asthma or chronic obstructive pulmonary disease, should travel with an adequate supply of rescue medications and a plan to access care in the event of symptoms that are difficult to control. Depending on their underlying medical condition, patients may need to adjust the dose or use alternative agents for acute altitude illness prophylaxis or treatment (**Table 10.4**).

Individuals at risk for severe hypoxemia or adverse consequences from the pulmonary vascular responses to hypoxia should consider using supplemental oxygen during the sojourn. In light of the logistical difficulties associated with air travel with supplemental oxygen, the best options for this would be to travel with a small, battery-powered portable oxygen concentrator, which is allowed on most commercial airlines, or to travel with a prescription for supplemental oxygen that can be filled at the destination if the patient has significant symptoms and/or severe hypoxemia. Patients with pulmonary hypertension may also need to add or augment pulmonary vasodilator therapy to blunt the expected pulmonary vascular responses at high altitude. Other disease-specific approaches are described in many of the references at the end of this chapter.

On returning to home at the conclusion of the trip, individuals who added or adjusted their medications should return to their baseline medication regimen.

RETURN TRAVEL TO HIGH ALTITUDE

Many of the issues described above are of greatest relevance to the first-time traveler to high altitude who has no prior sense of their susceptibility to acute altitude illness or how any underlying medical problems will be affected by this environment. As individuals make repeated trips to high altitude, however, they will gain greater understanding of their personal tolerances of hypoxia, which should carry several benefits. They will better understand their ability to acclimatize to hypobaric hypoxia and, as a result, can adjust their ascent profiles and trip itineraries accordingly. The person who acclimatizes well, for example, may be able to move somewhat faster than the recommended rates, while highly susceptible individuals will learn they need to move slower than recommended and to consider pharmacologic prophylaxis. Individuals with underlying medical problems will also gain a greater understanding of how control of that problem is affected at high altitude and become better at adjusting their therapeutic regimen during their travels.

FURTHER READING

General High-Altitude Medicine

Bartsch, P., Mairbaurl, H., Maggiorini, M., et al., 2005. Physiological aspects of high-altitude pulmonary edema. J. Appl. Physiol. 98, 1101–1110.
This review provides a comprehensive overview of the clinical features and management of high-altitude pulmonary edema and the underlying pathophysiology of the disease.

Bartsch, P., Swenson, E.R., 2013. Clinical practice: acute high-altitude illnesses. N. Engl. J. Med. 368, 2294–2302.
This is a comprehensive review of the clinical aspects of the three main forms of acute altitude illness by leading experts in the field. It is a more up-to-date version of the review by Hackett and Roach below.

Hackett, P.H., Roach, R.C., 2001. High-altitude illness. N. Engl. J. Med. 345, 107–114.
This is a comprehensive review of the clinical aspects of the three main forms of acute altitude illness by leading experts in the field.

Hackett, P.H., Roach, R.C., 2004. High altitude cerebral edema. High Alt. Med. Biol. 5, 136–146.
This is a comprehensive review of the clinical aspects and underlying pathophysiology of high-altitude cerebral edema.

Hackett, P.H., Roach, R.C., 2012. High altitude medicine. In: Auerbach, P. (Ed.), Wilderness Medicine. Elsevier Mosby, Philadelphia, pp. 2–33.
This chapter is the most comprehensive overview of all aspects of high-altitude medicine, including the physiologic responses to hypoxia; the clinical features, management, and pathophysiology of the acute altitude illnesses; and other medical problems at high altitude and how to approach the high-altitude traveler with underlying medical conditions.

Luks, A.M., 2014. Physiology in medicine: a physiologic approach to prevention and treatment of acute high altitude illnesses. J. Appl. Physiol. (1985) 118 (5), 509–519. Epub ahead of print.
This review provides an overview of clinical high-altitude medicine with an emphasis on the physiologic basis for the approach to preventing and treating acute altitude illness.

Luks, A.M., Swenson, E.R., 2008. Medication and dosage considerations in the prophylaxis and treatment of high-altitude illness. Chest 133, 744–755.
This review describes the primary medications used in the prevention and treatment of acute altitude illness, including proper dosing, dose adjustments for patients with underlying liver and kidney disease, and other important issues to consider when placing travelers on these medications.

Luks, A.M., McIntosh, S.E., Grissom, C.K., et al., 2014. Wilderness Medical Society Practice Guidelines for the Prevention and Treatment of Acute Altitude Illness: 2014 update. Wilderness Environ. Med. 25, S4–S14.
This is a widely read set of expert guidelines outlining the recommended approach to the prevention and treatment of AMS, HACE, and HAPE, with grading of the evidence for those recommendations.

Swenson, E.R., Bartsch, P., 2013. High Altitude: Human Adaptation to Hypoxia. Springer, New York.
This is a very comprehensive overview of high-altitude physiology and medicine that includes the physiology of hypoxia in all major organ systems as well as clinical aspects of acute and chronic altitude illness.

West, J.B., Schoene, R.B., Luks, A.M., et al., 2013. High Altitude Medicine and Physiology, 5th ed. CRC Press, Taylor & Francis Group, Boca Raton, FL.
This textbook is another comprehensive textbook on high-altitude physiology and medicine that contains information on the physiologic responses to hypobaric hypoxia and the clinical aspects of both acute and chronic forms of altitude illness.

Travelers with Underlying Medical Conditions
Bartsch, P., Gibbs, J.S., 2007. The effect of altitude on the heart and lungs. Circulation 116, 2191–2202.
This review describes the physiologic responses to hypoxia in the heart and lungs and describes an approach to patients with underlying coronary artery disease, heart failure, hypertension, and pulmonary hypertension who want to travel to high altitude.

Doan, D., Luks, A.M., 2014. Wilderness and adventure travel with underlying asthma. Wilderness Environ. Med. 25, 231–240.
This is a comprehensive review of the evaluation and management of individuals with asthma who want to participate in wilderness activities, with particular attention focused on high-altitude travel and diving.

Latshang, T.D., Bloch, K.E., 2011. How to treat patients with obstructive sleep apnea syndrome during an altitude sojourn. High Alt. Med. Biol. 12, 303–307.
Drawing on research data from their own research group, the authors provide practical recommendations for managing obstructive sleep apnea during travel to high altitude.

Luks, A.M., 2009. Do lung disease patients need supplemental oxygen at high altitude? High Alt. Med. Biol. 10, 321–327.
This review article considers the issue of hypoxemia in patients with lung disease traveling to high altitude and discusses tools for predicting the degree of hypoxemia at high altitude, logistical issues associated with travel with supplemental oxygen, and recommendations for assessing need and providing oxygen on a trip.

Luks, A.M., Hackett, P., 2014. High altitude and common medical conditions. In: Swenson, E.R., Bartsch, P. (Eds.), High Altitude: Human Adaptation to Hypoxia. Springer, New York, pp. 449–478.
This is one of the most comprehensive, up-to-date reviews of travel to high altitude with underlying medical problems. Building on an earlier review by the senior author, this chapter covers a broad range of diseases across multiple organ systems and provides practical recommendations for the approach to these patients.

Luks, A.M., Swenson, E.R., 2007. Travel to high altitude with pre-existing lung disease. Eur. Respir. J. 29, 770–792.
This is a comprehensive review of the issues associated with high-altitude travel in patients with a variety of lung diseases, including obstructive, restrictive, pulmonary vascular, and ventilatory control disorders.

Mieske, K., Flaherty, G., O'Brien, T., 2010. Journeys to high altitude—risks and recommendations for travelers with preexisting medical conditions. J. Travel Med. 17, 48–62.
This is a general review of high-altitude travel in patients with underlying medical problems across a variety of organ systems.

Richards, P., Hillebrandt, D., 2013. The practical aspects of insulin at high altitude. High Alt. Med. Biol. 14, 197–204.
This is a comprehensive review of travel to high altitude with diabetes mellitus that includes a lot of practical information on monitoring blood glucose and traveling with insulin.

Rimoldi, S.F., Sartori, C., Seiler, C., et al., 2010. High-altitude exposure in patients with cardiovascular disease: risk assessment and practical recommendations. Prog. Cardiovasc. Dis. 52, 512–524.
This is a comprehensive review of the challenges of high-altitude travel in patients with various forms of cardiovascular disease.

CHAPTER 11

Dive Medicine

Edmond Kay

One thorn of experience is worth a whole wilderness of warning.
James Russell Lowell

In diving, the predominant forces of nature are the gas laws, and the two most important ones are Boyle's law and Henry's law. Simply stated, Boyle's law refers to a pressure–volume relationship. As a diver descends in the water, each 33 ft of seawater (fsw) adds approximately one additional atmosphere of pressure. At that pressure (33 fsw = 1 bar = 1 atm = 760 mmHg = 14.7 psi) the volume in a closed space (e.g., the middle ear) is reduced by half. Descending to 66 fsw, the volume is reduced by half again, and divers affectionately call this "The Squeeze." Henry's law governs gas distribution in the body. At increasing pressure (and depth), the amount of gas dissolved in tissues of the body will increase proportionately. The diver absorbs extra nitrogen and oxygen, delivered by a pressure gradient that forces the gases into tissues of the body at a rate that is proportional to the partial pressure of the gas. This is the reason a diver cannot stay down indefinitely without incurring a penalty called decompression sickness (DCS). A third hazard present on virtually all dives is not actually related to a gas law. This is the inherent narcotic potential of dissolved inert gas at pressure. Inhaled gases under pressure have different characteristics, and the most important one for our purposes is the solubility of the gas. The higher the solubility of the gas, the greater the tendency for a given gas such as nitrogen to cause "narcosis" at high partial pressures. This is the so-called rapture of the deep and is one of the reasons deeper diving is so much more hazardous. Narcosis has been equated (approximately) to the effect of alcohol, and quantitatively the potency of the effect can be described by "Martini's law." This approximation of the narcotic potential of nitrogen on the central nervous system was devised by the US Navy to warn the uninitiated that at a depth of 50 ft a diver will feel the effects of narcosis approximately equal to drinking one martini. Double that to 100 fsw, and the effect is approximately equal to two martinis. By 150 ft of depth, this becomes an extreme hazard to all but the most experienced diver. Even breath-hold divers can be affected adversely by narcosis. An alcohol intoxication-like effect is just part of the experience, however, and many other changes in mood and perception also occur. A deep-diving individual can feel elated or high but is just as likely to feel confused, tense, and anxious, with a deep foreboding sensation that ominous shadows lurk everywhere. Without exception, everyone has difficulty concentrating, but with advanced training a diver can compensate for this mental clouding. This is one of the reasons why deep diving, beyond the 100-ft recreational depth limit, is hazardous, particularly for the novice diver.

PREPARATION FOR DIVE TRAVEL

The Divers Alert Network (dan.org) provides a valuable service to the dive traveler. Over the years the network has been updating dive injury and fatality statistics. The information is clearly useful in determining who might be at greater risk for dive injury. Fortunately, we as medical providers are also blessed with data that can be found in the subscriber-funded newsletter *Undercurrent*. The number of dive accidents is on the rise, according to last year's report, but fatalities have remained approximately the same. DCS incidents are down from the previous year's high of 91, and now DCS is hovering at 56 incidents (2014 statistics). *Undercurrent* goes on to reference statistics related to older divers:

Five deaths involved divers who suffered heart attacks while in the water (out of 16 fatalities), and the average age of these divers was 60. In the last 2 years, nine in-water diving fatalities were attributed to medical causes in divers aged 50 or over. This number is significantly higher than the average age of non-medical fatalities, which is 42 years.

The British Sub-Aqua Club (BSAC) quoted these statistics in its Annual Diving Incident Report for 2014. The report goes on to say, "Older divers are advised to take account of the increased likelihood of a medical event when considering the type of diving in which they engage, and those diving with them should be more aware of the increased risk." The physician advising a dive traveler is in an excellent position to help reduce this number.

Divers usually do not ask for medical clearance unless it is required by the dive resort. Issues such as asthma, obesity, heart disease, and physical disability may limit a diver's tolerance for unanticipated adversity encountered on a dive, and there are well-defined parameters a physician can use to determine who may be at risk. That said, "fitness to dive" is a notoriously difficult issue to determine with certainty. Dr. Tom Neuman, of San Diego, California, has been quoted as saying, "It is probably more important to ask if someone has ever run out of gas on the freeway than to ask about most medical conditions." This comment is in reference to the well-known fact that some divers will run out of breathing gas in their SCUBA tank while diving due to inattention to air consumption. The ensuing emergency ascent is often not survived due to pulmonary barotrauma leading to air embolism. What is needed is a no-nonsense approach to dive fitness that could be applied to all divers whether they travel or not. It is essential to know what type of diving the traveler has planned. Will it be a low-stress dive vacation in warm, clear, tropical waters or is it going to be adventure diving in a cave or in deep shipwrecks in the North Atlantic using rebreather technology?

The most recent dive accident statistics indicate a number of other near-miss incidents. The most recently compiled causes of death include rapid ascent due to problems with buoyancy control or out-of-air situations, equipment problems, and solo diving or snorkeling. Medical history obtained after a fatality has revealed surprisingly consistent findings over the years. Cardiovascular disease is always the most prevalent, present in over 10% of all fatalities (13.6% in 2009, 12% in 2010) and this is still true today.

Most reports list "drowning" as a cause of death because that is all the coroner can confirm at autopsy. It takes experience and skill to tell the difference between a fatality in the water caused by drowning and one that is caused by air embolism. If the diver makes an emergency ascent due to an out-of-air situation or other problem causing panic in the water, air in the lung expands at a faster rate than can be safely exhaled. Pulmonary barotrauma, sometimes called "pulmonary overpressure injury," allows a small amount of air to enter the pulmonary arterial system. Within three heartbeats this air is transmitted to the brain, causing momentary confusion or loss of motor control. The diver can no longer protect the airway, and the final common pathway for death is indeed drowning, but the antecedent cause is "air embolism," and before that it is running out of air to breathe.

Scuba diving can be divided into several categories depending on the physical and technical demands of the anticipated dive and the remoteness of the dive location. This easily breaks down into three manageable categories:

- Recreational diving for the beginner or occasional diver in warm, clear water breathing compressed air, the maximum depth limited to 100 ft of seawater.
- Advanced deeper, multiday diving often using Nitrox (also known as enriched air nitrox). Nitrox refers to a modified breathing gas with a higher concentration of oxygen than is found in air (21%). The oxygen concentration is higher in order to lower the concentration of inert gas and lower the risk of DCS. The diver gets to dive longer, but the trade-off is that diving must be done at a shallower depth due to the potential for CNS oxygen toxicity.

- Technical diving, usually done with either multiple tanks or rebreather technology and requiring long decompression times before surfacing. Often the dives are deep and penetrate into caves or sunken vessels where there is no possibility of direct return to the surface. The dive sites are often in remote locations with virtually no access to medical care or a hyperbaric treatment facility.

In actuality there are many other subsets of diving. To name a few, there is the instructor, commercial diver, scientific diver, engineer, seafood harvester, public safety diver (usually performed by police and fire departments), military diver including marine mammal training for guard duty, and unexploded ordinance removal diving. The care of most of these fall under the general category of occupational medicine, and physical requirements are much more rigorous and are usually specified by the agency responsible for certification of the diver. It is beyond the scope of this chapter to review the requirements of each one.

Concerning a diver's "fitness to dive," Dr. Richard Moon has stated that:

1. A diver should be able to do the "work" of diving. That is, to breathe, swim, and exercise underwater. Note here that some dives are more work than others, but if a diver is called on to rescue his or her partner, intense physical exertion will be required. This is why the minimum standard of physical fitness for any type of diving is the ability of the diver to achieve 13 metabolic equivalents (METS) or better of exercise, running on a treadmill. This is only one of many different ways in which physical fitness can be assessed. Each test of cardiovascular fitness has its strengths and weaknesses; one of the easier, cost-effective tests to administer in a medical clinic is the Harvard step test. This test is designed to work best for healthy individuals of normal weight. One of the weaknesses of the test is that it does not accurately predict fitness swimming or diving or apply to anyone with a partial disability or who is markedly overweight. Disadvantages include Biomechanical characteristics. They vary between individuals. For example, considering that the step height is standard, taller people are at an advantage as it will take less energy to step up onto the step. Body weight has also been shown to be a factor. Testing large groups with this test will be time consuming. Those in the latter categories will have trouble performing up to their physical potential with a Harvard step test. A bicycle ergometer can also be used, but its availability is somewhat limited.
2. A diver should not be unusually susceptible to barotrauma, which is pressure-related damage to the ears, lungs, or gastrointestinal tract. Barotrauma is the most common injury for any class of diving but happens most often to the novice diver.
3. A diver should not be susceptible in any way to loss of consciousness caused by seizures, hypoglycemia related to insulin-dependent diabetes, or heart block.
4. A diver should not have any disease that diving (exercising underwater) could make worse. This includes sinus or middle-ear disease, previous labyrinthine window rupture, or heart failure.
5. If female, a diver should not be pregnant, as the risk of bubble-related birth defects (decompression injury) is thought to be significant.
6. A diver should not be "overly" susceptible to DCS. There are 24 known variables that affect an individual's susceptibility to DCS at any given time. Some of these factors are increasing age, first day of menses, previous undeserved DCS, fatigue, dehydration, vigorous exercise at depth underwater, or heart disease such as an atrial septal defect or a patent foramen ovale.

DECOMPRESSION SICKNESS

DSC goes hand in hand with physical fitness and an individual's "fitness to dive." Microscopic bubbles are formed constantly in the body under normal circumstances from heterogeneous sources and are known to be present to a greater extent when a diver becomes fully saturated with inert gas. It has been known for many years that clinical symptoms of decompression sickness are determined by the body's ability to withstand and tolerate the effect of bubbles and not by the presence of bubbles themselves. Vascular bubbles produced by "provocative diving" (diving in a manner more likely to produce DCS) can cause disruption of the vascular endothelium. This in turn triggers a cascading sequence of events, the first of which is believed to be activation of white blood cell (WBC) adhesion molecules on the surface of the endothelium. WBCs adhere at the site of injury and trigger a chain of events resulting in increased permeability of the vessel, localized tissue edema, and intravascular plasma loss. Vessel occlusion ultimately results from a combination of bubble obstruction and circulatory sludging (localized intravascular dehydration). This in turn results in tissue hypoxia and release of inflammatory cytokines (signaling molecules), including the very important class of molecules called eicosanoids. The inflammatory cascade caused by WBC adhesion also fosters the production of newly discovered microparticles (MPs) in the bloodstream. These MPs are small fragments of membranes and nucleic acids (also termed "cellular dust") that arise from the damaged endothelial tissue. The magnitude of MP production is highly variable and to some extent genetically mediated. This means that some individuals are more likely to get DCS on any given dive due to genetic variability. This finally explains the phenomenon of the "bends prone" individual. It is known but not well understood that diving leads to the activation of genes that are mainly triggered by hyperoxia. While some individuals are more prone to DCS, others (especially those who dive frequently) are rather immune to the effect of bubbles in the circulatory system. This is termed "DCS acclimatization" or the "work-up" dive effect. In some individuals, repeated exposure to high levels of inert gas can trigger an adaptive immunoinflammatory response by modulation of nuclear factors.

If tissue damage occurs and progresses, excitatory neurotransmitters are released, and ultimately reperfusion injury occurs. This is progressively irreversible tissue damage from reactive oxygen species (chemically reactive molecules containing oxygen). If DCS is allowed to progress untreated, the injury also triggers apoptosis (programmed cell death), the final and irreversible outcome of untreated DCS.

Overt DCS is an outward manifestation of this highly variable and multifaceted inflammatory disorder. Aerobic exercise can reduce bubble formation in animals and humans. The mechanism for this is probably the effect of nitric oxide liberated by exercise, but this is not known with certainty. What is known for certain is that the addition of nitric oxide in test animals who have been subjected to potentially lethal dives results in survival with no neurological injury. Nitric oxide has the ability to remove vascular bubbles; this raises the question of whether medication can potentially help treat DCS.

A thorough diving history and physical examination might uncover risk factors, but the examining provider needs to know what to look for. Certainly, a genetic predisposition for the inflammatory response associated with bubble formation is something that could be suspected only after multiple episodes of undeserved DCS. Fortunately, there are many guidelines available for determining a diver's fitness, and to a large extent the risk to any individual diver depends on the type of diving he or she will be doing.

A helpful strategy for quickly assessing a diver's risk is simply to review the medications the diver has taken recently. Certain medications are not recommended during diving, but, more importantly, some drugs signal the presence of medical or psychological conditions that should be taken into account when clearing someone for diving. **Table 11.1** lists potentially problematic drug classes along with specific problems encountered in each class. The author has used this table for a number of years at the National Oceanic and Atmospheric Administration (NOAA) Physicians Training Course in Undersea and Hyperbaric Medicine lecture on the effect of medications and diving.

If a diver has normal exercise tolerance for age, a normal pulmonary function test with no evidence of significant reversible obstruction, low risk of heart disease, and no evidence of diabetes or other chronic or debilitating diseases, then you are well on the way to granting unrestricted clearance. A diver's psychological profile should be included in your assessment; the diver should not have a history of disabling anxiety, psychosis, or suicidal ideation. Psychological fitness to dive is much more difficult to define in some individuals, and occasionally it is necessary to get clearance from a mental health provider when unsure of the diver's safety in the water. Of course, the diver should not be taking any significantly problematic medications.

Some dive resorts provide appropriate warnings regarding possible dangers encountered while diving at the resort, but more often than not it is difficult to actually obtain

TABLE 11.1 Various Drugs and Their Effects on Diving

Class of Drugs	Drug Effects Adverse to Diving
Anticoagulants	Hemorrhage from barotrauma or spinal DCS
Narcotics, marijuana, and alcohol	Impaired judgment and problem solving; aggravation of nitrogen narcosis
Tranquilizers	Impaired judgment and problem solving; aggravation of nitrogen narcosis
Antidepressants	Risk of seizures with bupropion (Wellbrin)
Decongestants and antihistamines	Sleepiness and nasal rebound congestion; risk of ear barotrauma and oxygen toxicity with pseudoephedrine (Sudafed)
Motion-sickness drugs	Sedation, impaired judgment, and aggravation of nitrogen narcosis
Beta-blockers	Reduced ability to respond to needs of stress; aggravation of Raynaud phenomenon and asthma
Antimalarials	Mefloquine (Lariam) psychological and neurological side effects are similar to symptoms of DCS. Doxycycline causes disabling photosensitivity
Sympathomimetics	Amphetamines, methylphenidate, and, to a lesser extent, pseudoephedrine (CNS stimulants) increase risk of CNS oxygen toxicity. Amphetamines can distort or amplify self-confidence (grandiosity) or increase risk of panic during frightening narcosis.

CNS, Central nervous system; *DCS*, decompression sickness.

up-to-date information. Some resorts suppress bad or conflicting news so as not to deter potential customers. It is well known that the Centers for Disease Control (cdc.gov) offers advice regarding food and water precautions and malaria prophylaxis, but it is more difficult to get information regarding in-water hazards such as serious marine envenomation, which is the fourth highest cause of dive injury as reported by DAN. Assessing the safety of dive sites for the beginner, disabled, or older diver is not possible until the diver is actually at the location. To stay up-to-date on a host of other dive safety issues, it is useful to have access to the monthly DAN newsletter, *Safety Stop*. Another monthly publication, *Undercurrent* (www.undercurrent.org), is probably the best source for this type of information and has a large, searchable database online with specific information about most dive resorts. There is also region-specific jellyfish information, constantly updated with an online database for Mediterranean waters, that is free for all interested users: the CIESM Jellywatch Program (www.ciesm.org/marine/programs/jellywatch.htm). The Commission Internationale pour l'Exploration Scientifique de la Mer Méditerranée, or simply the Mediterranean Science Commission, is an intergovernmental body with 23 member states that border the Mediterranean coast; using Jellywatch anyone can easily track population blooms of stinging jellyfish in a region of interest during a specified period of time. This is quite significant in light of fatal or severely disfiguring aquatic envenomation from jellyfish such as the Sea Nettle and the Box Jellyfish to name a few.

I find it valuable to remind travelers about dive accident insurance and travel insurance before the trip. Dive accident insurance can be literally purchased at the last minute from several sources, but this is not the case with travel insurance. Just to remind you, if a dive accident were to occur, especially if hospitalization, hyperbaric treatment, and a pressurized air ambulance is needed, the cost would be in the hundreds of thousands of dollars. Travel insurance is also useful to have, as it is not unusual for travel to an exotic dive location to cost many thousands of dollars. Divers often do not recognize that once the first arrangement for a trip has been made, whether a payment is involved or not, that day becomes what the insurance industry terms "the deposit date." Travel insurance needs to be purchased immediately once the first arrangement has been made or else it is often simply not available.

An up-to-date diver's first-aid kit is highly recommended, especially when diving in remote locations. This is a fairly comprehensive list; the actual contents needed may vary depending on where the diving will take place. The following items are recommended (★ indicates items that requires doctor's prescription):

1. Concise medical problem list of the individual diver for emergency use (with emergency phone numbers)
2. Assortment of water-resistant generic adhesive dressings, moleskin, chlorhexidine 4% surgical soap, 2-inch-wide elastic bandage, mupirocin★ ointment, folding scissors
3. White wine vinegar and disposable razor for jellyfish stings
4. Prophylactic eardrops for swimmer's ear (otitis externa) containing acetic acid 2% (many over-the-counter products are available for this). Drops are best applied before and after a day of diving, as long as the drops are allowed to stay in the ear for a contact time of 5 minutes
5. Neomycin★, polymyxin B, hydrocortisone generic otic drops or ofloxacin otic★ for treatment of swimmer's ear
6. Melatonin for jet lag (circadian rhythm sleep disorder)
7. Loperamide for traveler's diarrhea. Azithromycin★ (for treatment of severe symptoms or infection)
8. Sunscreen with sun protection factor (SPF) 15 for normal sun sensitivity and SPF 30 or above for those unusually sensitive to the sun or who have a history of skin cancer (reapply often if swimming)
9. Insect repellent containing greater than 35% N,N-diethyl-meta-toluamide (DEET) or CDC recommended equivalent. Reapply three times a day
10. Hand sanitizer
11. Personal medications and 1% hydrocortisone ointment or stronger if allergic reaction to bug bites have occurred in the past. Consider acetaminophen and diphenhydramine
12. Birth control (condoms).

PREVENTION OF SWIMMER'S EAR (OTITIS EXTERNA)

Swimmer's ear is a very painful bacterial infection of the external auditory canal. It occurs suddenly and progresses rapidly in swimmers and divers. It can be caused by swimming in polluted waters, but the most crucial factor is maceration of the external ear epithelium caused by constant moisture, breaking down the skin barrier to infection. Infections are usually caused by *Pseudomonas aeruginosa* (the most common pathogen), although many different organisms can contribute to ear inflammation, including fungi.

The person who gets all the credit for devising a workable prophylactic strategy for swimmer's ear is Dr. Edley Jones, who was a YMCA summer camp physician who noticed this condition occurring in his camp swimmers in the 1920s. Dr. Jones found that 5% acetic acid in 85% isopropyl alcohol worked well to inhibit pathogenic bacterial growth as long as a contact time in the ear of 5 minutes was maintained prior to swimming. This was reported in 1971 and provides us with the gold standard prophylaxis for swimmer's ear we use today. The Navy adopted Dr. Jones' technique utilizing a 2% acetic acid solution (pH of 3.0) and found that this mixture dropped the ear canal pH to 4-5 and confirmed that this level of acidity (applied over 5 minutes) was bactericidal to *Pseudomonas*. Straight white wine vinegar alone is too irritating to be used on external ear tissues by itself, but in the absence of commercial products, a 50/50 mixture of vinegar in isopropyl alcohol should work well. The key to success is a 5-minute contact time.

RECREATIONAL DIVING

Scuba diving is a demanding sport, and the underwater environment is unforgiving. This is why training in local waters (before travel) with fully certified dive classes utilizing local dive instructors and with opportunity to learn skills such as buoyancy control critical for dive safety is recommended. Resort courses are usually short, introductory sessions that rarely provide the training necessary for a diver to respond to unexpected emergencies. Learning how to manage gear problems, gas consumption, effective underwater communications, and emergency ascent techniques takes time and takes practice to perfect. As long as everything goes according to plan, warm, clear water can be very enticing. It is the unexpected issues that one has to train for, and this is where the injuries often occur. The DAN has been keeping dive injury statistics for more than 20 years, and that database has proved to be invaluable, as it can focus attention on the most frequent and most deadly of the injuries that divers sustain. The two groups that seem to have emerged as having the most problems with diving are newly introduced divers (<10 dives) and older, more experienced divers (>60 years of age). Of the medical problems that can be predicted and prevented, heart disease stands out as the most glaring example of a preventable tragedy. A cardiac event underwater is usually fatal; in 2010 (the last year statistics were available) well over 30% of the fatalities were due to some type of coronary event (arrhythmia or infarct). The striking detail to remember is that this is often a preventable issue. Cardiac risk factors should always be assessed in every older diver.

Immersion has a large effect on the cardiovascular system, but when immersion, cold water, and exercise during a dive are combined, the effects can be dramatic and widespread. From a physiological perspective, not only is cardiac preload increased (central venous pressure increased) due to the redistribution of fluids, but also we find that cold water and exercise increase arterial tone and virtually all pulmonary pressure parameters. Dr. Richard Moon explains in his lecture entitled "Fitness to Dive and Return to Diving after an Incident" given to the Undersea and Hyperbaric Medical Society (UHMS) in 2009 that "Immersion causes a displacement of approximately 500-800 mL of blood from the legs into the central circulation. This effect is even greater during cold water immersion. If a diver's heart is unlikely to tolerate a sudden transfusion of fluid, diving and swimming should be restricted". Dr Moon goes on to say that a diver must have clean coronary arteries and an ejection fraction greater than 40% to be declared fit to return to diving after myocardial infarction (MI).

BAROTRAUMA

The most common preventable injury while diving is middle-ear barotrauma. A middle-ear squeeze will curtail all diving activities and even make the trip home painful. It is not well appreciated, but hearing may be permanently impacted. In the worst-case scenario, permanent hearing loss and vertigo can ensue, and if the injured diver is also a musician, the impact on hearing can easily impair professional musical ability. With few exceptions musicians are not warned that permanent, irreversible high-frequency hearing loss could occur with a single diving mistake. Armed with this knowledge, a travel medicine consultation should include examination of the ears and verification that the diver knows how to compensate for the pressure he or she will be experiencing during a dive.

Boyle's law describes the pressure–volume relationship affecting a diver on descent. Simply stated, pressure and volume of a gas are inversely related. When descending in the water at the beginning of a dive, pressure increases in a linear fashion. At the same time, the volume of that gas in a closed space such as the middle ear or a sinus is compressed in a linear but inverse fashion. This pressure–volume relationship is most significant in the first 33 fsw, as the magnitude of volume change in a closed space is one-half at a depth of 33 ft and is half again at 66 ft. Every 33 ft the remaining volume in a closed air space decreases by half unless the diver finds a way to compensate for this volume change as pressure increases. Novice divers usually underestimate the effect of Boyle's law, and severe middle-ear injuries can occur even while training in a swimming pool.

The volume change under pressure occurs in all closed spaces of the body. This includes sinuses and even under dental fillings and caps if airspace is present. This effect is particularly devastating in facial sinuses. If effective equalization of pressure does not occur, that volume change becomes excruciating for the diver. If the airspace gradually equalizes in a sinus during a dive but causes bleeding and swelling, then when the diver attempts to ascend the volume expansion becomes excruciating in the reverse direction. This is termed a "ball-valve" effect (also known as one-way valve) and will prevent air from leaving the sinus altogether. Facial bones can become grotesquely swollen in some unfortunate individuals. The diver is then experiencing what is termed "reverse block" as air expands at the end of the dive. "Reverse block" can be so painful it becomes debilitating. The effect can last minutes, hours, and, in some cases, weeks. This condition requires specialty consultation and, if medical treatment is ineffective, occasionally surgical correction of enlarged turbinates to avoid recurrences.

During a pre-dive physical examination the physician should look in the ear and directly visualize the tympanic membrane with an otoscope. If cerumen is present, blocking the view of the tympanic membrane, it should be removed. The patient should be asked to "pop" the ears. If the patient instinctively pinches the nose, building up a modest amount of pressure in the nasopharynx, and the tympanic membrane bulges out slightly as seen with an otoscope, this change in appearance signals a successful Valsalva maneuver and should be recorded in the chart as (+) Valsalva.

The Valsalva technique is easy and intuitive for most people, but there are many ways it can be done incorrectly. A moderate amount of pressure is first built up in the chest. Fingers keep the air from escaping through pinched nostrils. If the soft palate is not preventing the air pressure from reaching the nasopharynx, the pressure will also be transmitted to the soft tissues of the nose. A slight bulge of the nose can be visualized if the procedure is performed correctly. A Valsalva maneuver should be a short maneuver with a moderately quick upstroke of pressure to the opening pressure of the eustachian tube. It is held for a second to allow the tissues of the eustachian tube to dilate, and then the pressure should be allowed to escape as the middle ear returns to ambient pressure. If the pressure builds up too quickly, the lumen of the eustachian tube often will not have time to dilate. If the pressure is held too long, venous engorgement of the middle ear can occur, and diminished cardiac return of venous blood to the heart is well documented, lowering the cardiac output and blood pressure.

A Valsalva maneuver can be safely performed only when the ear is not squeezed by pressure. It is very safe to use as a pre-pressurization technique, but dangerous once a squeeze has occurred. If a middle-ear squeeze is present, a forceful Valsalva maneuver can create an "air-hammer" effect. Delicate tissues such as the round window and the hair cells of the cochlea can be damaged with this forceful maneuver. Interestingly, the reverse situation is most often the cause of ear injury while diving. Instead of trying too hard, a timid diver may never generate enough pressure to open the eustachian tube under any circumstances, and that is why visualization of the tympanic membrane movement is essential to verify adequacy of middle-ear pressurization. There are so many ways to perform the Valsalva incorrectly that I call it the "Much Maligned Valsalva."

Luckily, there are many other ways to compensate for pressure changes while diving, and most of these are much safer to perform. It is actually quite rare for a diver to truly be unable to equalize pressure with any technique. I estimate that as many as two-thirds of new divers are able to pressurize their middle ear effortlessly without specific training once they are informed of the need to do so. For those individuals, merely puffing into a snuggly fitted diver's face mask or gently puffing with pinched nostrils will do the trick. Those individuals rarely get in trouble with ear squeeze, but for the other recreational divers who do have difficulty equalizing, help will be needed. Middle-ear pressurization can be challenging, and for those divers, equalization techniques must be tailored to the individual. Swallowing is a good, simple, and safe technique that often helps the diver equalize pressure to the middle ears, but side effects occasionally limit the usefulness, as a diver can swallow large amounts of air. When pressurization alone is ineffective, it can be combined with another method such as swallow, yawn, or maximal jaw thrust to enable air flow through the eustachian tube. Once an effective technique has been found, the diver should be encouraged to practice it several times a day. I always encourage new divers to listen to the sounds that their ears make with various maneuvers. This simple form of biofeedback will help a novice diver perfect the technique before he or she damages their ears in the pool.

TABLE 11.2 Ear-Clearing Techniques[a]

	Valsalva	Frenzel	Toynbee	BTV[b]
Nose	Pinched	Pinched	Pinched	No restriction
Mouth	Closed	No restriction	Closed	No restriction
Glottis	Opened	Closed	Closed	No restriction
Action	Puff in the nose	Throat piston	Swallow	Tubal opening
Air Flow	Active	Active	Passive	Passive
Result	Overpressure from lungs	Overpressure from nasopharynx	Sinusoidal pressure changes	Balanced pressure
Achievement	Easy	Moderate	Easy	Difficult
Safety	Danger	Good	Good	Excellent
Complications	Hypotension, tympanic membrane or round window rupture	None	Flatus	None

[a]This table first appeared in the French language journal referenced below. Translation is provided along with additional information on risks associated with each technique for middle-ear equalization.
[b]Béance tubaire volontaire (BTV) was first described by G. Delonca in Prévention des accidents: la plongée santé-sécurité [Prevention of Accidents: Diving Safety and Health, FRUCTUS (X) / SCIARLI (R), Publisher: Atlantic 1980 1980, p.118.

The faint clicking sound heard during swallowing is caused by the moist membranes of the eustachian tube separating as the tube dilates. Hearing that clicking sound and voluntarily manipulating the sound is what may be termed developing "eustachian tube awareness." New divers who have trouble equalizing can also practice tubal aerobics as described in the *Manual of Freediving* by Pelizzari and Tovaglieri. The exercise techniques described are designed to improve awareness and control of the eustachian tube and middle ear.

In all cases, pre-pressurization of the middle ear is far superior to "clear as you go" techniques. This is especially true for the diver who is a bit squeamish and reluctant to adequately pressurize the middle ear. One of the worst things that can happen to a diver while equalizing is a round window rupture (inner ear barotrauma), also known as a labyrinthine fistula. If the diver does not seek prompt remediation or if the diagnosis is not made promptly, permanent vertigo and hearing loss can ensue. Verification of an adequate ear-clearing technique (middle-ear pressurization) is a requirement for any type of dive physical examination.

There are volumes written about ear-clearing techniques. **Table 11.2** is provided as a baseline. It underscores the multitude of possible techniques for ear-pressure equalization while diving. The technique chosen must always be optimized for the diver who has trouble clearing his or her ears.

Not everyone is comfortable performing a Valsalva maneuver. I call this phenomenon "ear fear," and it is often caused by memory of painful events in the past, perhaps an episode of otitis. To fully understand what is happening, attention must be paid to the effort displayed by the diver while attempting to pressurize the ears. Some individuals will grimace and struggle in a manner that I call the "excessive effort sign." No matter how hard they try, no pressure reaches the soft tissues of the nose or middle ear. Another tipoff that the individual is not performing a Valsalva maneuver correctly is to look for what I call the "Dizzy Gillespie sign." If a diver's cheeks are bulging but the nose is not, the diver is involuntarily blocking pressure from reaching the opening of eustachian tubes in the nasopharynx. A reluctance to build up adequate pressure in the nasopharynx can also be caused by retrograde inflation of the lower tear duct. This inflation usually causes an itchy, fizzing sensation as air bubbles exit through the lacrimal puncta of the lower lid. The diver is usually concerned that this will somehow cause an infection or simply does not like the sensation. Retrograde inflation of the tear duct is totally harmless, except that it is one of the causes of "ear fear"; this anxiety while pressurizing almost always leads to a middle-ear squeeze.

The astute provider will also occasionally note rather dramatic expressions that accompany successful inflation of the middle ear. If the person wrinkles his or her nose in disgust or shakes the head from side to side with a sad or angry expression, exclaiming, "I hate that!" you will have a better understanding of their risks of barotrauma. If they hate the feeling of middle-ear pressurization, it is unlikely that they will generate enough pressure to prevent middle-ear barotrauma. Worse yet, they may decide to forcefully pressurize while the squeeze is present and thus set up the necessary conditions for inner-ear barotrauma (round window rupture). Most providers who recognize this will simply tell the traveler not to dive rather than spend the time necessary to teach the proper technique.

Another technique that I call the "throat piston" is formally known as the Frenzel maneuver and was developed during World War II to help dive-bomber pilots equalize their ears while preparing to release their munitions on a bombing run. In this technique, the larynx and tongue can be turned into a "piston" and used to pressurize air in the nasopharynx. The diver must first gain control of the larynx, voluntarily moving it up and down at will. This can be first achieved with vocalization and easily practiced in a repetitive manner while watching in a mirror. Bobbing the thyroid cartilage (Adam's apple) up and down while the nose is pinched closed is a good way to learn the technique.

The most challenging technique, béance tubaire volontaire (voluntary tubal opening), was first reported by the French diver Georges Delonca. Some divers seem to be anatomically gifted with control over the tissues in the back of the throat and the soft palate. Those divers can voluntarily raise the soft palate so that the uvula almost completely disappears upward. At the same time the diver must tense the tongue so as to create a solid base in the back of the throat that can then be used to tug on nasopharyngeal tissues. A natural yawn can accomplish the same thing—opening the eustachian tube orifice—but the yawn itself is too prolonged and cumbersome to be functionally useful while diving. Commercial divers can develop the ability to perform this maneuver by first thrusting the jaw forward in a maximal manner while tensing the tongue and opening the back of the throat. Practicing the maneuver can be accomplished if one rides an elevator in a tall building up and down, gradually gaining control through repetition.

Sinus barotrauma also occurs, but for different reasons. Unlike the middle ears, which are constantly drained and pressure equalized by the undulating motion of the eustachian tube, the sinus ostia are fixed openings buried underneath the turbinates. It is through these ostia that ventilation of the sinuses is accomplished. Turbinate hypertrophy can be due to chronic allergies or anatomical distortion from a deviated sinus, and there might not be an adequate opening for equalization of the sinus to occur. Chronic nasal congestion, chronic allergies, frequent sinus infections, or previous facial fractures are all risk factors. Unfortunately there is no easy way to tell whether air will move easily into and out of a sinus. This is why the novice diver should always be trained in local waters to ensure adequate supervision. If a diver has never had sinus problems and can clear ears and sinuses easily with air travel, it is not likely that he or she will have a problem, but it still can occur. Nasal decongestants should never be used at the start of a dive vacation. Decongestants such as oxymetazoline have a rebound effect, termed "tachyphylaxis." This means the drug will last for shorter and shorter durations, and intranasal tissues will become engorged (hypercongestion) much more rapidly when the drug wears off. If necessary to ensure that a diver can travel safely on the homeward leg of a vacation, it is certainly acceptable to use a generous amount of oxymetazoline (only for the trip home), but it never should be used at the start of a dive vacation. Chronic use of nasal decongestants will result in permanent changes in the nasal mucosa. The natural vasoactive signals of nasal mucosa gradually become lost by chronic decongestant use. Mild chronic intranasal and turbinate hypertrophy can be dealt with by using intranasal corticosteroids but at times require surgical intervention. Fortunately we now have office procedures such as radiofrequency tissue reduction (somnoplasty) to shrink tissues with relatively short healing time.

AFTER THE TRIP

A diver returning from a tropical dive vacation will occasionally have coral abrasions that are slow to heal or painful sea urchin punctures. Recalcitrant infections can occur, as the ocean is full of opportunistic bacteria. The incidence of multidrug-resistant bacterial infections is on the rise, and it is prudent to culture any infection in a diver. Treat any injury in the water with caution and follow up closely until it is clear that the condition is under control. If there is no improvement, prompt referral to a dermatologist is warranted.

Stings and scratches that burn should be treated on-site with full-strength vinegar as soon as the injury occurs. Jellyfish tentacles have stinging cells (nematocysts) but jellyfish stings due to the occasional encounter with floating jellyfish debris are usually simply an annoyance. Unfortunately, some very small jellyfish carry very potent venom. The most potent and dangerous of these are the box jellyfish: in particular, Irukandji. If one encounters these miniscule jellyfish, a characteristic syndrome will occur that usually results in hospitalization of the diver. Symptoms include severe headache, backache, muscle pains, chest and abdominal pain, nausea and vomiting, sweating, hypertension, and extreme pain characterized by the sensation that your skin is being ripped off. Local information on jellyfish risks will help a diver stay out of trouble, but as the waters of the earth warm, the distribution of tropical species of all types will continue to change; that change has already started. In the future, changes to venomous jellyfish habitat may be more widespread.

Invasive species of fish are also a problem for the diver, as lionfish are now present in all of the world's oceans. A puncture from the poisonous spines of a lionfish causes acute pain and local swelling, occasionally causing systemic symptoms. The site of envenomation can be treated with applications of very hot water, but this should be applied promptly if it is to be effective. Heat denatures the poison delivered by the lionfish via thermolysis, but the hot water must be just below scalding, approximately 113-114°F for it to be of any use. Often this either is not available on the dive boat or is too dangerous to be safe. Weakness, vomiting, shortness of breath, or loss of consciousness may require immediate stabilizing measures. More extensive blistering wounds will require topical antiseptics such as silver sulfadiazine, bacitracin, or mupirocin ointment, along with dressing changes. Large wounds from a lionfish may require months to heal.

For those interested in pursuing a career in diving medicine, it is best to start with a strong foundation in your chosen medical field. Internal medicine or family medicine are excellent choices, but there is no one approved pathway. For dive medical training, start with a four-day introductory course. Several of these are available from well-known providers, variously called either "fitness for diving" or "fitness to dive." The best (most comprehensive) civilian course is actually a 2-week training course called Physician Training in Diving and Hyperbaric Medicine, held every year by NOAA. The Navy has a pathway for the Diving Medical Officer in the Submarine Service for those so inclined. Ongoing physician education is crucial, as the pace of scientific advances in the field is often mind boggling. For this, the Undersea and Hyperbaric Medical Society (UHMS) offers a yearly scientific meeting where exchange of ideas flows freely. Duke University offers a fellowship in hyperbaric medicine, which is highly desirable for a physician who is just starting out in his or her professional career. This combination of a solid scientific foundation in diving medicine coupled with regular updates when new science is available makes this field challenging and rewarding. The UHMS website (UHMS.org) has all the information a provider might need in terms of educational opportunities.

FURTHER READING

Anderson, B., Farmer, J.C., 1978. Hyperoxic myopia. Trans. Am. Ophthalmol. Soc. 76, 116–124.
Recommended as the original reference describing the effects of high partial pressure oxygen on the eye.

Bennett, M.H., Lehm, J.P., Mitchell, S.J., et al., 2012. Recompression and adjunctive therapy for decompression illness. Cochrane Database Syst. Rev. 5, CD005277.
Recommended state-of-the-art evidence-based review of treatment options for decompression sickness.

Brubakk, A.O., Neuman, T., Bennett, P., et al., 2003. Physiology and Medicine of Diving, fifth ed. Saunders, Edinburgh.
Highly recommended as the preferred desktop reference manual for dive-related medical issues.

Brubakk, A.O., Ross, J.A.S., Thom, S.R., 2014. Saturation diving; physiology and pathophysiology. Compr. Physiol. 4, 1229–1272.
Recommended as an excellent in-depth review of diving physiology.

Chandy, D., Weinhouse, G.L., 2015. Complications of Scuba Diving. Available at <UpToDate.com>.
Recommended as a description of the state-of-the-art approach to the complications of SCUBA diving.

Delonca, G., 1980. Prévention des accidents: La plongée santé-sécurité, FRUCTUS (X) / SCIARLI (R), Edité par Editions Maritimes et d'Outremer, 1980, Translated to English: Health and Safety of Diving, FRUCTUS (X) / SCIARLI (R), Publisher: Atlantic Publishing 1980 [Prevention of Accidents: Diving Safety and Health], 116–118.
In French. Recommended as the original description of the French method of equalizing middle-ear pressure while diving, béance tubaire volontaire (voluntary tubal opening).

Farmer, J.C. Jr., 1985. Eustachian tube function and otologic barotrauma. Ann. Otol. Rhinol. Laryngol. 120, 45.
Recommended, as Dr. Farmer was the original physician who described and categorized middle-ear barotrauma.

Hardy, K.R., 1997. Diving-related emergencies. Emerg. Med. Clin. North Am. 15, 223–240.
Recommended for its comprehensive handling of the various emergencies that can present while diving.

Isbister, G.K., 2014. Marine envenomation from corals, sea urchins, fish, or stingrays. Available at <UpToDate.com>.
Recommended as a description of the state-of-the-art knowledge concerning marine envenomation.

Marcus, E.N., Isbister, G.K., 2014. Jellyfish stings. Available at <UpToDate.com>.
Recommended as a description of the state-of-the-art knowledge concerning jellyfish stings.

Moon, R.E., Vann, R.D., Bennett, P.B., 1995. The physiology of decompression illness. Sci. Am. 273, 70.
Recommended as an excellent review of the issues regarding the physiology of decompression sickness.

National Oceanic and Atmospheric Administration (NOAA), 2013. Diving Manual, fifth ed. US Department of Commerce, Best Publishing Company (Author), NOAA Diving Office (Editor), 5th edition.
Excellent resource for up-to-date technical issues regarding commercial and military diving. This is complementary to the US Navy Diving Manual.

Neblett, L.M., 1985. Otolaryngology and sport scuba diving. Update and guidelines. Ann. Otol. Rhinol. Laryngol. Suppl. 115, 1–12.
Recommended as an excellent reference for ear and sinus barotrauma.

Nevo, B., Breitstein, S., Psychological and Behavioral Aspects of Diving. Best Publishing Co 1999.
Recommended as a review of the psychological aspects pertinent to the diver's behavior in the water.

Pelizzari, U., Tovaglieri, S., 2004. Manual of Freediving: Underwater on a Single Breath. Idelson-Gnochi, Reddick, FL.
Recommended as a detailed and comprehensive guide for anyone who wants to understand breath-hold diving. Specific chapters outline valuable techniques that can be found nowhere else but in this manual.

Roydhouse, N., 1993. Underwater Ear and Nose Care. Best Publishing, Flagstaff, AZ.

Recommended as an excellent introduction to the various techniques a diver may use to equalize middle-ear pressure.

Tetzlaff, K., Muth, C.M., Waldhauser, L.K., 2002. A review of asthma and scuba diving. J. Asthma 39, 557–566.
Recommended for understanding the additional risks associated with diving with reversible airway disease (asthma).

Undercurrent Newsletter. <http://www.undercurrent.org/>.
Recommended as the highly acclaimed source of up-to-date information regarding dive hazards and fatality statistics. This newsletter often contains information that is not available anywhere else on the Internet regarding a diver's health and safety.

US Department of the Navy, 2011. U.S. Navy Diving Manual, Rev 6. Available at <http://www .supsalv.org/00c3_publications.asp>.
Recommended as the Bible of current military diving techniques, often used in commercial diving and often referred to as the gold standard of technical data.

Wienke, B., 2008. Diving Physics with Bubble Mechanics and Decompression Theory in Depth. Best Publishing, Flagstaff, AZ.
Recommended as an in-depth review of the physics and physical properties of decompression sickness.

Wurtman, R., 2013. Physiology and Clinical Use of Melatonin. Available at <UpToDate.com>.

CHAPTER 12

Travel Advice for Pediatric Travelers

Sheila M. Mackell

Pediatric travelers present unique challenges to the travel medicine provider. Each facet of travel medicine has special caveats relating to the different developmental stages, sizes, and maturity levels of the infant, child, or adolescent traveler. In addition, children traveling to any destination require attention to basic pediatric issues. The pre-travel consultation provides an opportunity to highlight specific travel medicine issues and vulnerabilities in the pediatric population.

DEVELOPMENTAL ASPECTS AND TRAVEL

A journey with a child presents many opportunities and challenges. Travel with children opens many doors for cultural experiences that would not be readily available otherwise. Newborns can be easily transported; their schedules are easily adjusted to time zone changes; and they can be protected from many environmental and dietary risks of travel. Children thrive on routine. Toddlers are often the most challenging age. Their mobility presents safety and infectious exposure issues. They are more vulnerable to diarrhea due to hygiene and oral-fecal contact. Toddlers should be carefully labeled with identification that is carried in a waistpack or affixed to their clothing. The child's name, birth date, citizenship, and passport number should be included, along with the telephone number and address of the appropriate consulate or embassy in the destination country. An active, curious toddler can easily wander off in a crowded airport, train station, or market. The use of a chest harness on the child with a tether to an accompanying parent or adult is strongly recommended. Toilet training may be interrupted when a change in routine occurs. Lowering adult expectations of traveling toddlers is wise. Older children may be reluctant to use unfamiliar toilets, so carrying an extra change of clothing and toddler pants is recommended. Using the toilet on the airplane just before de-planing avoids the problem of unavailability or phobia of facilities in overseas terminals. Diaper availability may be limited in some developing countries. Diaper liners can be helpful for disposal of stool when in remote locations. Advise families traveling to Africa about the tumbu fly. Cloth diapers dried in the sun can have fly eggs deposited on them and later result in larval myiasis when used. Although work intensive, ironing cloth diapers and other articles of clothing dried in the sun will kill the eggs and ensure safety.

School-aged children need education about safety and traffic concerns. They should be aware of dangers of animal encounters such as bites, licks, or scratches and instructed to report any contact to a parent. The unfamiliar environment may be particularly challenging to certain youngsters. Bringing along familiar toys, blankets, or books from home may be comforting.

Traveling high school and college students are addressed in Chapter 13.

165

AIRLINE TRAVEL

Occupying children with activities during long airplane flights is intuitive for most parents. Pens, paper, playing cards, and books are essential elements of the carry-on bag. Water and snacks are helpful to have during long waits in hot airline terminals and can salvage difficult delays in customs terminals. Special meals can be ordered ahead of time for children when planning an airplane flight.

Airline regulations vary regarding children traveling alone on planes. Generally, children <5 years old are not permitted to travel unaccompanied by an adult. The child's age and maturity level should be taken into account when considering whether to send him or her alone. Nonstop flights are preferable, and contingency plans should be set up in case delays or cancellations occur. Special passes may be obtained at airline ticket counters for parents to accompany their minor child to the departure gate through security. The child should be comfortable with requesting help from the flight attendants and be told what to expect during a normal flight. Education on personal and stranger safety issues is best reinforced at this time.

Children under 40 pounds are safest in airplanes if riding in an approved child restraint system. Though not required, the Federal Aviation Administration (FAA) strongly recommends their use. Holding young children on the lap or buckling them in the same seat belt as the adult carrying them is hazardous during severe turbulence, rough landings, and crash situations. Federal safety standards have found that all child restraint seats manufactured after January 1, 1981 adequately protect children under 40 pounds on an airplane. A sticker stating that all applicable FAA standards have been met for airplane travel identifies appropriate seats. Child restraint systems without this sticker are not allowed on the plane. The airline's infant-seat policy should be checked at the time reservations are made. Some airlines offer discounted seats for children using restraint systems. Choosing off-peak flights may improve the chances of getting a free individual seat for the child or infant, but purchasing a full seat is the only guarantee.

Otitis media is not a contraindication to air travel. Tympanic membrane rupture is not a reported complication of flying in aircraft. Barotrauma is a theoretical concern when middle-ear equilibration fails. Have the child or infant swallow during ascent and, particularly, descent to help the eustachian tube equilibrate the middle ear. A pacifier may help the infant with equilibration. Older children can be taught pressure equalization techniques such as the Valsalva maneuver to relieve the discomfort of middle-ear pressure. Administering an antihistamine before the flight may help some children, but its benefit has not been conclusively reported.

Advice on sedating children with a weight-appropriate dose of over-the-counter antihistamine may be requested by the parent(s) and can be done as close to actual take-off time as possible. Paradoxical reactions to antihistamines occur in a small percentage of children and are best discovered at home, before the plane trip. Prescription sedatives should be avoided. An unanticipated side effect, such as respiratory depression, can be much more serious in-flight, where medical care is unavailable.

Past recommendations have suggested that infants <6 weeks old should not travel by air. No data exist to support the restriction of healthy infants flying on airplanes. The avoidance of infectious diseases between birth and 2 months old is of prime concern to parents and healthcare providers, as fever in a neonate <2 months old requires urgent medical evaluation at home or while traveling.

There is an expanding market of travel-related gear for children and their parents, from child-sized neck pillows to inflatable potties to breast pump backpacks. Convertible airplane-ready strollers that roll down aisles easily, then convert to car seats and, later, feeding booster seats make travel more convenient than in the past. Most vendors are easily located on the Internet. While electronic devices (DVD and MP3 players and handheld games) are useful entertainers at times, the battery requirements and electrical incompatibility may limit their overall usefulness during prolonged trips abroad.

TABLE 12.1 Medications for Motion Sickness		
	Dose	Comments
Over-the-counter		
Diphenhydramine	5 mg/kg per day p.o. divided q.i.d.	Strong sedative effect; available in liquid form
Dimenhydrinate	2-5 years: 12.5-25 mg p.o. t.i.d., to maximum 75 mg/day	Available in liquid form
	6-12 years: 25-50 mg p.o. t.i.d., to max. 150 mg/day	
	>12 years: 50 mg p.o. t.i.d. –q.i.d. Adult maximum: 400 mg/day	
Meclizine	>12 years: 25-50 mg p.o. once daily	Chewable tablet
Prescription		
Scopolamine (Transderm-Scop) 1.5-mg patch	>12 years: 1.5-mg patch behind the ear every 3 days	Apply at least 4 h before expected symptoms; wash hands after applying; do not cut patch
Promethazine	>2 years: 0.5 mg/kg per dose p.o. q12 h p.r.n.; max 25 mg/dose	Good for severe symptoms; may cause profound sedation. Do not use with other respiratory depressants. Contraindicated for those <2 years.

p.o., By mouth; *p.r.n,* as needed; *q.i.d.,* four times per day; *t.i.d.,* three times per day.

MOTION SICKNESS

Children suffering from motion sickness present particular challenges to mobile families. Nonpharmacologic treatment includes sitting susceptible children beside a window, facing forward, and avoiding heavy meals before travel. Wearing dark glasses and traveling at night may also reduce symptoms. Ginger preparations have not been tested in children.

Acceptable and safe medications for motion sickness in children are listed in **Table 12.1**. Over-the-counter preparations will usually suffice for mild to moderate symptoms. The use of promethazine should be reserved for children over 2 years with severe symptoms. Any of these medications are best given 1 hour before the anticipated symptoms occur.

VACCINE SCHEDULES FOR INFANTS AND CHILDREN

Immunization against common vaccine-preventable diseases occurs routinely throughout the first 24 months of life and mirrors routine pediatric health supervision visits. Routine vaccination schedules have changed yearly or more in the past 10 years. In the United States, the varicella vaccine is recommended for all children at 12 months of age and older. The measles, mumps, rubella (MMR) vaccine is recommended at 12 months. It can be administered to infants between 6 and 12 months in outbreak situations and for those whose travel itinerary poses risk. Second doses of both MMR and varicella vaccines are routine at 4-6 years of age. The second dose of MMR vaccine can be given as soon as 1 month after the first dose. The second dose of varicella vaccine can be given 3 months after the first dose if indicated. The injectable inactivated polio vaccination series has been in use in the United States since 2000. The 13-valent pneumococcal conjugate vaccine is recommended for infants and children 2-23 months of age and other defined older at-risk groups. Influenza vaccination is routinely recommended for all children older than 6 months, regardless of travel plans. Meningococcal meningitis conjugate vaccine is routinely recommended at age 11-12 years, with a booster 5 yrs after the first dose. Licensure of the conjugate vaccine has been extended down to 9 months of age if a travel indication exists. An adolescent booster for both tetanus and pertussis is given at age 10-11 years. The reduced pertussis/tetanus/diphtheria vaccine (Tdap) is given if 5 years have elapsed from the last tetanus shot. Further tetanus boosters should be given as Td (tetanus and diphtheria). Conjugate meningococcal vaccine, if indicated, is best administered at the same time as Tdap. Vaccinations against multiple strains of human papilloma virus (HPV) known to cause cervical cancer are available and recommended routinely in a two- or three-dose series (0, 2, and 6 months) for girls >11 years. Some are also licensed for use in males >11 years to prevent HPV genital infection.

Minor febrile illnesses are not a contraindication to any of the routine vaccines. Simultaneous administration of vaccines is acceptable and does not diminish antibody response. Give live viral vaccines together or, if separate, at least 30 days apart. Current recommendations for childhood vaccination are summarized in **Figure 12.1**.

International travel increases the risk of exposure to communicable diseases. It is important for a young infant or child going abroad to receive as much protection as possible against preventable diseases. Unique vaccine considerations exist for children, which guide choices before travel. Routine vaccines may have to be given on an accelerated schedule, with recommendations for extra booster doses. An acceptable schedule for accelerating routine vaccines is found in **Table 12.2**. Some travel vaccines, such as yellow fever vaccine, have serious complications in the young infant and are not recommended until a certain age is attained (9 months for yellow fever vaccine). Other vaccines, such as meningococcal polysaccharide vaccine, are not optimally immunogenic in children <2 years old, and more effective options exist in the conjugate vaccines. Still others, such as hepatitis A, are not approved for use in children under certain ages owing to the presence of interfering maternal antibody that limits vaccine response.

Hepatitis A is usually a mild disease in children <5 years old. Children, however, can serve as reservoirs and can infect adults and caretakers. Continuing to breast-feed traveling infants offers the advantage of added gastrointestinal immunity to enteric diseases. Immunization with the hepatitis A vaccine is recommended for child travelers >1 year without pre-vaccine serology testing. Foreign-born children from developing countries may be considered for serologic testing before vaccination. Recommendations have been made from the Centers for Disease Control and Prevention (CDC) in 2006 for universal childhood

TABLE 12.2 Accelerated Routine Immunization Schedules for Pediatric Travelers[a]

Vaccine	Schedule
DTaP (Diphtheria, tetanus, and acellular pertussis)	6, 10, 14 weeks, and 6 months after dose 3
Measles, mumps, rubella (MMR)	
MMR	6-11 months of age
MMR, two doses	12 months of age, 1 month after first MMR
Inactivated polio vaccine	6, 10, and 14 weeks of age
Haemophilus influenza type B conjugate vaccine	
HbOC, PRP-T	6, 10, 14 weeks, and 12 months
Hepatitis B vaccine	0, 1, 2 months. Give a booster dose at 12 months

[a]Give as many doses as possible of a vaccine series following an accelerated schedule before departure.
HbOC, PRP-T, *Haemophilus* b conjugate.

These recommendations must be read with the footnotes that follow. For those who fall behind or start late, provide catch-up vaccination at the earliest opportunity as indicated by the green bars in Figure 1. To determine minimum intervals between doses, see the catch-up schedule (Figure 2). School entry and adolescent vaccine age groups are shaded.

Vaccine	Birth	1 mo	2 mos	4 mos	6 mos	9 mos	12 mos	15 mos	18 mos	19–23 mos	2–3 yrs	4–6 yrs	7–10 yrs	11–12 yrs	13–15 yrs	16–18 yrs
Hepatitis B[1] (HepB)	1st dose	← 2nd dose →			← 3rd dose →											
Rotavirus[2] (RV) RV1 (2-dose series); RV5 (3-dose series)			1st dose	2nd dose	See footnote 2											
Diphtheria, tetanus, & acellular pertussis[3] (DTaP: <7 yrs)			1st dose	2nd dose	3rd dose		← 4th dose →					5th dose				
Haemophilus influenzae type b[4] (Hib)			1st dose	2nd dose	See footnote 4		← 3rd or 4th dose, See footnote 4 →									
Pneumococcal conjugate[5] (PCV13)			1st dose	2nd dose	3rd dose		← 4th dose →									
Inactivated poliovirus[6] (IPV: <18 yrs)			1st dose	2nd dose	← 3rd dose →							4th dose				
Influenza[7] (IIV; LAIV)							Annual vaccination (IIV only) 1 or 2 doses				Annual vaccination (LAIV or IIV) 1 or 2 doses			Annual vaccination (LAIV or IIV) 1 dose only		
Measles, mumps, rubella[8] (MMR)					See footnote 8		← 1st dose →					2nd dose				
Varicella[9] (VAR)							← 1st dose →					2nd dose				
Hepatitis A[10] (HepA)							2-dose series, See footnote 10									
Meningococcal[11] (Hib-MenCY ≥ 6 weeks; MenACWY-D ≥9 mos; MenACWY-CRM ≥ 2 mos)					See footnote 11									1st dose		Booster
Tetanus, diphtheria, & acellular pertussis[12] (Tdap: ≥7 yrs)														(Tdap)		
Human papillomavirus[13] (2vHPV: females only; 4vHPV, 9vHPV: males and females)														(3-dose series)		
Meningococcal B[11]														See footnote 11		
Pneumococcal polysaccharide[5] (PPSV23)												See footnote 5				

Range of recommended ages for all children
Range of recommended ages for catch-up immunization
Range of recommended ages for certain high-risk groups
Range of recommended ages for non-high-risk groups that may receive vaccine, subject to individual clinical decision making
No recommendation

This schedule includes recommendations in effect as of January 1, 2016. Any dose not administered at the recommended age should be administered at a subsequent visit, when indicated and feasible. The use of a combination vaccine generally is preferred over separate injections of its equivalent component vaccines. Vaccination providers should consult the relevant Advisory Committee on Immunization Practices (ACIP) statement for detailed recommendations, available online at http://www.cdc.gov/vaccines/hcp/acip-recs/index.html. Clinically significant adverse events that follow vaccination should be reported to the Vaccine Adverse Event Reporting System (VAERS) online (http://www.vaers.hhs.gov) or by telephone (800-822-7967). Suspected cases of vaccine-preventable diseases should be reported to the state or local health department. Additional information, including precautions and contraindications for vaccination, is available from CDC online (http://www.cdc.gov/vaccines/recs/vac-admin/contraindications.htm) or by telephone (800-CDC-INFO [800-232-4636]).

This schedule is approved by the Advisory Committee on Immunization Practices (http://www.cdc.gov/vaccines/acip), the American Academy of Pediatrics (http://www.aap.org), the American Academy of Family Physicians (http://www.aafp.org), and the American College of Obstetricians and Gynecologists (http://www.acog.org).

NOTE: The above recommendations must be read along with the footnotes that follow.

Fig. 12.1 Recommended childhood and adolescent immunization schedules, United States, 2015. The tables in this figure are reproduced from the Centers for Disease Control and Prevention website. Consult the website for access to the complete footnotes. Available at http://www.cdc.gov/vaccines/schedules/hcp/imz/child-adolescent-compliant.html.

Continued

Footnotes — Recommended immunization schedule for persons aged 0 through 18 years—United States, 2016

For further guidance on the use of the vaccines mentioned below, see: http://www.cdc.gov/vaccines/hcp/acip-recs/index.html.
For vaccine recommendations for persons 19 years of age and older, see the Adult Immunization Schedule.

Additional information

- For contraindications and precautions to use of a vaccine and for additional information regarding that vaccine, vaccination providers should consult the relevant ACIP statement available online at http://www.cdc.gov/vaccines/hcp/acip-recs/index.html.
- For purposes of calculating intervals between doses, 4 weeks = 28 days. Intervals of 4 months or greater are determined by calendar months.
- Vaccine doses administered ≤4 days before the minimum interval are considered valid. Doses of any vaccine administered ≥5 days earlier than the minimum interval should not be counted as valid doses and should be repeated as age-appropriate. The repeat dose should be spaced after the invalid dose by the recommended minimum interval. For further details, see MMWR, General Recommendations on Immunization and Reports / Vol. 60 / No. 2; Table 1. Recommended and minimum ages and intervals between vaccine doses available online at http://www.cdc.gov/mmwr/pdf/rr/rr6002.pdf.
- Information on travel vaccine requirements and recommendations is available at http://www.cdc.gov/travel/destinations/list.
- For vaccination of persons with primary and secondary immunodeficiencies, see Table 13. Vaccination of persons with primary and secondary immunodeficiencies, in General Recommendations on Immunization (ACIP), available at http://www.cdc.gov/mmwr/pdf/rr/rr6002.pdf; and American Academy of Pediatrics. "Immunization in Special Clinical Circumstances," in Kimberlin DW, Brady MT, Jackson MA, Long SS eds, Red Book: 2015 report of the Committee on Infectious Diseases. 30th ed. Elk Grove Village, IL: American Academy of Pediatrics.

1. Hepatitis B (HepB) vaccine. (Minimum age: birth)

Routine vaccination:

At birth:
- Administer monovalent HepB vaccine to all newborns before hospital discharge.
- For infants born to hepatitis B surface antigen (HBsAg)-positive mothers, administer HepB vaccine and 0.5 mL of hepatitis B immune globulin (HBIG) within 12 hours of birth. These infants should be tested for HBsAg and antibody to HBsAg (anti-HBs) at age 9 through 18 months (preferably at the next well-child visit) or 1 to 2 months after completion of the HepB series if the series was delayed; CDC recently recommended testing occur at age 9 through 12 months, see http://www.cdc.gov/mmwr/preview/mmwrhtml/mm6443a3.htm.
- If mother's HBsAg status is unknown, within 12 hours of birth administer HepB vaccine regardless of birth weight. For infants weighing less than 2,000 grams, administer HBIG in addition to HepB vaccine within 12 hours of birth. Determine mother's HBsAg status as soon as possible and, if mother is HBsAg-positive, also administer HBIG for infants weighing 2,000 grams or more as soon as possible, but no later than age 7 days.

Doses following the birth dose:
- The second dose should be administered at age 1 or 2 months. Monovalent HepB vaccine should be used for doses administered before age 6 weeks.
- Infants who did not receive a birth dose should receive 3 doses of a HepB-containing vaccine on a schedule of 0, 1 to 2 months, and 6 months starting as soon as feasible. See Figure 2.
- Administer the second dose 1 to 2 months after the first dose (minimum interval of 4 weeks); administer the third dose at least 8 weeks after the second dose AND at least 16 weeks after the first dose. The final (third or fourth) dose in the HepB vaccine series should be administered no earlier than age 24 weeks.
- Administration of a total of 4 doses of HepB vaccine is permitted when a combination vaccine containing HepB is administered after the birth dose.

Catch-up vaccination:
- Unvaccinated persons should complete a 3-dose series.
- A 2-dose series (doses separated by at least 4 months) of adult formulation Recombivax HB is licensed for use in children aged 11 through 15 years.
- For other catch-up guidance, see Figure 2.

2. Rotavirus (RV) vaccines. (Minimum age: 6 weeks for both RV1 [Rotarix] and RV5 [RotaTeq])

Routine vaccination:
Administer a series of RV vaccine to all infants as follows:
1. If Rotarix is used, administer a 2-dose series at ages 2 and 4 months.
2. If RotaTeq is used, administer a 3-dose series at ages 2, 4, and 6 months.
3. If any dose in the series was RotaTeq or vaccine product is unknown for any dose in the series, a total of 3 doses of RV vaccine should be administered.

Catch-up vaccination:
- The maximum age for the first dose in the series is 14 weeks, 6 days; vaccination should not be initiated for infants aged 15 weeks, 0 days or older.
- The maximum age for the final dose in the series is 8 months, 0 days.
- For other catch-up guidance, see Figure 2.

3. Diphtheria and tetanus toxoids and acellular pertussis (DTaP) vaccine. (Minimum age: 6 weeks. Exception: DTaP-IPV [Kinrix, Quadracel]: 4 years)

Routine vaccination:
- Administer a 5-dose series of DTaP vaccine at ages 2, 4, 6, 15 through 18 months, and 4 through 6 years. The fourth dose may be administered as early as age 12 months, provided at least 6 months have elapsed since the third dose.
- Inadvertent administration of 4th DTaP dose early: If the fourth dose of DTaP was administered at least 4 months, but less than 6 months, after the third dose of DTaP, it need not be repeated.

3. Diphtheria and tetanus toxoids and acellular pertussis (DTaP) vaccine (cont'd)

Catch-up vaccination:
- The fifth dose of DTaP vaccine is not necessary if the fourth dose was administered at age 4 years or older.
- For other catch-up guidance, see Figure 2.

4. Haemophilus influenzae type b (Hib) conjugate vaccine. (Minimum age: 6 weeks for PRP-T [AC-THIB, DTaP-IPV/Hib (Pentacel) and Hib-MenCY (MenHibrix)], PRP-OMP [PedvaxHIB or COMVAX], 12 months for PRP-T [Hiberix])

Routine vaccination:
- Administer a 2- or 3-dose Hib vaccine primary series and a booster dose (dose 3 or 4 depending on vaccine used in primary series) at age 12 through 15 months to complete a full Hib vaccine series.
- The primary series with ActHIB, MenHibrix, or Pentacel consists of 3 doses and should be administered at 2, 4, and 6 months of age. The primary series with PedvaxHib or COMVAX consists of 2 doses and should be administered at 2 and 4 months of age; a dose at age 6 months is not indicated.
- One booster dose (dose 3 or 4 depending on vaccine used in primary series) of any Hib vaccine should be administered at age 12 through 15 months. An exception is Hiberix vaccine. Hiberix should only be used for the booster (final) dose in children aged 12 months through 4 years who have received at least 1 prior dose of Hib-containing vaccine.
- For recommendations on the use of MenHibrix in patients at increased risk for meningococcal disease, please refer to the meningococcal vaccine footnotes and also to MMWR February 28, 2014 / 63(RR01):1-13, available at http://www.cdc.gov/mmwr/PDF/rr/rr6301.pdf.

Catch-up vaccination:
- If dose 1 was administered at ages 12 through 14 months, administer a second (final) dose at least 8 weeks after dose 1, regardless of Hib vaccine used in the primary series.
- If both doses were PRP-OMP (PedvaxHIB or COMVAX), and were administered before the first birthday, the third (and final) dose should be administered at age 12 through 59 months and at least 8 weeks after the second dose.
- If the first dose was administered at age 7 through 11 months, administer the second dose at least 4 weeks later and a third (and final) dose at age 12 through 15 months or 8 weeks after second dose, whichever is later.
- If first dose is administered before the first birthday and second dose administered at younger than 15 months, a third (and final) dose should be administered 8 weeks later.
- For unvaccinated children aged 15 months or older, administer only 1 dose.
- For other catch-up guidance, see Figure 2. For catch-up guidance related to MenHibrix, please see the meningococcal vaccine footnotes and also MMWR February 28, 2014 / 63(RR01):1-13, available at http://www.cdc.gov/mmwr/PDF/rr/rr6301.pdf.

Vaccination of persons with high-risk conditions:
- Children aged 12 through 59 months who are at increased risk for Hib disease, including chemotherapy recipients and those with anatomic or functional asplenia (including sickle cell disease), human immunodeficiency virus (HIV) infection, immunoglobulin deficiency, or early component complement deficiency, who have received either no doses or only 1 dose of Hib vaccine before 12 months of age, should receive 2 additional doses of Hib vaccine 8 weeks apart; children who received 2 or more doses of Hib vaccine before 12 months of age should receive 1 additional dose.
- For patients younger than 5 years of age undergoing chemotherapy or radiation treatment who received a Hib vaccine dose(s) within 14 days of starting therapy or during therapy, repeat the dose(s) at least 3 months following therapy completion.
- Recipients of hematopoietic stem cell transplant (HSCT) should be revaccinated with a 3-dose regimen of Hib vaccine starting 6 to 12 months after successful transplant, regardless of vaccination history; doses should be administered at least 4 weeks apart.
- A single dose of any Hib-containing vaccine should be administered to unimmunized* children and adolescents 15 months of age and older undergoing an elective splenectomy; if possible, vaccine should be administered at least 14 days before procedure.

Fig. 12.1. cont'd

For further guidance on the use of the vaccines mentioned below, see: http://www.cdc.gov/vaccines/hcp/acip-recs/index.html.

4. Haemophilus influenzae type b (Hib) conjugate vaccine (cont'd)

- Hib vaccine is not routinely recommended for patients 5 years or older. However, 1 dose of Hib vaccine should be administered to unimmunized* persons aged 5 years or older who have anatomic or functional asplenia (including sickle cell disease) and unvaccinated persons 5 through 18 years of age with HIV infection.
  - *Patients who have not received a primary series and booster dose or at least 1 dose of Hib vaccine after 14 months of age are considered unimmunized.

5. Pneumococcal vaccines. (Minimum age: 6 weeks for PCV13, 2 years for PPSV23)

Routine vaccination with PCV13:
- Administer a 4-dose series of PCV13 vaccine at ages 2, 4, and 6 months and at age 12 through 15 months.
- For children aged 14 through 59 months who have received an age-appropriate series of 7-valent PCV (PCV7), administer a single supplemental dose of 13-valent PCV (PCV13).

Catch-up vaccination with PCV13:
- Administer 1 dose of PCV13 to all healthy children aged 24 through 59 months who are not completely vaccinated for their age.
- For other catch-up guidance, see Figure 2.

Vaccination of persons with high-risk conditions with PCV13 and PPSV23:
- For children 2 through 5 years of age with any of the following conditions: chronic heart disease (particularly cyanotic congenital heart disease and cardiac failure); chronic lung disease (including asthma if treated with high-dose oral corticosteroid therapy); diabetes mellitus; cerebrospinal fluid leak; cochlear implant; sickle cell disease and other hemoglobinopathies; anatomic or functional asplenia; HIV infection; chronic renal failure; nephrotic syndrome; diseases associated with treatment with immunosuppressive drugs or radiation therapy, including malignant neoplasms, leukemias, lymphomas, and Hodgkin disease; solid organ transplantation; or congenital immunodeficiency:
  1. Administer 1 dose of PCV13 if any incomplete schedule of 3 doses of PCV (PCV7 and/or PCV13) were received previously.
  2. Administer 2 doses of PCV13 at least 8 weeks apart if unvaccinated or any incomplete schedule of fewer than 3 doses of PCV (PCV7 and/or PCV13) were received previously.
  3. Administer 1 supplemental dose of PCV13 if 4 doses of PCV7 or other age-appropriate complete PCV7 series was received previously.
  4. The minimum interval between doses of PCV (PCV7 or PCV13) is 8 weeks.
  5. For children with no history of PPSV23 vaccination, administer PPSV23 at least 8 weeks after the most recent dose of PCV13.
- For children 6 through 18 years who have cerebrospinal fluid leak; cochlear implant; sickle cell disease and other hemoglobinopathies; anatomic or functional asplenia; congenital or acquired immunodeficiencies; HIV infection; chronic renal failure; nephrotic syndrome; diseases associated with treatment with immunosuppressive drugs or radiation therapy, including malignant neoplasms, leukemias, lymphomas, and Hodgkin disease; generalized malignancy; solid organ transplantation; or multiple myeloma:
  1. If neither PCV13 nor PPSV23 has been received previously, administer 1 dose of PCV13 now and 1 dose of PPSV23 at least 8 weeks later.
  2. If PCV13 has been received previously but PPSV23 has not, administer 1 dose of PPSV23 at least 8 weeks after the most recent dose of PCV13.
  3. If PPSV23 has been received but PCV13 has not, administer 1 dose of PCV13 at least 8 weeks after the most recent dose of PPSV23.
- For children aged 6 through 18 years with chronic heart disease (particularly cyanotic congenital heart disease and cardiac failure), chronic lung disease (including asthma if treated with high-dose oral corticosteroid therapy), diabetes mellitus, alcoholism, or chronic liver disease, who have not received PPSV23, administer 1 dose of PPSV23. If PCV13 has been received previously, then PPSV23 should be administered at least 8 weeks after any prior PCV13 dose.
- A single revaccination with PPSV23 should be administered 5 years after the first dose to children with sickle cell disease or other hemoglobinopathies; anatomic or functional asplenia; congenital or acquired asplenia; HIV infection; chronic renal failure; nephrotic syndrome; diseases associated with treatment with immunosuppressive drugs or radiation therapy, including malignant neoplasms, leukemias, lymphomas, and Hodgkin disease; generalized malignancy; solid organ transplantation; or multiple myeloma.

6. Inactivated poliovirus vaccine (IPV). (Minimum age: 6 weeks)

Routine vaccination:
- Administer a 4-dose series of IPV at ages 2, 4, 6 through 18 months, and 4 through 6 years. The final dose in the series should be administered on or after the fourth birthday and at least 6 months after the previous dose.

Catch-up vaccination:
- In the first 6 months of life, the minimum age and minimum intervals are only recommended if the person is at risk of imminent exposure to circulating poliovirus (i.e., travel to a polio-endemic region or during an outbreak).
- If 4 or more doses are administered before age 4 years, an additional dose should be administered at age 4 through 6 years and at least 6 months after the previous dose.
- A fourth dose is not necessary if the third dose was administered at age 4 years or older and at least 6 months after the previous dose.

6. Inactivated poliovirus vaccine (IPV). (Minimum age: 6 weeks) (cont'd)

- If both OPV and IPV were administered as part of a series, a total of 4 doses should be administered, regardless of the child's current age. If only OPV were administered, and all doses were given prior to 4 years of age, one dose of IPV should be given at 4 years or older, at least 4 weeks after the last OPV dose.
- IPV is not routinely recommended for U.S. residents aged 18 years or older.
- For other catch-up guidance, see Figure 2.

7. Influenza vaccines. (Minimum age: 6 months for inactivated influenza vaccine [IIV], 2 years for live, attenuated influenza vaccine [LAIV])

Routine vaccination:
- Administer influenza vaccine annually to all children beginning at age 6 months. For most healthy, nonpregnant persons aged 2 through 49 years, either LAIV or IIV may be used. However, LAIV should NOT be administered to some persons, including 1) persons who have experienced severe allergic reactions to LAIV, any of its components, or to a previous dose of any other influenza vaccine; 2) children 2 through 17 years receiving aspirin or aspirin-containing products; 3) persons who are allergic to eggs; 4) pregnant women; 5) immunosuppressed persons; 6) children 2 through 4 years of age with asthma or who had wheezing in the past 12 months; or 7) persons who have taken influenza antiviral medications in the previous 48 hours. For all other contraindications and precautions to use of LAIV, see MMWR August 7, 2015 / 64(30):818-25, available at http://www.cdc.gov/mmwr/pdf/wk/mm6430.pdf.

For children aged 6 months through 8 years:
- For the 2015-16 season, administer 2 doses (separated by at least 4 weeks) to children who are receiving influenza vaccine for the first time. Some children in this age group who have been vaccinated previously will also need 2 doses. For additional guidance, follow dosing guidelines in the 2015-16 ACIP influenza vaccine recommendations, MMWR August 7, 2015 / 64(30):818-25, available at http://www.cdc.gov/mmwr/pdf/wk/mm6430.pdf.
- For the 2016-17 season, follow dosing guidelines in the 2016 ACIP influenza vaccine recommendations.

For persons aged 9 years and older:
- Administer 1 dose.

8. Measles, mumps, and rubella (MMR) vaccine. (Minimum age: 12 months for routine vaccination)

Routine vaccination:
- Administer a 2-dose series of MMR vaccine at ages 12 through 15 months and 4 through 6 years. The second dose may be administered before age 4 years, provided at least 4 weeks have elapsed since the first dose.
- Administer 1 dose of MMR vaccine to infants aged 6 through 11 months before departure from the United States for international travel. These children should be revaccinated with 2 doses of MMR vaccine, the first at age 12 through 15 months (12 months if the child remains in an area where disease risk is high), and the second dose at least 4 weeks later.
- Administer 2 doses of MMR vaccine to children aged 12 months and older before departure from the United States for international travel. The first dose should be administered on or after age 12 months and the second dose at least 4 weeks later.

Catch-up vaccination:
- Ensure that all school-aged children and adolescents have had 2 doses of MMR vaccine; the minimum interval between the 2 doses is 4 weeks.

9. Varicella (VAR) vaccine. (Minimum age: 12 months)

Routine vaccination:
- Administer a 2-dose series of VAR vaccine at ages 12 through 15 months and 4 through 6 years. The second dose may be administered before age 4 years, provided at least 3 months have elapsed since the first dose. If the second dose was administered at least 4 weeks after the first dose, it can be accepted as valid.

Catch-up vaccination:
- Ensure that all persons aged 7 through 18 years without evidence of immunity (see MMWR 2007 / 56 [No. RR-4], available at http://www.cdc.gov/mmwr/pdf/rr/rr5604.pdf) have 2 doses of varicella vaccine. For children aged 7 through 12 years, the recommended minimum interval between doses is 3 months (if the second dose was administered at least 4 weeks after the first dose, it can be accepted as valid); for persons aged 13 years and older, the minimum interval between doses is 4 weeks.

10. Hepatitis A (HepA) vaccine. (Minimum age: 12 months)

Routine vaccination:
- Initiate the 2-dose HepA vaccine series at 12 through 23 months; separate the 2 doses by 6 to 18 months.
- Children who have received 1 dose of HepA vaccine before age 24 months should receive a second dose 6 to 18 months after the first dose.
- For any person aged 2 years and older who has not already received the HepA vaccine series, 2 doses of HepA vaccine separated by 6 to 18 months may be administered if immunity against hepatitis A virus infection is desired.

Catch-up vaccination:
- The minimum interval between the 2 doses is 6 months.

Continued

Fig. 12.1, cont'd

For further guidance on the use of the vaccines mentioned below, see: http://www.cdc.gov/vaccines/hcp/acip-recs/index.html.

10. Hepatitis A (HepA) vaccine (cont'd)

Special populations:
- Administer 2 doses of HepA vaccine at least 6 months apart to previously unvaccinated persons who live in areas where vaccination programs target older children, who are at increased risk for infection. This includes persons traveling to or working in countries that have high or intermediate endemicity of infection, men having sex with men, users of injection and non-injection illicit drugs; persons who work with HIV-infected primates or with HIV in a research laboratory setting; persons with clotting-factor disorders; persons with chronic liver disease; and persons who anticipate close personal contact (e.g., household care or regular babysitting) with an international adoptee during the first 60 days after arrival in the United States from a country with high or intermediate endemicity. The first dose should be administered as soon as the adoption is planned, ideally 2 or more weeks before the arrival of the adoptee.

11. Meningococcal vaccines. (Minimum age: 6 weeks for Hib-MenCY [MenHibrix], 9 months for MenACWY-D [Menactra], 2 months for MenACWY-CRM [Menveo], 10 years for serogroup B meningococcal [MenB] vaccines; MenB-4C [Bexsero] and MenB-FHbp [Trumenba])

Routine vaccination:
- Administer a single dose of Menactra or Menveo vaccine at age 11 through 12 years, with a booster dose at age 16 years.
- Adolescents aged 11 through 18 years with human immunodeficiency virus (HIV) infection should receive a 2-dose primary series of Menactra or Menveo with at least 8 weeks between doses.
- For children aged 2 months through 18 years with high-risk conditions, see below.

Catch-up vaccination:
- Administer Menactra or Menveo vaccine at age 13 through 18 years if not previously vaccinated.
- If the first dose is administered at age 13 through 15 years, a booster dose should be administered at age 16 through 18 years with a minimum interval of at least 8 weeks between doses.
- If the first dose is administered at age 16 years or older, a booster dose is not needed.
- For other catch-up guidance, see Figure 2.

Clinical discretion:
- Young adults aged 16 through 23 years (preferred age range is 16 through 18 years) may be vaccinated with either a 2-dose series of Bexsero or a 3-dose series of Trumenba vaccine. The two MenB vaccines are not interchangeable; the same vaccine product must be used for all doses.

Vaccination of persons with anatomic or functional asplenia (including sickle cell disease):

Children with anatomic or functional asplenia (including sickle cell disease):

Meningococcal conjugate ACWY vaccines:
1. Menactra
   o Children who initiate vaccination at 8 weeks: Administer doses at 2, 4, 6, and 12 months of age.
   o Unvaccinated children who initiate vaccination at 7 through 23 months: Administer 2 doses, with the second dose at least 12 weeks after the first dose AND after the first birthday.
   o Children 24 months and older who have not received a complete series: Administer 2 primary doses at least 8 weeks apart.
2. Menveo
   o Children who initiate vaccination at 8 weeks: Administer doses at 2, 4, 6, and 12 months of age.
   o If the first dose of Menveo is given at or after 12 months of age, a total of 2 doses should be given at least 8 weeks apart to ensure protection against serogroups C and Y meningococcal disease.
3. Menactra
   o Children 24 months and older who have not received a complete series: Administer 2 primary doses at least 8 weeks apart. If Menactra is administered to a child with asplenia (including sickle cell disease), do not administer Menactra until 2 years of age and at least 4 weeks after the completion of all PCV13 doses.

Meningococcal conjugate ACWY vaccines:
1. Bexsero or Trumenba
   o Persons 10 years or older who have not received a complete series: Administer a 2-dose series of Bexsero, at least 1 month apart, or a 3-dose series of Trumenba, with the second dose at least 2 months after the first and the third dose at least 6 months after the first. The two MenB vaccines are not interchangeable; use the same vaccine product must be used for all doses.

Children with persistent complement component deficiency (persons with inherited or chronic deficiencies in C3, C5-9, properdin, factor D, factor H, or taking eculizumab [Soliris]):

Meningococcal conjugate ACWY vaccines:
1. Menactra
   o Children who initiate vaccination at 8 weeks: Administer doses at 2, 4, 6, and 12 months of age.
   o If the first dose of Menveo is given at or after 12 months of age, a total of 2 doses should be given at least 8 weeks apart to ensure protection against serogroup C and Y meningococcal disease.

11. Meningococcal vaccines (cont'd)

3. Menactra
   o Children 9 through 23 months: Administer 2 primary doses at least 3 months apart.
   o Children 24 months and older who have not received 2 primary doses: Administer 2 primary doses at least 8 weeks apart.

Meningococcal B vaccines:
1. Bexsero or Trumenba
   o Persons 10 years or older who have not received a complete series: Administer a 2-dose series of Bexsero, at least 1 month apart, or a 3-dose series of Trumenba, with the second dose at least 2 months after the first and the third dose at least 6 months after the first. The two MenB vaccines are not interchangeable; the same vaccine product must be used for all doses.

For children who travel to or reside in countries in which meningococcal disease is hyperendemic or epidemic, including countries in the African meningitis belt or the Hajj:
- administer an age-appropriate formulation and series of Menactra or Menveo for protection against serogroups A and W meningococcal disease. Prior receipt of Hib-MenCY vaccine is not sufficient for children traveling to the meningitis belt or the Hajj because it does not contain serogroups A or W.

For children at risk during a community outbreak attributable to a vaccine serogroup:
- administer or complete an age- and formulation-appropriate series of MenHibrix, Menactra, or Menveo.
   Bexsero or Trumenba.

For booster doses among persons with high-risk conditions, refer to MMWR 2013 ; 62(RR02):1-22, available at http://www.cdc.gov/mmwr/preview/mmwrhtml/rr6202a1.htm.

For other catch-up recommendations for these persons, and complete information on use of meningococcal vaccines, including guidance related to vaccination of persons at increased risk of infection, see MMWR March 22, 2013 ; 62(RR02):1-22, and MMWR October 23, 2015 ; 64(41):1171-1176 available at http://www.cdc.gov/mmwr/pdf/rr/rr6202.pdf and http://www.cdc.gov/mmwr/pdf/wk/mm6441.pdf.

12. Tetanus and diphtheria toxoids and acellular pertussis (Tdap) vaccine. (Minimum age: 10 years for both Boostrix and Adacel)

Routine vaccination:
- Administer 1 dose of Tdap vaccine to all adolescents aged 11 through 12 years.
- Tdap may be administered regardless of the interval since the last tetanus and diphtheria toxoid-containing vaccine.
- Administer 1 dose of Tdap vaccine to pregnant adolescents during each pregnancy (preferred during 27 through 36 weeks' gestation) regardless of time since prior Td or Tdap vaccination.

Catch-up vaccination:
- Persons aged 7 years and older who are not fully immunized with DTaP vaccine should receive Tdap vaccine as 1 (preferably the first dose in the catch-up series; if additional doses are needed, use Td vaccine. For children 7 through 10 years who receive a dose of Tdap as part of the catch-up series, an adolescent Tdap vaccine dose at age 11 through 12 years should NOT be administered. Td should be administered instead 10 years after the Tdap dose.
- Persons aged 11 through 18 years who have not received Tdap vaccine should receive a dose followed by tetanus and diphtheria toxoids (Td) booster doses every 10 years thereafter.
- Inadvertent doses of DTaP vaccine:
   o If administered inadvertently to a child aged 7 through 10 years may count as part of the catch-up series. This dose may count as the adolescent Tdap dose, or the child can later receive a Tdap booster dose at age 11 through 12 years.
   o If administered inadvertently to an adolescent aged 11 through 18 years, the dose may be counted as the adolescent Tdap booster.
- For other catch-up guidance, see Figure 2.

13. Human papillomavirus (HPV) vaccines. (Minimum age: 9 years for 2vHPV [Cervarix], 4vHPV [Gardasil] and 9vHPV [Gardasil 9])

Routine vaccination:
- Administer a 2-dose series of HPV vaccine on a schedule of 0, 1, 2, and 6 months to all adolescents aged 11 through 12 years. 2vHPV, 9vHPV, 4vHPV or 2vHPV may be used for females, and only 9vHPV or 4vHPV may be used for males.
- The vaccine series may be started at age 9 years.
- Administer the second dose 1 to 2 months after the first dose (minimum interval of 4 weeks).
- Administer the third dose 24 weeks after the first dose (minimum interval of 12 weeks) and 24 weeks after the first dose.

Catch-up vaccination:
- Administer the vaccine series to females (2vHPV or 4vHPV or 9vHPV) and males (4vHPV or 9vHPV) at age 13 through 18 years if not previously vaccinated.
- Use recommended routine dosing intervals (see Routine vaccination above) for vaccine series catch-up.

Fig. 12.1. cont'd

vaccination against hepatitis A. Parents of children <1 year old can be given the option of immune globulin for the infant, although it is not essential, given the mild nature of the disease in young children.

Typhoid vaccination is similarly complicated by the choices available. The oral typhoid vaccine (Ty21a) in capsule form is approved for use in children >6 years. A lyophilized vaccine preparation that reconstitutes to a liquid oral suspension is available in Canada and Switzerland. This preparation can be used in children >3 years. The injectable typhoid Vi polysaccharide vaccine is an approved alternative in all countries for children >2 years. For younger infants, prudent and cautious food and water advice needs to be emphasized. **Table 12.3** indicates the recommended ages and intervals for travel immunizations. **Table 12.4** lists important vaccine interactions.

Yellow fever vaccination, an attenuated live virus vaccine, is absolutely contraindicated in infants <6 months old. There is a risk of vaccine-associated encephalitis in this age group. Vaccination should be delayed until 9 months old. In infants 6-9 months of age, the yellow fever vaccine should be considered only if epidemic exposure exists and in consultation with experts. A letter of waiver for infants and egg-allergic children can be provided before travel. Infants unable to receive the yellow fever vaccine due to age contraindications should be advised to delay travel to yellow fever-endemic areas if possible until the vaccine can be safely given. Intradermal testing of egg-allergic travelers can be performed prior to vaccination. The vaccine is not recommended for immunocompromised individuals.

Rabies vaccination (**Table 12.4** and Chapter 5) is recommended for ambulatory children who will travel extensively (1-3 months) or live in rural villages in countries where rabies is endemic or for anyone who desires maximal protection for the itinerary. Consideration for vaccination should be given to the availability of rabies immune globulin in case post-exposure prophylaxis is needed. The initial treatment of animal bites with soap and water and first-aid measures must be emphasized, along with the importance of obtaining post-exposure rabies prophylaxis within 24 hours.

A tuberculosis (TB) skin test is recommended for children before, if the TB status is unknown, and after extended travel in tropical and developing countries. Bacillus Calmette-Guérin (BCG) vaccine administration in the United States is controversial. Some advocate its use for infants <1 year old if high-risk travel to rural, endemic areas is planned. BCG vaccine decreases the incidence of TB meningitis in this age group. Official US recommendations for BCG vaccine administration are limited to (1) continuous exposure to an untreated or ineffectively treated person with infectious TB or multidrug-resistant (MDR) TB when the child cannot be removed from the environment or (2) healthcare workers in settings with a high percentage of MDR TB and an unsuccessful TB control program. It is contraindicated in immune-deficient persons.

MALARIA PREVENTION

Personal Protective Measures

Protecting the traveling child from insect bites will decrease exposure to malaria and other serious infections spread by biting insects. Many insect-borne infections, including malaria, dengue fever, chikungunya, encephalitis, filarial diseases, leishmaniasis, trypanosomiasis, and cutaneous myiasis, are not vaccine preventable, so minimizing exposure is critical.

Malaria is transmitted by biting female *Anopheles* mosquitoes, which feed mainly between the hours of dusk and dawn. The risk of exposure to malaria in an infant or child can be greatly reduced by the following precautions: (1) limit outdoor exposure during the hours between dusk and dawn; (2) wear protective clothing that covers most of the body when outdoors (a hooded "bug suit" that covers head, arms, body, and legs can be made out of mosquito netting or is commercially available); (3) use diethyltoluamide (DEET)-containing insect repellent of ≤35%, sparingly, on exposed areas of skin when outdoors (see Chapter 6); (4) spray a permethrin-containing insecticide on external clothing (see Chapter 6); and (5) sleep under a permethrin-impregnated mosquito net at night (see Chapter 6). The use

TABLE 12.3 Travel Vaccinations for Children

Vaccine	Age	Primary Series	Booster Interval; Comments
Cholera, oral (CVD103-HgR)[a,b]	>2 years	1 dose oral, in buffered solution	Optimal interval not established, manufacturer recommends 6 months
Hepatitis A	>1 year	Havrix (GSK): two doses (0.5 mL i.m.) at 0, 6-18 months later VAQTA (Merck): two doses (0.5 mL i.m.) at 0 and 6 months	See text
Immune globulin	Birth	0.02 mL/kg i.m.	Lasts 6 weeks; see text
Japanese B encephalitis (IXIARO®)	2 mos through 2 yrs	2 doses (0.25 mL i.m.) at 0 and 28 days	No data for booster to date
	>3 years:	two doses (0.5 mL i.m.) at 0 and 28 days	No data for booster to date
Meningococcal meningitis, conjugate[c]	9 mos	2 doses: (0.5 mL i.m.) – 0 and 3 mos	3 yrs after primary series, then every 5 yrs if exposure risk
Menactra®	11-55 yrs	1 dose	5 yrs after first dose
Menveo®	2 mos	4 doses: 2,4,6 and 12 mos	3 yrs after primary series, then every 5 yrs if exposure risk
	11-55 yrs	1 dose (0.5 mL i.m.)	5 yrs after first dose
Meningococcal meningitis, polysaccharide	>2 years	1 dose (0.5 mL s.c.)	Boost after 2-3 years if first dose was given before 4 years old
Plague vaccine	>18 years	Not for use in children	
Rabies vaccine	Any age	Three doses (1 mL i.m., deltoid [or anterolateral thigh in infants] or 0.1 mL i.d.) at 0, 7, and 21 or 28 days	Only HDCV approved for intradermal (i.d.) use
Typhoid, Ty21a,[b] oral	>3 years[a]	Three doses: 1 sachet p.o. in 100 mL water every other day	Liquid vaccine[a] booster: 7 years
	>6 years	Four doses: 1 capsule p.o. every other day	Capsule vaccine booster: 5 years
Typhoid, Vi polysaccharide, parenteral	>2 years	One dose (0.5 mL i.m.)	Boost after 2 years for continued risk of exposure
Yellow fever[b]	>9 months	1 dose (0.5 mL s.c.)	10 years; see text

[a]Not approved in the United States. Available in Canada and Switzerland.
[b]Caution: may be contraindicated in patients with any of the following conditions: pregnancy, leukemia, lymphoma, generalized malignancy, immunosuppression resulting from HIV infection or treatment with corticosteroids, alkylating drugs, antimetabolites, or radiation therapy.
[c]See reference CDC Health information for international travel 2016. Hib-MenCY-TT(MenHibrix not indicated for traveling infants).
HDCV, Human diploid cell rabies vaccine; *i.d.*, intradermally; *i.m.*, intramuscularly; *p.o.*, by mouth; *s.c.*, subcutaneously.

TABLE 12.4   Vaccine Interactions

Vaccine	Interaction	Precaution
Measles, mumps, rubella (MMR) vaccine and varicella vaccine	Immune globulin or other antibody containing blood products	Give vaccines at least 2 weeks before immune globulin (IG) or 3-11 months after IG, depending on dose and product received.
Oral typhoid vaccine	Antibiotics	Delay vaccine administration at least 24 h after antibiotics.[a]
Virus vaccines, live (MMR, OPV, varicella, yellow fever vaccine)	Other live virus vaccines	Give live virus vaccines on the same day, or separate the doses by at least 28 days.
Virus vaccines, live (MMR, OPV, varicella, yellow fever vaccine)	Tuberculin skin test (PPD)	Do the skin test before or on the same day as receipt of a live virus vaccine, or 4-6 weeks after; virus vaccines can impair the response to the PPD skin test.
Varicella	Salicylates	Avoid salicylates 6 weeks after vaccine due to theoretical risk of Reye syndrome

[a]These recommendations are based on theoretical considerations; efficacy studies are in progress.
OPV, Oral polio vaccine; *PPD,* purified protein derivative.
From: CDC. Health Information for International Travel 2016.

of permethrin-impregnated bed nets has been studied in many rural malarious areas, with a dramatic decrease in the transmission of malaria, even when chemoprophylaxis is not being used.

The active ingredient in recommended mosquito repellants is DEET. DEET has been approved by the Environmental Protection Agency (EPA) for use in humans but with specific warnings and directions. Child safety claims were removed from labeling in 1998. Brief exposure, following the label directions, is not believed to pose a health concern. DEET is recommended for use in children at concentrations of ≤35%. Although extremely rare, reported toxicities include seizures, subacute encephalopathy, and local skin or eye irritation. Advise parents to apply it sparingly, avoiding the palms, and do not allow children to handle it directly. It should not be applied under clothing and should be washed off once indoors. A patch test on the antecubital fossa can identify children with skin sensitivity. Combination DEET/sunscreen products have not received EPA approval pending further assessment of potentially unnecessary DEET exposures. Specific EPA updates can be obtained at the website http: www.epa.govpesticides and at the National Pesticide Information Center at 800-858-7378. If using both products, apply the sunscreen product to the skin first, then the insect repellent.

Some insect repellants containing citronella, lemon eucalyptus, and neem oil and the Avon bath oil Skin So Soft, have been shown to have some limited effectiveness as repellants but no significant action against the *Anopheles* mosquito that transmits malaria. Their use is not recommended for insect protection when traveling to malarious areas.

The scratching of mosquito bites also predisposes children to impetigo in the tropics.

Chemoprophylaxis

Drug choices to prevent malaria in children are similar to those available for adults, with specific weight and formulation caveats. Chloroquine is used to prevent chloroquine-sensitive malaria. Chloroquine can be used in any sized infant; however, its pill form makes dosing small infants difficult. Splitting pills is cumbersome for certain child weights and often requires pre-weighing and packaging by a pharmacist. Chloroquine can be obtained abroad as a pediatric suspension but is not available in the United States or Canada in this form. An alternate drug is hydroxychloroquine (Plaquenil), which offers the same protection in chloroquine-sensitive areas as chloroquine. In the United States, hydroxychloroquine is significantly less expensive than chloroquine.

For prevention of chloroquine-resistant malaria, mefloquine can be given to children using a weight-adjusted dose. It is currently recommended for use in infants of any size. Contraindications to the use of mefloquine (seizure disorders, cardiac conduction defects, and neuropsychiatric disorders) are identical to those for adults. Doxycycline should not be used in children <8 years old due to dental staining. The fixed-drug combination atovaquone/proguanil is highly effective as chemoprophylaxis against chloroquine-resistant malaria and may be used in infants weighing >5 kg.

Primaquine phosphate is used for eradication of latent incubating *Plasmodium vivax* or *Plasmodium ovale* malaria parasites in the liver after intense exposure in endemic areas (**Table 12.5** and Chapter 6). The glucose 6-phosphate dehydrogenase level must be checked

TABLE 12.5 Drugs Used for Malaria Chemoprophylaxis in Children

Drug	Weight (kg)	Dose	Comments
Chloroquine phosphate (Aralen)[a]	Any	8.3 mg/kg per week (salt) = 5 mg/kg(base); max. 500 mg/week (salt), 300 mg/week (base)	Use 250-mg tablets if available; very bitter; liquid preparation available in some countries
Hydroxychloroquine sulfate (Plaquenil)[a]	Any	6.5 mg/kg per week (salt) = 5 mg/kg (base); max. 400 mg/week (salt), 310 mg/week (base)	200-mg tablet; liquid preparation may be available
Mefloquine (Lariam)[b]	<15	5 mg/kg per week	250-mg tablet; no liquid form available
	15-19	¼ tablet q week	
	20-30	½ tablet q week	
	31-45	¾ tablet q week	
	>45	1 tablet q week	
Atovaquone/proguanil (Malarone)[c]	5-8	½ pediatric tablet	62 mg atovaquone and 25 mg proguanil = pediatric tablet; 250 mg atovaquone and 100 mg proguanil = adult tablet; take with food or milk
	8-10	¾ pediatric tablet	
	10-20	1 pediatric tablet/day	
	20-30	2 pediatric tablets/day	
	30-40	3 pediatric tablets/day	
	>40	4 pediatric tablets (or 1 adult tablet)/day	
Doxycycline (Vibramycin, Doryx, others)[d]	Any	2 mg/kg per day, up to 100 mg/day	100 mg tablet; contraindicated in <8 years old
Primaquine phosphate	Any	0.5 mg/kg salt = 0.3 mg/kg base daily × 14 days	26.3-mg (15-mg base) tablet; must check G6PD status; post-exposure terminal prophylaxis for *Plasmodium vivax*

[a]Start 2 weeks before entering malarious area and continue 4 weeks after returning.
[b]Start 2 weeks before entering malarious area and continue 4 weeks after returning
[c]Start 1-2 days before entering malarious area and continue 7 days after returning.
[d]Start 1-2 days before entering malarious area and continue 4 weeks after returning.
G6PD, Glucose 6-phosphate dehydrogenase.

prior to prescribing primaquine, as it is a potent red blood cell oxidizer in those who have inadequate or deficient levels of this enzyme present. No studies have been done on loading doses of antimalarials in children, and such practices are not recommended in pediatric age groups at this time. A summary of antimalarial drugs and pediatric dosing is found in **Table 12.5**.

Children <6 years old usually have difficulty swallowing pills. Parents of the traveling child can purchase a pill splitter available in many pharmacies. After splitting a mefloquine or chloroquine tablet into the appropriate-sized pieces, the tablet fragment can be crushed to a fine powder with the back of a spoon or with a pill crusher also available in many pharmacies. The correct dose of powdered medication can then be mixed into a spoonful of chocolate syrup or jelly (to mask the bitter taste) and given to the child. For older children, the portion of a crushed pill can be embedded in a candy bar, cream-filled sandwich cookie or other sweet food. For infants weighing between 5 and 10 kg, one-quarter of a tablet can be finely crushed and mixed in a measured aliquot (10 mL) of breast milk or formula. The calculated milliliter dose can then be given by syringe, with the remainder being discarded.

Alternatively, if the correct dose for weight is calculated and prescribed, a pharmacist can pulverize the medication and dispense the proper weekly dose (with the addition of inert filler) into capsules. The capsules can be opened up and suspended into a spoonful of chocolate syrup for the weekly dose. Enteric-coated tablets of chloroquine (500 mg) are difficult to crush and prepare. Generic chloroquine phosphate tablets (250 mg), if available, lend themselves more readily to pediatric preparations.

Antimalarial drugs are not secreted in the breast milk at therapeutic levels, so nursing infants of mothers taking antimalarials must also be given appropriate chemoprophylaxis. Parents should be warned that antimalarial drugs are extremely toxic and that the tablets should be stored in childproof containers out of reach of small children. Ingestion of one 500-mg (salt) tablet of chloroquine resulted in the death of a 12-month-old toddler. Chloroquine overdose in children has a reported 80% mortality rate.

Drug dosing for standby therapy of malaria in children can be found in **Table 12.6**. The treatment with atovaquone/proguanil should be given if this drug is not being taken for prophylaxis. The lower weight limit for treatment dosing is 5 kg. Parents should be urged to seek medical evaluation of any ill child and not to treat this potentially life-threatening disease without medical guidance. An important aspect of the pre-travel visit is to discuss the availability of medical care while away.

DIARRHEA PREVENTION AND TREATMENT

Prevention of diarrhea in children is especially important during travel in hot, tropical climates, since children rapidly become dehydrated during diarrheal illnesses. Safe food and

TABLE 12.6	Drugs Used for standby therapy of Malaria in Children	
Medication	**Weight (kg)**	**Dose[a]**
Atovaquone/proguanil	5-8	2 pediatric tablets
	9-10	3 pediatric tablets
	11-20	1 adult tablet
	21-30	2 adult tablets
	31-40	3 adult tablets
	>40	4 adult tablets

[a]Once daily dose for 3 consecutive days.
Adapted from CDC 2016.

water selection is the same as for travelers in general and is outlined in Chapter 8 and discussed in detail in Chapter 9. Breast milk is ideal for the traveling infant. Other milk should be boiled, pasteurized, or irradiated. Ultra-high temperature labeled milk, sterilized by flash heating to 137°C for 2-4 s, is an alternative that does not require refrigeration until opening. In addition to preventing diarrheal illness, meticulous attention to safe food and water selection will also decrease exposure to intestinal parasites. The worldwide burden of *Ascaris* and hookworm is carried mainly by children through ingestion of these pathogens. Hand washing, especially before eating; nail trimming; and wearing shoes are simple ways to interrupt transmission of these common parasites. The use of alcohol-based hand sanitizer is encouraged.

Preventing dehydration by oral rehydration with appropriate fluids is the first-line treatment of diarrhea in children. The World Health Organization's recipe for oral rehydration solution (ORS) is recommended. The molecular basis for ORS relies on a 1:1 ratio of sodium to glucose transport at the intestinal epithelial level. A powdered formula is commercially available in inexpensive foil packages that can be suspended in 1 L of purified water to yield the correct solution (see Chapter 8). Cereal-based oral rehydration therapy is also available. The rice cereal base offers a lower osmolarity and provides continued nutrition during the illness. Once the starch base is absorbed, twice the amount of glucose is released to promote intestinal reabsorption of electrolytes. In patients with cholera, the cereal-based ORS has been shown to provide clinically significant reductions in 24-hour stool output compared with standard ORS. In acute, noncholeric diarrhea, the effect is less pronounced. ORS should be used in place of milk-based formula and other fluids until the child is fully recovered from the initial dehydration phase of the illness. One half to 1 cup of ORS is recommended for each diarrheal stool passed in a 10-kg child. Practical recommendations for giving the required volume of ORS include using a syringe or a spoon, adding pre-sweetened drink mix as some of the glucose source for both the color and flavor, and making it into frozen treats. The only contraindications to ORS are intractable vomiting, ileus, and abnormally low level of consciousness. Slow and steady administration of oral fluids to the vomiting child avoids overdistention of the stomach. Parental education regarding early signs of dehydration (decreased urine output and tears) and quantities of ORS to use is an important part of counseling about traveler's diarrhea.

Recommendations regarding medications for prevention and treatment of pediatric traveler's diarrhea differ from those for adults. Bismuth subsalicylate (BSS) and antibiotics are not recommended for prevention of traveler's diarrhea in pediatric patients. BSS may be considered for symptomatic treatment of watery diarrhea in infants and small children. It should be avoided if fever or bloody diarrhea is present. The use of BSS is contraindicated in persons with aspirin allergy. It should not be used in children and teenagers who have varicella or influenza or who have had recent exposure, because of the theoretical risk of Reye syndrome. Each tablespoon (15 mL) of commercial BSS suspension (Pepto-Bismol) contains 130 mg of salicylate. Several studies have reported that relief of diarrhea was safely obtained in hospitalized infants and young children with a weight-adjusted dose of BSS equal to 100-150 mg/kg per day given orally in five doses for up to 5 days without adverse side effects. Both the salicylate and the bismuth levels were well below toxic ranges.

Antimotility medications (loperamide, diphenoxylate) are not recommended in infants or young children. One investigation on the use of loperamide at the standard dosage (0.2 mg/kg per day) in infants and young children did not show a statistically significant difference in duration or outcome of illness when compared with placebo. In another study, high-dose loperamide (0.8 mg/kg per day) was shown to reduce stool output in hospitalized infants. Adverse central nervous system events, abdominal distention, and ileus have been reported in infants and young children taking loperamide. This evidence precludes routine recommendation for its use as a self-administered medication in children <6 years old. Because it is readily available to parents over the counter, discussion of its indications and side effects is warranted in pre-travel counseling. Loperamide may be considered for occasional use in older children if symptoms of dysentery are absent and a prolonged journey is necessary.

Bulking agents, such as kaolin and pectin, have little effect on overall disease and are not recommended. Probiotics including various species of the genus *Lactobacillus* have been studied for their effect in children, with favorable results. Antibiotic-associated diarrhea and viral diarrhea have been shown to be reduced to varying degrees by probiotics. The US Food and Drug Administration (FDA) does not currently regulate these supplements; thus, precise dosing and recommendations have not been published to date. The exact role of these supplements in traveling children has not been delineated, but it points to an interesting direction in diarrhea intervention.

Safety and efficacy influence antibiotic treatment of traveler's diarrhea in infants and young children. Choices for treatment in children differ slightly from those for adults. The antibiotics that are considered safe for pediatric use are not necessarily effective against some of the emergent drug-resistant strains of bacterial pathogens implicated in traveler's diarrhea (Chapter 8). Azithromycin is considered the first choice for pediatric traveler's diarrhea. Quinolones are approved by the FDA for use in children <18 years old for specific infections (resistant urinary tract and bone infections). While experience with quinolones in children has not borne out the potential risk of the joint toxicity seen in experimental animals, widespread recommendations on using this class of drugs in children have not been made. Many advocate that the benefits of a 3-day course off label of quinolones for children with traveler's diarrhea outweigh the risks for this potentially severe disease. Nalidixic acid, a nonfluorinated quinolone, has a long history of use in children for urinary tract infections. It is used in many countries for pediatric traveler's diarrhea and is effective against some strains of *Escherichia coli* and *Shigella* resistant to other drugs. Arthropathy has not been reported in children taking nalidixic acid. However, it has the same theoretical contraindications as fluoroquinolones and is not approved by the FDA for use in children <18 years old unless the potential benefit justifies the risk. Obtaining informed consent is recommended if quinolones are prescribed for pediatric patients.

Given these constraints, a practical recommendation is to prescribe a therapeutic course of azithromycin in the travel medical kit for first-line antibiotic treatment of pediatric diarrhea. There have been no studies done to date to evaluate the duration of treatment needed for pediatric traveler's diarrhea. A 3-day course of treatment using 10 mg/kg per day is standard practice. Instituting therapy in children with frequent diarrheal stools while away is currently recommended. Fever and bloody stools necessitate antibiotic treatment as well. If a second-line drug is deemed necessary because of allergy, ciprofloxacin should be considered. For areas of *Campylobacter* predominance, azithromycin is preferable. Alternatively, parents should be informed that if prompt improvement after first-line treatment does not occur, medical evaluation is indicated. The proposed treatment plan should be discussed in detail with the parents. Any medications prescribed should be labeled with the indication for use. Families should be instructed to seek medical care for the child with severe dehydration, vomiting that prevents oral rehydration, fever lasting >24 hours (especially in malarious areas), grossly bloody stools, and symptoms that continue or become worse. Empiric antibiotic treatment of infants >2 months can be considered, though young infants require a conservative approach with medical evaluation early in the illness. Febrile infants <2 months old should have an urgent medical evaluation and are thus not candidates for empiric antibiotic treatment of diarrhea while traveling.

Dietary energy intake improves nutritional outcome in pediatric diarrheal disease. Early enteral feeding stimulates intestinal cell renewal. Parents can continue breast feeding or restart full-strength lactose-free or lactose-reduced formula in bottle-fed infants as soon as rehydration has occurred. Cow's milk products should be reintroduced gradually. The incidence of true post-diarrheal lactose intolerance varies. Severe rotaviral illness is the pediatric enteritis most likely to be associated with lactose intolerance and malabsorption, with rates reported as high as 60-80%. Most infants with mild to moderate rotaviral illness can return directly to cow's milk-based formula. The "BRAT" diet—bananas, rice, applesauce, and toast—has traditionally been advised for diarrheal illness, despite the lack of protein and energy. No evidence exists that this restrictive diet is necessary or advantageous for diarrhea treatment. Starches, cereals, yogurt, fruits, meats, and low-fiber vegetables are good alternatives. Foods high in simple sugars and fats should be avoided in favor of complex carbohydrates until intestinal recovery has occurred.

Diaper dermatitis is an under-recognized complication of diarrhea in young infants. Discomfort, pain, and parental and child distress accompany this condition. Advise parents to be prepared with barrier cream (zinc oxide and petrolatum) for use on raw diaper areas. Hydrocortisone 1% can be used sparingly on broken-down skin in the diaper area. Anti-fungal cream is often necessary for secondary yeast dermatitis. Pustular rashes may need local antibacterial coverage. Prepare for frequent diaper changes and cool compresses if rashes become severe with frequent stooling. Avoid commercially available diaper wipes and use paper towel or cloth with liquid soap to ease the sting of cleaning-sensitive diaper areas.

GENERAL SAFETY FOR TRAVELING CHILDREN AND ADOLESCENTS

In many developing countries, the car seat will need to be fastened to the automobile or bus seat for the small child who will do extensive land travel. A nylon webbing strap or length of climbing rope should be taken along to use with the car seat.

Accidental poisoning occurs commonly at home, even with close supervision, and increased vigilance is needed during travel. Contents of the travel medical kit, particularly antimalarial medications, are potential sources of poisoning when a toddler explores a new environment. All medications should be kept in childproof containers and out of the reach of small children. New accommodations need careful inspection to make sure that contact with matchbooks, chemicals, cleaning solutions, and insecticide pads or coils can be supervised at all times or that these items are removed from easy access. Poisonous plants should be removed from easy reach. Electrical outlets should be covered. Supervision around swimming pools is vital.

All travelers to tropical and developing countries need advice about rabies prevention. The natural curiosity and friendliness that many children have toward animals should be discussed with parents. Children should be monitored closely to prevent animal contact while traveling. Older children should be warned to be cautious with all animals. Animal bites, particularly dog bites, in tropical and developing countries warrant medical attention. Monkey bites may transmit rabies and macaque bites may expose the child to simian herpes virus, a potentially fatal infection. In addition to the physical trauma and risk of bacterial wound contamination, rabies post-exposure prophylaxis should be discussed and a plan made in the event of an exposure.

ALTITUDE

Children who accompany their parents to high-altitude destinations are at risk of developing altitude-related illnesses. The diagnosis of altitude illness is more difficult to recognize in young children. Nonspecific symptoms that cannot be verbalized, like irritability, anorexia, and headache, mark the onset of potential altitude illness. Rapid descent is critical if any questionable illness or behavioral change occurs. Several studies have shown that infants and young children born at sea level are perhaps more at risk of high-altitude pulmonary edema than adults. Viral respiratory illnesses appear to increase this risk. Children with chronic lung disease, cardiac lesions with increased pulmonary blood flow, or sickle cell disease have been shown to have a predisposition to develop altitude illness. Children with Down syndrome are particularly vulnerable to altitude illness, especially pulmonary edema.

Precautions against altitude illness in children are identical to those for adults: acclimatization by slow ascent and sleeping at altitudes below maximum daily altitudes (see Chapter 10). If air travel to high altitude precludes slow acclimatization, rest and avoidance of dehydration and over-exercise in the early stages of the trip are best advised. Preventive medications, such as acetazolamide, have not been conclusively studied in children. For children who have demonstrated past acute mountain sickness or who are traveling to a high-altitude location without the ability to slowly acclimatize (i.e., flying to La Paz, Bolivia, or Cuzco, Peru), a weight-adjusted dose of acetazolamide (5 mg/kg per day divided b.i.d.)

can be considered. Likewise, there are no data on the use of pharmaceuticals to treat mountain sickness in children.

Infantile sub-acute mountain sickness is a distinct clinical entity that has been described in a small group of infants and young children several months after relocating from sea level to Tibet. Muscular hyperplasia of the pulmonary vascular bed occurs in an unpredictable subset of these children. The resultant pulmonary hypertension and right heart failure are severe enough to cause death. It is thought to be a complete failure of acclimatization.

MISCELLANEOUS ISSUES FOR YOUNG TRAVELERS

Children are vulnerable to the cumulative effects of sun exposure and damage. Lifetime risk of malignant melanoma and nonmelanoma skin cancers is related to sun exposure that occurs before the age of 18 years. Sunburns in childhood magnify the risk. Avoiding mid-day exposure, when the sun is strongest, is recommended. Clothing and brimmed hats are the first lines of defense. Clothing made from tightly woven fabric that absorbs ultraviolet light is available commercially. Standard clothing, however, affords considerable protection. Sunscreens with a sun protection factor (SPF) of ≥30 should be used on exposed skin. Sunblocks containing zinc oxide or titanium dioxide offer the advantage of a physical barrier, rather than chemical protection. Any sunscreen should be applied liberally to children >6 months at least 30 min before exposure. While infants <6 months should be covered while exposed to the sun, sunscreen use is safe. Reapplication is necessary every 2 hours, especially if swimming. When traveling overseas, advise bringing an adequate supply of sunscreen, as it may be unavailable while away. Sunglasses that block ultraviolet rays are also recommended to protect the retinas of children's eyes.

A suggested medical kit for travel with children is found in **Table 12.7**. Any essential medications, especially for asthma, anaphylaxis, or chronic disease, should be labeled and carried on board the airplane. Any child with a chronic disease should have a visit with the regular provider before travel. Children with asthma need to have their asthma management

---

TABLE 12.7 Recommended Medical Kit for Travel with Children

Medical card with age, weight, any important medical history, allergies, blood type if known, immunization records, and passport copy

Over-the-counter medications:

  barrier cream (zinc oxide and petrolatum) for use on raw diaper areas

  Acetaminophen

  Ibuprofen

  Antihistamine (e.g., diphenhydramine)

  1% Hydrocortisone cream

  Cough suppressant

  Antibacterial skin ointment

  Bismuth subsalicylate/loperamide, depending on age

  Antifungal cream

Prescription medications:

  Any regularly taken, with adequate supply

  Antibiotic treatment dose for traveler's diarrhea

  Antimalarial medication, if indicated

Consider:

  Antibiotic if child has recurrent otitis

  Injectable epinephrine kit, if there is a history of severe allergic reaction to insect stings or foods

  Antibiotic eye drops

  Medication for motion sickness, if susceptible

Continued

TABLE 12.7   Recommended Medical Kit for Travel with Children—cont'd

First-aid supplies/miscellaneous:
   Thermometer, safety pins, colorful adhesive bandages, ACE wrap
   Sunscreen, lip balm
   Disposable wipes
   Oral rehydration salts, pre-packaged
   Mosquito repellant
   Povidone iodine solution
   Nail brush for cleaning fingernails
For wilderness adventures, add:
   Thermal reflective blanket
   Structural aluminum malleable (SAM) splint
   Fingertip pulse oximeter

plan updated. It is advisable to review the management of asthma exacerbations and carry an adequate supply of inhalers and steroids in case of emergency. Evacuation insurance is a prudent purchase for all travelers, since medical evacuations are not a standard part of US health plans.

FURTHER READING

CDC, 2013. Use of Japanese encephalitis vaccine in children: recommendations of the advisory committee on immunization practices, 2013. MMWR Morb. Mortal. Wkly Rep. 62 (45), 898–900.
Information on dosing for young children.

Centers for Disease Control and Prevention (CDC), 2010. Transmission of yellow fever vaccine virus through breast feeding – Brazil, 2009. MMWR 59, 130–132.
Yellow fever virus can be transmitted through breastmilk to infants.

Centers for Disease Control and Prevention, 2016. CDC health information for international travel 2016. Oxford University Press, New York, NY.
Essential reference.

Chen, L.H., Zeind, C., Mackell, S., et al., 2009. Breastfeeding travelers: precautions and recommendations. J. Travel Med. 1195–1982.
Everything you wanted to know about breastfeeding and travel.

Committee on Injury, Violence, and Poison Prevention, American Academy of Pediatrics, 2011. Child passenger safety. Pediatrics 127, e1050–e1066.
Technical report on child passenger safety from the AAP. Specific recommendations on car seat use. There is a section pertaining to safety of children on commercial airlines.

Duster, M.C., Derlet, M.N., 2009. High-altitude illness in children. Pediatr. Ann. 38, 218–223.
A concise review of the topic.

Eren, M., Dinleyici, E.C., Vandenplas, Y., 2010. Clinical efficacy comparison of Saccharomyces boulardii and yogurt fluid in acute non-bloody diarrhea in children: a randomized, controlled, open label study. Am. J. Trop. Med. Hyg. 82, 488–491.
In this small study, probiotics appear to be beneficial in the treatment of acute non-bloody diarrhea in children.

Fox, T.G., Manaloor, J.J., Christenson, J.C., 2013. Travel-related infections in children. Pediatr Clin N Am 60, 507–527, Nice, simple review.

Hagmann, S., LaRocque, R.C., Rao, S.R., et al., 2013. Pre-travel health preparation of pediatric international travelers: analysis from the Global TravEpiNet Consortium. J Pediatr Infect Dis Soc 2, 327–334.
Our colleagues provide an important view of the challenges associated with the pediatric traveler. [See editorial in same journal: Omer SB, Orenstein WA. Vaccine refusal among pediatric travelers. J Pediatr Infect Dis Soc 2013;2:335-336.].

Hagmann, S., Schlagenhauf, P., 2011. Prevention of imported pediatric malaria – travel medicine misses the bull's eye. J. Travel Med. 18, 151–152.
A must-read editorial.

Hendel-Paterson, B., Swanson, S.J., 2011. Pediatric travelers visiting friends and relatives (VFR) abroad: illnesses, barriers and pre-travel recommendations. Trav Med Infect Dis 9, 192–203.
Review article on the pediatric VFR. Useful information.

Herbinger, K.H., Drerup, L., Alberer, M., et al., 2012. Spectrum of imported infectious diseases among children and adolescents returning from the tropics and subtropics. J. Travel Med. 19, 150–157.
Younger travelers are more likely to acquire an infectious diseases while traveling.

Hochberg, N.S., Barnett, E.D., Chen, L.H., et al., 2013. International travel by persons with medical comorbidities: understanding risks and providing advice. Mayo Clin. Proc. 88, 1231–1240.
While not a pediatric study, much of the findings have implications to the pediatric traveler with medical conditions.

Jost, M., Luzi, D., Metzler, S., et al., 2015. Measles associated with international travel in the region of the Americas, Australia and Europe, 2001-2013: a systematic review. Travel Med. Infect. Dis. 13, 10–18.
A nice analysis of measles transmission as relates to international travel.

Lafond, K.E., Englund, J.A., Tam, J.S., et al., 2013. Overview of influenza vaccines in children. J Pediatr Infect Dis Soc 2, 368–378.
New influenza vaccines reviewed.

Neumann, K., 2006. Family travel: an overview. Travel Med. Infect. Dis. 4, 202–217.
A comprehensive review.

Pitzinger, B., Steffen, R., Tschopp, A., 1991. Incidence and clinical features of traveler's diarrhea in infants and children. Pediatr. Infect. Dis. J. 10, 719–723.
The best description of the epidemiology of traveler's diarrhea in children.

Schlagenhauf, P., Adamcova, M., Regep, L., et al., 2011. Use of mefloquine in children-a review of dosage, pharmacokinetics and tolerability data. Malaria J 10, 292.
Mefloquine can still be a useful antimalarial agent in children.

Venturini, E., Chiappini, E., Mannelli, F., et al., 2011. Malaria prophylaxis in African and Asiatic children traveling to their parents' home country: a Florentine Study. J. Travel Med. 18, 161–164.
High-risk VFR children need attention to malaria prevention.

Warrell, M.J., 2012. Current rabies vaccines and prophylaxis schedules: preventing rabies before and after exposure. Travel Med. Infect. Dis. 10, 1–15.
Excellent review. Everything you wanted to know about rabies vaccines and preventive strategies against rabies.

CHAPTER 13

Students Traveling Abroad

N. Jean Haulman and Sarah Kohl

Students are traveling abroad in increasing numbers, with the largest increase observed in the university-student age group. Preparing the student for travel abroad encompasses the depth and breadth of travel medicine. The benefits of foreign travel and educational international exchange programs include cross-cultural knowledge and competency, international language development, leadership development, and personal growth.

Current data show shifting patterns of travel within the 13- to 17-year-old group. Information from the Council on Standards for International Educational Travel (CSIET) suggests that participation in semester-long or year-long study-abroad programs is decreasing for American students and increasing for those traveling to the United States from other countries. The statistical information from CSIET captures only data from school programs applying for CSIET listing; the exact number of students traveling abroad within this age group is currently unknown.

The number of American students traveling abroad in the university-age group has more than tripled in the last 20 years, and this trend appears to be accelerating. A recent study shows more students are traveling to Asia, Africa, the Middle East, and Latin America than in the past. University students often are more independent and travel more remotely than the younger students.

Students traveling abroad represent a distinct group within the travel medicine community due to rapid changes in physical and developmental maturation, propensity for risk-taking activities, and style of travel. Many students travel to remote locations for long periods of time and engage in activities with an increased likelihood of adverse health outcomes compared with older populations.

Due to their developmental maturation, traveling students often act like adults and children at the same time. In addition, students with the same chronologic age can be at different developmental ages. The wise practitioner will adjust his or her advice to the developmental level of the traveler.

Working with enthusiastic students can be a delight for the healthcare provider. But it requires subtlety to master the dual obligations to both the student and his or her parents. Having an open conversation at the outset of the appointment about what will and will not be disclosed often sets the tone for a successful visit. Many countries have specific regulations about how confidentiality about mental health and sexuality issues is handled.

Students traveling abroad will need the same counseling as other travelers regarding basic food and water precautions, insect bite avoidance, malaria prevention (when appropriate), and altitude precautions. It can be difficult to reach traveling students, as several studies show that they underutilize preventative travel health services. Additionally, this age group is likely to get health advice from nonprofessional sources such as guidebooks and travel websites.

The way in which the information is presented is likely to have a profound effect on how well the student understands and follows the recommendations. Practitioners working with university students often use a variety of formats, including group visits, educational videos, and questionnaires, to present the information in an engaging and relevant manner. If a chaperone is traveling with the group, he or she can reinforce healthy habits and behaviors, such as daily use of insect repellants, sun protection, and appropriate food choices.

THE PRE-UNIVERSITY STUDENT

Health-associated risk and specific disease entities in adolescent international travelers are underreported in the medical literature. Analysis of the GeoSentinel surveillance data shows that travel for tourism is the most common reason for travel in the 12- to 17-year-old group, but conclusions about diseases acquired while traveling cannot be drawn due to limitations created by the methods of data collection in this age group. In this age group, a case report of 29 female student New Zealand travelers (mean age 16) and six accompanying adults including one physician traveling to Peru found the following percentages of illness based on organ system: 37% gastrointestinal, 16% respiratory, 12% altitude, 7% dermatologic, 5% each for anxiety, genitourinary, neurologic, and musculoskeletal, and 3% adverse drug reactions.

UNIVERSITY STUDENTS

More information can be found in the literature for this group of travelers. University students traveling for pleasure often do so during designated school breaks, such as spring break, and travel for shorter periods of time (1-2 weeks), with "fun" being the driving force for the trip. Excessive alcohol consumption and risky sexual behavior have been associated with spring break vacations.

Students who travel for longer tourist excursions usually travel in the low-budget category, including backpacking and camping, which puts them at greater risk for various mosquito-, fly-, tick-, and water-borne diseases. These trips may include travel to more than one country. "Adventure" is often the driving force for travel in this population. The backpack traveler is more likely to take risks with personal safety; the lack of social norms, lack of an anchoring job or school responsibility, and freedom experienced in a new exotic environment lead to risky sexual behavior that may or may not be associated with alcohol and drug usage.

Another group of university students travel for study-abroad programs for 1-3 months at a time. This group often has a more formalized agenda than the adventure traveler; however, these students may seek adventure on the weekends or tack on an adventure trip at the end of their stay.

Students on longer trips for any reason are at risk for several additional health problems. Longer duration of stay is associated with chronic diarrhea, giardiasis, chronic fatigue, eosinophilia, cutaneous leishmaniasis (CLM), schistosomiasis, and *Entamoeba histolytica* diarrhea. Sometimes, traveler loneliness can precipitate a reactive depression. Anticipation of these problems and arrangement for post-travel follow-up may be needed.

HEALTH SCIENCE STUDENTS ABROAD

The advent of global health programs has spurred health science students' interest in participating in clinical programs in less developed countries. An interest in international health, a desire for increased cultural competency, the need for hands-on clinical experiences, and the desire to help have all been cited as reasons for the growth in electives abroad for health science students. These students are more mature than undergraduate students; however, they still may not perceive true risks in less developed countries. Surveys of medical students and nursing students with high-risk blood-borne pathogen exposure including human immunodeficiency virus (HIV) have shown that students rarely if ever report such injuries and do not take HIV post-exposure prophylaxis (PEP), even if they bring the medicines with them.

Many health science schools have developed specific curriculum criteria such that only experienced students participate in higher-level clinical activities. However the literature still reports that "junior" students participate in risky procedures such as surgeries and delivery of babies. In addition, provision of care in less developed countries exposes students to illnesses related to poverty and crowding, such as tuberculosis and meningococcal disease.

Counseling for health science students traveling internationally for clinical rotations should include the standard destination-specific travel advice: vaccine recommendation, malaria prophylaxis, medication for travelers' diarrhea, and insect precautions. Students in health science fields usually have already been vaccinated with hepatitis B vaccine. The counseling should include screening pre and post travel for tuberculosis either with a purified protein derivative placement or one of the interferon gamma-releasing assay (IGRA) blood tests. Meningococcal vaccine should be offered if the student is traveling to high-risk countries (e.g., the meningitis belt in Africa) or will have prolonged clinical contact with host populations.

Universal precautions, high-risk procedures (e.g., surgical procedures in regions with a high prevalence of HIV), and the need for HIV PEP should be discussed, offering HIV PEP if necessary. Due to the costs and side effects of such medications, students are often given a 3- to 5-day quantity with the understanding that the exposure necessitates an immediate trip back to the home country for more medication and monitoring. Current recommendations for HIV PEP can be found at http://nccc.ucsf.edu/clinical-resources/pep-resources/pep-guidelines.

Some studies show that despite their medical education, health science students are less likely to follow recommendations for malaria prophylaxis and insect precautions. This disparity between perceived and real risk is of paramount importance due to the intimate nature of contact with patients. As for all students traveling abroad, the risks of motor vehicle safety, drug usage, alcohol overconsumption, and unprotected sexual experiences should also be discussed.

VACCINES FOR STUDENTS

Routine childhood vaccinations vary by country. Recommended schedules for European countries can be found at http://vaccinews.net/vaccination_schedule.php. However, a review of actual vaccines received by the specific student is needed to avoid any gaps in coverage.

Students who are under-immunized present a unique problem for the travel medicine provider. Increasing rates of vaccine refusal in childhood puts this subset at risk of acquiring preventable illness while traveling. Healthcare providers encountering an under-immunized student will need to have a frank discussion about the suitability of travel to the desired destination without proper immunization and discuss strategies for "catch-up" immunizations (see http://www.cdc.gov/vaccines/schedules/hcp/imz/catchup.html). The risk of acquiring vaccine-preventable disease while traveling is not trivial; there are many reports of under-immunized travelers returning with vaccine-preventable diseases.

Students traveling to remote destinations or for long periods of time are more likely to need rabies pre-exposure prophylaxis and Japanese encephalitis vaccines than others. Students are typically unaware of the dangers of encounters of potentially rabid animals. Rabies avoidance precautions are essential, since the long-term traveler who is feeling lonely may want to pet an animal. Many students forego rabies vaccine due to the high cost in the developed world without realizing the difficulty of obtaining rabies immune globulin in the event of a bite. Students should be encouraged to purchase travel health insurance with evacuation to assist with obtaining appropriate wound care in a timely manner.

MEDICATIONS FOR TRAVELING STUDENTS

Pediatric dosing schedules for medications should be used for students between 12 and 17 years of age. Consult Chapter 8, on pediatric travelers, for advice about appropriate dosing of altitude and malaria medications. Traveler's diarrhea is treated with azithromycin

10 mg/kg/day for 3 days up to a maximum of 500 mg per day for 3 days. Some students will need their antibiotics in dry powder form with instructions for reconstitution, and others can manage tablets easily. Rifaximin or symptomatic care can be used for the azithromycin-intolerant adolescent.

University and graduate students use adult doses of medications. Obtaining the patient's medication list is very important when prescribing either ciprofloxacin or azithromycin. Given the stress of higher education, many students are taking medication for depression and/or mood stabilization. These drugs may cause prolongation of the QT interval when used in combination with azithromycin or ciprofloxacin. Consultation with a pharmacist is recommended. Rifaximin is an alternative for these patients. Also, one should always be mindful that unintended pregnancy is a possibility. Medications that are inappropriate for pregnant women should be avoided.

THE ROLE OF THE CHAPERONE

The challenge for the healthcare provider is to help students prepare to manage their health and safety while away from familiar surroundings and the assistance of their families. Students traveling abroad with a chaperone are often younger students, travel in groups, and typically visit well-traveled itineraries.

Since most chaperones are parents or teachers not trained in healthcare, ground rules need to be established about the role of a chaperone in a student's health. It is important for the student, the chaperone, and the sponsoring organization to have a clear understanding of what health information needs to be shared with the chaperone, privacy issues, and how to handle health problems that arise. Additionally, the student and family should be reminded that the chaperone is not typically trained in healthcare, and this should be kept in mind when planning to travel with a chronic illness. The student and/or family member may request a note from the specialist detailing additional precautions and emergency plans with the chaperone.

TRAVELING WITH CHRONIC ILLNESS

Helping the student with an underlying medical condition successfully travel is one of the joys of travel medicine. The secret to a successful trip is plenty of advance planning. The travel medicine provider will need to guide the traveler in examining what conditions at the destination are likely to either cause a flare-up of symptoms or impact the traveler's ability to respond to a flare-up of the underlying health problem. For example, discussions about travel with asthma might include exposure to possible triggers such as cigarette smoke, air pollution, mold in damp climates, cold air, respiratory infections, and animals in people's homes. In addition, the level of medical care available at the planned destination should be reviewed with regard to the student's particular health condition. With careful questioning many problems can be anticipated or avoided all together.

Travelers with chronic conditions such as diabetes, asthma, Crohn's disease, and other diseases often have predicable causes of flare-ups. Most have become quite adept at managing these episodes in their home country. Anticipatory guidance should include providing the student with a sufficient quantity of his or her maintenance medications for the duration of the trip along with the usual medications for flare-ups. It is also important to educate both the traveler and supervising adult about what to watch for, when it is okay to self-treat, and when to seek medical care locally.

Many advocacy organizations organized around a particular disease have informative "how to" tip sheets and travel guides available on their websites. National health services such as the Centers for Disease Control and Prevention, National Health Service, Health Canada, and Australian Department of Health also have informative web pages designed to assist travelers with questions about specific diseases. Chapter 16, on Travel with Chronic Medical Conditions, is an excellent resource for more detailed information.

Traveling with food sensitivities or allergies causes significant concern for the student and his or her family. Several organizations offer pre-printed cards in multiple languages to help avoid the offending items. Accidental exposure to the offending food often happens when traveling despite using the language cards. For this reason travelers with food sensitivities and allergies should be prepared to manage a severe reaction. If a student with anaphylaxis to certain foods is traveling with a chaperone, teaching the chaperone to use an epinephrine auto-injector and the importance of follow-up care at a local emergency room is essential. Unaccompanied students will need to educate their traveling companions about their severe reactions and what their companions should do to help the distressed traveler.

Students with compromised immune systems (immune-compromising illnesses or who take immunosuppressive medications) represent a distinct group. Modern medications may have normalized the lives of these patients so dramatically that they are now ready to join their peers studying abroad. These students may experience a significant flare-up of their underlying disease or an increased susceptibility to certain infections acquired at their destination. Their disease state and medication dosage may limit the ability to receive live attenuated vaccines such as yellow fever vaccine, thus limiting travel to certain geographic destinations. They are also harder to protect prior to departure since they are also more likely to have a weakened immune response to other vaccines.

Healthcare providers will need to provide advice for management of common health problems and/or significant flare-ups of the underlying condition and determine how to protect the student from infections and access the ability of local medical providers to provide appropriate and timely care. For example, some destinations are well equipped to manage a flare-up of organ transplant rejection or Crohn's disease, while others are not. Often this will require consultation with the healthcare providers at the destination; this is far easier to do now through use of the Internet access to colleagues in international professional societies. Some destinations may not be appropriate for a particular student based on conditions at the destination or level of available medical care. Frank discussions are often uncomfortable, but necessary, in these situations.

MENTAL HEALTH

Traveling with a mental health problem has its own set of unique uncertainties. Two issues need to be addressed: Is the condition stable enough to withstand the stresses of travel? and Are the routine medications used permitted in the host country? Many students do not disclose their underlying illness due to privacy or other concerns. This leaves the chaperone or supervising adult in a delicate position, one for which they are untrained, should there be an exacerbation of symptoms. Full disclosure and honest discussion of the underlying problem and management is essential in ensuring a successful trip.

There are no established guidelines to determine whether a mental health problem is stable enough to withstand the stressors of travel. A common rule of thumb is that it is okay to travel if the dose of medication has not been adjusted within the last 3 months and if the supervising mental health provider agrees that the student is ready for travel. It is important to discuss the role of maintaining routines in sleep, eating, and medication usage throughout travel.

Certain medications, including stimulants used for attention deficit hyperactivity disorder, may or may not be permitted at the destination. The student should be encouraged to contact the embassy or consulate of the host country to inquire about local laws and regulations for their specific medication. Many patients are unaware that they can receive up to 3 months of medication prior to departure from their home country with proper documentation from their supervising doctor. If time allows, some can be switched to nonregulated medications prior to departure.

The student should be discouraged from stopping medication while traveling. The stressors of travel are known to exacerbate underlying mental health problems. Additionally, some places and healthcare systems do not have the capacity to provide treatment of mental health problems. Therefore, prior to departure, contingency plans for repatriation in the event of worsening symptoms should be discussed. For this reason, purchase of travel health insurance should be strongly encouraged.

SOCIAL ISSUES

Traveling to other nations and cultures fosters deeper cultural understanding. This occurs at a time of increasing independence of the adolescent. At times students can be unsure of themselves, often looking to the group for acceptance and normative behaviors. Parents often express concern and anxiety as their son or daughter moves through this maturational process.

The separation created as the student travels abroad can temporarily increase this anxiety until both parents and children become more comfortable with this newfound independence. In some cases, this separation provokes the parent to request or demand inappropriate and somewhat smothering contact with their child. This limits the ability of the student to learn to travel independently. Discussing this with the family, especially of the younger student, by emphasizing the supervision provided by the sponsoring group and setting up guidelines for frequency of contact, allows for a successful transition.

Travel to another culture raises the possibility of experimentation with activities that are different from those in the student's home country. Students often interpret differences in rules and regulations, such as age of drinking alcohol, as tacit permission to participate. Alternatively, what may be permissible in the home country may have severe penalties in the host country, such as drug use or same-gender sexual encounters.

Alcohol use among university and graduate students is common. A study of university students found that, overall, university students traveling abroad drank twice as much as in their home country and reported negative consequences from this drinking. The degree of integration within the local culture had a protective effect against the negative effects of alcohol use. Clearly, counseling about alcohol overconsumption is needed, including its association with poor judgment and unprotected sexual encounters.

Students will need to become culturally aware of the customs and taboos of the host country. This becomes vitally important regarding issues of sexuality. In some locales, premarital sex or same-sex encounters are prohibited. Safer sexual practices, appropriate birth control, and follow-up care should be reviewed with the student. Familiarize the traveler with how to access information regarding emergency birth control in the event of unprotected sexual encounter (e.g., http://ec.princeton.edu/ecmaterials/).

PERSONAL SAFETY

Parents worry whether their child will be safe when studying abroad. This concern is validated by understanding that the adolescent brain does not fully mature until about age 25. As a group, adolescents have less executive function and fewer inhibitions. This leads to participation in more risky behavior. The desire for adventure coupled with the immature frontal lobes sets up a dynamic where the young adult traveler is at risk for personal safety issues.

In the United States the leading causes of death in the 12-29 age group are motor vehicle crashes, homicide, suicide, and other accidents; all are more common for men than women. Data about death of US citizens while abroad is not segregated by age but show motor vehicle crashes, homicide, suicide, and drowning as the leading causes of death while abroad. Of note, in one study 15% of motor vehicle crashes involved a motorcycle. The student should be actively counseled about the inherent risks of two-wheeled modes of transportation; this risk is amplified in low- to middle-income countries.

Drowning is almost as common as suicide among US travelers abroad. Caution the enthusiastic student to always check the depth of the pool or pond before jumping in and to never jump in head first. Unfamiliarity with the currents, inability to swim, and lack of lifeguards are thought to contribute to drowning. Personal flotation devices (life jackets) may be in short supply at water sport concessions. Those who wish to scuba dive should always search for a Professional Association of Diving Instructors (PADI)-certified dive shop and follow the buddy system and other best diving practices.

Water safety also includes counseling for schistosomiasis and leptospirosis prevention (when appropriate) and what to do in the event of an unanticipated exposure to potentially infectious fresh water. Numerous case reports of documented infections with only one exposure to water exist. If one member of a group tests positive, all should be tested, since up to 80% may test positive within the cohort. The advice to avoid fresh-water exposure can be confusing to the active student who may encounter water sports concessions that appear very similar to home. It cannot be emphasized enough that they must avoid all waters known to be infected.

The negative effect of alcohol consumption on judgment must be discussed in conjunction with accident reduction. As in the home country, death, accidents, unintended sexual encounters, and other risky behavior are all associated with alcohol consumption. Legal ages for alcohol consumption may be much lower than in the home country, which may lead to the traveler drinking at a younger age.

Many study-abroad programs include a home stay. No guidelines exist for evaluation the safety of these popular programs. The prudent traveler will investigate how the host families are vetted by the sponsoring agency.

The goal of effective counseling is to change behaviors and minimize risk to the traveler. At the time of this writing, the most effective techniques to counsel young travelers to reduce risk are not known; this is an ongoing area of active research. It is known that many students travel abroad without pre-travel professional healthcare.

CONTINGENCY PLANNING FOR EMERGENCIES

From time to time emergencies arise when studying abroad. Travel health insurance with repatriation in the event of severe illness is strongly advised. These policies are minimal in cost and can be purchased on behalf of the entire group. Each sponsoring organization has a different policy regarding decision making and parental consent for medical treatment in the event of an emergency. In some instances written permission is needed to allow the chaperone to make decisions on behalf of the parent. Encourage the traveling student and his or her family to learn how communication will be handled in the event of an emergency.

SUMMARY

Students traveling abroad are increasing in numbers. Researchers are gathering data on where students are traveling, for how long, and what they are doing there. Preliminary trends show an increase in complexity of travel plans to more remote locations and for longer periods of time. Students traveling abroad for vacation, cultural exchange, and scholastic studies are vulnerable to predictable safety and health concerns. The poor executive brain function associated with this age group is thought to contribute to the propensity for risk-taking behavior.

Preparing the student for a successful travel abroad experience requires addressing vaccinations, infections, and medications and managing any underlying illnesses at the destination. Ideally the first visit to the healthcare practitioner will be 4-6 weeks in advance of departure. Accident reduction counseling is essential due to the increase in risk-taking behaviors by this age group. Certain groups, such as long-duration travelers and health sciences students, require additional counseling for specific health problems related to the activities at the destination.

FURTHER READING

General Travel

Harvey, K., et al., 2013. Surveillance for travel-related disease – GeoSentinel Surveillance System, United States, 1997-2011. MMWR 62 (3).

This article reviews the diagnoses among 10,032 United States after-travel patients.

Pre-University Adolescent Student Traveler

Hagmann, S., et al., 2010. Illness in children after international travel: analysis from the GeoSentinel Surveillance Network. Pediatrics 125 (5), doi:10.1542/peds.2009-1951.

This study is the only systematic review of the demographics, travel related illness, and health care use of children after international travel.

University Student Travelers

Emergency contraception: <http://ec.princeton.edu/ecmaterials/>.

This website provides information on how to provide emergency contraception using a worldwide database of oral contraceptive pills.

Hartjes, L.B., et al., 2009. Travel health risk perceptions and prevention behaviors of US study abroad students. J. Travel Med. 16 (5), 338–343. doi:10.1111/j.1708-8305.2009.00322.x.

Demographic, sources of travel prevention information, and travel related problems are discussed in this retrospective cross-sectional web-based questionnaire for returned University of Wisconsin study abroad students.

Hunley, H.A., 2010. Students functioning while studying abroad: the impact of psychological distress and loneliness. Int. J. Intercult. Relat. 34 (4), 386–392. doi:10.1016/j.ijintrel.2009.08.005.

This article highlights the psychological stress that may occur in study abroad students.

Pederson, E.R., et al., 2010. Heavier drinking American college students may self-select into study abroad programs: an examination of sex and ethnic differences within a high-risk group. Addict. Behav. 35, 844–847. doi:10.1016/j.addbeh.2010.04.003.

Students selecting study abroad programs may be a subgroup of heavier drinkers.

Rhodes, G., et al., 2014. Study Abroad & Other International Student Travel, Chapter 8 Advising Travelers with Specific Needs, CDC Yellow Book.

This chapter in the CDC yellow book has excellent resources and information for international student travel.

Health Science Student Travelers

PEP @ UCSF.edu: <http://nccc.ucsf.edu/clinical-resources/pep-resources/pep-guidelines>.

This website has up-to-date recommendations on occupational HIV post-exposure prophylaxis.

Franklin, G.F., et al., 2001. Provision of drugs for post-exposure prophylaxis of HIV for medical students on overseas elective. J. Infect. 43 (3), 191–194. PMID 11798258.

37% medical students participating in overseas electives from one medical center reported significant exposure to potentially infective fluids. Strategies to provide PEP for HIV in regions where it is not readily available are discussed.

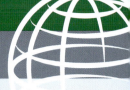

CHAPTER 14

Advice for Women Travelers

Susan Anderson

Travel health issues for women will vary according to the life stage and lifestyle of the women. Issues differ depending on whether the woman is in her second trimester of pregnancy or about to go on her first solo journey at age 80. To adapt the standard pre-travel health recommendations to the needs of a female traveler, one needs to consider potential gender- and age-related issues with regard to susceptibility and long-term sequelae of parasitic and other infectious diseases, safety of immunizations during pregnancy, and adaptation of the medical kit for health concerns relevant to the life stage of the woman. Other gender-related issues that may be important relate to environmental risks, such as altitude or climate, and sports-related concerns.

Gender-related issues in travel and tropical and wilderness medicine are important to consider when we counsel female travelers regarding possible risks of disease before travel. For example, are the immunizations and medications recommended for a specific itinerary contraindicated in pregnancy? Can a woman on estrogen replacement trek safely over an 18,000-ft pass? What is a woman's risk of female genital schistosomiasis and future infertility if she is a Peace Corps volunteer working on a water conservation project for 2 years in a country endemic for schistosomiasis?

GENDER-BASED MEDICINE

In 2001, the Institutes of Medicine released a landmark report that studied the basic biochemical differences in the cells of males and females as well as the health variability between the sexes from conception throughout life. The report confirmed the differences between the sexes in the prevalence and severity of a broad range of diseases, disorders, and conditions. In 2004, the Society for Women's Health Research persuaded the US Congress to include language in a 2005 appropriations bill demanding the National Institutes of Health to "include sex-based biology as an integral part" of all medical research.

GENDER-RELATED ISSUES IN TROPICAL DISEASE

Although there is a growing body of research in developed countries with regard to the interrelationships between gender and health, few studies in developing countries have focused on gender differences with regard to the biomedical, social, or economic impact of tropical diseases, much less their impact at the personal level. For this reason, the World Health Organization (WHO) section of Tropical Diseases Research formed the Gender and Tropical Disease Task Force to stimulate research on gender determinants and consequences of tropical disease. The focus of WHO is on women living in endemic countries. We also need to consider the possible gender-related effects of tropical disease on female travelers living in endemic areas for extended periods and/or female adventure travelers involved in high-risk activities.

For many diseases endemic to the developing world, differences between female and male prevalence rates in indigenous people are difficult to measure, as cases in women are more likely to be undetected. When incidence rates in women and men are equal, there are still significant differences between the sexes in both the susceptibility and impact of tropical disease. Even when tropical diseases are shared by both sexes, they may have different manifestations, natural histories, or severity. For example, exposure to malaria is similar in women and men, with a slightly higher incidence in men. Biologically, however, a woman's immunity is compromised during pregnancy, making her more likely to become infected and implying a different severity of the consequences. Malaria during pregnancy is an important cause of maternal mortality, spontaneous abortion, and stillbirths.

Similarly, both sexes are susceptible to schistosomiasis, but genital schistosomiasis in women has been associated with a wide range of pathobiologic manifestations such as infertility, abortion, and preterm delivery. Thus physicians may be confronted more often with parasitic infections causing infertility, not only in patients originating in tropical countries but also in Western women as a result of a tendency to travel and work in exotic and subtropical countries.

Further research is needed to clarify the general question of sex differences in susceptibility and differential severity of the sequelae of tropical infectious diseases. These issues are important when we advise women on pre-travel issues, especially the long-term or adventure traveler. Knowledge of gender-specific risks for tropical disease is also important when we evaluate returned female travelers and recent female immigrants for health problems related to their history of travel and/or living in countries endemic for tropical diseases.

GENERAL HEALTH ISSUES OF WOMEN TRAVELERS

Basic questions related to health include the following: What is the woman's reproductive stage of life? Is she using contraception? Is her contraceptive method appropriate for her travel itinerary? Does she have emergency contraception? Is she prepared to treat the usual women's health problems, such as urinary tract infections (UTIs), vaginitis, and menstrual cramps? Is she pregnant, planning to get pregnant, or breast feeding? If menopausal, does she have estrogen replacement therapy or herbal medications for symptoms? A format for obtaining a pre-travel health history for women is given in **Table 14.1**.

Women's Travel Medicine Kit

Women travelers, especially those embarking on adventure travel itineraries or planning extensive travel abroad, may find it beneficial to augment the basic travel medical kit (see Chapter 1) with supplies and medications specific to a given woman's life stage and reproductive health. **Table 14.2** lists items that might be included in a travel medical kit for women, and **Table 14.3** provides some Internet resources for further information on health issues of women travelers.

Menstruation

Women between 12 and 55 years old menstruate, on average, once a month, with a high degree of variability among women. During travel, a woman should be prepared for either the worst menstrual period of her life with more cramping and more bleeding than usual or for her periods to actually cease. Menses may cease or become irregular during travel for a number of reasons other than pregnancy. For example, the mere stress of traveling, including changes in sleep patterns, diet, activity, illness, and time zones, can easily disrupt a woman's menstrual cycle. Recommendations can be made regarding measures to take depending on whether she uses oral contraceptives, her previous history, and the result of a self-pregnancy test. A woman should be warned that just because she is not menstruating while traveling does not mean she is not ovulating. She still needs a method of contraception to prevent unplanned pregnancy. Self-pregnancy tests are also important in the evaluation of a sexually active woman of reproductive age to help determine whether her abdominal pain and/or abnormal vaginal bleeding could be related to a pregnancy.

TABLE 14.1 Pre-Travel History for Women

Current age
Menstrual history
    Date of last menstrual period
    Irregular menses/dysfunctional uterine bleeding
    Menstrual products: tampons, pads, alternative options
    Premenstrual syndrome
    Postmenopause
        Symptoms
        Issues regarding hormonal vs. nonhormonal prescription drugs
Reproductive history
    Previous pregnancies, births, abortions
    Need for contraception/emergency contraception
    Pregnancy issues during travel
    Lactation
Sexually transmitted infections
    Male partners
    Female partners
    Both
    Diagnosis and treatment card
    HIV post-exposure prophylaxis for high-risk encounters
Health maintenance
    Vital signs: blood pressure, heart rate, and respiration
    Breast self-examination
    Mammogram
    Pap smear
    Bone density
    Electrocardiogram

HIV, Human immunodeficiency virus.

It is important to carry sufficient disposable sanitary napkins or tampons, since they are not available in many countries. Menstrual cups are another option. There are also reusable tampons made out of sea sponges and a variety of washable pads. Reusable products are ideal for the environmentally concerned backpacker and the long-term traveler. Pre-moistened towelettes for personal hygiene and plastic bags to dispose of sanitary supplies are also useful.

Some women prefer not to have a menstrual cycle while traveling. One option to control the menstrual cycle is through the use of a hormonal contraceptive method, such as the combined oral contraceptive pill, patch, or vaginal ring. By skipping the "hormone free" week and continuing the active hormone component (pill, patch, or ring) as directed, no withdrawal bleeding occurs, until the woman is ready to stop the active hormone and get withdrawal bleeding.

Medication for menstrual cramping and other symptoms of premenstrual syndrome should also be carried in the medical kit (**Table 14.2**).

Urinary Tract Infections
Women are prone to UTIs during travel as a result of multiple factors, including dehydration, less frequent urination because of a lack of convenient toilets, fewer available facilities

TABLE 14.2   Medical Kit for Women

Menstrual supplies
  Calendar to keep track of menses
  Supplies/devices
    Pads, tampons, menstrual cups (disposable vs. reusable)
    Towelettes/plastic disposal bags
  Premenstrual syndrome
    Ibuprofen, other
  Dysfunctional uterine bleeding
    Premarin, estradiol
    Oral contraceptive pills
    Ibuprofen, other
Urinary tract infections
  Ciprofloxacin
  Macrobid
  Pyridium
  Optional: urinary dipstick to check for leukocytes and nitrites
Urinary voiding
  Toilet tissue, towelettes
  Funnels, paper or plastic
  Disposable personal urinal bag ("portable john")
Vaginitis caused by *Candida*
  pH paper: pH <4.5
  Acidophilus dietary supplements
  Vaginal creams: miconazole vaginal cream
  Vaginal suppositories: Mycostatin
  Oral medication: fluconazole
  Mild soaps
Hydrocortisone cream for pruritus
Loose-fitting clothes
Bacterial vaginosis
  pH paper: pH >4.7
  Vaginal creams: metronidazole, clindamycin
  Oral: metronidazole, clindamycin
Trichomoniasis
  Metronidazole
Contraception
  Chart to keep track of pills if using them, menstrual periods
  Timer: special wrist watch alarm or smartphone app to use for oral contraceptive dosing when
    changing time zones
  Male/female condoms
  Diaphragm/cap/sponge
  Spermicides/contraceptive creams, jellies, films
Emergency contraception
  Review options in country of destination
  Ulipristal acetate (Ella)
  Levonorgestrel and combined pill regimens
  Anti-emetic tablets or rectal suppositories

Continued

TABLE 14.2   Medical Kit for Women—cont'd

Emergency post-exposure HIV prophylaxis for high-risk unprotected sexual encounter
Pregnancy tests
  Carry extras, depending on length of trip
Sexually transmitted infections
  Preventive measures: condoms, dental dams, Saran wrap, gloves, barrier methods
  Magnifying glass
  Chart for identifying basic lesions, symptoms, recommendations for treatment
  Medications for treatment
Perimenopausal/menopausal issues
  Vaginal dryness: vaginal moisturizers, estrogen: creams, pill, or ring
  Menstrual cycle irregularity: consider low-dose oral contraceptive
  Stress incontinence: vaginal moisturizers and lubricants, Kegel exercises
  Hot flashes and night sweats
  Estrogen replacement therapy (ERT)
  SSRIs, progestins, gabapentin
Insomnia
  Avoid stimulants (caffeine, other), exercise, eat food with tryptophan
  Irritability/moodiness: exercise, ERT vs. antidepressants
  Osteoporosis: weight-bearing exercise, calcium, vitamin D, medications
  Headaches: may be triggered by changes in hormones
Pregnancy supplies
  Blood pressure cuff
  Urine protein/glucose strips
  Leukocyte esterase strips
Personal safety
  Alarms
  Pepper spray
  Lessons in self-defense before trip

SSRI, Selective serotonin re-uptake inhibitor.

for hygiene, an increase in sexual activity, and other changes in exercise, diet, and clothing. Preventive measures include instructions for female travelers to stay well hydrated and to urinate wherever there is convenient access to a public toilet whether or not the bladder is full.

A number of plastic and paper funnel devices have been designed so that a woman may urinate in the standing position. Another option to try for a cold night in a tent or when there is no bathroom facility is a "portable john." This is a unisex funnel that empties into a biodegradable plastic bag with biodegradable filler that turns the urine into a solid so it will not spill. The personal urinal bags can be used until full (800 cc or 28 oz), then disposed of.

To maintain hygiene, it is important to carry a supply of paper tissues or toilet paper and some packets of pre-moistened towelettes in a fanny pack or backpack. If an older woman is experiencing vaginal dryness and urinary frequency or urgency without dysuria, recent data suggest that estrogen vaginal creams, a vaginal ring, or even an oral contraceptive pill intravaginally once a week may decrease urogenital dryness and frequency symptoms. Vaginal moisturizers (e.g., Replens) can also be used. If a woman experiences increased frequency, urgency, and dysuria, she should be advised how to diagnose and treat herself for a UTI with an antibiotic and an analgesic.

TABLE 14.3   Internet Resources for Women Travelers

	Website	
Contraception		
International Consortium for Emergency Contraception	www.cecinfo.org/ www.cecinfo.org/country-by-country -information/status-availability-database/	Emergency contraception options worldwide
Emergency contraception options	http://ec.princeton.edu/worldwide/	Information about emergency contraception and what is available worldwide, searchable by country
International Planned Parenthood	http://www.ippf.org/ www.ippf.orgwww.contraceptive.ippf.org/	Information on contraceptive methods available worldwide, searchable by composition, brand name, type, manufacturer
Contraceptive technology	www.contraceptivetechnology.org/	Resource on contraceptive technology
Sexual health	http://www.cdc.gov/sexualhealth/	
		Information for women travelers on issues related to sexual health and contraceptive options worldwide
HIV post-exposure prophylaxis	http://nccc.ucsf.edu/ http://nccc.ucsf.edu/clinician-consultation/ pep-post-exposure-prophylaxis/ http://nccc.ucsf.edu/clinical-resources/ pep-resources/pep-quick-guide/	Non-occupational PEP guidelines; PEP hotline 888-448-4911
Pregnancy		
Pregnant traveler	www.pregnanttraveler.com	Resource for clinicians and pregnant travelers
Lactation		
Thomas Hale	http://neonatal.ttuhsc.edu/lact/	Resource on issues relating to breast feeding and medication use
International Lactation Association	http://gotwww.net/ilca/	Resource for an international lactation consultant for women
Evacuation insurance		
International SOS	www.internationalsos.com	
MEDEX	www.medexassist.com	
Travel kit		
Female urinary directors	www.freshette.com www.travelmateinfo.com www.traveljohn.com	Options for female urinary directors
Menstrual supplies	www.divacup.com/www.keeper.com/ www.softcup.com/www.gladrags.com/	Reusable menstrual products for travel
Travel guide for women	http://travel.gc.ca/travelling/ publications/her-own-way	Travel information for women travelers throughout the lifespan

If an older woman has a problem with stress incontinence or bladder control, she should consult with a physician specializing in female urinary tract problems in advance of the anticipated trip. For minor problems, a woman can be taught to do Kegel exercises and should bring a supply of panty liners.

Vaginitis

Women are at risk for vaginitis during travel, secondary to many of the same reasons as for UTI. One of the most common causes of vaginitis is *Candida albicans*. This organism usually causes a thick cottage cheese-like white discharge with vulvar and vaginal itching. The risk of yeast vaginitis may be greater if doxycycline is used for malaria chemoprophylaxis or if other broad-spectrum antibiotics are used for the treatment of traveler's diarrhea or other medical problems.

Several topical preparations against yeast are available over the counter, including nystatin, miconazole, and clotrimazole vaginal creams or troches. Prescriptions for resistant cases can be recommended, such as tetrazole vaginal cream (3 days) or fluconazole (150 mg as a single oral dose). Many women prefer to use the oral medication, as the vaginal creams can be messy during travel. Other women feel the vaginal creams help with the symptoms of itching. A hydrocortisone cream may also be used if needed for vulvar itching. Any persistent symptoms should be evaluated by a gynecologist when returning home. Even if a woman has never had vaginitis, it is important to prepare her for the possibility, especially for extended travel.

Another common cause of vaginal discharge is bacterial vaginosis. This is caused by overgrowth of the bacteria in the vagina, which can be due to many of the same causes listed previously. The discharge is usually more of a grayish color with a fishy odor. Bacterial vaginosis is treated with metronidazole tablets taken orally or clindamycin vaginal cream applied topically. If a female traveler develops a discharge and pelvic pain after a new sexual encounter, she may have a sexually transmitted disease and should follow the recommendations discussed in Chapters 41-44.

Contraception

Contraceptive advice should be included in the pre-travel counseling for all women of reproductive age at risk for pregnancy. It should also be included in the pre-travel counseling for men who might put women at risk for pregnancy. This is especially important if the man's partner might be in a country where she might not have easy access to contraception.

Women may become pregnant as a result of a lack or misuse of contraception, and women travelers are no exception. In the United States, over 50% of pregnancies are unplanned. If a woman is already using contraception, the method should be evaluated for its ease of use and reliability during travel along with any special recommendations concerning its use during travel. If a woman wishes to try a new contraceptive method, ideally she should begin months before travel, especially if she is planning to be overseas long-term or will be living in a remote area. Back-up plans for what the woman should do if she loses her present method should be discussed. The International Planned Parenthood Federation (IPPF) keeps a worldwide guide to contraceptives and an address list of family planning agencies available on the Web (**Table 14.3**).

Special Considerations for Women on Oral Contraceptives

Women should be advised to take extra supplies of their oral contraceptives with them, since it may be difficult to find the identical brand in another country. It may be difficult to remember to take an oral contraceptive pill when traveling because of changes in time zones and schedule. However, keeping on schedule is especially important for women taking the low-dose combined and progestin-only pills. It is advised that women on such regimens consider wearing a special wristwatch with alarm, dedicated to signaling when the 24-hour scheduled oral contraceptive dose is due, or to download one of the smartphone apps available to help remember medication dosing.

Another problem is pill absorption during illness. Nausea and vomiting and/or diarrhea may cause decreased pill absorption. If vomiting occurs within 3 hours of taking a pill, the woman should take another one. If nausea and vomiting and/or diarrhea are persistent, the woman should consider using another contraceptive method for the rest of the month. Another option might be to insert the oral contraceptive pill in her vagina for absorption. A number of studies have demonstrated vaginal absorption of hormones in either the pill or the ring form as a method of contraception or estrogen replacement. A woman might choose the contraceptive patch or vaginal ring as a good alternative contraceptive method for travel.

Drug Interactions That May Affect Oral Contraceptive Efficacy

A big concern among women travelers taking oral contraceptives is whether antibiotics affect oral contraceptive efficacy. Antibiotics have been shown in animal studies to kill intestinal bacteria responsible for the deconjugation of oral contraceptive steroids in the colon. Without such deconjugation and subsequent reabsorption, decreased hormone levels may result, leading to a decrease in hormone efficacy. Despite numerous case reports of penicillins, tetracyclines, metronidazole, and nitrofurantoin causing contraceptive failure in humans, no large studies have demonstrated that antibiotics other than rifampin lower steroid blood concentrations.

To date, there are no known drug interactions between oral contraceptives and malaria chemoprophylaxis such as atovaquone/proguanil and mefloquine. Doxycycline and other broad-spectrum antibiotics temporarily reduce colonic bacteria, thus inhibiting the entero-hepatic circulation of ethinyl estradiol. The importance of this effect on the enterohepatic circulation varies from woman to woman. This is not thought to be clinically significant, and a back-up method of contraception is not routinely recommended. A more conservative approach would be to recommend a back-up method of contraception for the first 3 weeks a woman is taking both doxycycline and oral contraceptives. If the hormone-free week occurs during this time, she should continue her contraception with a new package of hormonally active pills so as not to let her blood levels fall. After 3 weeks, the enterohepatic circulation should be restored and the back-up method of contraception stopped.

Contraceptive Failure: Emergency Contraception

The potential for being or becoming a pregnant traveler exists for most women of reproductive age. Contraceptive failures are common. Condoms break, diaphragms slip, oral contraceptives may be missed due to changes in time zones, or malabsorption of the pill may occur as a result of vomiting and diarrhea. The contraceptive method could also be lost or stolen. A woman may experience a rape or assault.

Emergency contraception (EC) is defined as a method of contraception that a woman can use after unprotected intercourse to prevent pregnancy. For maximum effectiveness EC treatment should be started as soon as possible after unprotected intercourse. Treatment is most effective if initiated within the first 12-24 hours and definitely within 120 hours. Thus it is important for the travel medicine clinician to include a recommendation for emergency contraception for all women who may be at risk for pregnancy and/or how to access EC.

Ulipristal acetate (Ella) was approved by the US Food and Drug Administration (FDA) in 2010 and is the most effective EC pill. It is a progesterone receptor modulator and is effective for up to 5 days after unprotected intercourse. It is available by prescription or on the Web. In Europe it is known as ellaOne.

The easiest method for a female traveler to obtain is Plan B, consisting of two tablets of levonorgestrel (750 μg). Plan B is approved by the FDA for over-the-counter sale. Other options for EC include regimens using progestin-only mini- or low-dose pills to provide a dose comparable to the branded Plan B product or using regular oral contraceptives containing ethinyl estradiol and either norgestrel or levonorgestrel (**Table 14.4**). Recent data suggest that the progestin-only EC treatment (two tablets of 750 μg levonorgestrel taken together as one dose) is more effective and causes less vomiting than does treatment with

TABLE 14.4   Emergency Contraceptive Methods

Brand	First Dose	Second Dose (12 h later)	Ulipristal Acetate per Dose (mg)	Ethinyl Estradiol per Dose (μg)	Levonorgestrel per Dose (mg)
	Ulipristal Acetate Pills				
Ella	1 white pill	None	30		
	Progestin-only pills				
Levonorgestrel	2 white pills	none			1.5
Plan B one step	1 white pill	none		0	1.5
	Combined estrogen and progestin pills				
Levora	4 white pills	4 white pills		120	0.60
Lo/Ovral	4 white pills	4 white pills		120	0.60
Nordette	4 light orange	4 light orange		120	0.60
Seasonal	4 pink pills	4 pink pills		120	0.60

Adapted from <http://ec.princeton.edu/>; more options on the Web.

combined estrogen-progestin tablets (100-120 μg ethinyl estradiol and 500-600 μg levonorgestrel in each dose). Nausea and vomiting are common with the combined pill regimen, so antiemetic tablets may be prescribed to be taken 30 min before the second dose of oral contraceptive. Mifepristone (RU-486) is an antiprogesterone drug that can be used for EC in lower doses than used for medical abortion. It prevents the release of an egg from the ovary and makes the uterine lining inhospitable to implantation. Studies have shown it to be more effective, safer, and with fewer side effects than either levonorgestrel or the combined pill regimen. It is available in Europe and China.

Worldwide, there is great variability in the availability of EC. If a woman loses her prescription or it is stolen, it would be important to advise her of the methods that might be available in the areas she is traveling. The Emergency Contraception Website (http://ec.princeton.edu/) has information on EC methods and a searchable database for options available worldwide. There also is an Emergency Contraception 24-hour hotline (1-888-NOT-2-LATE). If a traveler becomes pregnant and wishes to terminate the pregnancy, it may be best for her to return home. More than half of the 128 countries listed by the IPPF prohibit abortion except in extreme circumstances, such as rape and life-threatening illness.

Sexually Transmitted Infections

Sexually transmitted infections (STIs) are of special importance to women due to gender-related pathophysiology that leads to an increased rate of transmission from an infected male to an uninfected female. In addition, women suffer more serious sequelae from a sexually transmitted disease, such as pelvic inflammatory disease or infertility, than do men.

To prevent STIs, one should avoid casual sex or practice safe sex by using condoms, regardless of concomitant use of another method of birth control. High-quality latex condoms are an essential part of the personal medical kit of adult travelers, regardless of gender and whether or not sexual activity during travel is planned or unplanned. A female condom made out of polyurethane is an effective alternative for persons allergic to latex. Travelers may be provided with an information card or sheet summarizing STI signs and symptoms for use in self-diagnosis and possible treatment if remote from professional medical care. One resource is the sexual health website at the Centers for Disease Control and

Prevention (CDC; www.cdc.gov/sexualhealth/). Women travelers should be informed about the availability of antiretroviral drugs and their use in post-exposure human immu-nodeficienty virus (HIV) prophylaxis (termed non-occupational post-exposure prophylaxis [NPEP]) following a high-risk sexual exposure or sexual assault. The rate of HIV transmis-sion from an infected male to an uninfected female is estimated to be equivalent to a high-risk needle stick. Thus, NPEP should be started preferably within 1 hour and no later than 72 hours after a high-risk exposure.

In certain cases, a woman traveler may be given an NPEP "starter kit" of a 3- to 5-day supply of antiviral drugs. This can be used in an emergency until the situation can be further evaluated and/or more medication can be obtained. As the drugs can be associated with significant adverse effects, ongoing NPEP treatment should be administered under medical supervision. These medications are not available in most developing countries.

Gynecologic Concerns at Altitude

Women taking oral contraceptives may continue them at moderate altitudes (<3600 m, or 12,000 ft), since the risk of pregnancy may be greater than the risk of thrombosis. Women on oral contraceptives have a higher risk of deep vein thrombosis (DVT)/pulmonary embo-lism (PE) at any altitude, estimated to be about 5/100,000. Pregnancy increases the risk of DVT/PE 12-fold to about 60/100,000. Women on oral contraceptives should be advised to consider other contraceptives for extended stays at very high altitudes (>5500 m), because of a theoretical increased risk of thrombosis and PE.

TRAVEL DURING PREGNANCY

Pregnant women of all ages and at all stages of pregnancy travel for business, professional, and personal reasons. First, the past medical and obstetric history should be reviewed with the woman in conjunction with her obstetrician (**Table 14.5**). Travel during the last month of pregnancy and travel that may pose a serious risk to the mother or the fetus should be avoided. Possible risk factors and potential contraindications to travel are listed in **Table 14.6**. If a woman has had a previous adverse pregnancy outcome or has had a difficult time becoming pregnant and is in her late 30s or 40s, she should weigh the possible risks with particular caution.

The complete itinerary should be evaluated with attention to the quality of medical care possible both during transit and at the final destination. Access to high-quality care during travel is essential in case of pre-term labor or an unexpected complication of pregnancy. The itinerary should also be reviewed for possible risks of exposure to certain infections, for example, chloroquine-resistant *Plasmodium falciparum* malaria, hepatitis E, typhoid, ame-biasis, influenza, polio, and yellow fever, as these travel-associated diseases may have more severe or even fatal complications in a pregnant woman because of her altered immune status during pregnancy compared with a nonpregnant individual. In addition, there are special considerations concerning the use of malaria chemoprophylactic drugs and certain immunizations during pregnancy. The potential exposure to specific health risks may be improved by adjusting certain destinations and activities on the trip route.

It is important for a woman to check her health insurance plan regarding coverage. Many plans do not cover pregnant women overseas, and many have gestation cutoff dates for travel beyond which they will not cover delivery out of the area. She may have to buy additional coverage and emergency evacuation insurance. All pregnant travelers should carry a copy of their medical records (including current gestational age, expected date of delivery, blood type and Rh, and a copy of fetal ultrasound report) in case of emergency.

Basic Questions to Answer When Counseling Pregnant Women

Pregnant women anticipating travel to remote places need to have the following questions answered before confirming their itinerary:
1. What medical, obstetric, social, and demographic risks are associated with travel?
2. Are the required and recommended immunizations for the itinerary safe in pregnancy?

TABLE 14.5   Pre-Travel Evaluation for Pregnant Woman

Step	Content
History	Review past medical and past obstetric and gynecologic history
Physical examination	Obstetrician to assess gestational age, fetal growth performance, coexistent medical, obstetric, social, and demographic risks
Laboratory tests	Ultrasound
	Serology for hepatitis A and B, E, CMV, measles, rubella, varicella, and toxoplasmosis, depending on history
Review planned itinerary	Access to care
	OB/GYN care during transit and at destination
	Health insurance coverage
	Evacuation insurance
	Risk/benefit analysis for mother and fetus for exposure to:
	Infectious disease: usual and exotic
	Recommended immunizations
	Recommended chemoprophylaxis against malaria
	Risk of treatment if acquire the disease along itinerary
	Environmental risks
	Water/food
	Transportation
	Insects
	Altitude
	Scuba diving
	Pollution
	Heat
	Sports activity
	Other
Specific recommendations	Immunizations
	Environmental risks
	Transportation
	Insects
	Water/food
	Altitude
	Self-treatment measures for minor complaints (nausea, bloating, reflux, urinary frequency, hemorrhoids, pedal edema, other)
	Review emergency signs and symptoms
	Medical kit: see Chapter 1
	Carry copy of medical history including blood type and Rh factor, ultrasound results, and other pertinent data

CMV, Cytomegalovirus; *OB/GYN,* obstetric/gynecologic.

3. What drugs against malaria and other parasitic illnesses are safe in pregnancy?
4. What prophylactic or therapeutic measures against traveler's diarrhea are safe in pregnancy?
5. What medical services are available in the area(s) of destination?
6. What does her health insurance cover if she is out of area for delivery or pregnancy-related complications?
7. What are signs of serious pregnancy-related illness for which emergency medical help should be sought?

TABLE 14.6   Potential Contraindications for Travel during Pregnancy

Absolute contraindications	Relative contraindications
Abruptio placentae	Abnormal presentation
Active labor	Fetal growth restriction
Incompetent cervix	History of infertility
Premature labor	History of miscarriage or ectopic pregnancy
Premature rupture of membranes	Maternal age <15 or >35
Suspected ectopic pregnancy	Multiple gestation
Threatened abortion, vaginal bleeding	Placenta previa or other placental abnormality
Toxemia, past or present	Medical conditions: heart disease, diabetes, lung disease, thrombosis, kidney disease, other systemic illnesses
Destination risk considerations	Postpone travel if risks outweigh benefits.
Malaria	
Outbreak of disease requiring live vaccine	
Outbreak of a disease for which no vaccine is available but there is a high risk of fetal and maternal morbidity	
Medical services during transit and at destination	
Environmental risk considerations: altitude, heat, water, other	

Adapted from: Centers for Disease Control and Prevention. CDC Health Information for International Travel 2016. New York: Oxford University Press; 2016.

8. What are some general guidelines to follow for the medical management of illness that will safeguard the pregnant woman and her fetus?

Cultural aspects of traveling while pregnant or nursing should also be researched prior to travel. Customs vary in different cultures. Breast feeding an infant in public areas may not be allowed in some cultures.

Transportation Risks during Pregnancy

Airlines

Airline policies regarding pregnancy and flying vary, so it is best to check with them when booking a flight. Some may require medical forms to be completed. Most airlines do not allow pregnant women to travel if they are at more than 35-36 weeks' gestation without a letter from a physician. Commercial aircraft cruising at high altitudes are able to pressurize only to 5000-8000 ft (1524-2438 m) above sea level. Women with moderate anemia (Hgb <8.5 g/dL) or with a compromised oxygen saturation may need oxygen supplementation. The fetal circulation and fetal hemoglobin protects the fetus against desaturation during air flight (see Chapter 4).

Certain precautions should be taken by pregnant women during flight. During pregnancy, alterations in clotting factors and venous dilation predispose these women to superficial and deep thrombophlebitis, or "economy class syndrome." Pregnant women have a rate of acute iliofemoral venous thrombosis that is six times more frequent than that of nonpregnant women. Contributing factors to this risk may be (1) compression on the inferior vena cava and iliac veins by the enlarged uterus and/or (2) an increase in the coagulation factors and fibrinolysis inhibitors. The pregnant traveler should request an aisle seat and should walk in the aisles at least once every 30 min during long airplane flights, whenever it is safe to do so, to increase the circulation. General stretching and isometric leg exercises should be encouraged on long flights.

The low humidity of pressurized flights leads to significant insensible water loss. The humidity in cabins is low. Hydration is crucial for placental blood flow. Women should be encouraged to drink non-alcoholic beverages. Seat belts should be worn low around the pelvis and should be worn throughout the flight.

Intestinal gas expansion can be particularly uncomfortable for the pregnant traveler. She should avoid gas-producing foods and airline food. Women should bring their own healthy snacks and bottled water.

Jet lag is an important phenomenon for travelers heading eastward over several time zones. Pharmacologic therapy for jet lag is not recommended during pregnancy. Pregnant women should get enough fluids, food, and rest whether or not they use planned schedules to avoid jet lag. A program of daily exercise and alteration of sleep pattern that can minimize disturbances in circadian rhythm and mentation that occur as a result of jet lag are recommended. Melatonin has not been found to cause toxicity during pregnancy, but it has not been well studied.

Radiation exposure during airport security is minimal and has not been found to increase adverse outcomes. These are magnetometers and are not harmful to the fetus.

Automobile Travel

A pregnant woman should not sit for prolonged periods when traveling in an automobile or bus because of the risk of venous stasis and thromboembolism. Varicose veins of the perineum and legs are also common pregnancy-related problems exacerbated by prolonged sitting or a supine posture. Thus, pregnant women should wear elastic hose and avoid prolonged periods of immobilization. The usual recommendation is driving for a maximum of 6 hours/day, stopping at least every 1-2 hours for 10 minutes, to walk and increase venous return from the legs.

Motor vehicle accidents account for most severe blunt trauma to pregnant women. The American College of Obstetricians and Gynecologists (ACOG) has recommended that pregnant women wear three-point restraints when riding in automobiles. Travelers should be warned that in many parts of the world, taxicabs and other automobiles and buses do not have safety restraints.

Sea Travel

Most cruise liners will carry pregnant women up to the seventh month of pregnancy and have reasonably well-equipped medical facilities aboard. A woman should research the availability of medical care, equipment, and trained personnel on board. Lack of access to medical care may be an issue on sailboats operated by smaller tour companies or on self-designed tours. One of the main health risks during sea travel is the exacerbation of nausea and vomiting associated with pregnancy. Caution must be observed when walking on deck to avoid accidents caused by the motion of the ship and the general imbalance imposed by pregnancy.

FDA Use-in-Pregnancy Ratings

The FDA has established a system that classifies drugs on the basis of data from humans and animals, ranging from class A drugs, which are designed as safe during pregnancy, to class X drugs, which are contraindicated in pregnancy because of proven teratogenicity. The system has resulted in ambiguous statements that not only may be difficult for physicians to interpret and use for counseling but may cause anxiety among women. It is also been found that the classification is not updated when new data are available.

Category A	Adequate and well-controlled studies in women show no risk to the fetus.
Category B	No evidence of risk in humans. Either studies in animals show risk but human findings do not or, in the absence of human studies, animal findings are negative.

Category C	Risk cannot be ruled out. No adequate and well-controlled studies in humans, or animal studies are either positive for fetal risk or lacking as well. Drugs should be given only if the potential benefit justifies the potential risk to the fetus.
Category D	There is positive evidence of human fetal risk. Nevertheless, potential benefits may outweigh potential risks.
Category X	Contraindicated in pregnancy. Studies in animals or humans or investigations or post-marketing reports have shown fetal risk that far outweighs any potential benefit to the patient.

The Teratology Society has proposed that the FDA abandon the current classification in terms of more meaningful, evidence-based narrative statements. Other countries, such as Sweden, Australia, the Netherlands, Switzerland, and Denmark, have different classification systems based on a hierarchy of estimated fetal risk.

All clinicians advising pregnant travelers should have access to references such as *Drugs in Pregnancy and Lactation* by Briggs et al. (2011) and online sources such as the Organization of Teratology Information Services (http://otispregnancy.org/) and the Teratogen Information Service (http://depts.washington.edu/~terisweb/teris/). The clinician must help the pregnant woman to weigh the risk to benefit ratio of travel on both the developing fetus and maternal health. This includes evaluating the risks for the woman or her fetus with regard to the recommended immunizations, need for chemoprophylaxis, and exposure to malaria, traveler's diarrhea, or other parasitic and infectious diseases and environmental concerns. If the women must travel, physicians and other health practitioners involved in travel advice should be aware of the following guidelines and precautions that will help to ensure the safety of the mother and her unborn traveler.

Travel Vaccines for Women

Recommendations, cautions, and contraindications regarding vaccines may change depending on a woman's life stage. Ideally, women who are planning pregnancy should consider pre-conceptional immunization to prevent disease in their offspring. It is estimated that over 50% of all pregnancies are unplanned, so it makes sense to update the travel and routine immunization status of all women on a regular basis. If a woman receives a live virus vaccine, she should defer pregnancy for at least 4 weeks due to the theoretical risk of transmission to the fetus. If a woman receives a live virus vaccine and later finds out she is pregnant, it is not an indication to terminate the pregnancy. Vaccine registries collecting post-exposure data have found no increase in fetal anomalies in pregnant women inadvertently vaccinated with a live virus vaccine to date. Breast feeding is not a contraindication to vaccination. Post partum is an ideal time to update any vaccinations a woman may need.

Vaccination during Pregnancy

The risk to benefit ratio of each immunization should be carefully reviewed with regard to its potential effect on the fetus versus risk of contacting the actual disease and its subsequent effect on the mother or fetus. Vaccination during pregnancy usually outweighs any theoretical risk of the vaccine when the risk of exposure to the disease is high. Ideally, vaccination should be avoided in women during the first trimester, owing to uncertain effects on the developing fetus. The presence of protective serum antibodies against hepatitis A, hepatitis B, varicella, measles, and rubella could be checked to assess the traveler's susceptibility (www.cdc.gov/vaccines/adults/rec-vac/pregnant.html).

Toxoid vaccines, such as tetanus, diphtheria, and pertussis vaccines; inactivated vaccines, such as inactivated polio vaccine, inactivated typhoid vaccine, hepatitis A and hepatitis B vaccines, viral influenza vaccine, and rabies vaccine; and polysaccharide vaccines such as meningococcal and pneumococcal vaccines are all probably safe in pregnancy, as well as immune globulin or specific globulin preparations. These vaccines are classified as Pregnancy

Category B or C because there are insufficient scientific data to evaluate the safety and use of these vaccines in pregnancy. Indications for vaccination during pregnancy are listed in **Table 14.5**.

Live, attenuated-virus vaccines are generally contraindicated in pregnant women or those likely to become pregnant within the next month after receiving vaccine(s). Measles, mumps, rubella and varicella vaccines are absolutely contraindicated during pregnancy. Yellow fever and Japanese encephalitis vaccine may be given if high-risk exposure is unavoidable, because the theoretical risks of the vaccine are outweighed by the potential risks of the actual disease on the mother and/or fetus.

Certain travel vaccines are discussed next in the context of the pregnant traveler. The reader should consult Chapter 5 for a detailed review of vaccines for travelers.

Cholera

Two oral vaccines are available outside the United States: Dukoral (www.crucell.com) and Shancol (www.shanhabiotect.com). Because cholera during pregnancy is a serious illness due to the effects of dehydration, exposure during pregnancy should be minimized whenever possible.

Hepatitis A Vaccine

Hepatitis A virus (HAV) infection of the mother is not associated with perinatal transmission; however, placental abruption and premature delivery of an infected infant have been reported during acute HAV infection. The safety and efficacy of the inactivated hepatitis A vaccines in pregnant women have not been established, and the vaccine is classified as FDA pregnancy category C by the manufacturer. Because this is not a live virus vaccine, the main concern is a febrile response. If a high-risk itinerary is planned, hepatitis A vaccine or immune globulin should be given. Serology should be checked before travel if the patient has lived in or was born in a developing country.

Hepatitis B Vaccine

Hepatitis B virus (HBV) vaccine is recommended for a pregnant woman if she is a long-term traveler planning delivery overseas, if there is a possibility she will be sexually active with a new partner, or if she is working in a healthcare clinic, refugee camp, or similar setting. HBV vaccine should be considered in all sexually active women including pregnant women visiting areas where blood is not routinely screened for hepatitis B. Hemorrhage after miscarriage or delivery could require transfusion with possibly infected blood. If the mother carries the hepatitis B surface antigen or e-antigen, the newborn should receive the HBV vaccine and hyperimmune globulin at birth. The recombinant (inactivated) HBV vaccine series can be administered to pregnant women who are at risk, preferably after the first trimester. Immunization for HBV also prevents hepatitis D.

Hepatitis A/B Combination Vaccine

No data in pregnancy. May be considered if indicated.

HPV Vaccine

Human papilloma virus (HPV) lesions in the genital area can proliferate during pregnancy and may be transmitted to the fetus during delivery. Data on the quadrivalent HPV vaccine are limited, and it is not recommended during pregnancy. Women should be encouraged to get vaccinated prior to pregnancy. Lactating women may receive HPV vaccine.

Japanese Encephalitis Vaccine

Relatively little is known about the risk of Japanese encephalitis (JE) virus acquired in pregnancy and the consequences of intrauterine infection; however, infection acquired during the first two trimesters has resulted in miscarriage. The safety of the currently available JE vaccines in pregnant women has not been determined. If travel to an at-risk area is not mandatory, travel should be delayed. The natural reservoirs for JE include pigs and aquatic birds; infections are transmitted by mosquitoes. Precautions for all travelers to

JE-endemic areas include prevention of mosquito bites and avoiding travel to rural agricultural areas where pig farming and rice paddies are present.

Meningococcal Vaccines

Immunization against meningococcal disease is required for travelers to Saudi Arabia during the Hajj and is recommended for travelers to high-risk areas, including the sub-Saharan African epidemic belt for meningococcal disease from December through June, or to epidemic foci such as Kenya, Uganda, Tanzania, Nepal, and India year round. Pregnancy is not a contraindication. The quadrivalent meningococcal conjugate vaccine (MCV4) against serogroups A, C, Y, and W-135 is safe and immunogenic among nonpregnant women 11-55 years of age, but no data are yet available on the safety of MCV4 during pregnancy. It may be used if clearly indicated. If a pregnant woman received MCV4, she should be registered with the pregnancy registry (800-822-2463). Studies of vaccination during pregnancy with the quadrivalent (A, C, Y, W-135) meningococcal polysaccharide vaccines (MPSV4) have not documented adverse effects. In a number of other countries, a bivalent meningococcal vaccine against serogroups A and C is commonly used. An A/C bivalent vaccine has been evaluated in pregnant women and infants during an epidemic of meningitis in Brazil and appeared to be safe. Meningitis B vaccines may be used in pregnancy and breast feeding if clearly indicated in outbreak situations

Polio

The pregnant traveler needs adequate protection against polio. Paralytic disease may occur with greater frequency when infection develops during pregnancy. Anoxic fetal damage with maternal poliomyelitis has been reported. There is a 50% mortality rate in neonatal disease contracted transplacentally during the third trimester. If the traveler has received the primary immunization and the last dose was within 10 years, she is considered protected (although some experts would recommend a booster within 5 years of traveling to a highly endemic area). The inactivated polio vaccine is recommended for adult travelers including pregnant women who need primary immunization or a booster dose for travel to endemic areas. Oral polio vaccine may be administered if inactivated polio vaccine is not available in a high-risk situation. Several thousand pregnant women in Finland received the oral polio immunization during a nationwide immunization campaign, and there was no increase in the occurrence of congenital malformations.

Rabies Vaccines (Diploid Cell Culture)

Rabies vaccine may be given during pregnancy for pre-exposure or post-exposure prophylaxis. A recent review of the literature found 24 cases of pregnant women exposed to rabid animal bites. The exposures occurred during all trimesters. The women received equine rabies immune globulin and Vero cell vaccine or duck embryo vaccine. Among the infants, two were born prematurely and there was one spontaneous abortion. There were no physical or mental abnormalities except in a case described where the child did well after surgical repair of transposition of the great vessels. In this case, the bite occurred after the heart would have been formed embryologically, so the congenital malformation was not thought to be vaccine related.

Vaccination pre-exposure or post-exposure to rabies is considered safe with modern tissue culture-derived rabies vaccine products. If a woman is at high risk or visiting an endemic country for >30 days, she can receive pre-exposure vaccination. Post-exposure vaccination should be administered as soon as possible after a scratch or bite of an infected mammal, including monkeys and bats. In a mother with rabies, a viable infant should be delivered as soon as possible and given rabies hyperimmune globulin and the post-exposure vaccine regimen.

Tetanus, Diphtheria (Td) and Tetanus, Diphtheria, and Pertussis (Tdap) Vaccines

Immunization with Td and Tdap is safe in pregnant women. Tdap allows high levels of antibody to be transferred to newborns during the first 2 months of life when the morbidity and mortality from pertussis infection in infants is the highest. Pregnant women at 26 weeks of pregnancy or later should be encouraged to received a dose of pertussis-containing vaccine such as Tdap.

Typhoid Vaccines

Two vaccines are available for the prevention of typhoid. Information is not available on the safety of either of these vaccines during pregnancy. The Vi capsular polysaccharide parenteral vaccine is recommended during pregnancy only if clearly indicated. The live-attenuated Ty21A bacterial oral vaccine is not recommended on theoretical grounds.

Varicella

Varicella during pregnancy can lead to severe maternal illness, and it appears to be five times more likely to be fatal than in nonpregnant women. Varicella infection during pregnancy usually leads to birth of a healthy infant; however, in utero infection may lead to congenital abnormalities or severe varicella of the newborn.

Post-exposure prophylaxis of varicella is indicated for pregnant women with a history of varicella exposure. VariZIG is a purified immune globulin made from plasma containing high levels of antivaricella antibodies (immunoglobulin class G [IgG]). If a woman is given VariZIG prophylaxis, she should also receive the varicella vaccine 5 months later, to assure immunity. If a pregnant women exposed to varicella cannot receive VariZIG or immune globulin within 96 hours, treatment with acyclovir could be considered. VariZIG may be obtained by calling 800-843-7477 or online at http://www.fffenterprises.com.

Yellow Fever

YF vaccine is a live virus vaccine and should not be given routinely to pregnant women. If a pregnant woman is traveling to an endemic area of very low risk and a certificate of yellow fever vaccination is required by the destination country, an official letter of waiver will meet the requirement (in lieu of actual vaccination) according to WHO regulations. If travel to a YF high-risk endemic area is necessary, the benefits of the vaccine are thought to outweigh the small theoretical risk to the fetus and the mother, and the vaccine should be given.

There are some conflicting data on the immunogenicity of the YF vaccine during pregnancy. The YF vaccine (17d vaccine) was administered to 101 pregnant women during the 1986-1987 outbreaks in Nigeria without any untoward effects to the fetus or the mother. Antibody responses of pregnant women and mothers who were vaccinated mainly during the last trimester were much lower than those of nonpregnant women vaccinated with YF in a comparable control group.

A more recent study has demonstrated a better immune response to the YF vaccine during pregnancy. The YF vaccine was given to 480 pregnant women at a mean of 5.7 weeks' gestation during a mass campaign in Brazil 2000. After a minimum of 6 weeks, 98.2% were IgG positive. Thus, the seroconversion rate for pregnant women to the YF vaccine was found to be 98% (425/433 pregnant women immunized early in pregnancy). Maternal seroconversion to the YF vaccine given during the first trimester did not appear to cause malformations.

There are a number of registries that are collecting outcome data on women exposed to certain vaccines during pregnancy. Thus, women who receive vaccination during pregnancy should be registered with the appropriate registry in order to develop more data on the safety of a vaccination during pregnancy.

Vector-Borne Diseases during Pregnancy

Personal protection measures to prevent vector-borne diseases are important during pregnancy, because some of these illnesses may have a more accelerated course during pregnancy. Mosquitoes have been found to be more attracted to pregnant women. Thus, it is imperative that pregnant travelers wear clothing that covers most of their body, apply permethrin to clothes and bed nets, and be meticulous about applying DEET-containing repellants to exposed skin. Use of insect repellants is reviewed in Chapter 6.

Malaria Chemoprophylaxis in Pregnancy

Prevention of malaria in travelers, including pregnant women, is discussed in detail in Chapter 6. In brief, the weekly doses of chloroquine phosphate used for chemoprophylaxis of chloroquine-sensitive strains of malaria appear to be safe during pregnancy. Chorioretinitis has been reported in newborns of mothers given daily doses of chloroquine and is a theoretical risk.

The chemoprophylaxis of malaria in areas where chloroquine-resistant malaria is present is more of a problem for the pregnant traveler, because of concerns about the safety of the other antimalarial drugs with regard to fetal growth and development. The CDC has issued a statement that mefloquine can be used in all trimesters for malaria prophylaxis and for treatment of malaria. Doxycycline is contraindicated due to teratogenic effects on the fetus. Primaquine is contraindicated as the fetus cannot be screened for glucose 6-phosphate dehydrogenase deficiency. Atovaquone-proguanil is not recommended because of the lack of safety data. (See Chapter 6 for a detailed consideration of alternative chemoprophylactic regimens for chloroquine-resistant *P. falciparum* malaria.)

Treatment of diagnosed malaria during pregnancy is indicated because the potential adverse effects of the antimalarial drugs to the mother and fetus are far outweighed by the potential morbidity and mortality of untreated malaria. Maternal malaria can cause profound anemia, predispose to serious intercurrent illness, cause intrauterine infection and placental insufficiency, and contribute to intrauterine growth retardation, prematurity, low-birth weight, abortion, and stillbirth. (The treatment of malaria is discussed in detail in Chapter 6.)

Prevention of Traveler's Diarrhea during Pregnancy

Antimicrobial prophylactic therapy is not recommended for prevention of traveler's diarrhea. Preventive measures include boiling water or purifying it chemically, drinking only bottled carbonated water, bottled or canned fruit juices or soft drinks, and hot liquids; and avoiding ice, salads, and raw vegetables. The iodine-based methods of chemical water purification (Chapter 7) by a pregnant woman could result in adverse effects on the fetal thyroid gland and are not recommended

Treatment of traveler's diarrhea is challenging. The typical illness causes 4-5 days of watery diarrhea and is self-limited but can lead to significant weakness and malaise in both the pregnant and nonpregnant traveler. Bismuth subsalicylate (Pepto-Bismol) is not recommended during pregnancy. Bismuth in large doses is a known teratogen in sheep, and in humans salicylates have been both teratogenic and the cause of fetal bleeds throughout pregnancy. The antiperistaltic medications loperamide and diphenoxylate have been used without complication in pregnant women and are not known teratogens. Diphenoxylate has a known narcotic-like effect, and loperamide a theoretical one, which could cause respiratory depression if given to the mother in high doses toward term. Both these antiperistaltic agents should be used with caution for control of frequent watery diarrhea and intestinal cramps in the traveler.

The usual antibiotic of choice for treatment of traveler's diarrhea is one of the fluoroquinolones; however, these have been contraindicated during pregnancy because of an association with fetal cartilage abnormalities in animal studies. The FDA has approved ciprofloxacin for use in pregnant and lactating women for anthrax prophylaxis. More data are needed. Some travel medicine clinicians will consider the use of ciprofloxacin for pregnant women for short-term use if indicated in the second or third trimester.

The best option for use in pregnancy for the treatment of enteric pathogens is azithromycin (Zithromax). Third-generation cephalosporins may also be considered. Doxycycline is thought to stain both fetal teeth and bones and is contraindicated in pregnant women and neonates. Rifaximin is non-absorbed; however, there are insufficient data to make an assessment regarding its safety during pregnancy.

In summary, it appears that the safest course for pregnant women is to take all preventive measures possible, and if diarrhea occurs, to have with them a supply of loperamide, oral rehydration solution (see Chapter 8), azithromycin, and a cephalosporin. If fever or bloody diarrhea occurs, immediate medical care should be sought.

Other Parasitic Diseases

All travelers can decrease the risk of acquiring parasitic infections in tropical areas by following general insect precautions (Chapter 6), by selecting safe food and water, and by wearing shoes in rural areas (Chapters 7 and 45).

The effects of parasitic disease, including protozoan, nematode, trematode, and cestode infections, on pregnancy and the fetus are summarized in **Table 14.7**. There are no absolutely safe antiparasitic drugs for use during pregnancy. Decisions for medical intervention must be made on the basis of serious risk to either fetal or maternal health by the disease itself. It is important to note that in the case of mild infection (light parasite loads), it is best to delay treatment until the postpartum period.

Other Infections

Hepatitis E virus (HEV) is a major cause of hepatitis in Nepal, India, Burma, Pakistan, China, and Africa. Transmission of the virus occurs through fecal–oral exposure. HEV acquired during pregnancy has a particularly high fatality rate of 15-30%. The reasons why

TABLE 14.7　Potential Effects of Parasitic Infections on Reproduction[a]

Parasitic Infections	Impaired Fertility	Failure to Carry to Term	Fetal Infection
Protozoans			
Entamoeba histolytica	X	X	X
Giardia lamblia	X	X	X
Leishmania species	X	X	X
Plasmodium species (malaria)	X	X	X
Trypanosoma species	X	X	X
Toxoplasma gondii		X	X
Pneumocystis carinii		X	X
Intestinal nematodes			
Ascaris lumbricoides	X	X	X
Enterobius vermicularis (pinworm)	X		
Trichuris trichiura (whipworm)			
Hookworm species	X	X	X
Extraintestinal nematodes			
Strongyloides stercoralis	X	X	
Trichinella spiralis	X	X	X
Filaria species	X	X	X
Trematodes			
Schistosoma species	X	X	
Clonorchis sinensis	X	X	
Paragonimus westermani	X	X	
Cestodes			
Echinococcus species	X	X	
Taenia species	X	X	

[a]See text for discussion.
Adapted from MacLeod, C.L., Lee, R.V., 1988. In: Burrow, G.N., Ferris, T.F. (Eds.), 2013. Medical Complications during Pregnancy, second ed. Saunders, Philadelphia.

the infection is more severe in pregnancy are not known. Prevention of HEV is dependent on strict food and water precautions. Pregnant women should avoid travel to areas with known outbreaks of HEV (Chapter 22).

Toxoplasma gondii is an intracellular coccidian parasite found throughout the world. Infection is spread through the ingestion of oocysts in undercooked meat, exposure through handling cat litter, and consumption of foodstuffs contaminated with oocysts. The most important factor is eating raw or undercooked meat. Cats excrete up to 10 million oocytes a day post-infection. Oocytes become infective 1-5 days after excretion and are spread by surface water. Oocytes can survive up to 1 year. Thus, contact with soil and water and eating undercooked meat are greater risk factors than exposure to cats. Fetal infection occurs as a result of primary maternal infection. Infection acquired prior to conception is not a risk to the fetus. The risk during pregnancy is that the infection will cross the placenta and cause spontaneous abortion, stillbirth, hydrops fetalis, or congenital infection. Preventative measures are important: pregnant women should avoid contact with cat feces, wear gloves when gardening, avoid eating raw or undercooked meat, and wash vegetables and salads thoroughly.

Exercise

For a woman with a normal pregnancy, there are no known contraindications to exercise. Pregnant women may plan to trek at altitude, ski, or go on extended bicycle trips. The ACOG guidelines state that pregnant women should tailor their exercise to their needs and abilities. The woman should exercise within a comfort zone. If the woman is healthy and accustomed to vigorous exercise, there is no reason that she cannot exceed the ACOG guidelines as long as she does not become hyperthermic, hypoglycemic, or dehydrated. In general, a pregnant woman should avoid any vigorous physical activities that she did not regularly participate in before pregnancy. Limitations and/or contraindications to an exercise program during pregnancy would include any of the following: a history of spontaneous abortion or miscarriage, premature labor, multiple gestation, incompetent cervix, unusual bleeding, placenta previa, and severe cardiac or pulmonary disease.

Temperature control is important. In general, a pregnant woman should avoid extreme exercise in hot and humid climates because of the possible effect of raising the maternal and fetal temperature. The concern is an increase in neural tube defects. Hot tubs and saunas should be avoided for the same reason.

The effects of altitude are discussed in Chapter 10. A medical commission from the International Climbing and Mountaineering Federation (UIAA) reviewed the research to date on women and altitude and in 2008 published a consensus paper as well as official recommendations at their website (www.theuiaa.org). There are limited studies on short-term exposure to altitude during pregnancy. Altitude-associated effects such as fetal growth retardation, pregnancy-induced hypertension, and neonatal hyperbilirubinemia have been documented in studies on permanent residents at altitude. Women with risk factors for pre-eclampsia or placental abruption or whose babies are at risk for intrauterine growth retardation should not go to high altitude. A healthy, non-acclimatized, sedentary pregnant women should not exceed an altitude of 2500 m (8250 ft) during the first few days of a short-altitude exposure and should allow a few days to acclimatize before exercising. A woman with a normal pregnancy may have no contraindication to short-term moderate exercise at 2500-3600 m (8000-12,000 ft) after acclimatizing for 2-3 days. Exercise may cause fetal hypoxia or pre-term labor at high altitude if competition occurs for blood supply between the skeletal muscles and the already compromised uteroplacental junction. Elite athletes, skiers, and mountain climbers should discuss their risk with their personal physicians. Pregnancy may increase a woman's risk of injury during sport-related activities due to a change in the center of gravity and joint laxity. Access to emergency care should also be considered when planning skiing or hiking activities in mountain areas.

There is no difference in the incidence of acute mountain sickness (AMS) between pregnant and nonpregnant women. There are few data on the treatment of AMS during pregnancy. Strict guidelines for acclimatization should be followed to prevent AMS. Acetazolamide and other sulfonamides are contraindicated during the first trimester due to animal studies demonstrating teratogenicity and, after 36 weeks, due to a risk of neonatal jaundice. If a pregnant woman has symptoms of AMS, the risks of the medication must be weighed against the symptoms. Descent and oxygen are preferred treatment. Use of acetazolamide or dexamethasone may be considered on an individual basis.

Scuba diving during pregnancy is absolutely contraindicated, since the fetus is at risk from nitrogen bubbles and gas embolism in the fetal placental circulation during decompression on ascent. If a woman inadvertently completes a dive before she knows she is pregnant, the present evidence is not to recommend an abortion, since normal pregnancies have been documented. Snorkeling can be practiced during pregnancy. Water skiing or other water sports that might force water and air in the vagina or injure the uterus are contraindicated for all pregnant women.

Medical Service Available in the Area of Destination

Travel during the last 4 weeks of pregnancy should be limited to travel that is absolutely necessary, to avoid delivery in an unfamiliar hospital without medical records. Domestic airline regulations stipulate that no travel at >36 weeks' gestation is allowed, and most foreign airlines have a cut-off point of 35 weeks' gestation. In addition, a note signed by the patient's physician specifying the expected date of confinement is required by most airlines. Pregnant travelers should ask their doctors for referral to colleagues in the destination countries. Listings of medical services available can be obtained from some travel agencies and airlines. A list of English-speaking physicians around the world is available from the International Association of Medical Assistance to Travelers.

Health Insurance Coverage When Out of Area

Each health insurance company has different stipulations about coverage when out of area. Many have gestational-date cut-offs for travel, beyond which they will not cover delivery out of area, and this information should be ascertained during trip planning, a long way in advance of departure.

Signs of Serious Pregnancy-Related Illness for Which Emergency Medical Help Should be Sought

These signs and symptoms should be learned before departure. Travel should be avoided, particularly in the last trimester, if multiple births are expected or if there is a history of pregnancy-induced hypertension or bleeding. Home blood-pressure cuffs and urine dipsticks for urine sugar and protein should be carried by pregnant women traveling to remote places during the third trimester. Signs of serious pregnancy-related illness for which medical attention should be sought include:

1. Vaginal bleeding
2. Severe abdominal pain
3. Contractions
4. Hypertension
5. Proteinuria
6. Severe headache or visual complaints
7. Severe edema or accelerated weight gain
8. Suspected rupture of membranes.

TRAVEL ISSUES AND BREAST FEEDING

A woman should be encouraged to travel with her nursing infant. Nursing reduces the risk of many enteric diseases in the infant. Resource information to facilitate travel with a nursing infant can be found in **Table 14.3**.

Women who are breast feeding may safely receive all vaccinations. With the exception of attenuated rubella virus, strains of live virus are not known to be transmitted in breast milk. Breast feeding is a precaution for the administration of YF vaccine due to at least three cases of YF vaccine neurologic disease in breast-fed infants.

There have been no large-scale, randomized clinical trials on the use of various medications during breast feeding. Most routinely prescribed medications are safe for use during breast feeding, but the clinician should check current sources on medication safety during pregnancy and breast feeding for new information.

The American Academy of Pediatrics publishes a list of drugs and chemicals that transfer into human milk (www.aap.org). "Medications and Breastfeeding Mothers" (Thomas Hale; http://neonatal.ttuhsc.edu/lact/) reviews the basic physiology of lactation and the current data on the degree of transfer of medications into human milk, the effect on mother and infant, and the relative risks to the infant.

Drugs used for malaria chemoprophylaxis are all excreted into human milk in small amounts. The amount of these drugs is insufficient to protect the nursing infant, therefore the infant must be adequately protected with antimalarial medications (see Chapter 6).

Meticulous breast hygiene should be practiced by the nursing mother while traveling. The signs and symptoms of mastitis and methods of self-treatment should be reviewed, such as more frequent nursing and/or pumping, warm compresses, and an antistaphylococcal antibiotic, such as cephalexin, for self-treatment. She should be warned about the possibility of a drug-resistant infection such as methicillin-resistant *Staphylococcus aureus* and the need for further assessment if there is no prompt improvement of her symptoms with her self-treatment measures.

A woman traveling without her nursing infant will need to take measures to maintain her milk supply while she is traveling. This would include using an electric or a manual pump to express the milk on a schedule similar to her nursing infant and a consideration of the supplies needed for milk storage during travel and at destination. Milk may be pumped and discarded if adequate refrigeration is not available. Milk may be stored and transported in refrigeration or frozen in dry ice. Freshly expressed milk is safe for infant consumption for up to 6-8 hours at room temperature, or up to 72 hours if refrigerated.

OLDER WOMEN TRAVELERS

Women are living longer, appear to look younger, and have more energy than their chronological age suggests, in spite of background medical problems. Breast cancer survivors have scaled major mountain peaks. Many octogenarians have free time and disposable income to trek in the Himalayas, kayak in the South Pacific, or volunteer in a refugee camp in Africa. There are data to support regular exercise and travel as being important to psychological health, well-being, and aging gracefully. Aging can also lead to a change in the response to immunizations, a change in metabolism of certain medications, and changes in response to environmental extremes.

Practical issues important to address with an older woman would be a history of osteoporosis and a risk for hip or other fractures. Risks for STIs and the need for hepatitis B (and A) vaccines and/or other health educational materials related to STIs should be discussed. Studies have shown that women over 50 do not always practice safe sex strategies and can be naïve about their risk for an STI. Symptoms related to the urinary tract, such as urgency, frequency, incontinence, dysuria, and more frequent UTIs, should be reviewed along with self-treatment measures and recommendations for helpful paraphernalia, such as female urinary directors, portable johns, and pads that could be included in the travel medical kit (**Table 14.2**).

Postmenopausal vaginal symptoms of vaginal dryness, discomfort, itchiness, and dyspareunia occur in 50% of older women. These symptoms can be treated with a vaginal moisturizer (Replens) and/or an estrogen preparation (cream, tablet, or ring). Pre-travel evaluations with an electrocardiogram, mammogram, and Pap smear are important prior to extended travel. Arranging medical and evacuation insurance is imperative.

Although there has not been much evidence-based research on travel medicine issues related to older women travelers, as the baby boomers age more data will be obtained.

PERSONAL SECURITY AND SAFETY ISSUES

All women should learn basic self-defense techniques before travel. Other advice might include the following: assess risks in new areas carefully, dress moderately and respect local customs, talk to other travelers, use common sense, and avoid walking in unknown areas at night. Individuals may carry pepper spray or a personal alarm to scare an assailant, depending on regulations at a destination.

SUMMARY

Pre-travel and post-travel evaluation of women should consider the life stage and lifestyle of the woman along with possible gender and age-related issues regarding the risks, prevention, and treatment of travel and tropical diseases. More research and data are needed in this area.

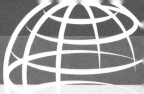

CHAPTER 15

The Immunocompromised Traveler

Shireesha Dhanireddy, Yuan Zhou, and Susan L.F. McClellan

As the world becomes increasingly interconnected, more people have the opportunity to travel outside their home communities and thus be at risk for novel and unexpected infections. The immunocompromised host requires special attention in pre-travel planning. This chapter will review travel preparations for immunocompromised patients, including human immunodeficiency virus (HIV)-infected individuals, solid organ or hematopoietic transplant recipients, and persons taking immunosuppressive medications.

THE IMMUNOCOMPROMISED TRAVELER

People with compromised immune systems require special preparation for travel to many geographic areas. The reasons are many and include increased risk of infection with common and unusual pathogens, failure of usual therapy to cure infection, atypical manifestations of infection, drug reactions and disease mimickers, diminished immune response to vaccines, and (especially in the case of HIV/acquired immune deficiency syndrome [AIDS]) political, social, and legal issues that may complicate movement from one country to another. Given the ease of administration of many current medications (e.g., monthly biologic agent injections, once-daily dosing of highly active antiretroviral therapy [HAART]) and improved side-effect profiles, many people are able to travel to both industrialized and developing nations. This raises additional issues about potential drug–drug interactions and the need for regular laboratory monitoring. **Table 15.1** lists drugs commonly used for immunosuppression and antiretroviral regimens and indicates potential interactions with drugs commonly used by travelers.

The immunocompromised traveler who becomes ill after returning home also poses special challenges. He or she may present with unusual manifestations of travel-related illnesses or develop complications from travel-acquired illness long after the exposure. Opportunistic infections may also occur in a time frame that mimics travel-related illness. With the complexities of such infections, both the travel medicine practitioner and the traveler's specialized care provider should coordinate prevention efforts and manage and coordinate care of the returned ill, immunocompromised traveler.

Infectious Disease Risks

Travelers frequently encounter pathogens that are absent or uncommon in their country of residence. In addition, their risk of infection with ubiquitous pathogens, such as *Salmonella* species, is greater during travel than during daily activities at home. Many of these pathogens can potentially cause increased morbidity and mortality in immunocompromised persons. In persons infected with HIV/AIDS (PHAs), a number of pathogens may be asymptomatic or cause mild symptoms in a traveler with a high CD4$^+$ T-cell count but manifest as a significant opportunistic infection if the person's CD4$^+$ T-cell count later falls. Three general

215

TABLE 15.1 Potential Drug Interactions of Frequently Used Travel-Related Medications[a]

Drug	Potential Interaction with Common Immunosuppression Medications[b]	Potential Interaction with HIV Medication
Acetazolamide	May increase potassium levels with prednisone	No specific contraindications
Atovaquone-proguanil		Decreased atovaquone and proguanil levels with atazanavir, lopinavir/ritonavir, and efavirenz, leading to less protection against malaria. No dose adjustment established
Azithromycin	May increase QT interval with prednisone	No specific contraindications
Chloroquine	Avoid with tacrolimus due to QT prolongation and risk for cardiac arrhythmias	No specific contraindications
DEET	No specific contraindications	No specific contraindications
Doxycycline	No specific contraindications	No specific contraindications
Loperamide	No specific contraindications	No specific contraindications
Proton pump inhibitors	May increase methotrexate level	Dose 12 h apart from atazanavir. Avoid with rilpivirine
H2 blockers	No specific contraindications	Dose at least 2 h before or 10 h after atazanavir. Dose at least 12 h before or 4 h after rilpivirine
Mefloquine	Contraindicated with cyclosporine due to QT prolongation and cardiac arrhythmias	May lower ritonavir levels (no recommendations to change dosing)
Pepto-Bismol (bismuth subsalicylate)	Monitor CBC if on methotrexate and salicylates	No specific contraindications
Quinolones	Avoid with cyclosporine due to increased cyclosporine levels and nephrotoxicity	Administer quinolone at least 2 h before didanosine

[a]Information obtained from pharmaceutical company package insert and communication with company representatives.
[b]Common immunosuppression medications reviewed in table: corticosteroids, calcineurin inhibitors (tacrolimus, cyclosporine), mycophenolate, nonbiologic disease-modifying antirheumatic drugs (DMARDs) (methotrexate, sulfasalazine, hydroxychloroquine, leflunomide, azathioprine), biologic DMARDs (infliximab, adalimumab, etanercept, rituximab, anakinra).
CBC, Complete blood count.

groups of infections merit special attention: enteric infections, respiratory infections, and vector-borne infections.

Enteric Infections

Pathogens that enter via the gastrointestinal tract pose considerable threat to the immuno-compromised traveler, as both intestinal mucosal and systemic defenses against gut pathogens are diminished. Decreased gastric acid and diminished local immune response mean that a smaller inoculum may be needed to establish infection. Once established, infection may be more severe and difficult to cure. The consequences of even typical traveler's diarrhea may be more profound for the immunocompromised patient. For PHAs taking antiretroviral therapy, nausea may be significant and interfere with the tolerability of their usual drug regimen. Infections with *Salmonella*, *Shigella*, and *Campylobacter* species tend to be chronic and relapsing and can lead to bacteremia. Salmonellosis in particular may be characterized by recurrent bacteremias. Campylobacteriosis, cryptosporidiosis, and microsporidiosis may extend into the biliary tree, making clearance more challenging. An important opportunistic pathogen to be aware of is *Strongyloides* (see Chapter 45). This infection is commonly found in tropical climates including the southeastern United States, acquired through the skin when travelers come into direct contact with fecally contaminated soil. *Strongyloides* is usually asymptomatic or causes mild diarrhea symptoms and a transient recurrent rash called larva currens. In immunosuppressed individuals, however, it can more readily cause acute hyperinfection syndrome. *Strongyloides* can also lie dormant for years to decades after initial infection. Cases of reactivated strongyloidiasis hyperinfection may happen after patients receive immunosuppression with even short courses of corticosteroids; most of these cases have been fatal. **Table 15.2** summarizes some of the enteric infections frequently encountered by travelers and indicates increased morbidity in immunocompromised persons, relative to the general population. Of note, increased risk was most notable in the pre-HAART era and likely reflects risk in patients with advanced HIV. Risk in relatively immunocompetent patients on effective ART may be similar to that of the general population.

Respiratory Infections

Respiratory tract infections are common during travel, although the etiology is usually undefined. Several outbreaks of influenza in travelers have been documented, necessitating vaccination and early treatment (both will be discussed later in this chapter). Legionnaires' disease is acquired from stagnant or poorly cleaned water sources and has infected travelers

TABLE 15.2   Enteric Infections in Travelers

Disease	Estimated Incidence in General Travelers[a]	Estimated Morbidity/Mortality in Immunocompromised Persons[b]
Amebiasis	Uncommon in most areas	Same or increased
Campylobacteriosis	Common	Increased
Cholera	Rare	Probably increased; no data
Cryptosporidiosis	Probably common	Increased; may become chronic and debilitating
Cyclospora	Probably common	Possibly increased
Escherichia coli diarrhea	Common	Possibly increased
Giardiasis	Uncommon in most areas	Same or increased; may become chronic and resistant to therapy
Isosporiasis	Uncommon in most areas	Increased
Microsporidiosis	Unknown	Increased
Salmonellosis	Common	Increased
Shigellosis	Common	Increased
Strongyloides	Common	Increased
Typhoid fever	Rare or uncommon in	Increased most areas
Vibrio parahaemolyticus and other noncholera *Vibrio* species	Uncommon	Possibly increased

[a]*Common* indicates pathogens reported to cause at least 5% of cases of diarrhea in travelers in multiple studies in different geographic areas; *uncommon* refers to pathogens causing <5% of diarrheal cases. *Rare* describes infections not found as a cause of diarrhea in most studies of travelers. For nondiarrheal illnesses, *rare* indicates incidence in travelers is <10 cases/100,000 per month.
[b]Estimated morbidity and mortality in immunocompromised persons represents a composite of greater frequency and severity of disease relative to normal hosts.
Adapted from Wilson, M.E., von Reyn, C.F., Fineberg, H.V., 1991. Infections in HIV-infected travelers: risks and prevention. Ann. Intern. Med. 114:582.

staying at resort hotels and using spa facilities in several locations, including Europe and the Caribbean. Outbreaks of influenza and legionellosis on cruise ships document another possible place of transmission.

Two geographically focal fungal infections, histoplasmosis and coccidioidomycosis, can be progressive and disseminate in immunocompromised persons. Infection occurs via inhalation of air-borne organisms. The endemic area for coccidioidomycosis includes the southwestern United States, Mexico, and Central and South America. Although the largest number of reported cases of histoplasmosis has been in the United States, the disease has been reported in all continents, and the organism is an important cause of disseminated disease in PHAs in the Caribbean and parts of Central and South America. Another soil-associated fungal pathogen, *Penicillium marneffei*, found in Southeast Asia and China, is one of the most common opportunistic infections in northern Thailand. Travelers to this region who become infected may manifest symptoms as early as 4-5 weeks and as late as 10 years or more after exposure. Immunocompromised travelers to areas where these fungi are endemic should take precautions to avoid inhaling dust or entering caves; if heavy or long-term exposure is unavoidable, prophylaxis with fluconazole (100 mg/day) for coccidiomycosis or itraconazole (200 mg/day) for histoplasmosis and penicilliosis may be used.

Immunodeficient persons are exquisitely susceptible to tuberculosis. Patients receiving anti-tumor necrosis factor (TNF) therapy are at particularly higher risk of tuberculosis reactivation. Up to 10% of HIV-infected persons with latent tuberculosis will develop active infection. The likelihood of exposure to tuberculosis in many developing countries (where annual incidence rates may exceed 100/100,000 population) is substantially higher than in the United States (with annual incidence rates <10/100,000 population). Rarely, transmission has also been documented during travel (e.g., airplane, bus, train, boat). Vaccination with attenuated bacillus Calmette-Guérin (BCG) is neither routine nor recommended in the United States, so avoidance of infection and early identification of latent tuberculosis infection are paramount. Tuberculin skin testing (TST) should be done routinely in all immunosuppressed persons, regardless of travel plans (see Chapter 25). An induration of 5 mm is considered positive in HIV-infected persons, organ transplant recipients, and those on immunosuppressive medications (equivalent of 15 mg prednisone). The TST should be repeated 2-3 months after prolonged stays in high-incidence areas, which include many parts of Africa and Asia. A period of 4-12 weeks after exposure is generally required for development of delayed-type reactivity to the TST; however, some patients may develop primary clinical disease prior to skin test conversion. Immunocompromised persons should avoid prolonged stays in areas where ventilation is poor, tuberculosis rates are high, and multidrug resistance is common. Newer interferon gamma release assays (IGRA) to detect latent tuberculosis infection are being used with increasing frequency. Neither the TST nor the IGRA is entirely reliable in any population, but they are of particularly limited utility in those with severe immune deficiencies, because of the increased possibility of anergic responses.

Vector-Borne Infections

Animals and insects transmit vector-borne diseases. While immunocompromised patients are not necessarily at higher risk for acquiring these infections than the general traveler, symptomatic disease can be more severe. Malaria is the most common cause of febrile illness in travelers. Data linking severe malaria and compromised immune systems are limited, but there is concern for severe manifestations of the disease in these patients. The interaction between HIV-1 infection and malaria is complex, although research confirms that HIV-1 infection increases the likelihood of both asymptomatic parasitemia and clinical malaria in persons from endemic areas. In areas of unstable *Plasmodium falciparum* malaria transmission, some studies have suggested more severe malaria and higher mortality from malaria in HIV-1 infected individuals, especially those with CD4+ T-cell counts <200 cells/mm^3. There is also evidence that HIV-1 infected persons are more likely to suffer treatment failure, which may be true for other immunocompromised populations. Prophylaxis against malaria would therefore be of utmost importance to the immunocompromised traveler, which will be reviewed later in this chapter.

A weakened immune system may dramatically change the clinical course of visceral leishmaniasis and likely also cutaneous leishmaniasis, leading to more severe and disseminated disease, especially in HIV-positive and transplant patients. In visceral leishmaniasis, mortality is high, not only due to delayed diagnosis, but also because of a poor immunological response to the pathogens. Typical clinical features, such as splenomegaly and hyperglobulinemia, may be absent, and antibodies, often sought for diagnostic purposes, may be absent or delayed in appearance. Infection may manifest months or years after exposure in endemic areas; these include popular tourist destinations, such as Spain and other parts of southern Europe.

American trypanosomiasis or Chagas disease is also more likely to disseminate in the immunocompromised individual. In HIV-positive persons, *Trypanosoma cruzi* has been recognized as a cause of acute meningoencephalitis and central nervous system (CNS) mass lesions, which are not typical presentations. Fortunately, few travelers stay in accommodations (i.e., straw-thatched dwellings) where they are at risk for being bitten by infective reduviid bugs, and reports of American trypanosomiasis in visitors to endemic areas have been rare.

Interestingly, dengue has not been reported to cause a more severe illness in immunocompromised patients, though this may be due to lack of recorded data. Similarly, there is a lack of studies on chikungunya in these patients, although it is a rapidly emerging disease found in many tropical areas around the world.

PREPARATION OF THE IMMUNOCOMPROMISED TRAVELER

Given a number of increased risks, it is important for immunocompromised travelers to seek the advice of a knowledgeable travel health practitioner prior to embarking; however, this need is not always recognized. A study of 267 transplant patients showed that one-third of patients traveled outside the United States and Canada following transplant; of these patients, only 66% sought pre-travel counseling from a medical provider. Another study in Canada of HIV-positive travelers showed that only 44% of PHAs sought health advice before traveling, and half of these patients did not disclose their HIV status.

The approach to the immunocompromised traveler involves a series of steps, outlined in **Table 15.3**, and should typically include communication with the patient's specialized care provider (e.g., HIV physician, oncologist, transplant coordinator). Some steps may be omitted or abbreviated, but evaluation and preparation of the immunocompromised traveler in most instances will require extra time. Essential to the evaluation is an estimate of the degree of immunosuppression or stage of HIV disease; this will help assess the types of infections and other complications that are most likely. The first 6-12 months post-transplant or initiation of immunosuppressive medications is generally the riskiest time period for infection and patients, who are usually advised to not travel far from their home medical center. For the HIV-infected patient, a recent CD4$^+$ T-cell count and HIV RNA level are the most helpful, along with a realistic assessment of the traveler's compliance and comfort with his or her current antiretroviral regimen. Persons with a CD4+ T-cell count <200 cells/mm^3 (or CD4% < 15) and a high viral load are at highest risk for acquiring new

---

TABLE 15.3 Preparation and Education before Departure

- Review feasibility of planned travel
- Identify medical resources abroad
- Anticipate legal and immigration issues
- Review itinerary and area-specific risks
- Educate regarding risk reduction (e.g., prudent dietary habits)

infections, travel-related or otherwise. In some cases, it may be appropriate to counsel the patient to delay travel to certain areas until an effective antiviral regimen has been started and the viral load controlled. In general, an HIV-positive patient on antivirals should be on a stable and successful regimen for at least 8 weeks before departure. By that time, problematic side effects have usually been identified, and the time of peak incidence of an immune reconstitution event passed.

One goal of a pre-travel visit is to identify specific risks, assess their magnitude, and educate the traveler in ways to reduce them. Destination-related risks for the immunocompromised traveler may influence decisions about whether to undertake all or part of a proposed trip. The healthcare provider should review area-specific risks and consider available means to reduce them. Guidelines for prevention of disease and bureaucratic difficulties should be provided, preferably accompanied by written information. The traveler will have to decide whether the estimated risks are worth taking. Under some circumstances, the traveler may decide to change an itinerary if risk of serious disease cannot be eliminated or reduced.

Destination and duration of stay will affect recommendations. For persons with more severe disease or those planning a prolonged stay, it is especially important to identify medical resources before departure. All travelers should have medical insurance that will provide coverage for care during the trip. For travel to developing countries (or any place where good medical facilities may be unavailable), travelers should also have special insurance that will cover evacuation in the event that local medical facilities are inadequate to provide good care for an acute illness or injury. It may be necessary to arrange in advance for the continuation of special therapy or laboratory testing, and of course for the availability of necessary medications.

Some countries require screening for HIV for any extended travel. Specific regulations vary among countries, and requirements for testing are often tied to duration of expected stay. Knowledge of updated regulations in the destination countries can help avoid aggravating, disruptive, and unpleasant experiences. Test results from the United States are accepted in some countries but not in others. In these countries, entering travelers can be required to undergo testing at the demand of government officials. This evokes all of the concerns about quality control in testing, reliability of confirmatory tests, and sterility of needles and syringes.

It is important to stress the need for immunocompromised travelers to continue their usual immunosuppressive or antiviral regimen during travel. The Canadian study referenced above also found that a large proportion of HIV-infected travelers discontinued or interrupted therapy during travel, for reasons ranging from convenience or the desire for a "holiday" to intercurrent illness. Despite the lure of combining a travel holiday with a "drug holiday," studies have documented an increased risk of untoward events, including death, in HIV-positive patients who interrupted therapy, even under the close monitoring conditions of a study and with CD4$^+$ T-cell counts >250 cells/mm^3. For transplant recipients, the risk of graft rejection due to stoppage of immunosuppression can be equally as disastrous, even if the break is brief.

Potential drug interactions can become an issue, especially for certain drug classes (e.g., protease inhibitors). The traveler should bring the package inserts for his or her medications and carefully review potential interactions for any medication given or prescribed while overseas; of particular importance are proton pump inhibitors or H2 blockers given for gastric distress, which can interfere with medication absorption. Cisapride, no longer available in the United States, may be prescribed overseas and contribute to potential arrhythmia. Also to be reviewed is the feasibility of appropriate storage of medications, especially if the destination is a tropical, developing country, where refrigeration may be unavailable or erratic. It is important to keep in mind that "room temperature" in the tropics may be considerably warmer than the temperature at which the stability of any of the medications was tested. If necessary, the travel health provider can work with the specialized care provider to develop the most convenient and appropriate regimen for travel.

For the long-term traveler, it is essential to assess the need for periodic laboratory testing and the availability of specialized tests (e.g., complete blood count, comprehensive metabolic panel, T-cell subsets, HIV RNA level, immunosuppressive drug levels) in the destination country. Many patients on immunomodulary medications may not need routine laboratory monitoring if they are otherwise well, but even stable HIV-infected patients on a anti-retroviral therapy usually require monitoring tests every 6 months.

Infection Prevention Strategies

Preventive strategies for travel-associated infectious diseases include general precautions, as well as immunoprophylaxis and chemoprophylaxis. Basic safeguards include hand hygiene, respiratory precautions, and proper food preparation. The importance of hand washing and sanitation cannot be stressed enough, as it is the single most effective method of preventing infection. If soap and clean water are not easily accessible, immunocompromised patients should plan to keep portable hand sanitizer with them at all times. Respiratory infections are commonplace, but immunocompromised individuals should try to avoid contact with persons suffering from respiratory symptoms. Viral illnesses such as influenza may seem out of season, but depending on one's travel destination, they may be at the peak of transmission. Food safety practice is an area of travel medicine that should be emphasized in pre-travel counseling. Any food that is not thoroughly cooked should be avoided altogether, while cooked food should be eaten immediately and not allowed to sit out. Undercooked meat and seafood can lead to infections with bacteria (e.g., *Escherichia coli*, *Salmonella*, *Campylobacter*, *Vibrio* species), parasites (e.g., *Toxoplasma*, *Entamoeba*, tapeworms, paragonimiasis), and viruses (e.g., hepatitis A and norovirus). Unpasteurized dairy products are common in many developed and developing countries, which can place immunocompromised travelers at risk for infections with *Listeria* and *Brucella*. Bottled or boiled drinking water is recommended, and ice should be avoided. In summary, the same recommendations for all travelers apply here, with added vigilance and compliance because the risk and consequences of respiratory and gastrointestinal illnesses are higher in this immunosuppressed population.

Vaccinations

With respect to vaccines, two basic questions are relevant:
- What extra vaccines should be given or considered because of the increased need for protection?
- What routine vaccines should be avoided or given with caution to the immunocompromised person because of increased risk of adverse events from the vaccines?

Efficacy of vaccines is an issue in immunocompromised individuals. In general, administration of vaccines after immunosuppression leads to antibody levels that are lower and less durable and may be less potent than in the populations included in published trials. Most vaccines thus should be given months in advance of immunosuppression, if possible. In HIV-positive persons, response to vaccination improves in those on a successful antiviral regimen. If vaccination can be deferred until such time as the viral load is suppressed and the CD4$^+$ T-cell count is >200 cells/mm^3, the efficacy is likely to be increased further.

Serious adverse events associated with vaccine administration are a concern in immunocompromised individuals, and the appropriateness of live vaccines in these patients is variable. Many live vaccines are contraindicated in transplant recipients; however, as experience grows, this recommendation may change in the future. A small study in pediatric renal transplant patients of a live attenuated varicella vaccine has shown efficacy and safety. The measles, mumps, rubella vaccine can be given 2 years post-transplant if patients are otherwise stable and without signs of graft versus host disease. In HIV-positive patients, some live vaccines are considered safe in patients with CD4$^+$ T-cell counts >200 cells/mm^3. Interestingly, a number of studies have documented transient increases in plasma levels of HIV RNA after vaccination with influenza and pneumococcal vaccines and tetanus toxoids; however, there has been no clear evidence that the antigenic stimulus from vaccines leads to a sustained increase in HIV replication or hastens progression of HIV disease.

Four general recommendations follow from these observations: (1) The potential benefits from many vaccines seem to outweigh their risks; (2) one may choose to measure antibody titers to assess vaccine response; (3) appropriate timing of vaccination may increase efficacy; and (4) where different routes or schedules are available, the most immunogenic should be used. Specific recommendations are given below.

Table 15.4 lists vaccines to consider giving an HIV-infected person before travel. These assume the patient received the full primary series of immunization with vaccines usually given in childhood in the United States. Many PHAs receiving HIV care will also have received additional immunizations as recommended for the care of PHAs. The pre-travel

TABLE 15.4   Immunizations for Adult HIV-Infected Travelers

Indication	Vaccine[a]	Comments
Routine	Tetanus and diphtheria (Td)	Booster interval 10 years
	Tetanus, diphtheria, and acellular pertussis (Tdap)	Once regardless of interval between last Td. Repeated with each pregnancy
	Haemophilus influenzae b, conjugate	Not routinely recommended for HIV care
	Hepatitis B[b]	Recommended as routine care. Assess antibody level 1 month following vaccine series
	Influenza	Yearly
	Pneumococcal	PCV13 once, then PPSV23 at least 8 weeks following PCV13. PPSV23 should be repeated 5 years later
Standard for travel to developing countries	Hepatitis A[c]	Preferably at least 4 weeks before departure
	Measles or MMR[d]	Avoid in patients with HIV with CD4+ T-cell counts <200 cells/mm^3
	Polio, enhanced inactivated	Avoid live oral polio vaccine
	Typhoid, inactivated Vi polysaccharide	Booster interval 2 years; avoid live oral typhoid vaccine (Ty21a)
For selected destinations or circumstances	Japanese encephalitis	Assess risks and benefits; no efficacy data
	Meningococcus	No efficacy data; conjugate vaccine probably more effective
	Rabies	Use IM vaccine series; no efficacy data
	Yellow fever[e]	Do not give if CD4+ T-cell counts <200/mm^3; no data on efficacy. Booster interval 10 years
	Bacille Calmette-Guérin (BCG)	Avoid BCG in all HIV-positive patients, regardless of CD4+ count or viral load

[a]Recommendations assume a history of routine childhood immunizations.
[b]Omit if person is already immune to hepatitis B.
[c]Omit if person has serologic evidence of immunity to hepatitis A.
[d]May be omitted if patient has serologic evidence of measles immunity.
[e]Required by many countries in Africa and South America and by other countries for travelers who have visited or been in transit through countries where yellow fever is endemic.
HIV, Human immunodeficiency virus; *IM*, intramuscular; *MMR*, measles, mumps, rubella; *PCV*, Pneumococcal conjugate Vaccine; *PPSV*, pneumococcal polysaccharide vaccine.
Adapted from Wilson, M.E., von Reyn, C.F., Fineberg, H.V., 1991. Infections in HIV-infected travelers: risks and prevention. Ann. Intern. Med. 114:582.

visit offers an opportunity to review such routine vaccines as well as the exotic ones. Annual influenza vaccination is recommended for HIV-infected persons, even when no travel is planned. Because influenza occurs during April through September in the Southern Hemisphere and throughout the year in tropical countries, it may be prudent to give travelers the vaccine outside the usual North American influenza season, although availability of the vaccine can be a problem in the off-season. Prophylaxis or self-treatment with oseltamivir is another option if there is a poor match between the circulating influenza strains and the current vaccine and the traveler is going to an area with extensive influenza transmission.

Pneumococcal infections are more common and more likely to result in bacteremia in HIV-infected persons. Rates may be >100-fold higher than in an age-matched non-HIV–infected population. Thus vaccination against pneumococcal disease is recommended in HIV-infected persons, preferably early in the course of HIV infection. Asymptomatic HIV-infected persons with CD4$^+$ T-cell counts <500 cells/mm^3 are less likely to respond to the pneumococcal capsular polysaccharide (PPSV23) than healthy young adults, although even with advanced stages of immunosuppression, some HIV-infected persons are able to mount an antibody response. Pneumococcal conjugate vaccine (PCV13) is now recommended for all HIV-infected adults in addition to PPSV23. Pneumococcal infections may not be more common during travel, but penicillin-resistant strains are more prevalent in many areas of the world than they are in the United States, and any serious illness during travel can be disruptive.

Because hepatitis B and HIV share similar routes of transmission, and because immunization is recommended as routine HIV care, many HIV-infected persons will already be immune to hepatitis B or be chronic carriers of hepatitis B surface antigen (HBsAg). The hepatitis B vaccine appears to be safe to use, and strong consideration should be given to vaccinating all hepatitis B-susceptible, HIV-infected persons. HIV-infected persons are more likely to become chronic carriers of HBsAg if they become infected with hepatitis B virus. They also respond less well to the vaccine, with only 50-70% developing antibody titers that are considered protective. Anti-HB surface antibody titer should be assessed 1 month after completion of series.

Rates of invasive *Haemophilus influenzae* infections are higher in HIV-infected persons than in the general population, but the organism remains a relatively rare cause of invasive disease in this population. Because many of the strains causing invasive disease are not serotype B (e.g., only 33% of strains were serotype B in one study in HIV-infected men), the conjugate vaccine directed against type B disease in common use may have limited benefit and is not currently recommended as part of routine HIV care.

Vaccines for Travel to Developing Countries

A second group of vaccines listed in **Table 15.4** are frequently administered before travel to developing countries. Because of the increased risk of vaccine-associated poliomyelitis in immunosuppressed persons, the enhanced inactivated parenteral polio vaccine should be used instead of oral live polio vaccine in HIV-infected persons and their household contacts. The inactivated Vi polysaccharide typhoid vaccine should also be used in preference to the oral typhoid vaccine (Ty21a), although no cases of progressive infection with this attenuated strain of *Salmonella typhi* have been reported. Travelers who lack immunity to hepatitis A should be given one of the inactivated hepatitis A vaccines, ideally at least 4 weeks before departure. The commercially available serologic tests for hepatitis A antibody assess whether a person is immune because of past infection but are not sufficiently sensitive to pick up vaccine-induced antibodies. Hence, routine serologic testing after hepatitis A vaccination is not recommended.

Recommendations about the measles vaccine in HIV-infected persons differ from advice about other live vaccines. This live vaccine is recommended for HIV-infected persons, unless they have severe immunosuppression (CD4$^+$ T-cell counts <200/mm^3 or clinical AIDS). A case of fatal giant cell pneumonitis associated with measles vaccine virus has been reported in a young man with late-stage AIDS. The following observations underlie the current recommendation: (1) Measles infection in HIV-infected persons can be atypical, severe, and sometimes fatal; (2) measles vaccine has generally been safe (with exception noted previously), although most of the experience in HIV infection has been in young children; (3) treatment modalities for measles are limited; (4) measles is highly contagious and exposure is often inapparent; and (5) risk of exposure is greater during travel to many developing countries than it is in the United States. The measles cases in the United States now are imported or related to imported cases. The current recommendation is for two doses of measles vaccine (the first dose usually given at age 12-15 months, with a second dose in childhood). Some adults who never experienced natural infection because of measles vaccination in infancy have not received a second vaccine dose and may be candidates for the second dose before travel. It may be worthwhile to assess measles antibody status in HIV-infected persons even if born before 1957, if they have no history of natural measles, or to consider proceeding with vaccination.

Special Vaccines for Specific Destinations or Activities

Other vaccines listed in **Table 15.4** are recommended only for specific destinations or special circumstances. The traditional inactivated cholera vaccine is safe, but it is no longer available in the United States. HIV-infected persons may be at increased risk for cholera because gastric acid is an important barrier to infection, and PHAs often have reduced gastric acidity. Education about the need for rehydration for severe diarrhea and the availability of oral rehydration salts is important for all travelers.

Rabies vaccine should be given to HIV-infected persons who meet the usual criteria for the vaccine. The more immunogenic intramuscular route and dose (1 mL) should be used (instead of 0.1 mL dose via intradermal route, which is currently not available in the United States), because it offers a greater potential for efficacy.

The yellow fever vaccine often poses the most difficult dilemma: infection with yellow fever may be lethal and effective treatment is unavailable; the vaccine contains live virus; and proof of vaccination is required for entry into many countries. There are three main options for an HIV-infected person who plans to travel to yellow fever-endemic countries. Transmission of yellow fever is focal in endemic areas, and many travelers to countries requiring yellow fever vaccine are at no risk of infection. A reasonable option for a person visiting an area without current yellow fever transmission is to provide a letter of waiver stating that the vaccine is contraindicated for medical reasons. Another approach is to change the itinerary to avoid countries requiring the vaccine. The third option is to give the vaccine. HIV-infected persons with CD4$^+$ T-cell counts >200/mm^3 who cannot avoid exposure to the yellow fever virus should be offered the vaccine. No reports have been published of recognized yellow fever vaccine-related disease in PHAs, and several reports have indicated the general safety of the vaccine in this population. In persons with lower CD4$^+$ counts, the possible risks and benefits should be considered on an individual basis. For HIV-infected persons who receive the vaccine and who will be at moderate or high risk of exposure, it may be prudent to assess levels of neutralizing antibodies after vaccination (consult the state health department or Centers for Disease and Control and Prevention at 970-221-6400). Whether or not the vaccine is given, the traveler should be given explicit instructions in ways to avoid mosquito bites. Insect-control maneuvers can help prevent many infections in addition to malaria and yellow fever. Use of permethrin sprayed on clothing is a useful adjunct to other approaches to preventing bites.

Although the possibility of testing for antibody response to various vaccines has been mentioned above, the cost of such testing and the time required to receive the results may be prohibitive. As there are no clear guidelines on how to proceed if the antibody response is low in this situation (with the exception of hepatitis B immunization), a rational approach should be taken.

Chemoprophylaxis for Traveler's Diarrhea

All travelers should be given advice and written materials, if possible, describing strategies to avoid risky food and beverages. Immunocompromised persons should be scrupulous about following dietary guidelines to avoid enteric pathogens, in particular, inadequately treated water, undercooked meats, and raw, unpeeled fruits and vegetables. Those traveling to developing countries should be given a prescription for an antimicrobial agent, either to be taken as prophylaxis or to be used as empiric therapy in the event of acute diarrheal illness (see Chapter 8). Because immunocompromised persons have a higher risk for diarrhea than other travelers, the threshold for recommending prophylactic antibiotics may be lower. This issue should be discussed and individual preferences considered. Some considerations in the decision to use prophylaxis versus early empiric therapy include destination and duration of stay, available medical facilities at the destination, allergies, and other concurrent medications. If the traveler is already taking trimethoprim/sulfamethoxazole for *Pneumocystis* prophylaxis, a different agent should be chosen for early self-treatment of diarrhea. A quinolone, such as norfloxacin or ciprofloxacin, is a reasonable choice, although azithromycin is preferred in areas with resistant *Campylobacter*, such as Southeast Asia. The non-absorbable antimicrobial rifaximin is licensed for the treatment of traveler's diarrhea due to *E. coli*, but has been found to be effective as a prophylaxis as well and may be a consideration. Since the drug is not absorbed into the systemic circulation, there should be no drug interactions.

Antimalarial Prophylaxis

Antimalarial agents and advice about personal protective measures to prevent mosquito bites should be given to all travelers. General precautions are first lines of defense, which include appropriate bed-net use, skin-covering clothing preferably treated with permethrin, and topical DEET or picaridin solutions. Mefloquine is currently a first-line drug recommended for most chloroquine-resistant malarious areas. Because of the high frequency of underlying neurologic problems, especially in HIV-infected persons, it is important to review any history of seizures or current signs or symptoms of CNS disease before prescribing this agent. Atovaquone-proguanil (Malarone®) is another first-line drug for malaria chemoprophylaxis that may be considered. Malarone is still an option even if the traveler is already taking atovaquone for the prevention of *Pneumocystis jiroveci*, because the atovaquone dose can be reduced while on Malarone. For example, adults using atovaquone-proguanil 250 mg/100 mg who normally take 1500 mg of atovaquone for daily *Pneumocystis* pneumonia prophylaxis should change to 1250 mg of daily atovaquone. Alternatively, if the traveler has access to proguanil alone (not available in the United States), that can be taken in addition to his or her regular atovaquone. Doxycycline also remains an acceptable option for malaria prophylaxis, with the caveat that those prone to thrush should also carry clotrimazole troches or fluconazole tablets for pre-emptive treatment.

Sexual Precautions

Persons living with HIV/AIDS should be reminded that they remain at risk of acquiring sexually transmitted diseases while away from home and that these infections may have particularly significant implications for their health. Certainly, HAART should continue without interruption during the journey. But this does not remove the importance of responsible sexual behavior. Although there are little data on the efficacy of HAART in preventing secondary HIV acquisition among infected overseas travelers, there is concern that the regimen used by these patients may not protect them fully from acquiring a new infection due to drug-resistant HIV strains. And, of course, barrier protection greatly reduces the risk of transmitting HIV to uninfected partners, regardless of viral load.

FURTHER READING

Alvar, J., Cañavate, C., Gutiérrez-Solar, B., et al., 1997. Leishmania and human immunodeficiency virus coinfection: the first 10 years. Clin. Microbiol. Rev. 10, 298–319.

Angel, J.B., Walpita, P., Lerch, R.A., et al., 1998. Vaccine-associated measles pneumonitis in an adult with AIDS. Ann. Intern. Med. 129, 104–106.

Cetron, M.S., Marfin, A.A., Julian, K.G., et al., 2002. Yellow fever vaccine. Recommendations of the Advisory Committee on Immunization Practices (ACIP). MMWR Recomm. Rep. 51 (RR-17), 1–11.

Chariyalertsak, S., Sirisanthana, T., Supparatpinyo, K., et al., 1997. Case-control study of risk factors for *Penicillium marneffei* infection in human immunodeficiency virus-infected patients in northern Thailand. Clin. Infect. Dis. 24, 1080–1086.

Colebunders, R., Bahwe, Y., Nekwei, W., et al., 1990. Incidence of malaria and efficacy of oral quinine in patients recently infected with human immunodeficiency virus in Kinshasa, Zaire. J. Infect. 21, 167–173.

Fleming, A.F., 1990. Opportunistic infections in AIDS in developed and developing countries. Trans. R. Soc. Trop. Med. Hyg. 84, 1–6.

Fuller, J.D., Craven, D.E., Steger, K.A., et al., 1999. Influenza vaccination of human immunodeficiency virus (HIV)-infected adults: impact on plasma levels of HIV type 1 RNA and determinants of antibody response. Clin. Infect. Dis. 28, 541–547.

Gamester, C.F., Tilzey, A.J., Banatvala, J.E., 1999. Medical students' risk of infection with blood-borne viruses at home and abroad: questionnaire survey. BMJ 318, 158–160.

Godofsky, E.W., Zinreich, J., Arnstrong, M., et al., 1992. Sinusitis in HIV-infected patients: a clinical and radiographic review. Am. J. Med. 93, 163–170.

Gotuzzo, E., Frisancho, O., Sanchez, J., et al., 1991. Association between the acquired immunodeficiency syndrome and infection with *Salmonella typhi* or *Salmonella paratyphi* in an endemic typhoid area. Arch. Intern. Med. 151, 381.

Goujon, C., Touin, M., Feuillie, V., et al., 1995. Good tolerance and efficacy of yellow fever vaccine among carriers of human immunodeficiency. J. Travel Med. 2, 145.

Hawkes, S., Hart, G.J., Johnson, A.M., et al., 1994. Risk behavior and HIV prevalence in international travelers. AIDS 8, 247.

Hess, G., Clemens, R., Bienzle, U., et al., 1995. Immunogenicity and safety of an inactivated hepatitis A vaccine in anti-HIV positive and negative homosexual men. J. Med. Virol. 46, 40–42.

Kaplan, J.E., Masur, H., Holmes, K., 1995. USPHS/IDSA guidelines for the prevention of opportunistic infections in persons infected with human immunodeficiency virus: an overview. Clin. Infect. Dis. 21, S12.

Kassalik, M., Monkemuller, K., 2011. *Strongyloides stercoralis* hyperinfection syndrome and disseminated disease. Gastroenterol Hepatol (NY) 7, 766–768.

Kaul, D.R., Cinti, S.K., Carver, P.L., et al., 1999. HIV protease inhibitors: advances in therapy and adverse reactions, including metabolic complications. Pharmacotherapy 19, 281.

Kemper, C.A., Linett, A., Kane, C., et al., 1995. Frequency of travel of adults infected with HIV. J. Travel Med. 2, 85.

Lopez-Velez, R., Perez-Molina, J.A., Guerrero, A., et al., 1998. Clinicoepidemiologic characteristics, prognostic factors, and survival analysis of patients coinfected with human immunodeficiency virus and *Leishmania* in an area of Madrid, Spain. Am. J. Trop. Med. Hyg. 58, 436–443.

Patel, R.R., Liang, S.Y., Koowal, P., et al., 2015. Travel advice for the immunocompromised traveler: prophylaxis, vaccination, and other preventative methods. Ther Clin Risk Manag 11, 217–228.

Rhoads, J.L., Birx, D.L., Wright, D.C., et al., 1991. Safety and immunogenicity of multiple conventional immunizations administered during early HIV infection. J. Acquir. Immune Defic. Syndr. 4, 724–731.

Rocha, A., de Meneses, A.C., da Silva, A.M., et al., 1994. Pathology of patients with Chagas' disease and acquired immunodeficiency syndrome. Am. J. Trop. Med. Hyg. 50, 261–268.

Salit, I.E., Sano, M., Boggild, A.K., et al., 2005. Travel patterns and risk behavior of HIV-positive people travelling internationally. CMAJ 172, 884–888.

Schippers, E.F., Hugen, P.W., den Hartigh, J., et al., 2000. No drug–drug interaction between nelfinavir or indinavir and mefloquine in HIV-1-infected patients. AIDS 14, 2794–2795.

Stanley, S.K., Ostrowski, M.A., Justement, J.S., et al., 1996. Effect of immunization with a common recall antigen on viral expression in patients infected with human immunodeficiency virus type 1. N. Engl. J. Med. 334, 1222–1230.

Taburet, A.-M., Singlas, E., 1996. Drug interactions with antiviral drugs. Clin. Pharmacokinet. 30, 385.

Tattevin, P., Depatureaux, A.G., Chapplain, J.M., et al., 2004. Yellow fever vaccine is safe and effective in HIV-infected patients. AIDS 18, 825–827.

US Department of State, 2008. Human immunodeficiency virus testing requirements for entry into foreign countries. Updated annually. For copy, send self-addressed stamped envelope to: Bureau of Consular Affairs, CA/PA, Room 5807, Department of State, Washington DC, 20520. Also available at <http://travel.state.gov>.

Wilson, M.E., 1991. A World Guide to Infections: Diseases, Distribution, Diagnosis. Oxford University Press, New York.

Wilson, M.E., von Reyn, C.F., Fineberg, H.V., 1991. Infections in HIV-infected travelers: risks and prevention. Ann. Intern. Med. 114, 582.

World Health Organization, 2005. Malaria and HIV Interactions and Their Implications for Public Health Policy. Technical Consultation on Malaria and HIV Interactions and Public Health Policy Implications. Geneva, Switzerland.

Zurlo, J.J., Feuerstein, I.M., Lebovics, R., et al., 1992. Sinusitis in HIV-1 infection. Am. J. Med. 93, 157–162.

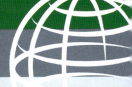

CHAPTER 16

Travel with Chronic Medical Conditions

Mari C. Sullivan

 Access evidence synopsis online at ExpertConsult.com.

In addition to travel by rail, ship, and automobile, almost 2 billion people travel by air annually. It is generally expected that primary care providers as well as travel medicine clinic personnel will identify individuals who are unfit for air travel and provide them with advice. Studies show that more than 95% of travelers with health problems who travel by air would like to receive additional medical advice from their providers prior to travel. The age of travelers is ever increasing as the population ages. Currently in the United States 14% of people are over 65 years of age. A recent Swiss study, by Boubaker, et al. 2016, reported that 10% of visits to a travel medicine clinic for pre-travel advice were made by travelers over the age of 60; 40% of these travelers reported a chronic medical condition.

It is important for the elderly traveler or those with chronic medical conditions to consider factors such as access to medical care, the possible increased demands for aerobic exercise, changes in diet, availability of medical supplies, and the effects of altitude when planning a trip to a foreign destination; thus, advance planning is essential for persons in this category of travelers. Another factor that could make a significant difference in the success of a journey is the ability to travel with a companion. The traveling companion need not be medically trained but could provide invaluable help in getting professional assistance should an urgent medical need arise. There are also commercial companies, such as Accessible Journeys, that maintain a directory of healthcare professionals willing to use vacation time from their jobs to accompany a traveler. It is important to advise the traveler to check the professional credentials and references of travel companion programs. A website that features a number of companies and travel agents that can assist with special travel services is www.disabledtravelers.com. Additionally, the US Transportation Security Administration (TSA) has a website that offers helpful information for travelers with medical conditions, as well as a TSA Cares Help Line. They advise that callers call at least 72 hours prior to travel, thus allowing the TSA Customer Service Manager advance notice that a specific traveler may need assistance. This information can be found at www.tsa.gov/traveler-information/travelers-disabilities-and-medical-conditions.

There are many remote areas of the world where medical care may be hours or days away from a traveler stricken by illness or complications of a pre-existing condition. If an elderly individual or one with a chronic disease is very stressed by the thought of remote travel and lack of access to care, it may be justified to counsel that traveler to adjust his or her itinerary to one that includes the availability of adequate medical care. The traveler with chronic medical conditions has to consider whether the anticipated benefits of the planned travel experience are worth the potential health risks associated with a given itinerary. This said, travel can be an extremely rewarding and confidence-building exercise for those limited by a chronic condition. The clinician advising the traveler must take into account the positive impact travel can have on an individual's sense of well-being while being realistic and practical when providing travel advice. The clinician advising the elderly traveler should recognize that the aging process brings with it changes that necessitate careful planning prior to travel. For example, it is prudent to advise the elderly traveler to get a thorough dental exam prior to embarking on a long trip. More than 50% of people will develop hypertension by the age of 65. Muscles begin to atrophy after the age of 40, and by the age of 80, one has lost between one-quarter and one-half of one's muscle mass. When advising the traveler at the far end of the lifespan on appropriate travel itineraries, their current state of health should be kept in mind; whether the individual has been relatively healthy or an infrequent user of health services, he or she may have underlying issues that could impact health without being aware of these based on the aging process alone. Aging can lead to immunosenescence, which impairs the host's ability to develop adequate immune responses to vaccines. Additionally, for the same reason teeth and bones are at risk due to lack of mineralization. Lack of bone mass, or osteopenia, is a major risk factor for fractures. A fracture on a trip can certainly ruin a trip, prolong disability for many months, and be a lifelong affliction in the elderly. Advise the elderly traveler to have a bone scan and assessment of risk for osteoporosis, and make recommendations based on the study. There is little we can do medically to slow the aging process, so prudent thought should go into the advice one gives elderly travelers, who may not readily want to admit their limitations or, indeed, may not even know they have them. On the other hand, research by Shitrit and Chowers (2010) reveals that because elderly travels tend to comply with health recommendations and are more careful about health-risk behaviors such as eating street food or drinking open drinks while abroad, their risk for illness during travel was significantly lower than that of younger travelers.

The Air Carrier Access Act of 1986 resulted in the US Department of Transportation developing regulations to assure that persons with disabilities and chronic medical conditions are treated without discrimination. However, air travel can be stressful because of noise, turbulence, crowding, limited seating space, and psychological factors (fear of flying, fear of terrorism, etc.). Air travel may present high-altitude barometric and oxygen stresses (Chapter 4), as well as rapidly transport the traveler across many time zones, necessitating special changes in the timing of medications. Travel by land or sea routes may be less stressful for people with medical conditions but still requires advanced planning. Regardless of mode of transportation, if special medical equipment must be taken along (wheelchairs, dialysis equipment and fluids, oversize or excess baggage for supplies, etc.), travelers should contact the medical departments of major airline, railroad, or cruise ship companies for specific information and guidance before confirming reservations. Travelers with mobility issues may have additional concerns as they plan their travel itinerary. The Centers for Disease Control and Prevention recommends that travelers with medical conditions or mobility issues due to age or other factors should seek pre-travel consultation at least 4 weeks before departure (2016, CDC Yellow Book, chapter 8).

Some commonsense approaches to pre-planning for travel with a medical condition will go a long way toward the prevention of problems while en route as well as at one's destination. It is important to advise the traveler to have an updated list of medications and doses as well as an adequate supply of medications to cover the duration of their journey.

CHRONIC OBSTRUCTIVE PULMONARY DISEASE, ASTHMA, AND OTHER RESPIRATORY CONDITIONS

The effects of exercise, exposure to cold, altitude, and extreme heat can be significant stressors for the traveler with underlying lung disease. The presence of environmental allergens and pollution in various cities of the world, such as Delhi, Beijing, Mexico City, and Kathmandu, to name a few, are additional significant considerations.

The Federal Airline Regulations require that airlines maintain a cabin pressure simulating an altitude between 5000 ft (1524 m) (e.g., Denver) and 8000 ft (2438 m) (e.g., Mexico City). Healthy passengers can tolerate this change in altitude, but patients with pulmonary disease may have increased hypoxemia owing not only to diminished oxygen pressure, but also to impaired hypoxic ventilatory drive, decreased cardiac reserve, and mechanical limitations. A study of adults in a simulation of a 20-hour flight revealed that the frequency of reported complaints associated with acute mountain sickness (fatigue, headache, light-headedness, and nausea) increased with increasing altitude and duration of flight. This peaked at 7498 ft (2438 m) and became apparent between 3 and 9 hours of exposure (Muhm et al. 2007).

The relatively low humidity inside the passenger cabin (10-12%) may cause difficulty for patients with thick pulmonary secretions or tracheostomies, so adequate individual hydration must be maintained. Water is the best beverage to maintain hydration while in the air or at altitude.

In general, overeating, alcoholic beverages, sedatives, and cigarette smoking should be avoided by patients with respiratory conditions during air travel and once at destination. While smoking on commercial aircraft is illegal, it is important that travelers who are concerned about environmental exposure to tobacco smoke be aware that smoking by others could present a problem in restaurants, hotels, banks, conference rooms, and other public places of business, as well as on buses and other modes of public transportation. The prevalence of smoking among the residents of the areas to be visited and the existence of smoke-free environments may influence the choice of itinerary for this group of travelers. Fortunately, smoking is prohibited in eating establishments and bars in the United Kingdom and Europe, but this does not apply to the many outdoor cafes or seating areas.

Table 16.1 presents some pulmonary contraindications to air travel. However, these contraindications are general, and certain individuals with chronic lung disease who fall into one of these categories may be able to travel on the advice of their medical providers. Most experts recommend supplemental oxygen during air travel for people with a baseline oxygen

---

TABLE 16.1　Respiratory Contraindications to Air Travel[a]

Conditions adversely affected by hypoxia
　Active bronchospasm
　Cyanosis
　Dyspnea at rest or during exercise
　Pneumonia or acute upper respiratory tract infection
　Pulmonary hypertension with or without cor pulmonale
　Severe anemia (hemoglobin level 7.5 g/dL) or sickling hemoglobinopathies
　Unstable coexisting cardiac disorders, such as arrhythmias, angina pectoris, and recent myocardial infarction (within 3-4 weeks)
Conditions adversely affected by pressure changes
　Thoracic surgery in the preceding 3 weeks
　Noncommunicating lung cysts
　Otitis media, sinusitis, or recent middle-ear surgery
　Pneumothorax or pneumomediastinum
Inadequate pulmonary function (as evidenced by one or more of the following)
　Diffusing capacity <50% of predicted
　Hypercapnia ($PaCO_2$ >50 mmHg)
　Hypoxemia while breathing room air (PaO_2 >50 mmHg)
　Maximum voluntary ventilation less than 40 L/min
　Vital capacity <50% of predicted
Other contraindications
　Contagious diseases, including active tuberculosis

[a]These contraindications are relative, since patients may significantly improve with appropriate therapy and supplemental oxygen.
From: Gong, H. Jr., 1990. Advising COPD patients about commercial air travel. J. Respir. Dis. 11, 484–499.

TABLE 16.2   Decline in Blood Oxygen Tension with Increase in Altitude in Two Patient Groups

Group	PaO$_2$ Sea Level	PaO$_2$ 5500 ft	PaO$_2$ 8000 ft[a]
Healthy young adults	98 mmHg	68 mmHg	60-63 mmHg
Patients with COPD	72.4 mmHg	–	47.7 mmHg[b]

[a]A given cruising altitude of 35,000 ft above sea level will result in a cabin altitude varying from 5000 to 8000 ft among different aircraft models, according to pressurization schedules.
[b]After 45 min steady-state hypobaric exposure, equivalent to 8000 ft above sea level.
COPD, Chronic obstructive pulmonary disease.
From: Dillard, T.A., Berg, B.W., Rajagopol, K.R. et al., 1989. Hypoxia during air travel in patients with chronic obstructive pulmonary disease. Ann Intern Med 111, 362–367.

saturation of 95% or less. Several methods and equations are available to assess the need for in-flight oxygen, and some guidelines suggest a hypoxic challenge test in individuals with an oxygen saturation of 92-95%. Predictive equations do not always accurately estimate the need for in-flight oxygen. Sea-level blood gas or pulmonary function testing with a hypoxic challenge remain the gold standard, with oxygen recommended for those with a PaO$_2$ of 70 mmHg or less or with an in-flight PaO$_2$ expected at 55 mmHg or less. Guidelines established by the British Thoracic Society in 2002 suggest that in-flight oxygen is not needed if the patient's resting SpO$_2$ (O$_2$ saturation) measured with room air is >95% and there are no additional risk factors. If a patient has a resting room air SpO$_2$ <92% at sea level, he or she will require in-flight oxygen. These studies are ideally performed on a clinically stable subject as close to the travel date as possible. **Table 16.2** shows the drop in the arterial PO$_2$ going from sea level to an altitude of 8000 ft in healthy young adults and in a group of patients with chronic obstructive pulmonary disease (COPD) Anyone requiring oxygen supplementation on the ground will obviously need it for air travel. British Thoracic Society or Aerospace Medical Association guidelines should be used for patients affected by pulmonary or cardiac disease who desire to travel by air.

Supplemental Oxygen

Passengers who require supplementary oxygen during flight can now bring their own Department of Transportation-approved portable oxygen-concentrating devices on-board most airlines. These must be "approved devices" and currently include a variety of portable oxygen concentrators. Passengers are responsible for making oxygen arrangements with the airplanes. At the time of writing, domestic airlines no longer provide supplemental oxygen, and one must utilize a third party supplier, such as Oxygen to Go, which will facilitate all of the procedures necessary and provide rental units and supplies. A company such as this, which arranges all aspects of the oxygen needs and has been in the business of doing so for more than 10 years, may be an excellent starting place for the traveler requiring supplemental oxygen (www.oxygentogo.com). Most carriers require an advance notice of 48-72 hours, but some can require 10 days to 2 weeks advance notice. Passengers should also consider the need for oxygen use during any layover stop(s) and at their final destination. They must also make arrangements (with the airline, friends, or relatives) with a local supplier for removal of the canister from the originating airport's gate area immediately after the gate is exited to board the aircraft. FAA regulations require that for all passengers requesting supplemental oxygen, airlines must obtain a signed physician's statement (specific to each airline), which must be provided by the traveler at least 48 hours prior to travel. This statement will include information such as the desired flow rate, type of mask, and whether the oxygen is to be used intermittently or continuously. The fees for rental of portable oxygen concentrators and the associated batteries and services can range from US$350 for a short flight and 1-week rental upward to US$1200 depending on the length of the trip. Airlines require that passengers requiring oxygen have 150% additional battery power above that supplied with the unit. Other respiratory equipment such as mechanical ventilators or nebulizers may be allowed on board, but their use must be pre-approved. These supplies must conform to applicable FAA regulations in order to avoid interference with sensitive aviation electronic equipment. Additional information on airline accommodations for supplemental oxygen can be found at the National Home Oxygen Patient's Association website (www.homeoxygen.org).

Special arrangements have to be made with oxygen distributors at each airport for supplies of oxygen needed on the ground during layovers and airport transfers to connecting flights, and even for the final destination if it is more than 5000 ft above sea level. Passengers should contact a local full-service oxygen supplier that can deliver oxygen not only at the home origin but at the destination and layover city with advance notice of at least 72 hours to ensure delivery. Travelers with moderate to severe COPD who are hypoxic at ambient conditions at home should not plan trips to high altitudes. The risk for high-altitude pulmonary edema is significant in these individuals.

The traveling companion should be instructed that visual impairment, fatigue, headache, sleepiness, dizziness, personality changes, and impaired memory, judgment, and/or coordination may be signs of oxygen deficiency and that medical assistance may be needed.

Travelers with Asthma

In 2007, the National Heart, Lung, and Blood Institute estimated that 22 million people, more than 6 million of them children, have chronic asthma in the United States. Respiratory infections are among the common ailments of travelers, with personal stress, air travel, contact with strangers, and environmental contamination all contributing to the risk of exposure. Thus, it is important for the traveler with asthma and other chronic respiratory conditions to have annual immunization against influenza and to be up-to-date on all other recommended vaccines (including pneumococcal vaccine and pertussis [DTaP]). Travelers over the age of 65 should have the pneumococcal pneumonia vaccine at least 1 month before travel as well as the shingles vaccine.

It is essential the clinician assure that the patient with asthma wishing to travel have stable and well-controlled asthma before embarking on a journey. Travelers with any remote history of asthma or reactive airway disease should be warned that travel to a new place could trigger asthma, even if they have been asymptomatic for years. Molds and pollens may present new or unidentified triggers for exacerbations of asthma. Dust mites and cockroaches are prevalent in some regions of the world, and exposure to byproducts of these could pose increased risks for triggering asthma attacks in hotel rooms and other dwellings. Air pollution is a significant problem in urban areas of the developing world (Chapter 2) and may cause exacerbations of asthma. Patients with asthma traveling to colder environments should be instructed to wear hats with a face mask or scarf to rewarm inhaled air, and appropriate clothing. Unlike patients with COPD, patients with asthma generally do well at altitude. Some theories for this are that they are less exposed to allergens and other etiologic factors responsible for triggering asthma exacerbations. In addition, patients with asthma may be more sensitive to declines in their respiratory function and may spontaneously limit or decrease their activity levels as this occurs. This may have a protective effect when trekking to altitude and while engaging in other types of physical activities.

Travelers with asthma should hand-carry an adequate supply of medications. Medications should not be placed in checked baggage during travel. All medications should be transported in their original containers, showing medication name, dose, dosing schedule, pharmacy, and prescribing physician. Asthma is a problem worldwide, and while it is best for patients to use medications acquired at home, traveling patients should be informed in case of lost or missing supplies that certain common medications may be available abroad under different brand names but similar formulation. For example, albuterol may be available as salbutamol, and Advair may be available as Seretide in other countries. International equivalents of common prescription drugs can be looked up by the healthcare provider utilizing a reference source, such as MD Consult (www.drugs.com/international) or other online databases.

Travelers with asthma should have a peak flow meter (PFM) and know how to use this device for self-assessment of subtle exacerbations of their condition while traveling. Recent evidence-based research has determined that β2-agonists and systemic corticosteroids remain the cornerstone of emergency treatment. Specific instructions on when and how to self-treat an exacerbation, based on PRM measurement, should be given. Depending on the travel itinerary and circumstances, the traveling patient should include short-acting bronchodilator multidose inhalers (MDIs), one or more courses of an oral steroid, and an adequate supply of leukotriene modifiers, if appropriate, as this medication is often unavailable in many countries outside the United States and Europe. National Asthma Education and Prevention Program Guidelines (2007) state there is no evidence to suggest that oral antibiotics are useful in the treatment of acute asthma. Medications for treatment of viral influenza (e.g., oseltamivir) and extra steroid MDIs and oral steroids should be carried in the travel medicine kit (Chapter 1).

To summarize:

- All patients with underlying significant pulmonary disease such as COPD, sarcoidosis, or pulmonary hypertension who will be traveling on flights longer than 1.5 hours in duration should be evaluated for in-flight supplemental oxygen.
- Any patient who uses oxygen at home, even if only at night, will likely require in-flight oxygen supplementation.
- Airlines are no longer required to carry oxygen on board for use in emergencies, and when they do have oxygen, it is often a small canister that would not last very long.
- Third-party oxygen distributers are capable of organizing all aspects of supplemental oxygen, from advising on the correct physician-generated paper work to delivery and collection of oxygen concentrators.

CARDIOVASCULAR DISEASE

In patients with cardiopulmonary disease, the hypoxemia that develops during travel by jet may produce symptoms during prolonged commercial flights. Cardiac events are the most common cause of in-flight emergencies, causing up to 20% in some studies. Supplemental oxygen will be required for any cardiac patient requiring supplemental oxygen at sea level. A recent study of travel safety perceptions and awareness in patients with cardiopulmonary disease revealed that only 19% were aware that the aircraft is pressurized to a cabin altitude of 5000-8000 ft, yet 50% of those studied had symptoms of hypoxia when they traveled by air. Some 81% had dyspnea, and almost 20% some degree of chest discomfort. It is important for the clinician to educate cardiopulmonary patients on the health risks of air travel and assure they are fit to fly and prepared.

Patients should be sure to carry their prescribed medications in their carry-on baggage, as well as copies of recent medical records (electrocardiogram, vital signs, list of diagnoses, list of prescription medication and doses, and names and telephone numbers of their medical providers). Salty foods, carbonated beverages, immoderate consumption of alcoholic beverages, and fatty or spicy foods should be avoided during flight. Bringing healthy snack foods from home is a good precaution against unsuitable airline food. Passengers should walk around the aircraft cabin periodically and/or flex and extend their lower extremities while seated at least once an hour to decrease venous stasis and pooling, keeping in mind that light exercise during air flight can actually worsen hypoxemia in those at risk.

A study of medical emergencies among commercial air travelers by Peterson et al. (2013) found that the flight tower communications center received calls for about 11,920 in-flight medical emergencies among an estimated 744 million airline passengers during the 30-month study period, for a rate of 16 medical emergencies per 1 million passengers, or one in-flight emergency per 604 flights. The most common medical issues were syncope or presyncope (37.4%), respiratory symptoms (12.1%), and nausea or vomiting (9.5%), with some variation across airlines. Approximately 7.9% of flights were diverted due to an in-flight emergency.

Of individuals requiring assistance for a medical problem during travel, the majority of emergencies among air travelers occurred within the air terminal. Only 25% experienced their problem during the flight. Although the rate of medical emergencies for inbound passengers was low, studies suggest that given the volume of passengers involved, a large number of people can be anticipated to experience medical problems requiring emergency assistance during air travel or in the hours immediately before or after the flight. Thirty-eight in-flight cardiac arrests were reported in the Peterson et al. study, and 31 of these resulted in death. Despite the low rate of medical emergencies, almost 1000 lives are lost annually from cardiac arrest in commercial aircrafts and airport terminals. Most of these individuals do not have a prior history of cardiac disease. In June 2001, the FAA mandated that all commercial air carriers carry automated external defibrillators (AEDs) on each aircraft. Since April 2004, all commercial aircraft now have AEDs on-board.

Given the physical and emotional stress on passengers in air terminals as they rush to cover relatively long distances on foot to make connecting flights, and the often lengthy pre-departure security checks, several commonsense tips for air travelers could be given:

1. Allow plenty of time for travel to the airport, airport parking, standing in line at the ticket counter to check in, and passage through security checks to get to the departure gate. Arrive at the airport at least 2 hours ahead of departure time for domestic flights and 3 hours or more ahead of departure time for international flights.
2. At the time the ticket is booked, request an aisle seat, for increased mobility and leg room (although the aisle seat places a passenger at increased risk of injuries from baggage falling out of overhead bins, should the aircraft experience severe turbulence, compared with a window seat).
3. Request special in-flight meals (low salt, vegetarian, etc.) in advance, at the time the ticket is booked. Special meals are almost always delivered prior to the regular food service.
4. Request assistance by wheelchair or airport motor cart for transport within the airport terminal if there are problems with ambulation, exercise tolerance, or any other disabilities.
5. Pack lightly and utilize luggage with wheels or a baggage cart for transport of carry-on bags within the terminal.
6. Wear comfortable clothing in layers that can be added for warmth or removed for cooling, and comfortable "broken-in" low-heeled walking shoes for travel. Loosen laces on footwear when settling in for the flight or change into slippers or airline socks. For long-haul flights, special socks that are designed to decrease venous stasis (e.g., T.E.D. antiembolism stockings) are recommended.
7. Do not place medications or products that may require immediate access in the overhead bins. Medicines such as bronchodilators, insulin, glucose tablets, and nitroglycerin should be placed under the seat or in the seat pocket in front of the traveler where they can be easily accessed if needed.

Patients with a history of cardiac disease may want to consider purchasing medical emergency evacuation insurance. They should review the policy to ensure that they will be covered for pre-existing conditions and should determine if the level of evacuation will meet their needs. Some of these companies will provide a fully equipped and staffed air ambulance (fixed-wing or helicopter) to evacuate a cardiac patient to the nearest regional medical center that could provide a level of care similar to the standard of care available in the patient's home country. Other companies will evacuate a patient to the nearest in-country medical center, where the care may or may not approximate prevailing Western standards. Sometimes the outcome of the evacuation is determined by weather, environment, availability of aircraft and fuel, and political factors.

Guidelines of the Aerospace Medical Association state that commercial airline flight is contraindicated within 3 weeks of an uncomplicated myocardial infarction (MI), within 6 weeks of a complicated MI, within 2 weeks of coronary artery bypass surgery, and within 2 weeks of a cerebrovascular accident. Other contraindications to commercial flights include unstable angina, uncontrolled congestive heart failure, and/or uncontrolled cardiac dysrhythmias and severe symptomatic valvular heart disease. Travelers with acute onset of these conditions should defer travel until these conditions have been stable for 3 months.

Cardiac Pacemakers and Implantable Cardiac Defibrillators

Travelers with implanted cardiac pacemakers and implantable cardiac defibrillators (ICDs) should have a thorough cardiac evaluation before extended overseas travel. The model and lot number of the device, as well as a copy of the patient's electrocardiogram with and without the pacemaker activated, should be carried on the trip along with the other important documents (passport, immunization booklet, traveler's health history; see Chapter 1). Identification of potential medical resources along the planned itinerary is advised, as not all types of medical facilities stock replacement batteries, pacemaker units, and electrodes. When undergoing airport security clearances, the traveler with an ICD or pacemaker should request a hand search, if possible, due to theoretical risk that the magnetic field created by handheld wands may be detected by an ICD and inadvertently lead to a defibrillator shock or inhibit a pacemaker's output. If security personnel insist on using a magnetic wand, ask that they avoid placing or waving the wand over the heart device.

Regarding pacemaker checks for integrity, travel within the continental United States is usually without problems, since many pacemaker patients can have their units checked via electronic telephone diagnostic programs. Medtronic, one of the manufacturers of ICDs, offers local support for their devices in more than 120 countries. Major pacemaker manufacturers and distributors maintain websites that list hospitals and physicians overseas who can evaluate pacemakers and other ICDs. A pacemaker or ICD identification code form is available from local branches of the American Heart Association. Prior to traveling with implanted heart devices the traveler should discuss his or her plans with the cardiologist and ask about specific activity restrictions or recommendations, steps to take if discomfort or symptoms occur, and location of a heart center or specialist at the travel destination.

DIABETES MELLITUS

Travelers with diabetes need to consider how to adapt their treatment programs to unfamiliar foods, irregular schedules, and varying amounts of exercise. Good planning and advance preparation are key to avoiding stress and problems arising as a result of traveling with diabetes. It is important to make plane and hotel reservations in advance and to allow reasonable time between connecting flights. Organize assistance ahead of time if the connection time will be a problem. Schedule necessary travel immunizations several weeks before travel. In addition to the usual travel vaccines, patients with diabetes should be encouraged to receive an annual flu shot, as well as the pneumococcal polysaccharide vaccine.

Table 16.3 lists supplies and medications that patients with diabetes need to assemble before departure. The American Diabetes Association is an excellent additional source of information for the traveler with diabetes. They distribute *The Diabetes Travel Guide*, by Davida F. Kruger. The second edition, published in 2006, includes information about diabetes supplies and a guide to insulin manufactured in the United States and abroad. Insulin manufactured in the United States is sold as U-100 strength, but it can be sold as U-40 or U-80 overseas.

The goal of management of diabetes while traveling is actually very simple: to avoid hypoglycemia. Clinical expertise of experienced diabetes clinicians indicates that complicated medication adjustment plans are unhelpful and can confuse patients. It is best to aim for a plan that will involve a single dose change. The management of diabetes is usually based on a 24-hour medication schedule. When traveling north or south, no adjustments in the 24-hour schedule are needed. Traveling westward results in a longer day, and traveling eastward results in a shorter day. When five or fewer time zones are crossed, no change is

TABLE 16.3   Checklist of Supplies for Insulin-Dependent Patients

Insulin sufficient to last the entire trip plus at least 1 extra week

Disposable U-100 syringes and needles to last entire trip plus 1 week

At least 1 bottle of Humalog (lispro) or other rapid-acting insulin analog

Reagent strips and lancets for blood glucose testing

Two blood glucose monitors with extra batteries, one carried on board and the other elsewhere

Ketone-detecting urine test strips (for use during illness or at altitude)

Glucose tablets and glucose gels

Glucagon emergency kit

Snacks: PowerBars, peanut butter crackers, and fruit juice, to take on board

Diabetes identification tag or bracelet (MedicAlert)

Billfold card detailing insulin dose and doctor's name and telephone number

Signed statement from personal physician on letterhead stationery documenting medical diagnosis and necessity for carrying supply of insulin, syringes, and needles for diabetic treatment, as well as original prescription labels on syringes and medications

Prescription from personal physician detailing insulin dose, in case supplies from home are lost, damaged, or stolen

All oral medications, including antibiotics, antiemetic and antidiarrheal agents, as well as essential over-the-counter medications

required in the usual insulin routine. However, when six or more time zones are crossed, adjustment in the usual schedule is advisable. The timing for oral diabetic medication is not as critical as that for insulin. People taking pills for their diabetes should simply take their medicine at the prescribed time, using local time. Patients wearing an insulin pump (continuous subcutaneous insulin infusion therapy) usually will *not* have to make adjustments in their basal insulin rates as they travel. However, it is important for patients with diabetes who use an insulin pump that they continue to check their blood sugars frequently after they arrive. It takes approximately 3-4 days for the body to adjust to a new time zone, and therefore, on the third day, the time on the insulin pump should be set to the local time. All the other settings should remain the same. Most airport security personnel in major international airports are familiar with insulin pumps. The events of 9/11 have increased security to the point that often the security agent will ask the pump wearer to open the back of the pump. This is a reasonable and easy request for some, but not all pumps, so it is often easiest to simply disconnect the device and let it be scanned through the screening machine. To facilitate easy removal of the pump, it should be stored in an easily accessible place such as a front pants or skirt pocket. It may be useful to carry a letter from one's physician explaining the need to travel with diabetes supplies and to provide a list of the supplies for airport security personnel. It is important to assure adequate pump supplies are carried with the traveler or split between carry-on and checked luggage. Many pump manufacturers have a back-up pump lending program; having a back-up pump is always recommended when traveling for an extended amount of time. Additionally, it is essential that those using a pump learn how to convert to a basal-bolus insulin regimen in the event of pump failure. They should have stored on paper as well as their smartphone or other device the amount of insulin they use in their pump as basal insulin as well as the amount they typically use as a pre-meal bolus. This information will allow a smooth conversion to a basal-bolus injection regimen. The basal rate can be substituted with a long-acting basal insulin (glargine or detemir), if needed.

Security regulations require that syringes, infusion sets, and other sharps retain the original pharmacy label stating the health provider's name. Frequent blood sugar monitoring is essential for safety. In addition to the typical measurements before breakfast, lunch, and dinner, travelers should check blood glucose levels every 3-4 hours while awake and whenever their daily routine is disrupted. Individuals who are normally lax about home glucose monitoring should *not* be while traveling. Most significant problems associated with fluctuations in blood sugars can be avoided by frequent checking of blood sugars. It is essential that travelers with diabetes have an adequate supply of the proper blood glucose strips for their particular meter and that they have batteries and even a back-up meter to use should they have a problem with their meter. Because the traveler will be ideally checking blood sugars more frequently, the healthcare provider may need to write a new prescription to take into account an increased number of glucose monitoring strips. Medical providers in former British colonies as well as the United Kingdom use meters and strips based on the millimoles per liter system and not on the more familiar milligrams per deciliter system that US meters report. A patient unfamiliar with this system of reporting would not be able to adequately interpret the data, so it is best to bring an extra meter and strips from home. The patient should have clear instructions regarding the management of high blood sugars while flying.

Diabetes and High Altitude

It is important to note that meters are not quite as accurate at altitude, but a study by Olateju et al. (2012) determined that while slight overestimation of blood glucose concentrations was found among various meters tested, no results obtained would have resulted in a failure to detect and treat blood glucose results requiring intervention. A study by de Mol et al. (2010) looked at a number of factors affecting the accuracy of handheld blood glucose meters at high altitude both simulated and on Mt. Kilimanjaro and found that of the nine different meters tested, the Accu-Chek Compact Plus and Accu-Chek Contour meters were the most accurate. A review article by Richards and Hillebrandt in 2013, found that highly motivated trekkers with type 1 diabetes who were free from long-term complications had metabolic and cardiovascular profiles comparable to those of control subjects, even though metabolic control was slightly worse. Despite the shortcomings in accuracy of blood glucose meters at altitude, frequent monitoring of blood glucose is required to remain safe from acute complications at altitude.

Traveling East across Six or More Time Zones

Traveling east shortens the day. There are a number of references dealing with the adjustment of insulin doses during travel through multiple east-to-west or west-to-east time zones. Studies demonstrate that straightforward and simple advice with regard to insulin management while traveling is preferred to elaborate protocols to alter insulin dosages, and usually adequate blood glucose control can be maintained with just one change in protocol. Regardless of the protocol used to adjust medications, patients should be advised to check blood glucose levels frequently during the flight and carry a quick-acting carbohydrate source that can be reached without having to leave the seat. Airline diabetic meals are not standardized, and therefore it is not necessary to order these. However, ordering a "Hindu," "low salt," or "vegetarian" meal will likely guarantee that the meal will be delivered prior to the regular meal service. More importantly, all insulin-using patients should be taught how to count carbohydrates and adjust rapid-acting insulin injections based on the quantity of carbohydrates to be consumed. There are excellent resources available for counting carbohydrates, and many of these are apps that can be downloaded to a smartphone or other handheld electronic device. A Certified Diabetes Educator or nutritionist can instruct the patient contemplating travel in how to master this task, which will go a long way to improving diabetes control while traveling. This teaching should occur well in advance of the planned trip.

Patients planning a long trip across many time zones may be greatly benefited by switching from regular insulin to one of the recombinant insulin analogs—Humalog (Lispro), NovoLog (insulin aspart), or Apidra (glulisine)—if they have not already done so. They should initiate this change at least 2 months before the trip so that baseline doses can be well established prior to travel. These agents have a rapid onset of action and can be taken with a meal, unlike regular insulin that must be injected at least 30 min before a meal to avoid postprandial hypoglycemia. Another significant advantage of recombinant insulin analogs is that it remains in the body for a maximum of 2-4 hours, thereby decreasing the likelihood of between-meal hypoglycemia.

Humalog or NovoLog insulin pen injection devices make administration of insulin extremely easy. Insulin pens look like large pens with cartridges. They can be used with small pen-tip needles instead of syringes and needles for giving insulin injections. A fine short needle, like the needle on an insulin syringe, is screwed onto the tip of the pen. Users turn a dial to select the desired dose of insulin and press a plunger on the end to deliver the insulin just under the skin. NovoLog Insulin pens are made by Novo-Nordisk and Humalog Insulin pens by Lilly. Pen needle tips are manufactured by Becton Dickinson.

The patient should be advised to work with a diabetes educator to determine the amount of quick-acting insulin that should be used to conservatively lower blood glucose if it is above the target range. For example, if a person is told to take one unit of insulin to lower the blood glucose by 50 points, he or she should use this ratio to correct hyperglycemia 3-4 hours after eating, while traveling.

When flying east, the day becomes shorter, so the basal dose of insulin should be adjusted using the formula:

$$\text{Travel dose} = \text{Normal dose} \times \left(0.9 - \frac{\text{Number of time zones crossed}}{\text{Hours between basal insulin doses}} \right).$$

This formula calculates the amount of insulin required to bridge the gap between the departure dose on the day of travel and the dose given after arrival, and takes into consideration the shortened day. It reduces the amount of insulin by a factor of 10-20% depending on the length of travel. For example: Jane has insulin-dependent diabetes and is traveling home from Nome, Alaska to New Jersey. She takes 20 units of Lantus (glargine) insulin at 8 p.m. every night as basal insulin. Using the formula above, which is fully explained in **Figure 16.1**, she would take her normal 20 units of Lantus the night before travel while in Nome. She would keep her watch on Nome time at 8 p.m. While flying, she would take 13 units. She would then change her watch to Eastern Standard Time at her destination. The next dose of Lantus is due at 8 p.m. EST after she arrives in New Jersey, which turns out to be only 18 hours after the last dose. The reduced time between doses is why the patient took just under three-quarters of her usual Lantus (glargine) dose on the flight. An excellent full explanation of these simple adjustments, including superb patient handouts, freely available to clinicians, can be found in Pinsker et al. (2013).

Traveling West Across Six or More Time Zones

Individuals on a basal-bolus insulin regimen flying west across six or more time zones should keep their watches set on their home time zone and should take their half of their basal insulin dose at the time they normally do. On arrival at their destination they should change the time on their watch to local time and take the remainder of their basal insulin at the time they normally would back home. By splitting the dose in half and at two different times, the Lantus (glargine) dose is extended to cover the entire day and will then put them back on schedule. On a twice-dosing basal regimen, the same protocol can be adopted with the same "one change" protocol. The patient would take their total dose of basal that they normally take in the morning prior to flying. The second dose would be due in-flight, so they should take half of that dose at the time they normally would. Then on arrival at their destination, they adjust their watch to local time and take the second half of their basal dose at the usual time. For example: Joe takes detemir 10 units twice per day at 9 a.m. and 9 p.m. He would take the full 10 units at 0900 and keep his watch on Newark time, his departure location. At 2100 in-flight, he would take half (5 units) of his detemir, and then when he arrives at his destination, take the additional 5 units at 2100 local time. At 0900 the next day, he is back on his regular schedule. He can continue to bolus before meals based on blood sugar results and carbohydrate intake, as always. Using a smartphone

WESTWARD travel
Basal Insulin Adjustment

STEP 1

Departure Info	Arrival Info
City: **New York**	City: **Honolulu**
Time Zone: **EST**	Time Zone: **HST**
Date / Time: **10 AM on May 15**	Date / Time: **3 PM on May 15**

STEP 2

DAY BEFORE TRAVEL (date **May 14**)
- Be sure to pack adequate supplies in your CARRY-ON bag -

Last dose of basal insulin: 20 units @ 8 am/pm

STEP 3

DURING TRAVEL
- Start travel with your watch set to your Departure Time Zone -
- Take your bolus insulin as needed for meals -
- Check your blood sugar frequently and watch for hypoglycemia! -

At 8 am/pm DEPARTURE TIME ZONE
take ½ of your "usual" basal insulin dose = 10 units

- Then set your watch to **2** am/pm (Arrival Time Zone) -

At 8 am/pm ARRIVAL TIME ZONE
take ½ of your "usual" basal insulin dose = 10 units
(This may be while still traveling or after arrival depending on the time)

STEP 4

AFTER ARRIVING (date **May 16**)
- Resume normal basal insulin dosing in the Arrival Time Zone -

Next dose of basal insulin: 20 units @ 8 am/pm

Free for non-commercial use, from Tripler Army Medical Center, Honolulu, HI, USA
Intended for use under supervision of a licensed diabetes care provider

Fig. 16.1 Formula for westward travel. (Reprinted with permission from Pinsker, J.E., et al., 2013. Extensive clinical experience: a simple guide to basal insulin adjustments for long-distance travel. J. Diabetes Metabol. Disord. 12, 59.)

application or checking www.worldtimezones.com can help one determine how many time zones will be crossed.

Regardless of the method used to adjust insulin dosages while traveling, it is essential that the person on insulin therapy understands how to recognize and treat hypoglycemia, how to monitor and interpret blood glucose results, and how to adjust insulin for a decrease or increase in the amount of carbohydrate present in the meal. A visit to a Certified Diabetes Educator or an endocrinologist with a special interest in diabetes prior to travel can be invaluable. These professionals can suggest individualized programs of insulin management to address changes in time zones, exercise levels, and illnesses while traveling. They can assist the Type 1 DM patient in switching from their pump to a long-acting insulin for basal needs with short-acting insulin alalogs for pre-pradial boluses and management of high blood sugars. With the improvements in insulin products available today, there is no reason that the individual with type 1 diabetes needs to suffer poor control of blood sugars while traveling.

Prevention of Hypoglycemia

Travel usually involves a drastic departure from daily routines. Meals may be delayed or unavailable. Physical activity is often greatly increased. These factors increase the risk of hypoglycemia. The principle of eating extra food when engaged in extra activity becomes especially important when traveling. Suitable snacks, such as crackers, dried fruits, or nuts, should be carried for use if meals are delayed or to supplement meals if necessary. Concentrated commercially available food bars such as Clif Bars, Luna Bars, or PowerBars suit this purpose very well, and for those counting carbohydrates, it is easy to calculate the amount of insulin required per carbohydrate as they are quantified on the label of the food bar.

Persons with diabetes should receive instruction from their diabetes care provider on recognition and treatment of hypoglycemia. A person with hypoglycemia may feel weak, drowsy, dizzy, or confused. Paleness, headache, trembling, sweating, rapid heartbeat, and a cold, clammy feeling are also signs of low blood sugar. The best method for treating very low blood sugar is with commercially available Gluco-Gel or Glucose Gel. These tubes are very quick acting. For low blood sugar levels that are only slightly below target, it is safe to use commercially available glucose tablets. One tablet is the equivalent of 4 g of glucose, so it will take three to four to raise a blood sugar level of 50 mg/dl into a safe zone. These commercially available products to treat hypoglycemia are highly recommended because they have a measured amount of concentrated carbohydrate content and are very stable. Liquid products such as Gluco-Gel or GU Energy Gel tend to work much faster and can be inserted into the patient's mouth, with no chewing necessary.

Traveling companions should be advised of the early signs of hypoglycemia and should understand the importance of administering sugar-containing drinks, or one of the products described above, if the person becomes glassy-eyed, grows confused or irritable, or is noted to be sweating inappropriately. If the person is too confused to swallow, food or fluid should not be administered, but Gluco-Gel can safely be administered into the mouth. If the situation worsens or cannot be treated orally, glucagon should be administered by injection.

Anyone using insulin as part of his or her diabetes treatment should travel with a glucagon emergency kit. Traveling companions should be briefed on proper use of the glucagon emergency kit. If the patient on insulin is traveling with a tour group, then the tour group leader or the person assigned to deal with medical problems for the group should be briefed on the use of glucagon and should be familiar with the kit and where the traveling patient is carrying it. For a lengthy trek, it is good to have more than one kit: one to be carried by the patient and one by the trip leader or medical support.

The traveler with diabetes who becomes stuporous or unconscious needs skilled medical care as soon as possible. However, one should *not* delay the administration of glucagon while attempting to obtain skilled medical care. Giving glucagon to a person with diabetes who does not need it may cause a significant rise in blood sugar, but this can be corrected relatively simply. Delaying glucagon administration in a diabetic person with severe hypoglycemia could result in severe medical complications. Glucagon can be administered by injection, even if the person of concern is stuporous or seizing. Any route of administration is reasonable, including intramuscularly or subcutaneously in an emergency situation. Once glucagon is administered, if the person regains full consciousness and is able to take food orally, a carbohydrate-protein snack should be given.

Names of English-speaking physicians overseas can be obtained from a number of sources listed in the Appendix. In addition, the Consulate of the American Embassy will have a list of physicians available to American citizens traveling abroad. It is important for all American citizens, particularly those with chronic medical problems, to register through the Smart Traveler Enrollment Program, a free service to allow US citizens and nationals traveling abroad to enroll their trip with the nearest US Embassy or Consulate. This service can be accessed at https://step.state.gov and can be completed before travel. Addresses and phone numbers of American Embassies overseas can be found at www.state.gov.

ARTIFICIAL HIP JOINTS AND OTHER ORTHOPEDIC HARDWARE

The metal components in artificial hip replacements and metal pins used for internal fixation of bone fractures may trigger the electromagnetic security alarms at airport passenger check-in stations. A traveler with an implanted orthopedic device or hardware should download the pdf "Disability Notification Card for Air Travel," which is available at www.tsa.gov. It is a card that can be presented to the security staff and simply states the medical condition and that alternate screening methods such as imaging or manual pat-down can be used. A passenger with metal implants can also request screening by imaging technology if it is in use at check-point. This may avoid lengthy explanations and delays in departure.

INTERNET RESOURCES

Access-Able Travel Source (www.access-able.com)
American Diabetes Association (www.diabetes.org)
American Lung Association (www.lungusa.org)
American Thoracic Society (www.thoracic.org)
British Thoracic Society (www.brit-thoracic.org.uk)
The International Society of Travel Medicine (www.istm.org)
The Oxygen Traveler (www.theoxygentraveler.com)
US Department of State (www.state.gov)
US Transportation Security Administration (www.tsa.gov)

REFERENCES AND FURTHER READING

Aerospace Medical Association, Medical Guidelines Task Force, Alexandria, VA, 2003. Medical Guidelines for Airline Travel, second ed. Aviat. Space Environ. Med. 74, A1–A19.

Boubaker, R., et al., 2016. Traveller's profile, travel patterns and vaccine practices-a 10-year prospective study in a Swiss Travel Clinic. J. Travel Med. 1–9. doi:10.1093/jtm/tav017.

Buhler, S., et al., 2014. A profile of travelers: an analysis from a large Swiss travel clinic. J. Travel Med. 21, 324–331.
Describes the demographics and health problems seen in a large cohort of travelers at a Swiss government travel clinic.

Centers for Disease Control and Prevention Yellow Book. 2014. Available at <wwwnc.cdc.gov/travel/yellowbook/2014> (accessed January 13, 2015).
The definitive book on issues related to travel and immunizations.

Coker, R.K., et al., 2002. Managing passengers with respiratory disease planning air travel: British Thoracic Society recommendations. Thorax 57, 289–304.

De Mol, P., Krabbe, H.G., de Vries, S.T., et al., 2010. Accuracy of handheld blood glucose meters at high altitude. Ludgate M, ed. PLoS One 5 (11), e15485. doi:10.1371/journal.pone.0015485.

Gawande, A., 2014. Being Mortal: Medicine and What Matters in the End. Metropolitan Books, H. Holt, New York.
Through compelling research, Dr. Atul Gawande examines the realities of aging and death and provides gripping stories of his own patients and family as they cope with these inevitabilities. He carefully explains the aging process in early chapters in this monumental work.

Gurgle, H.E., et al., 2013. Impact of traveling to visit friends and relatives on chronic disease management. J. Travel Med. 20, 95–100.

Iszadi, M., et al., 2014. Air travel considerations for the patients with heart failure. Iran Red Crescent Med. J. 16 (6), e17213.

Kruger, D.F., 2006. The Diabetes Travel Guide, second ed. American Diabetes Association, Alexandria, VA.

A comprehensive guide for those with diabetes planning a trip to anywhere in the world, with numerous sources for further information.

Muhm, J.M., et al., 2007. Effect of aircraft-cabin altitude on passenger discomfort. New Engl. J. Med. 357, 18–27.

Olateju, T., Begley, J., Flanagan, D., et al., 2012. Effects of Simulated Altitude on Blood Glucose Meter Performance: Implications for In-Flight Blood Glucose Monitoring. J. Diabetes Sci. Technol. 6 (4), 867–874.

Peterson, D.C., et al., 2013. Outcomes of medical emergencies on commercial airline flights. New Engl. J. Med. 368, 2075–2083.

Pinsker, J.E., et al., 2013. Extensive clinical experience: a simple guide to basal insulin adjustments for long-distance travel. J. Diabetes Metab. Disord. 12, 59.

This informative article based on a literature review and anecdotal experience from work at an Army Medical Center in Hawaii provides great hand-outs available to assist travelers with insulin dosing across multiple time zones.

Richards, P., Hillebrandt, D., 2013. The practical aspects of insulin at high altitude. High Alt. Med. Biol. 14 (3), 197–204. doi:10.1089/ham.2013.1020.

Shitrit, A.D., Chowers, M., 2010. Comparison of younger and older adult travelers. J. Travel Med. 17, 250–255.

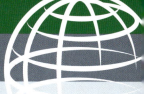

CHAPTER 17

Travel and Mental Health

Samuel B. Thielman

MEDEVAC STATISTICS

Although mental health is often an afterthought in travel medicine, in fact, the psychiatric impact of travel is an area of growing interest, not only because of the prevalence of international travelers from all sectors of the population, but also because of the changing nature of international travel. A recent Swiss travel clinic study of 22,584 travelers seeking pre-travel advice revealed the purposes of travel as follows: tourism, 81.5%; visiting friends and relatives, 7.8%; business, 5.6%; other (volunteer work, study, pilgrimage and so on), 5.1%. Although the majority of travel is still for tourism, increasingly, medical providers are called on to support people traveling for mission work, disaster relief, or military and para-military purposes. These changes make it critical for health providers involved in the support of travelers to be aware of common mental health problems that emerge during travel so that they can advise travelers on risks and offer effective support when problems emerge.

The World Health Organization recently drew attention to the importance of mental health issues for travel medicine, placing mental health disorders among the three major reasons for medical evacuation during travel (the other two being injury and cardiovascular accidents). Though statistics vary, the percentage of medevacked travelers who come back for psychiatric causes is between 6% and 11%.

In one large telephone survey of young travelers returning after travel to tropical countries, 11.3% reported some sort of psychiatric or psychological symptoms during travel. Unremarkably, the most common symptoms experienced were nonspecific symptoms such as sleep disturbance (53.1%), fatigue (48.7%), and dizziness (39.3%). But 2.5% of these people had had psychological symptoms they described as severe, and 1.2% had symptoms that lasted more than 2 months after return. Travelers who reported these symptoms were significantly ($p < .001$) more likely to have been on mefloquine prophylaxis for malaria. Consideration of the psychiatric impact of mefloquine (and chloroquine) on travelers should certainly be a factor in evaluating patients returning with psychiatric symptoms, especially symptoms of anxiety and/or psychosis.

A study of British diplomats found that 11% of all medevacs of travelers were for mental disorders. The most common causes for medevac were depression (41.2%), family crisis or "welfare" problems (23.5%), and debriefing following a critical incident (17.6%). In this study 5.9% were medevacked for alcohol-related problems.

PRE-DEPARTURE ASSESSMENT AND ADVICE: RISK FACTORS

While current knowledge does not allow us to make reliable predictions about the exact risk of the emergence of various mental health conditions, the destination, duration, and purpose of travel must be considered when advising patients at risk for mental disorder. For short-term travelers with a history of mental health disorders, the most important preparation

243

would be a review of prior psychiatric history, consideration of recurrence and how it might be managed, and education on the risks of casual sex (which is common among travelers and has mental health implications) and excessive alcohol use. For longer-term travelers, more extensive pre-travel assessment can be helpful. This would involve a more detailed psychiatric and substance abuse history, a history of prior exposure to trauma, discussion of how needed medications will be obtained, and consideration of the closest available mental health support in the traveler's native language. It should also give consideration to "resilience factors" (see below). Helping travelers think these issues through in advance helps mitigate the effect of problems that arise during travel.

Aside from prior psychiatric history, the most important risk factor for the emergence of psychiatric disorders during travel is level of stress experienced, and international travel is often stressful. Psychosocial stressors have long been known to exacerbate psychiatric conditions in travelers, especially depression, bipolar disorder, and psychosis. People with a history of depression are vulnerable to a number of the stresses of travel, especially international travel with duration of more than a few weeks. The sleeplessness caused by travel across many time zones, unexpected delays, misunderstandings due to language and culture barriers, and interpersonal stresses created by travel can all contribute to depression, so travelers vulnerable to depression should be prepared to anticipate stressors, have a game plan for dealing with the unexpected, and know where to turn in case problems arise.

Anxious patients who are traveling to malarious areas must use alternatives to mefloquine and chloroquine for malaria prophylaxis. Travelers with a history of anxiety or panic who are headed for stressful circumstances should be not only warned of the increased risk presented by stressful circumstances but counseled to assess the level of support available to them during travel and to determine how they will be supported should problems arise.

Alcohol-use disorders are also exacerbated by the stress of travel, and people are known to drink more freely during travel. As a result, alcohol-use disorders are a common focus of mental health concern among both short- and long-term travelers. Evaluation of travelers should include inquiry as to a history of an alcohol-use disorder along with guidance for moderate use of alcohol while traveling abroad and the importance of keeping in touch with friends or relatives during travel.

Patients on medications for chronic psychiatric conditions should be sure they have adequate medication and that it is located in more than one place, so that even if one portion is lost, a backup interim supply will be available. **Box 17.1** contains additional useful advice for patients with chronic psychiatric problems.

PRE-TRAVEL EVALUATION OF RESILIENCE

Classically, mental health evaluations have focused primarily on the risk factors discussed above. In recent years, however, there has been an additional focus on assessing resilience, since resilience factors seem to play an important role in assessing the likelihood of the development of mental health problems. "Resilience" in this context refers to a person's ability to recover after lengthy periods of adversity or after a traumatic event.

Increasingly, resilience assessment and training has become a part of preparation for people going on humanitarian travel of medium-term (3-12 months) duration. The resilience factors, as identified by Southwick and Charney, are factors that the traveler can start incorporating into his or her way of life in order to maximize the chances of a successful travel experience. Some of the resilience factors identified by Southwick and Charney include identifying sturdy role models, seeking out a resilient mentor, using cognitive flexibility as a coping style (e.g., humor, acceptance, reframing), active problem solving, drawing from religious and spiritual resources, and finding meaning in adversity. Travel preparation oriented around resilience may lessen vulnerability to traumas during travel where there is a significant risk of exposure to hardship or traumatic events. Southwick and Charney's summary of 10 factors that they observed in resilient individuals can also inform evaluation of travelers (**Box 17.2**).

Box 17.1 Practical advice for short-term travelers at risk for exacerbation of a psychotic disorder

1. Make sure you have travel insurance and that it covers medevac for psychiatric disorders.

2. Be sure you have an adequate supply of medicine, carry extra medication, and keep medicines in more than one place.

3. Educate yourself on where and how you can obtain medication in case you lose your medications.

4. Do not take travel medicines that may exacerbate psychiatric conditions unless your physician approves. Take an alternative to mefloquine if you need malaria prophylaxis; be cautious about chloroquine as well. Avoid taking modafinil or similar drugs for jet lag; be sparing in the use of zolpidem and other sleep-inducing medications that can affect memory and perception.

5. Attend to sleep; minimize the effects of jet lag by exposure to light and assuming the local sleep schedule as quickly as possible on arrival.

6. Pay special attention to prepare yourself for cultural changes to minimize a sense of cultural displacement.

7. If indicated, be sure to carry antianxiety medication to use in case of a panic attack.

8. Plan for consultation with your psychiatrist on return.

(Adapted from Vermersch, C., Geoffroy, P.A., Fovet, T., et al, 2014. Voyage et troubles psychotiques: clinique et recommandations pratiques. Presse Med. 43, 1317–1324.)

Box 17.2 The "resilience factors"

1. Identifying and emulating sturdy role models

2. Maintaining cognitive flexibility

3. Using active problem solving

4. Adopting an attitude of realistic optimism

5. Seeking social support

6. Following the inner moral compass

7. Drawing from religious/spiritual resources

8. Exercising intentional physical, mental, and emotional training

9. Exercising the ability to find meaning in adversity

10. Assuming responsibility for one's own emotional well-being

(Adapted from Southwick, S.M., Charney, D.S., 2012. Resilience: The Science of Mastering Life's Greatest Challenges. Cambridge University Press, New York.)

A final component of helping patients with psychiatric vulnerabilities to travel safely involves assessment of possible resources for the patient at the destination. Making such an assessment can be a complex process, not only because psychiatric resources can be extremely difficult to locate in the developing world, but also because, even in the developed world, such resources may well be suitable only for short-term travelers. Long-term travelers will need psychiatric care delivered in their native language and even developed countries in Europe may not have clinicians willing to cater to English speakers for ongoing care. Patients should be cautioned that, if they plan to be in a foreign country for an extended period of time, arrangements must be made in advance for the support of chronic psychiatric problems.

COMMON MENTAL HEALTH PROBLEMS AMONG TRAVELERS AND HOW THEY ARISE

Sleep, Travel, and Psychiatric Problems

There are a number of psychiatric problems that can affect travelers. One of the most common is sleep disruption, which is problematic for most people traveling across many time zones. It has mental health implications even for those without a prior mental health history, and sleep disruption can also exacerbate a pre-existing condition. International travel affects sleep in a variety of ways; jet lag, high altitude, alcohol, overnight flights, change in bedroom surroundings, climate, allergies, and pollution all can affect sleep. Sleep deprivation impairs normal cognition in a variety of ways. The decreased attention and vigilance create an increased risk for accidents and misunderstandings. Also affected are working memory, short-term memory, and processing speed. Thus, sleep deprivation interferes with adaptation and adjustment. In addition, extended sleep deprivation, most likely during long-haul travel, negatively affects mood and even emotional intelligence.

Sleep abnormalities are part of numerous psychiatric conditions (major depression, bipolar disorder, attention deficit hyperactivity disorder, schizophrenia), and there is evidence that the disruption of circadian rhythms may precipitate and escalate psychiatric disorders.

A recent study of jet lag and psychiatric disorders reviewed current evidence on this topic and noted an association between jet lag and depression, hypomania, schizoaffective disorder, and psychotic disorders. Interestingly, direction of travel was also found to be important: the emergence of depression is more likely to be associated with traveling in an eastward direction, while the emergence of hypomania is more likely to be associated with westward travel. Efforts to mitigate the effect of jet lag on psychosis with medication have been attempted, and in a small study, the use of melatonin to promote sleep seemed to maintain stability, but this approach needs further substantiation.

Careful attention to management of jet lag is particularly important with patients who have a history of psychiatric disorder, especially an affective disorder. Jet lag is usually managed with a combination of practical measures (exposure to light at appropriate times of day, adjusting to the local schedule), and short-term use of sleep medications (see Chapter 9). Use of zolpidem or zaleplon for 3-4 days after travel across multiple time zones is a common and often effective pharmacological approach to the situation. Patients with a history of psychiatric disorders should be warned against the use of alcohol as a remedy for jet lag, as this may contribute to mood instability and inhibit adjustment.

Alcohol-Use Disorders and Their Consequences

Abuse of alcohol during travel is a common occurrence. There are many reasons for this. Airlines and airports promote alcohol, and alcohol is often cheaper on the local market. Some feel that drinking alcohol is safer than drinking the local water, and alcohol use sometimes serves as a quick but ineffective fix for the loneliness and isolation of overseas living.

Because it is so readily available, alcohol use should be considered early on in the evaluation of any patient with altered mental status who has been traveling in an overseas setting. In certain countries, illegally produced alcohol can be a particularly vexing problem, since such brews can contain toxic substances that alter mental status markedly and are hard to identify. Further, intoxicated travelers may find themselves in situations in which there are no friends or relatives to inhibit heavy drinking. Travelers may come to medical attention after being found unresponsive in a hotel room or because of failure to pay a hotel bill or overstaying a reservation.

As noted, studies of medevacs indicate that alcohol abuse is a frequent cause for medevac, and transporting patients who are having alcohol withdrawal symptoms can be particularly problematic. Chronic heavy drinkers may develop alcohol withdrawal symptoms such as sweating, tachycardia, agitation, anxiety, insomnia, tremor, nausea, illusions, hallucinations, and seizures. Airlines will not knowingly transport patients who are psychiatrically unstable.

Therefore, it is usually necessary for such patients to be stabilized locally prior to transport. In the event that patients are able to travel, they must be accompanied by a medical attendant who can observe evidence of emerging withdrawal symptoms. A medical attendant may also be in a position to provide support with a benzodiazepine such as lorazepam or temazepam to prevent the emergence of a more serious alcohol withdrawal syndrome.

Use of licit or illicit drugs is also a frequent reason for mental health attention. Aside from problems with drugs of abuse common in the United States, travelers to some developing world countries have been known to participate in ceremonies that involve hallucinogenic drugs unfamiliar to medical providers (e.g., iboga in Gabon or yopo in Venezuela, and ayahuasca in the Peruvian Amazon).

Trauma- and Stressor-Related Disorders

For travelers who are staying in a new culture for an extended period of time, the difficulty of cultural adaptation can be dramatic. "Culture shock" is described in the *Diagnostic and Statistical Manual of Mental Disorders*, fifth edition (DSM-V), as a V code, Acculturation Difficulty (V62.4). Stressor-related disorders, that is, time-limited depression, anxiety, or a mixed state, are common in travel. In addition to the stresses of short-term travel, long-term travelers must adapt to a new culture, and even when the discomfort and dysphoria related to a new culture are of limited duration, patients sometimes seek out medical providers for information and reassurance. Adjustment disorders characterized by predominant emotions of anxiety or depression, but directly related to an identifiable stressor, do not meet the criteria for another psychiatric disorder and are presumed to be time limited. Information that is useful for patients with cultural adjustment issues is provided by intercultural trainer Ray Leki in his book *Travelwise* (2008): when in a new culture, focus on self-awareness, self-management, social awareness, and relationship management. Maintain a sense of humor and work hard at developing empathy toward your foreign contacts. Such advice can be reassuring to patients and provide a way forward for them.

Panic attacks and anxiety disorders are also stress sensitive and represent a major reason for psychiatric treatment following travel. In one study from Israel, anxiety disorders constituted almost half the psychiatric problems in returning patients who received psychiatric treatment.

The Psychological Sequelae of Exposure to Traumatic Events

Exposure to dangerous events is a hazard of many kinds of travel, and a recent meta-analysis found that exposure to intentional trauma produces posttraumatic stress disorder (PTSD) in 37% of exposed individuals. Additionally, travelers going out for disaster relief or refugee assistance frequently hear distressing stories from directly affected individuals, and this exposure, too, can create posttrauma symptoms of emotional numbing, avoidance of reminders, intrusive thoughts, hyperarousability, and negative thoughts and mood. If such symptoms persist beyond a month, referral for treatment for PTSD may be necessary. In current psychiatric practice, both psychological and psychopharmacological therapies have a role, and treatment by a knowledgeable clinician may markedly improve outcome after trauma exposure.

Psychosis

Psychosis is also precipitated by stressors, and the emergence of psychosis during travel is well documented. Patients with pre-existing disorders with a psychotic component, such as schizophrenia or bipolar disorder, may have exacerbations during travel. But psychosis can also emerge as a result of the strangeness of a different culture, and a brief reactive psychosis during travel can be a surprising occurrence. Such psychoses, if not indicative of an underlying disorder, may well be transient and remit on return to the home country. It appears that dramatic differences in cultures are particularly likely to precipitate such a psychotic episode (e.g., a rural Asian refugee placed in an urban US setting). In addition, certain destinations, such as Jerusalem or Machu Picchu, seem to put certain people at risk for the development of psychotic behavior.

Box 17.3 Antares/CDC mental health support recommendations for humanitarian organizations

1. An agency needs a written and active policy to prevent or mitigate the effects of stress.

2. There should be systematic screening and assessment of the capacity of personnel to respond to and cope with anticipated stresses of a position or contract.

3. All staff should have appropriate pre-assignment preparation and training in managing stress.

4. Staff response to stress should be monitored on an ongoing basis.

5. There must be provision for training and support on an ongoing basis to help staff deal with daily stresses.

6. There should be specific and culturally appropriate support in the wake of dramatic incidents and other unexpected periods of stress.

7. There should be practical emotional and culturally appropriate support for staff at the end of an assignment or contract.

8. There must be a clear understanding and written policies with respect to the ongoing support offered to staff who have been adversely impacted by exposure to stress and trauma during an assignment.

(From the Antares Foundation, Managing Stress in Humanitarian Workers: Guidelines for Good Practices.)

THE ROLE OF THE CLINICIAN: ORGANIZING SUPPORT

Mental Health Support for Humanitarian and Other Overseas Workers

The Centers for Disease Control and Prevention (CDC) and the Antares Foundation have recently released updated standards for mental health support for humanitarian workers (see **Box 17.3**). Medical providers who support humanitarian workers should familiarize themselves with these standards and, where appropriate, make sure that such workers have access to preparation that helps them understand the nature of their assignment, common reactions, and where to go for psychological help when it is needed. The standards also document the need for a good plan for support during deployment as well as information on issues of repatriation and adjustment on return. Although these recommendations target humanitarian organizations, they also represent best practices for those responsible for the care of any people being deployed to difficult assignments.

For certain high-risk groups, such as journalists, humanitarian workers in war zones, and diplomatic and military personnel who have been in violent areas, some sort of debriefing is increasingly seen to be necessary. Although the older types of psychological debriefing have been discredited as ineffective or even harmful (i.e., those involving emotional catharsis and universally administered protocol), an educationally oriented debriefing individually or with a small group of peers can be helpful. Such debriefings normally involve allowing the traveler to discuss whatever aspects of the trip were of special importance or concern to them, followed by information on repatriation, description of commonly occurring psychological and adjustment issues, and guidance as to where to get help if needed. Even a brief medical debriefing/outbriefing with travelers who are at risk can be very helpful with adjustment, and early attention is crucial to reducing the risk of emerging mental health problems.

INTERNET RESOURCES

http://www.who.int/ith/other_health_risks/psychological_health/en/
https://www.antaresfoundation.org/guidelines#.VVJXyfm-UZg
http://wwwnc.cdc.gov/travel/yellowbook/2014/chapter-2-the-pre-travel-consultation/mental-health-and-travel
http://www.nctsn.org/content/psychological-first-aid

FURTHER READING

Allison, G., Harvey, P.D., 2008. Sleep and circadian rhythms in bipolar disorder: seeking synchrony, harmony, and regulation. Am. J. Psychiatry 165, 820–829.

Beny, A., Paz, A., Potasman, I., 2001. Psychiatric problems in returning travelers: features and associations. J. Travel Med. 8, 243–246.

Boden, J.M., Fergusson, D.M., Horwood, L.J., 2014. Associations between exposure to stressful life events and alcohol use disorder in a longitudinal birth cohort studied to age 30. Drug Alcohol Depend. 142, 154–160.

Buhler, S., Ruegg, R., Steffen, R., et al., 2014. A profile of travelers: an analysis from a large Swiss travel clinic. J. Travel Med. 21, 324–331.

Charney, D.S., 2004. Psychobiological mechanisms of resilience and vulnerability. Focus 2, 368–391.

Chen, L.H., Wilson, M.E., Schlagenhauf, P., 2007. Controversies and misconceptions in malaria chemoprophylaxis for travelers. JAMA 297 (20), 2251–2263.

Eriksson, C., Lopes Cardozo, B., Foy, D., et al., 2012. Predeployment mental health and trauma exposure of expatriate humanitarian aid workers: risk and resilience factors. Traumatology 19, 41–48.

Flinn, D.E., 1962. Transient psychotic reactions during travel. Am. J. Psychiatry 119, 173–174.

Ifield, 1977. Current social stressors and symptoms of depression. Am. J. Psychiatry 134, 161–166.

Katz, G., Durst, R., Zislin, Y., et al., 2001. Psychiatric aspects of jet lag: review and hypothesis. Med. Hypotheses 56, 20–23.

Kehle, S.M., Ferrier-Auerbach, A.G., Meis, L.A., et al., 2012. Predictors of postdeployment alcohol use disorders in National Guard soldiers deployed to Operation Iraqi Freedom. Psychol. Addict. Behav. 26, 42–50.

Leki, R.S., 2008. Travelwise: How to Be Safe, Savvy and Secure Abroad. Intercultural Press, Boston.

Lopes Cardozo, B., Gotway Crawford, C., Eriksson, C., et al., 2012. Psychological distress, depression, anxiety, and burnout among international humanitarian aid workers: a longitudinal study. PLoS ONE 7, e44948.

Patel, D., Easmon, C.J., Dow, C., et al., 2000. Medical repatriation of British diplomats resident overseas. J. Travel Med. 7, 64–69.

Paykel, E.S., 2003. Life events and affective disorders. Acta Psychiatr. Scand. 108 (Suppl. 418), 61–66.

Post, R.M., Leverich, G.S., 2006. The role of psychosocial stress in the onset and progression of bipolar disorder and its comorbidities: the need for earlier and alternative modes of therapeutic intervention. Dev. Psychopathol. 18, 1181–1211.

Potasman, I., Beny, A., Seligmann, H., 2000. Neuropsychiatric problems in 2,500 long-term young travelers to the tropics. J. Travel Med. 7 (1), 5–9.

Putman, K.M., Lantz, J.I., Townsend, C.L., et al., 2009. Exposure to violence, support needs, adjustment, and motivators among Guatemalan humanitarian aid workers. Am. J. Community Psychol. 44, 109–115.

Sack, R.L., 2010. Jet lag. NEJM 362, 440–447.

Southwick, S.M., Charney, D.S., 2012. Resilience: The Science of Mastering Life's Greatest Challenges. Cambridge University Press, New York.

Strain, J.J., 1991. Stressors and the adjustment disorders. Am. J. Psychiatry 148, 1079-a-1081.

van Erp, K.J., Giebels, E., van der Zee, K.I., et al., 2011. Let it be: expatriate couples' adjustment and the upside of avoiding conflicts. Anxiety Stress Coping 24, 539–560.

Vermersch, C., Geoffroy, P.A., Fovet, T., et al., 2014. Voyage et troubles psychotiques: clinique et recommandations pratiques. Presse Med. 43, 1317–1324.

Weingarten, J.A., Collop, N.A., 2013. Air travel: effects of sleep deprivation and jet lag. Chest 144 (4), 1394–1401.

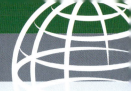

CHAPTER 18

Pre-Travel Assessment and Advice for Expatriates and Volunteers

Shawn Vasoo and Lim Poh Lian

 Access evidence synopsis online at ExpertConsult.com.

EXPATRIATES

Definitions

Expatriates are defined as travelers who reside abroad for work or volunteer reasons but intend to return eventually to their home country, in contrast to immigrants, who intend to stay in the destination country. They typically spend longer durations abroad than tourists or short-term business travelers.

Type of Expatriate

Exposures depend largely on the nature of work. This may range from executives in large cities to missionaries or relief workers in rural settings or disaster sites. Working in healthcare facilities, refugee camps, or orphanages increases infectious risks.

Expatriates employed by well-established organizations have better access to pre-travel preparation and may have extensive medical resources, including evacuation policies. By contrast, self-sponsored travelers or those sent by smaller organizations may limit their pre-travel preparation due to cost constraints and may have inadequate support if they fall ill abroad.

Destination

The most important factor to consider in pre-travel preparation is destination. Health exposures vary greatly by continent; for example, the risk of malaria is generally higher in sub-Saharan Africa compared with Asia or Latin America. Urban versus rural settings also modify exposure risks and access to care.

Decisions about vaccinations and advice about malaria prophylaxis also depend on which other countries or areas the expatriate is likely to go to while abroad, other than the stated destination country. This can include official or recreational side trips to rural areas, such as might occur for consular staff responding to emergencies.

Duration

Long-term residence abroad (>3-6 months) puts expatriates at risk for an extended range of health problems. First, longer duration mathematically increases exposure opportunities. Second, compliance with precautions becomes challenging to sustain over time. Third, long-term expatriates may have higher risk for specific exposures, depending on their work (humanitarian relief, medical, orphanages), and living conditions may approximate that of local or poorer populations (missionaries).

Emerging Trends

Although "expatriate" may conjure images of white-collar executives, it encompasses lower-income migrant workers from developing countries. These may include Indonesian domestic helpers in Hong Kong, Filipino nurses in Saudi Arabia, or Bangladeshi construction workers in Singapore. An emerging trend is south-to-south work migration, for example, the large influx of Chinese investment and construction in Africa. Pre-travel preparation and access to healthcare resources for these workers may be minimal.

PRE-TRAVEL CARE

Expatriates should undergo a comprehensive health assessment ideally 4-12 weeks pre-departure to identify previously undiagnosed disease, stabilize chronic illnesses, evaluate fitness for travel and risks, provide routine and travel-specific vaccinations, and educate regarding prevention and management of health issues while abroad.

History

A detailed medical and surgical history should be obtained with attention to those that need to be stabilized. Review of systems should include symptoms that may indicate undiagnosed problems, psychiatric issues, and substance abuse, because these may be exacerbated by the stress of travel abroad. Social history should elicit tobacco, alcohol/drug use, and sexual practices to guide advice about risk behaviors, with reference to the destination country.

Document medication allergies and review medications the patient is taking, their availability abroad, and any testing required. Patients on warfarin, insulin, injectable agents, or controlled substances will require detailed counsel on making prior arrangements for monitoring, safe supply, and legal access in the destination country.

Complete immunization records are required in order to provide appropriate advice about vaccinations. Specific forms, tests, or vaccinations may be required by the organization or the destination country. If accompanying children will attend school at the destination country, there may be additional school-related requirements.

Physical Exam

Perform a comprehensive physical examination, including vital signs, height, weight, and body mass index. Preventive health screening for women should include a breast exam (if ≥30 years), and a Pap smear for the sexually active or those ≥21. Men should have a testicular exam and, if ≥50 years, a digital rectal exam. A dental exam is recommended if dental care overseas may not be readily accessible.

Laboratory Tests

There are few evidence-based recommendations for screening laboratory tests for long-term expatriates. Health screening guidelines appropriate for age and occupation would be a minimum starting point. Additional screening tests for tuberculosis, human immunodeficiency virus (HIV), or syphilis may also be required by the destination country for long-term travelers.

These are screening tests to consider, based on age, risk factors, and destination:

- Complete blood count (CBC), chemistry, liver function tests, and fasting glucose and lipids
- Mammograms for women age >40
- Colonoscopy for men and women age >50
- Tuberculin skin test (TST) or interferon gamma release assay (IGRA)
- Baseline electrocardiogram (EKG) for persons age >45 and those with cardiovascular risk factors
- Baseline chest radiograph for patients with positive TST or pulmonary conditions
- HbA1c for diabetics
- HIV serology
- Hepatitis B and C serologies (HBsAg, HBsAb, HBcAb total, HCV Ab)
- Rapid plasma reagin and *Treponema pallidum* hemagglutination

For patients with specific risk factors or medical history, some of the following tests may also be required:

- β-human chorionic gonadotropin
- Thyroid stimulating hormone, free thyroxine
- Cardiac stress testing
- Pulmonary function testing

Test results should be reviewed, follow-up discussed, and a copy of the results provided. Baseline EKG or chest radiograph may be needed for comparison when residing abroad long term.

Assessing Fitness for Travel

Assessing fitness for travel may be required by the organization or requested for personal health reasons. Employer or country visa requirements can be quite specific. Information from the history, physical exam, and laboratory tests will help determine this. Stabilize newly diagnosed or pre-existing medical illness before departure.

Complex medical conditions in travelers should prompt a careful evaluation of availability at the destination for access to modern medical resources:

- Bleeding or clotting disorders (requiring blood products)
- Cancer (requiring treatment in the past 5 years or ongoing monitoring)
- Cardiovascular disease (symptomatic)
- Diabetes (HbA1c >8, end-stage organ disease)
- HIV (symptomatic or CD4 count <200)
- Renal failure (requiring renal replacement therapy)
- Rheumatologic disease (symptomatic in the last 6 months, on immunosuppression)
- Solid organ or bone marrow transplant recipient (within 2 years from transplant)
- Psychiatric disorder (symptomatic within the last 12 months)

These need not preclude travel. But if travel or assignment is to a remote location with poor access to appropriate medical care, travelers and their organizations should be made aware of the potential risks and options to mitigate those risks.

Depending on resources available, long-term travelers may need to make arrangements for medical follow-up at destination or else return home for this. Travelers need to check on availability of medications in the destination country. Local regulations may restrict the use of benzodiazepines and narcotics, and purchasing medications in-country may risk counterfeit medications or treatment interruptions due to stock-outs.

VACCINE-PREVENTABLE DISEASES (VPD)

For VPD, vaccine risk and cost should be balanced against a discussion of the risk of disease acquisition. **Figure 18.1** outlines the framework for risk assessment.

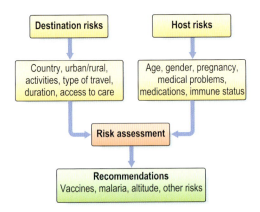

Fig. 18.1 Expatriate pre-departure assessment.

For long-term expatriates on their first extended posting abroad, the list of vaccines may be long and daunting. A useful framework for discussion is to group the vaccines into the following categories:

- Routine: vaccines they should be getting even if not traveling
- Recommended: vaccines appropriate for their exposure risk at the destination
- Required: vaccines required by the country or organization

These will vary based on the traveler's age, medical conditions, destination, work, or recreational exposures, and organizational policy. Another useful framework to discuss vaccines is by the main route of transmission:

- Food- and water-borne: hepatitis A, typhoid, rotavirus, polio
- Respiratory: measles, mumps, rubella (MMR), diphtheria, pertussis, chickenpox, influenza, pneumococcal, meningococcal
- Vector-borne: yellow fever, Japanese encephalitis
- Contact: tetanus, rabies
- Blood and body fluids/sexual: hepatitis B, human papillomavirus (HPV)

A careful vaccination history should be taken for travelers born in developing countries where vaccine uptake may be sub-optimal or for elderly travelers who were born before routine childhood vaccination programs.

All long-term expatriate travelers should receive routine vaccines. In today's increasingly mobile and globalized world, this sometimes requires discussion about whether to follow the national recommendations of:

- Their country of citizenship
- The country where they are receiving pre-travel care
- The destination country (for visa and school requirements)

For example, a healthy American family with two children (ages 5 and 13) seen in Singapore before their move to Mumbai for 3 years will need a nuanced discussion of influenza vaccine (universal in the United States but not in Singapore), meningococcal and HPV vaccine for the 13-year-old, and MMR number two (given at 15-18 months in Singapore but at 4-6 years in the United States) for the 5-year-old, in addition to whatever the international school in Mumbai may require of incoming students.

For recommended vaccines, long-term expatriates should receive as a minimum the same recommendations that short-term travelers get. However, the following vaccines deserve more detailed mention for long-term expatriates.

Typhoid Vaccine

Typhoid fever from *Salmonella typhi* is acquired by contaminated food or water. This risk is higher in developing countries, with the highest risk in South Asia (the Indian subcontinent). The incidence of typhoid among travelers is estimated at 3/100,000 per month. A longer duration of travel confers higher risk, although those who travel less than a week can still acquire typhoid infection.

Typhoid vaccine is available in the United States as a live attenuated oral vaccine and an injectable Vi polysaccharide vaccine. Protective efficacy is ~70%, so patients should be counseled to maintain food and water precautions. Duration of protection is about 2-3 years for the injectable vaccine and 5 years for the oral vaccine. Neither vaccine confers protection against *Salmonella paratyphi*.

Hepatitis B

Hepatitis B infection is transmitted via blood and body fluids (sexual intercourse, contaminated needles, or blood transfusions). It is present worldwide but endemic in Asia and the developing world. Expatriates may be exposed when seeking medical or dental care abroad. All long-term expatriates should receive hepatitis B vaccine at 0, 1, and 6 months. A four-dose rapid schedule of 0, 1, 2, and 12 months can be used as an alternative or the accelerated schedule of 0, day 7, day 21, and 12 months (not approved by the US Food and Drug Administration [FDA]). Checking antibody titers is not routine but may be considered for travelers with immunocompromise, on dialysis, with risk factors of being nonresponders, and with occupational exposures. Nonresponders should undergo a second primary series and have titers rechecked.

Japanese Encephalitis (JE) Vaccine

JE is a flavivirus infection transmitted by *Culex* mosquitoes. Incidence is estimated at 50,000 per year with transmission occurring in Asia, especially rural areas. There are four JE vaccines in use worldwide, but availability varies by country. We will discuss these so long-term expatriates can understand how newer vaccines compare with previous vaccines.

JE-MB Vaccine

This was a three-dose vaccine, given at 0, 7, and 28 days. Derived from mouse brain (MB), the Biken vaccine was discontinued in 2008. However, an equivalent JE-MB vaccine from Green Cross in South Korea was in use until 2015.

JE-VC Vaccine

A Vero cell (VC) vaccine, Ixiaro™, is FDA approved in the United States and available in Europe, Australia (Jespect™), and several sites in Asia (Singapore, Hong Kong). It is a two-dose series, given at 0 and 28 days. A booster is recommended at 12-15 months, with data suggesting immunogenicity for several years thereafter.

JE-CV Vaccine

A chimeric vaccine (CV), Imojev™ has been registered for use in Australia, Singapore, and several other countries (as of April 2015). It is a live attenuated vaccine approved for individuals 9 months of age and older. Protection is thought to be several years, but there are no recommendations for booster or timing at this time.

JE SA-14-14-2 Vaccine

This is a live attenuated viral vaccine using the SA-14-14-2 strain, produced by the Chengdu Institute of Biological Products in China. The schedule in China is a subcutaneous dose at age 8 months, followed by a booster at age 2 years, and another dose at 6-7 years.

Rabies

Rabies is an acute viral encephalitis that is primarily transmitted by mammal bites; dog bites are the most common mode of transmission. Long-term expatriates are at increased risk because of longer duration of exposure; they may also acquire pets, including stray animals. Young children may be at increased risk for high-risk animal bites to the head and neck region.

Pre-exposure vaccination consists of three doses given at day 0, 7, 21, or 28. This simplifies management after a bite—patients should be counseled to wash the wound with soap and water, then get two doses of vaccine: on the day of the bite and 3 days later. In those who have not received the pre-exposure vaccination, the patient receives four doses of rabies vaccine, on days 0, 3, 7, and 14 (US Advisory Committee on Immunization Practices schedule), or five doses of rabies vaccine on days 0, 3, 7, 14, and 30 (World Health Organization [WHO] schedule); a single dose of rabies immunoglobulin is also required, but this may not be readily accessible in low-income nations. There are currently no recommendations for routine boosters, unless the patient has frequent contact with animals, such as working as or with a veterinarian.

Yellow Fever

Yellow fever is an acute flavivirus infection, transmitted by infected *Aedes aegypti* mosquito bites. The International Health Regulations were amended in 2014 based on recommendations from the Strategic Advisory Group of Experts to WHO that a single dose of yellow fever vaccine would be sufficient to confer long-term protection. This change comes into effect in July 2016. For long-term expatriates moving to countries with yellow fever transmission, yellow fever vaccine should be recommended because of potential travel in-country during the extended period of their assignment.

On the Horizon

Several vaccines are in development for endemic populations but are not currently available commercially. Travel medicine practitioners should keep watch for these vaccines in late development:

- Inactivated yellow fever
- Dengue
- Malaria
- Hepatitis E

OTHER HEALTH PROBLEMS: INFECTIOUS

Nonvaccine-preventable illnesses, as applicable, should be discussed with individual travelers.

Malaria

Expatriates moving to malaria-endemic regions to work or live for extended periods are at risk for this protozoal infection transmitted by infected *Anopheles* mosquitoes. The risk of acquiring malaria depends on the country, rural versus urban location, duration of stay, seasonal transmission rates, practice of personal protective measures, and compliance with malaria prophylaxis. The risk of severe complications or death from malaria depends on patient and destination factors; children under 5 years, pregnant women, and asplenic patients are at higher risk. Access to medical care, antimalarial medications, and blood supply safety are other considerations. Glucose 6-phosphate dehydrogenase (G6PD) deficiency may also make the use of primaquine more difficult if infected with *Plasmodium vivax* or *Plasmodium ovale*.

Expatriates may opt not to take chemoprophylaxis because they perceive that malaria risk is low or because of concerns about side effects when taken for months or years or by very young children or women who may wish to conceive.

When prescribing chemoprophylaxis for long-term expatriates, the following factors should be considered: tolerability of side effects, frequency of dosing that affects compliance, interaction with concomitant medications, and comorbidities. Expatriates who wish to minimize their risk in malaria-endemic regions, who have limited access to care, or who are at risk of severe disease should be offered continuous prophylaxis. If the expatriate has access to good medical care and is in an area with seasonal risk of malaria, it may be possible to take prophylaxis only during seasons with highest transmission risk. However, it would be prudent to prescribe prophylaxis for the first several months until the traveler can establish a good local healthcare provider and learn about malaria transmission locally. Malaria medications should be supplied from home because of problems with counterfeit antimalarials in some developing countries. Chloroquine resistance is widespread, so in areas with resistance, options for prophylaxis include mefloquine, doxycycline, and atovaquone-proguanil. Primaquine is used by some clinicians for prophylaxis in areas where *P. vivax* is predominant, but G6PD levels should be checked before prescribing it.

Dengue

Dengue is an acute viral infection transmitted by infected *Aedes aegypti* mosquitoes. Expatriates relocating to dengue-endemic regions should be counseled about personal protective measures. Severe dengue infection is rare (<5% of all cases), but access to excellent supportive care is essential for such cases. There are four serotypes of dengue virus. Infection with confer serotype-specific protective immunity; more severe disease may occur if the traveler acquires an infection with another serotype.

Gastrointestinal (GI) Infections

GI infections are common among long-term expatriates, although some studies indicate that actual incidence may be lower compared with short-term travelers. Strict food and water precautions are difficult to maintain over a long period. Missionaries, Peace Corp volunteers, and humanitarian workers may be exposed to more risks. GI infections transmitted via food and water include cryptosporidiosis, giardiasis, amebiasis, liver flukes, tapeworms, salmonellosis, brucellosis, listeriosis, norovirus, and hepatitis E.

Safe water supplies can be ensured by bringing water to a rolling boil for 1-3 minutes, disinfecting with chlorine drops, or using water filtration systems (e.g., a 1-micron filter). Chlorination while killing bacteria and viruses has low to moderate efficacy in killing *Giardia* and *Cryptosporidium*; filtration does not remove viruses. Home-cooked food with attention to good sanitation and hygiene is generally safer. Household help should be instructed how to prepare, cook, and store food safely. Travelers should avoid undercooked meat and poultry and unpasteurized dairy products.

Sexually Transmitted Infections

Sexually transmitted infections include short incubation diseases, such as syphilis, gonorrhea, and chlamydia, or chronic infections such as HIV, hepatitis C, or HPV infection. Advice about abstinence, condom use, or pre-exposure prophylaxis may need to be addressed based on traveler risk factors.

Tuberculosis (TB)

TB is an airborne mycobacterial infection. Multidrug-resistant TB has increased in a number of developing countries. Expatriates going to countries with high TB prevalence should be tested for TB infection using a Mantoux test or IGRA pre-travel, on exposure to active TB, and after return. If the test is positive, perform a chest radiograph to exclude active disease. Isoniazid prophylaxis should be offered to travelers with latent TB infection. Household employees from countries with high TB incidence should be evaluated for active TB, especially if symptomatic.

Viral Hemorrhagic Fevers

In 2014, there was an unprecedented Ebola outbreak in West Africa, mainly in Guinea, Liberia, and Sierra Leone, with more than 28,000 cases and more than 11,000 deaths as of March 2016. This outbreak had a devastating impact on the economy and health services of the Ebola-affected countries. Long-term expatriates, especially healthcare workers, to countries at risk for Ebola and viral hemorrhagic fevers (such as Lassa and Marburg) need to be counseled about transmission risks and protective measures.

OTHER HEALTH PROBLEMS: NON-INFECTIOUS

Safety and Security

Personal safety from violent crime may be an issue depending on destination. Humanitarian workers in conflict areas may need more detailed evacuation and emergency plans. All doors and windows should have functioning locks. After arrival, expatriates should register with their respective embassies for travel warnings and security advisories. Missionaries need to be increasingly aware of religious conflict or ransom demands.

Traffic and Trauma

Road traffic accidents pose a serious health risk in many developing countries. Seat belts should be used at all times. Young children should travel in car seats where possible and not in the front passenger seat. If riding a motorcycle or bicycle, helmets should be worn. Expatriates should keep their windows up and doors locked when driving in higher risk neighborhoods.

Mental and Emotional Health

Psychiatric issues may be exacerbated or develop as a result of stresses related to living abroad, requiring repatriation home. Posttraumatic stress disorders may occur in volunteers in conflict areas and disaster zones. Competent psychiatric evaluation and medication access may be limited in certain settings. See Chapter 17.

Dental Problems

Dental-care needs for expatriates can range from emergency root canals to routine dental cleaning or orthodontics for accompanying children; high-quality dental care and disinfection for instruments may not be readily accessible at some destinations.

Cardiovascular

Cardiovascular events may occur in long-term expatriates. Individuals with risk factors such as diabetes, smoking, hypertension, or a strong family history should be advised regarding risk mitigation and should establish care with a competent healthcare provider at their destination.

MEDICAL CARE ABROAD

The most commonly reported problems that lead expatriates to seek medical care abroad include GI disorders, respiratory infections, and febrile illness with short incubation periods, such as influenza, dengue, or malaria. Acute injuries, including animal bites, road traffic accidents, and criminal violence, may require urgent medical attention.

In many developing countries, healthcare resources may be substandard. Seeking care may require navigating language and cultural barriers. Medication quality and blood transfusion safety may be considerations when deciding if one should seek medical care abroad. The adequacy of vaccine cold chains is a concern in developing countries where power outages occur frequently.

Medical evacuation home or to a regional center with advanced medical capabilities may become necessary in certain situations, depending on urgency, severity, and complexity. Expatriate volunteers should purchase insurance that provides access to a medical assistance company that can locate and coordinate quality healthcare and arrange for an evacuation if appropriate medical care is unavailable for life-threatening situations.

If expatriates die abroad, help from their embassy will be needed to address repatriation or burial abroad, notification of family, or care of accompanying children.

POST-TRAVEL CARE

When expatriates return home, they should receive a comprehensive history, exam and laboratory testing on their post-travel visit. History of exposure, destinations, and illnesses abroad will help guide further testing (**Table 18.1**). Screen for travel-related infections that

TABLE 18.1   Risk Exposures for Consideration at Post-Travel Visit

Risk Exposure	Diseases Possible	Screening and/or Treatment after Exposure
Food and water	Typhoid	Stool and blood culture
Unpasteurized dairy	Brucellosis	Brucella serology, blood culture
Respiratory	Influenza	Influenza PCR/DFA
Contact with ill persons, healthcare workers, or incarceration	Tuberculosis	Screening: IGRA, PPD Treatment: isoniazid for latent TB infection
Mosquito bites (endemic)	Malaria	Blood film for malaria
	Filariasis	Blood film for filaria, filarial serology
Fresh water contact	Schistosomiasis	Stool microscopy, *Schistosoma* serology
Walking barefoot	Hookworm	Stool microscopy
	Strongyloidiasis	Stool microscopy, *Strongyloides* serology
Animal bites	Rabies	Treatment: rabies post-exposure prophylaxis

Continued

TABLE 18.1   Risk Exposures for Consideration at Post-Travel Visit—cont'd

Risk Exposure	Diseases Possible	Screening and/or Treatment after Exposure
New sexual partners, contaminated needles, or blood transfusions	Hepatitis B	HBsAg, HBcAb, HBsAb
	Hepatitis C	HCV serology
	HIV	HIV serology
New sexual partners	Syphilis	RPR, TPHA, Syphilis IgG
	Gonorrhea	Urine or urethral swab for gonorrhea PCR
	Chlamydia	Urine or urethral swab for chlamydia PCR

DFA, Direct fluorescent-antibody; *HCV*, hepatitis C virus; *HIV*, human immunodeficiency virus; *IgG*, immunoglobulin G; *IGRA*, interferon gamma release assay; *PCR*, polymerase chain reaction; *PPD*, purified protein derivative; *RPR*, rapid plasma reagin; *TPHA*, *T. pallidum* hemagglutination.

may be asymptomatic or have long-term sequelae (TB, schistosomiasis, filariasis), address routine medical problems that have been diagnosed during their time abroad (e.g., diabetes, hypertension), update vaccinations, and reassess risk and preventive strategies for malaria and other issues if further travel is planned. A CBC should be performed for all returning travelers. Anemia may require evaluation for malaria, and stool microscopy may be required for hookworm and other GI parasites. Eosinophilia should prompt investigations for schistosomiasis, strongyloidiasis, and other causes. Eosinophilia may not be present in all cases, so all travelers who have had fresh water contact in endemic regions should be evaluated for schistosomiasis with stool microscopy and serology. More details about testing and treatment are available in other chapters.

FURTHER READING

Almuzaini, T., Choonara, I., Sammon, H., 2013. Substandard and counterfeit medicines: a systematic review of the literature. BMJ Open 3 (8), e002923. doi:10.1136/bmjopen-2013-002923.
Prevalence of counterfeit or substandard medications is 28.5%, highlighting a safety issue for long-term expatriates abroad.

Chen, L.H., Wilson, M.E., Davis, X., et al., GeoSentinel Surveillance Network, 2009. Illness in long-term travelers visiting GeoSentinel clinics. Emerg. Infect. Dis. 15 (11), 1773–1782.
Analysis of illness spectrum among returning travelers who spent 6 months or longer abroad.

Chen, L.H., Wilson, M.E., Schlagenhauf, P., 2006. Prevention of malaria in long-term travelers. JAMA 296 (18), 2234–2244.
Classic paper summarizing considerations for long-term malaria chemoprophylaxis.

Cunningham, J., Horsley, J., Patel, D., et al., 2014. Compliance with long-term malaria prophylaxis in British expatriates. Travel Med. Infect. Dis. 12 (4), 341–348.
This survey indicates that even well-informed employees self-reported poor adherence to malaria prophylaxis beyond the first 3 months.

Dahlgren, A.L., Deroo, L., Avril, J., et al., 2009. Health risks and risk-taking behaviours among International Committee of the Red Cross (ICRC) expatriates returning from humanitarian missions. J. Travel Med. 16 (6), 382–390.
Survey of Red Cross volunteers showing exposure to work stress, violence, and unprotected sexual contact.

Guse, C.E., Cortes, L.M., Hargarten, S.W., et al., 2007. Fatal injuries of US citizens abroad. J. Travel Med. 14 (5), 279–287.
Cross-sectional report of deaths in US citizens abroad with a higher proportion of fatalities from injuries, including motor-vehicle accidents and drowning.

Hoge, C.W., Shlim, D.R., Echeverria, P., et al., 1996. Epidemiology of diarrhea among expatriate residents living in a highly endemic environment. JAMA 275, 533–538.

Holtz, T.Z., Salama, P., Lopes Cardozo, B., et al., 2002. Mental health status of human rights workers, Kosovo, June 2000. J. Trauma. Stress 15 (5), 389–395.
Survey of emotional impact of hostility and violence on expatriate humanitarian relief workers.

Lim, P.L., Han, P., Chen, L.H., et al., for the GeoSentinel Surveillance Network, 2012. Expatriates ill after travel: results from the GeoSentinel Surveillance Network. BMC Infect. Dis. 12, 386.
Findings on post-travel illness for 2883 expatriates compared with 11,990 non-expatriate travelers presenting at GeoSentinel sites, showing exposure differences by destinations and type of expatriate traveler.

Pierre, C.M., Lim, P.L., Hamer, D.H., 2013, Expatriates: special considerations in pre-travel preparation. Curr. Infect. Dis. Rep. 15 (4), 299–306.
Review of literature on pre-travel preparations for expatriate travelers.

Shepherd, S.M., Shoff, W.H., 2014, Vaccination for the expatriate and long-term traveler. Expert Rev Vaccines. 13 (6), 775–800.
Review article on travel patterns and data on exposures to guide vaccinations for long-term expatriates.

Teichman, P.G., Donchin, Y., Kot, R.J., 2007. International aeromedical evacuation. N. Engl. J. Med. 356 (3), 262–270.
Review of medical evacuations.

Toovey, S., Moerman, F., van Gompel, A., 2007. Special infectious disease risks of expatriates and long-term travelers in tropical countries. Part I: malaria. J. Travel Med. 14, 42–49.
An excellent review of the challenges of malaria prophylaxis in the long-term expatriate.

Vaid, N., Langan, K.M., Maude, R.J., 2013. Post-exposure prophylaxis in resource-poor settings: review and recommendations for pre-departure risk assessment and planning for expatriate healthcare workers. Trop. Med. Int. Health 18 (5), 588–595.
Review of occupational exposures to blood-borne pathogens and recommendations for pre-departure planning of post-exposure prophylaxis.

Visser, J.T., Edwards, C.A., 2013. Dengue fever, tuberculosis, HIV, and hepatitis C virus conversion in a group of long-term development aid workers. J. Travel Med. 20 (6), 361–367. doi:10.1111/jtm.12072; Epub 2013 Oct 9.

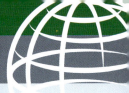

CHAPTER 19

Health Screening in Immigrants, Refugees, and International Adoptees

Douglas W. MacPherson and Brian D. Gushulak

It is much more important to know which sort of a patient has a disease than to know what sort of disease a patient has.
   William Osler

In an increasingly globalized world, migration and population mobility are important factors in the demographic makeup of national populations. In the United States, for example, recent estimates indicate that the foreign-born cohort comprises some 40 million people, or 13% of the total population. Many foreign-born individuals arrive as immigrants, refugees, or children adopted abroad. As such, and depending on their status, health screening may be a required or recommended component of their migratory process.

Migration-associated health screening is undertaken for two major purposes. First, screening may help identify medical conditions that have implications in terms of personal and community health. Second, foreign nationals seeking residence through organized immigration and refugee programs undergo screening due to legislative, regulatory, or administrative directives and mandates.

Similar epidemiologic principles govern the science and application of both screening processes. However, the rationale underlying these two screening approaches differs in terms of historical basis, operational characteristics, and ultimate goals.

- Screening for medical conditions of personal health significance is intended to improve health parameters or outcomes for the migrant and may not be legally required or mandated.
- Mandatory medical screening for immigration purposes is undertaken for regulatory reasons, such as the determination of admissibility on medical grounds under immigration legislation.

Reflecting the duality of screening related to migrants, this chapter on screening is presented in two parts.

MANDATORY IMMIGRATION SCREENING IN THE UNITED STATES: MEDICAL COMPONENT

The routine examination of travelers and migrants is one of the oldest recorded activities directed at civic administration and protecting the health of the public. The development of European quarantine practices in the mid-14th century was associated with the routine inspection of new arrivals, commercial goods, and conveyances in an attempt to prevent the introduction of epidemic infectious diseases. Those deemed to be at risk following inspection were contained, excluded, or expelled. These early public health activities accompanied the European settlement of the Americas.

Shortly after achieving nationhood, early legislative tools were introduced creating the US Public Health Service, whose initial role was to provide medical care to seafarers and to control the importation of serious diseases epidemic at the time, such as cholera and plague. A linkage to immigration later followed, with the screening of immigrants to exclude those with unwanted medical conditions such as certain loathsome diseases, individuals of suspected low moral behavior, and people with mental deficiencies who were likely to become wards of the state. In the United States, this process began in the late 1800s when the control of immigration was legally recognized as a congressional responsibility. Subsequently, the US Immigration Act of 1882 made specific reference to controlling the admission of immigrants on medical grounds. The routine medical inspection of immigrants was legislatively mandated in the United States in 1891.

Public health programs and policies designed to manage the major medical challenges of the day became linked to the routine medical inspection of immigrants on arrival. By the 1920s, the immigration medical inspection was extended to the European points of origin for the majority of migrants, creating a system of pre-departure immigration medical screening that continues to this day.

The legal basis governing inadmissibility to the United States because of health-related conditions and authorization to undertake medical examination to determine that admissibility is found in the Immigration and Nationality Act (INA) (Title 8 US Code). Under these provisions foreign aliens residing outside of the United States can be denied visas and rendered ineligible to enter the country. These provisions also extend to foreigners already residing in the United States who apply to become permanent residents.

The immigration medical examination provides the opportunity to determine whether the foreign national (known as an "alien" in the legislation) is ineligible for permission to enter the United States (known as Class A conditions) or has an illness or disorder that may interfere with independent self-care, education, or employment or may require future extensive medical treatment or institutional support (known as Class B conditions).

Health-related reasons that exclude admission (Class A conditions) to the United States include:

1. A communicable disease of public health significance
2. A physical or mental disorder or behavior posing a threat to property, safety, or welfare (either currently present or likely to recur)
3. Drug abuse or addiction
4. Failure to present documentation demonstrating having received recommended vaccinations.

The Department of Health and Human Services provides specific regulations (Medical Examination of Aliens 42 CFR, Part 34) to define and implement the health aspects of the INA. These regulations identify those who require medical examination, outline the process, define where and by whom the examinations are performed, and list the specific conditions associated with inadmissibility. The regulations also define conditions or disorders that, while not serious enough for exclusion, are significant enough (Class B conditions) that they must be brought to the attention of consular authorities. The Division of Global Migration and Quarantine at the Centers for Disease Control and Prevention (CDC) administers the regulations.

Currently, the regulations list the following as communicable diseases of public health significance:

- Active tuberculosis
- Infectious syphilis
- Gonorrhea
- Infectious leprosy
- Chancroid
- Lymphogranuloma venereum
- Granuloma inguinale
- Human immunodeficiency virus (HIV) infection

- Quarantinable diseases designated by any Presidential Executive Order
  - Current diseases include cholera, diphtheria, infectious tuberculosis, plague, smallpox, yellow fever, viral hemorrhagic fevers, severe acute respiratory syndrome, and influenza caused by novel or re-emergent influenza (pandemic flu)
- Any communicable disease that is a public health emergency of international concern reported to the World Health Organization (WHO) (under revised International Health Regulations of 2005)
  - For example, smallpox, poliomyelitis due to wild-type poliovirus, cholera, or viral hemorrhagic fevers (including Ebola)

Currently a medical examination is required for all refugees entering the United States and all those applying for an immigrant visa from outside the United States. Foreign residents in the United States applying to become permanent residents also require mandated medical examinations. Panel physicians, designated by consular officers of the US Department of State, perform medical examinations abroad, and civil surgeons, designated by the US Citizenship and Immigration Services, perform medical examinations for aliens who are already present in the United States. Both groups of physicians receive technical instruction and guidance from the CDC's Division of Global Migration and Quarantine.

Detailed medical history and physical examination are required for all individuals (see summary in **Table 19.1**). In addition, applicants who are ≥15 years undergo routine chest radiography and serologic testing for HIV and syphilis.

Those between 2 and 14 years of age who reside in a country where tuberculosis incidence rates (based on WHO data) are ≥20 per 100,000 have either a tuberculin skin test (TST) or an interferon gamma release assay (IGRA). If either the TST or IGRA are positive, the individual undergoes chest radiography. Depending on the clinical history, TST, IGRA, and radiological findings, supplementary screening requirements for tuberculosis include smears of respiratory secretions for acid-fast bacilli and cultures for tuberculosis. Any positive cultures undergo drug susceptibility testing.

Those rated Class A for tuberculosis (smear-positive infectious) generally must be treated until their sputum smears are negative before they are allowed to transit for immigration. Those rated Class B for tuberculosis are cleared for travel within certain time limits. Failure to journey to the United States within those time limits will require the individual to undergo rescreening.

Since 1996, individuals applying for immigrant visas to entry into the United States have had to demonstrate proof of vaccination for several vaccine-preventable diseases. Initially, these were general, routine vaccinations as recommended by the Advisory Committee for Immunization Practices (ACIP) for the domestic US population. In 2009, however, specific criteria for those requiring an immigration medical exam were adopted by the CDC.

Those criteria are:

1. The vaccine must be age appropriate (as recommended by the ACIP).

and

2. At least of these two conditions must be met:
   a) The vaccine must offer protection against a disease with the potential to cause an outbreak.
   b) The vaccine must protect against a disease that has been eliminated or is being eliminated in the United States.

At the time of the preparation of this chapter, required vaccines were:

- Diphtheria
- Tetanus
- Pertussis
- Polio
- Measles
- Mumps
- Rubella
- Rotavirus

TABLE 19.1 Mandatory Immigration Screening: Medical Component

Criteria	Conditions	Screening Tool	Exceptions
Communicable diseases of public health significance	TB Locations with TB incidence <20/100,000	Chest radiograph; ≥15 years of age	
	TB Locations with TB incidence ≥20/100,000	TST or IGRA; ≥2–14 years of age	Applicants who are asymptomatic, contacts of documented infected applicants
	Leprosy, chancroid, gonorrhea, granuloma inguinale, and lymphogranuloma venereum	History and physical examination; laboratory testing only if clinically indicated	
	Infectious syphilis	Serological tests; ≥15 years of age	Applicants who are contacts of documented infected applicants (e.g., children, spouse)
	Other communicable diseases of public health significance	Determined by HHS/CDC on a risk-based, case-by-case basis, depending on the situation	
Vaccinations	Diphtheria, tetanus, pertussis, polio, measles, mumps, rubella, rotavirus, *Haemophilus influenzae* type b, hepatitis A, hepatitis B, meningococcal, varicella, pneumococcal, influenza	Review of vaccination records	
Physical or mental disorder with harmful behavior	History of ever having caused serious injury to others or major property damage; or trouble with the law because of a medical condition, mental condition, or influence of alcohol or drugs; or having ever attempted suicide	History and physical examination; review of records	
Presence of drug abuse or drug addiction	Drug use: amphetamines, cannabis, cocaine, hallucinogenics, inhalants, opioids, phencyclidines, sedative-hypnotics, or anxiolytics		
	Other substance-related disorders, including alcohol addiction and at use, associated with other harmful behaviors such as driving under the influence of alcohol, domestic violence, or other alcohol-related criminal behavior		

CDC, Centers for Disease Control and Prevention; *HHS,* Department of Health and Human Services; *IGRA,* interferon gamma release assay; *TB,* tuberculosis; *TST,* tuberculin skin test.

- *Haemophilus influenzae* type b
- Hepatitis A
- Hepatitis B
- Meningococcal
- Varicella
- Pneumococcal
- Influenza

Immunizations recommended and required for US immigration purposes are summarized in the CDC's "Technical Instructions for Panel Physicians for Vaccinations," available at http://www.cdc.gov/immigrantrefugeehealth/exams/ti/panel/vaccination-panel-technical-instructions.html#status.

Pre-admission vaccination requirements do not apply for refugees or non-immigrant visa applicants. However, those individuals are required to meet the vaccination standards when they adjust their status in the United States after admission. As a procedural consequence, the immunization status of refugees is recorded during immigration process.

In the case of children adopted abroad, the vaccination requirements do not apply to those 10 years of age or younger. However, the adoptive parents must sign documentation stating that they are aware of US vaccination requirements and will ensure that all required vaccinations will be received within 30 days of the child's arrival in the United States.

The importance and cost-effectiveness of preventative medical interventions in the overseas environment, before transit to the United States, is receiving greater attention as a potential part of the immigration medical process. Currently, some refugee populations being resettled in the United States who are determined to be at increased risk for specific infections receive population-based treatment for malaria and intestinal parasites in addition to the routine immigration medical screening. Additionally, outbreaks of communicable diseases in refugee camps or transit facilities can trigger additional interventions or treatment prior to arrival.

In terms of harmful behavior, immigration medical screening is intended to identify those with neurologic or behavioral conditions associated with the risk of "ever causing serious injury to others, major property damage or having trouble with the law because of a medical condition, mental condition, or influence of alcohol or drugs" or "ever taken actions to end your [the applicant's] life." High-risk conditions in this group may be determined to be Class A (inadmissible) or Class B (admissible) conditions by panel physicians, depending on clinical findings, history, and situation.

Drug abuse or addiction (dependence) presents a Class A (inadmissible) situation. Those barred from admission are those who:
- Use a controlled substance (defined by the Controlled Substances Act)

and
- Meet the Diagnostic and Statistical Manual of Mental Disorders criteria for a mild, moderate, or severe substance use disorder.

It is sometimes possible for those individuals subject to medical examination who are determined to have a communicable disease of public health significance to still enter the United States. The legislation provides for a waiver process by which those determined to be inadmissible may request entry subject to conditions.

Documents providing further operational descriptions on the immigration medical screening process for both applicants abroad and those applying within the United States, including details on applicants seeking a change in immigration status, the use of Panel Physicians and Civil Surgeons, and reporting requirements, are available at http://www.cdc.gov/immigrantrefugeehealth/.

Summary

Mandatory medical screening to determine medical inadmissibility for immigration purposes is an important administrative process for applicants for permanent residency in the United States and may also be applied to certain temporary resident applicants.

Although the immigration medical examination does screen for some important medical conditions, it has clinical limitations. It is not designed to be a tool for identifying personal health risks, and it is procedurally limited to specific disorders and conditions of regulated public health concern. As a consequence, pre-existing medical conditions that do not fall under the immigration medical screening profile and other medical conditions of personal health significance may not be detected or reported during mandatory immigration screening. Those conditions, while not relevant for immigration purposes, can be significant for new arrivals, and their identification and clinical management in the United States is important in some migrant populations.

MEDICAL SCREENING OF NEW ARRIVALS IN THE UNITED STATES

In addition to an absolute increase in immigration, there has been a shift in source countries, with immigrants from Latin American nations other than Mexico, as well as Africa, Asia, and Oceania, increasingly contributing to the immigrant pool. The growing number and increasing diversity of foreign-born residents of the United States is important in numerous areas of clinical practice. Local health environments at their place of origin and relative disparity in health and disease indicators mean that some migrants may have disease exposure and acquisition patterns different from those at their new home.

In some communities, migrants represent rapidly increasing components of the population, and their specific health concerns may be different from those of the receiving community. International adoptions, for example, are now a major component of the adoption process in the United States. Of the approximately 1.5 million adopted children less than 18 years of age in the United States, 13% were foreign born, representing more than 200,000 individuals. Appropriately targeted and applied screening can assist in meeting the differential health challenges of these diverse foreign-born populations.

Increasing cultural and linguistic diversity can pose challenges to health systems and for physician and institutional healthcare service delivery. Health screening of immigrants and refugees can be done as part of primary care assessment in which routine immunizations should be documented and brought up-to-date if necessary; maternal-child health issues can be addressed; and specific health assessments for other defined populations (e.g., children, adolescents, women, and the elderly) can be performed.

In addition to language, some migrant groups experience difficulty accessing and utilizing healthcare services for other reasons. Cultural issues, including fear of interacting with official bureaucracies and concerns about affordability, may limit migrants' use of health prevention and promotional services. Services designed for the general populations often include health counseling and screening programs that may be unfamiliar to or underused by migrant populations.

Medical and health conditions of importance in new arrivals in the United States fall into two groups: those conditions for which existing screening programs are available for the local population that also occur in migrants, and those conditions not common or endemic in the United States affecting particular populations of migrants for which no routine screening programs exist in the United States.

Migrants may need special attention in terms of screening for:
- Risk behaviors, such as smoking, alcohol, and other substance abuse
- Health implications of diet and exercise
- Risks of sexual health practices
- Early recognition of mental and psychosocial health
- Impact of environmental risks presented by toxic substances, including lead in drinking vessels or paint
- Occupational exposures related to safe labor practices.

In addition, there are many targeted health promotion activities for specific groups, such as maternal-child care, which may not have been commonly available for many migrants in their home countries. Programs such as prenatal blood pressure monitoring, screening for gestational diabetes, and thyroid function may be unfamiliar to many migrants. Antenatal screening for infections such as rubella, syphilis, hepatitis B, and HIV can be important in migrant populations who originate from regions of the world where these diseases are more prevalent than they are in the United States and where screening practices are not uniformly available or are unfamiliar to women.

There are other important targeted screening programs of relevance to migrants. They may not have had access to genetic screening for inborn errors of metabolism or physical conditions such as congenital hip dysplasia and cataracts. Additionally, there are several diseases that may be more prevalent at the migrants' place of origin, such as malaria, thalassemia, and micronutrient deficiencies, for which screening may be indicated.

Finally, it is important to note that many migrants may be unfamiliar with the basis and rationale underlying health-screening programs. Common examples include screening programs for malignant disease such as uterine cervical dysplasia (Pap smear) and skin, bowel, breast, and prostate examinations. Depending on their location and status, many other migrants may have never been screened for common illnesses such as diabetes and hypertension. This is particularly true for vulnerable and disadvantaged migrant groups, such as refugees, asylum seekers, and migrants displaced by conflict.

Healthcare disparities affecting access due to language and culture can occur, but also in some health jurisdictions in the United States there are legislative initiatives that may create barriers to available healthcare services on "right of access" based on citizenship or "willingness to pay" (self-pay or Medicare entitlement). Migrants' use of unregulated medical service providers may be an important component in the subsequent health assessment of this population. Migrant populations may also be using traditional, herbal, alternative, or complementary medicines, some of which will be imported from abroad. Unregulated therapies and agents that do not meet standards of pharmacologic care in United States may not be revealed to attending healthcare professionals unless diligently sought. These alternate therapies may have the potential to complicate clinical presentations and in some cases may themselves be a source of illness.

Many migrants from diverse backgrounds also have significant disparities in health determinants (e.g., socioeconomics, behavior, genetics and biology, environment) directly related to the migration process. The pre-departure component of health determination is carried through the migration process and is affected by the transit conditions, particularly for irregular arrivals, the post-arrival period, and any return travel undertaken by migrants or their offspring.

For the healthcare professional providing services to migrants, this requires an in-depth knowledge of the geographic components of health determination and disease expression that will be carried over to low prevalence or non-endemic countries, such as the United States. The historical focus of immigration and international public health has tended to be on contagious diseases of epidemic potential such as trachoma, syphilis, tuberculosis, and, recently, HIV/acquired immune deficiency syndrome (AIDS). However, there has been a recent shift in attention to the personal health risks associated with immigration and other infectious and non-infectious diseases.

Summary

Table 19.2 presents some of the clinical screening issues for healthcare providers working with defined migrant populations. With globalization of economies and trade, rapidity of interregional transportation, and increasing international population mobility for temporary and permanent relocation, healthcare professionals will increasingly need both to recognize imported clinical syndromes and to be sensitive to quiescent conditions of both personal and public health significance when dealing with migrants.

Screening can be targeted at asymptomatic individuals or can be mass community screening of previously defined at-risk populations; both of these are based on demographic and biometric profiles representing disparity in frequency or severity of outcome. Increasingly in high-health service regions with low prevalence of any poor health indicators and excellent local public health programs, migrants and other mobile populations are becoming the

TABLE 19.2 Examples of Medical Screening of Migrants by Region, Population, Condition, and Intervention

Region	Population	Infectious Disease Conditions	Noninfectious Conditions	Intervention
Latin America	Migrant workers, agricultural	STD, TB, intestinal parasites, *Trypanosoma cruzi*	Substance use/abuse: alcohol, tobacco, others	Assessment and counseling, safer sex practices, HBV serology (HBsAg) and immunization of at-risk individuals; TST for children.
	Migrant workers, domestic	TB, intestinal tapeworm (*Taenia solium* and other parasites) Hansen disease, *T. cruzi*	Diet: caloric balance, micronutrient deficiencies; occupational risks: physical violence, psychological abuse, toxins, or dangerous environmental exposures	Immunization: routine, hepatitis B; perinatal care and screening for maternal-child health (all at-risk populations); preventative Rx for existing conditions (e.g., syphilis, HIV, hypothyroidism, diabetes, hypertension)
	Children of migrant laborers	TB	Physical and mental developmental milestones; educational participation and attainment	
Europe	Women smuggled or trafficked, particularly from Eastern Europe (also Asia and Africa)	Acquired risk environments and behaviors for STDs	Occupational risks: forced labor and commercial sex workers, physical and psychological abuse, violence, substance abuse	Assessment and referral to justice and immigration protection services
	The elderly	TB, tertiary syphilis, *Strongyloides* (southern Europe)	Common diseases of advancing age: renal failure, malignancies, diabetes, hypertension	Local standards of clinical practice need to be observed with a heightened suspicion of imported disease conditions that are of low or zero prevalence in the USA or Europe.
	Other workers		Previous occupational exposures: asbestos, radiation, trauma	
Asia	Migrants from rural environments	Intestinal parasites, including *Strongyloides*; tuberculosis, Hansen disease, chronic HBV carriage (most populations of Asia, sub-Saharan Africa, parts of Oceania)	Dietary deficiencies, acculturation effects on mental status	Stools for parasites; serology for *Strongyloides*; HBV (HBsAg) and immunization of at-risk individuals. TST (children)
			Occupational and environmental health risks	Clinical assessment for cultural norms: body mass, hematological and biochemical parameters
		Note: Pulmonary paragonimiasis can mimic TB. Liver flukes can lead to chronic hepatic scarring.		

Continued

TABLE 19.2 Examples of Medical Screening of Migrants by Region, Population, Condition, and Intervention—cont'd

Region	Population	Infectious Disease Conditions	Noninfectious Conditions	Intervention
Africa	Refugees	*Note:* Immigration medical waivers may have been given for screened Class A conditions (e.g., tuberculosis)	Victims of forced relocation, torture, rape, physical and psychological trauma, Posttraumatic stress disorders Nutritional deficiencies, particularly in children and women of childbearing potential Negative effects of acculturation	Intestinal, blood, and tissue parasites including *Strongyloides* (serology), schistosomiasis (urine), malaria TST (children) Iron status HBV serology (HBsAg) and immunization of at-risk individuals
Oceania	Immigrants	Hepatitis B, tuberculosis, Hansen disease		Serological screening: HBV (HBsAg) and immunization of at-risk individuals Skin examination. Heightened clinical suspicion
North America	Long-term expatriates (humanitarian/relief workers, business travelers, "overlanders" or backpackers) Sex tourists VFR: migrant return travel, with or without local-born children or next-generation travel	Communicable diseases endemic in the population and area of work or travel Consider exposures in those VFR; immune status, local access and use of healthcare services	Culture shock and other psychological adaptation disorders; acquired behavioral risks Cultural components of foreign exposures; VFR: female circumcision, scarification, tattooing, or piercing	Clinical assessment and management of post-exposure risks based on geographic environment and activities: tuberculosis, intestinal parasites, serology for *Strongyloides.* TST for long-term exposure in high-prevalence countries *Note:* eosinophilia correlates poorly to the presence or absence of invasive helminthic infections

HBV, Hepatitis B virus; *HIV,* human immunodeficiency virus; *Rx,* prescription; *STD,* sexually transmitted disease; *TB,* tuberculosis; *TST,* tuberculin skin test; *VFR,* visiting friends and/or relatives.

"at risk" populations. Many of the factors impacting on adverse health outcomes in migrants are amenable to screening, and there are effective interventions for health promotion or disease prevention.

High-risk populations of migrants, including refugees, workers, adopted children, victims of torture, and trafficked individuals, may require specialized medical care as well as specifically designed screening based on medical and sociological assessment of their needs. Professional healthcare providers, health educational, training, and professional societies, and governments and nongovernmental agencies will be challenged to develop policies and programs to respond to this emerging and dynamic challenge to address the health needs of internationally mobile populations.

FURTHER READING AND SALIENT REFERENCES

Advisory Committee on Immunization Practices. Available at: <http://www.cdc.gov/vaccines/schedules/hcp/index.html> (accessed March 23, 2015).
Reference on recommended immunizations.

Ampofo, K., 2013. Infectious disease issues in adoption of young children. Curr. Opin. Pediatr. 25, 78–87.
Review of communicable diseases that may be encountered in foreign adoptions.

Centers for Disease Control and Prevention. Technical Instructions for Panel Physicians and Civil Surgeons. Available at: <http://www.cdc.gov/immigrantrefugeehealth/exams/ti/index.html> (accessed April 2, 2015).
Detailed background and instructions related to US immigration medical screening practices.

Dallo, F.J., Kindratt T.B., 2015. Disparities in preventive health behaviors among non-Hispanic white men: heterogeneity among foreign-born Arab and European Americans. Am. J. Mens Health. 9, 124–131 [Epub April 29, 2014].
Article describing the differential knowledge and practice of preventive health measures by foreign-born and native-born populations.

Dang, K., Tribble, A.C., 2014. Strategies in infectious disease prevention and management among US-bound refugee children. Curr. Probl. Pediatr. Adolesc. Health Care 44, 196–207 [Epub 2014 Jun 25].
Recent overview of infectious disease challenges in pediatric refugee populations destined to the United States.

Grieco, E.M., Acosta, Y.D., de la Cruz, G.P., et al., 2012. The Foreign-Born Population in the United States: 2010. American Community Survey Reports, Number ACS 19. Available at: <http://www.census.gov/content/dam/Census/library/publications/2012/acs/acs-19.pdf> (accessed February 2, 2015).
Data on the demography of the scope and diversity of the US foreign-born cohort.

Gushulak, B.D., MacPherson, D.W., 2000. Population mobility and infectious diseases: the diminishing impact of classical infectious diseases and new approaches for the 21st century. Clin. Infect. Dis. 31, 776–780.
Review article outlining the importance of communicable diseases in migrant populations that are not usually subject to routine immigration medical screening.

Gushulak, B.D., MacPherson, D.W., 2004. Globalization of infectious diseases: the impact of migration. Clin. Infect. Dis. 38, 1742–1748.
Article describing and outlining the influence of population mobility on global disease epidemiology.

Lee, D., Philen, R., Wang, Z., et al., 2013. Disease surveillance among newly arriving refugees and immigrants—Electronic Disease Notification System, United States, 2009. MMWR Surveill. Summ. 62, 1–20.
Recent review of the scope and status of systems in the United States to identify and notify state health departments of diseases in migrants.

MacPherson, D.W., Gushulak, B.D., 2001. Human mobility and population health. New approaches in a globalizing world. Perspect. Biol. Med. 44, 390–401.
Review article that outlines how modern migration challenges traditional disease-control practices.

Passel, Jeffrey S., D'Vera, Cohn, 2014. Unauthorized Immigrant Totals Rise in 7 States, Fall in 14: Decline in Those from Mexico Fuels Most State Decreases. Pew Research Center's Hispanic Trends Project, Washington, DC. November. Available at: <http://www.pewhispanic.org/files/2014/11/2014-11-18_unauthorized-immigration.pdf> (accessed April 1, 2015).
Statistics and demographic analysis of the unauthorized/irregular foreign-born population in the United States.

Perla, M.E., Rue, T., Cheadle, A., et al., 2014. Population-based comparison of biomarker concentrations for chemicals of concern among Latino-American and non-Hispanic white children. J. Immigr. Minor. Health [Epub ahead of print].
An example of disparities in environmental health risks present in foreign-born populations.

Stauffer, W.M., Kanat, D., Walker, P.R., 2002. Screening of international immigrants, refugees, and adoptees. Prim. Care 29, 879–905.
Review article on recommendations for screening foreign-born migrants after arrival.

Swanson, S.J., Phares, C.R., Mamo, B., et al., 2012. Albendazole therapy and enteric parasites in United States–bound refugees. N. Engl. J. Med. 366, 1498–1507.
Article that describes enhanced pre-departure screening and treatment for high-risk migrant populations in certain circumstances.

US Department of Health and Human Services. Office of Minority Health. Minority Population Profiles. Available at: <http://minorityhealth.hhs.gov/omh/browse.aspx?lvl=2&lvlID=26> (accessed March 29, 2015).
Series of studies exploring diversity in health profiles among populations of differing ethnicity.

Walker, P.F., Barnett, E.D. (Eds.), 2007. Immigrant Medicine. Elsevier, Philadelphia.
Reference text on the health aspects of migration, with a US focus.

CHAPTER 20

Travel-Acquired Illnesses Associated with Fever

Andrea K. Boggild and W. Conrad Liles

 Access evidence synopsis online at ExpertConsult.com.

The evaluation of fever in travelers poses a diagnostic challenge to clinicians for many reasons. First, there are many possible etiologies, some of which are geographically localized and are, thus, unfamiliar (**Table 20.1**). Diagnosis may be delayed owing to lack of familiarity with routes of infection or clinical presentations of these geographically limited illnesses. Fever in travelers may be caused by infections that are potentially fatal if not recognized and treated expediently, the most common of which is malaria (**Table 20.2**). Furthermore, some infectious diseases that cause fever in travelers are highly communicable (**Table 20.3**). These infections represent a considerable public health danger, and some have been associated with fatal nosocomial transmission. However, most febrile illnesses in travelers are self-limited and remain unconfirmed microbiologically, such as viral upper respiratory infections and gastrointestinal infections. Thus the challenge facing the clinician in the evaluation of fever in travelers is the detection of serious treatable or communicable infections while not submitting the majority of travelers with benign, self-limited causes of fever to expensive or invasive diagnostic evaluations. To succeed, the clinician must know as much as possible about the epidemiology, distribution, mode of transmission, and clinical characteristics of the etiologies of fever in travelers.

EPIDEMIOLOGY

Studies of fever in travelers have been impaired by the highly mobile nature of travelers and by the fact that travelers seek help abroad or fail to present to physicians at all. Large, prospective surveillance databases such as the GeoSentinel surveillance network and TropNet provide aggregate multinational data on ill travelers returning from destinations around the globe who present for care at designated "sentinel" clinics. In the GeoSentinel analysis by Wilson et al. (2007), 28% of ill returning travelers reported fever as their chief complaint. A lack of pre-travel counseling was associated with acquisition of a febrile illness abroad, as was visiting friends and/or relatives (VFR) travel. While there was no age bias in fever presentation, male travelers were more likely than female travelers to present with fever.

In retrospective, questionnaire-based studies, the incidence of "high fever over several days" in short-term (<3 weeks) travelers was 1.9%. Of the prolonged fevers reported, 39% occurred only while the traveler was abroad, 37% occurred both abroad and at home, and 24% occurred at home only. Prolonged fever was significantly associated with longer stays (>4 weeks) in the tropics. Among a large cohort of American short-term travelers to the developing world, undifferentiated fever occurred in 3%.

Most causes of febrile illnesses remain undiagnosed in retrospective surveys of travelers. However, in the GeoSentinel analysis by Wilson et al. (2007), malaria was the most common specific cause of fever in ill returned travelers, accounting for 21% of cases, while acute diarrheal disease and respiratory illness accounted for 15% and 14% of cases, respectively. Dengue, while less common, was still an important cause of fever, occurring in 6%

TABLE 20.1 Relative Risk of Travelers Contracting Infectious Diseases in Developing Countries

High Risk	Moderate Risk	Low Risk	Very Low Risk
Escherichia coli enteritis	Cryptosporidiosis	Amebiasis	Anisakiasis
Upper respiratory infection	Cyclosporiasis	Ascariasis	Anthrax
Viral gastroenteritis	Shigellosis	Chancroid	Chagas disease
Campylobacteriosis	Chikungunya	Cholera	
Chlamydia		Enterobiasis	Clonorchiasis
Dengue		Hepatitis B	Crimean-Congo hemorrhagic fever
Epstein-Barr virus		HIV	Diphtheria
Giardiasis		Leptospirosis	Ebola/Marburg hemorrhagic fever
Gonorrhea		Lyme disease	Echinococcosis
Hepatitis A		Malaria (with prophylaxis)	Filariasis
Herpes simplex		Rubella	Gnathostomiasis
Malaria (without prophylaxis)		Rubeola	Lassa fever
Salmonellosis		Schistosomiasis	Legionellosis
		Strongyloidiasis	Lymphogranuloma venereum
		Syphilis	Melioidosis
		Trichuriasis	Paragonimiasis
		Tropical sprue	Pinta
		Tuberculosis	Plague
	Typhoid fever		Polio
			Psittacosis
			Q fever
			Rabies
			Relapsing fever
		Rickettsial spotted fevers	
			Toxocariasis
			Trichinosis
			Trypanosomiasis
			Tularemia
			Typhus
			Yaws
			Yellow fever

HIV, Human immunodeficiency virus.

TABLE 20.2 Selected Potentially Fatal Febrile Tropical Infections with Established Treatments

Infection	Treatment
Viruses	
Crimean-Congo hemorrhagic fever	Ribavirin
Lassa fever	Ribavirin
Bacteria	
Anthrax	Penicillin
Bartonellosis	Penicillin, tetracycline, chloramphenicol, or streptomycin
Brazilian purpuric fever	Ampicillin or chloramphenicol
Brucellosis	Rifampin plus doxycycline; Tetracycline plus aminoglycoside or TMP/SMX
Leptospirosis	Penicillin or ampicillin, or doxycycline
Melioidosis	Ceftazidime
Plague	Streptomycin or tetracycline
Rickettsial spotted fevers	Doxycycline
Tuberculosis	Isoniazid, rifampin, ethambutol, plus pyrazinamide
Tularemia	Streptomycin or gentamicin
Typhoid fever	Ciprofloxacin, ceftriaxone, or azithromycin
Tick typhus	Doxycycline
Parasites	
Amebiasis (liver abscess)	Metronidazole followed by a luminal agent
African trypanosomiasis	Suramin or pentamidine; melarsoprol or difluoromethylornithine for central nervous system infection
Malaria	Atovaquone-proguanil; artemether-lumefantrine; artesunate or quinine or quinidine plus doxycycline
Schistosomiasis	Praziquantel (consider corticosteroids)
Visceral leishmaniasis	Sodium stibogluconate or liposomal amphotericin B

TMP/SMX, Trimethoprim/sulfamethoxazole.

TABLE 20.3 Selected Tropical Diseases with Documented Potential for Nosocomial Transmission

Argentine hemorrhagic fever (Junin)
Bolivian hemorrhagic fever (Machupo)
Crimean-Congo hemorrhagic fever
Ebola virus disease
Lassa fever
Marburg virus disease
Meningococcal infection
MERS-CoV
Plague
Rubella
Rubeola
SARS
Tuberculosis
Varicella

MERS-CoV, Middle East respiratory syndrome coronavirus; *SARS*, severe acute respiratory syndrome.

of returned ill travelers; with increasing numbers of outbreaks of dengue in regions popular with tourists over the past 5 years, such as the Caribbean, dengue is becoming increasingly recognized as a specific cause of fever in the returned traveler. Enteric fever and acute hepatitis, both vaccine preventable, were less common, diagnosed in only 2% and 1%, respectively, of febrile returning travelers. Rickettsioses were also rare as a cause of fever, occurring in only 2% of cases. Rates of hospitalization due to post-travel fever range from 20 to 30%, with *Plasmodium falciparum* malaria being the most likely specific cause of hospitalization in this setting.

In general, high-risk areas for the acquisition of febrile illnesses include sub-Saharan Africa, Southeast Asia, and Latin America. Sub-Saharan Africa and Oceania are "hot spots" for malaria acquisition, whereas South Central Asia contributes many cases of travel-acquired enteric fever (i.e., typhoid fever and paratyphoid fever due to *Salmonella enterica* serotypes Typhi and Paratyphi, respectively). Travelers returning with rickettsial infections have traveled almost exclusively to sub-Saharan Africa, while dengue infections are most commonly acquired in Southeast Asia, Latin America, and, increasingly, the Caribbean. With the emergence of chikungunya in the Americas in late 2013, and Zika in late 2015, these viral infections remain on the differential diagnosis of fever in travelers returning from all parts of the Caribbean, and Central and South America, as well as areas of prior endemicity, such as the Indian Ocean islands.

MEDICAL HISTORY

The medical history, including pre-travel preparation and the details of activities and exposures during travel, is essential in identifying the differential diagnosis of fever in travelers.

Vaccinations and Prophylaxis

First, always establish the patient's vaccination status. No vaccination is 100% effective; efficacy ranges from the near-perfect, 10-year protection provided by yellow fever vaccine to the approximately 65% efficacy of both the injectable and oral typhoid vaccines. The efficacy of the current hepatitis A and hepatitis B vaccine series is >90%. When a dose of oral polio vaccine is repeated in adult life, as recommended for risk of exposure, vaccine efficacy approaches 90-100%. Thus, a documented history of recent vaccination administered appropriately renders the diagnosis of yellow fever, hepatitis A, hepatitis B, or polio unlikely, while illnesses with poorer vaccine efficacy, such as typhoid fever and influenza, remain more probable. Similarly, administration of immune globulin within 3 months of exposure makes hepatitis A highly unlikely.

A history of compliance with prophylaxis for malaria or traveler's diarrhea is helpful, although one should bear in mind that prophylaxis for malaria is not 100% effective (see Chapters 6 and 21). It is also important to inquire as to previous diagnostic tests and treatment, some of which may have occurred while traveling.

Exposures

It is important to learn the details of itinerary, duration, and style of travel, as well as the particular characteristics of a given trip, to ascertain the risk of serious disease presenting as fever. The travel itinerary is important because many diseases are limited in their geographic distribution (see **Tables 20.6, 20.8, 20.10, 20.11, and 20.12**). In addition to geographic exposure, there may be a significant association between length of travel and serious illness, and infections vary significantly between short-term travelers and immigrants exposed to similar conditions in the same geographic area.

For example, schistosomiasis may present as Katayama fever (acute schistosomiasis) among travelers, but this syndrome is rarely observed in individuals born and raised in endemic areas, who may present as immigrants with symptoms of chronic schistosomiasis, such as abdominal discomfort, ascites, and splenomegaly (Chapter 48). Age at time of exposure, underlying health, genetic factors, and intensity and duration of parasite exposure probably contribute to these differences.

Travel style can be associated with an increased risk of serious illness, especially if an individual resided with locals or participated in an "adventure tour" as opposed to staying in urban, first-class hotels. Travel on cruise ships is a notorious risk factor for norovirus infection and invasive bacterial gastroenteritis. Younger age and being a student also increase the risk of becoming ill while traveling.

Exposures are clues that can narrow the differential diagnosis (**Table 20.4**). It is important to inquire specifically about arthropod bites, animal contact, sexual behavior, blood- and body-fluid exposures from injections or transfusions of blood products, caring for ill individuals (see **Table 20.3**), and ingestion of unpurified water, unpeeled raw fruits, raw vegetables, raw or undercooked meat/seafood, or unpasteurized dairy products. One should inquire about bathing or swimming in fresh water in areas where schistosomiasis or leptospirosis are prevalent. Barefoot exposure to sand or soil establishes risk for geohelminth infections such as strongyloidiasis and hookworm infection. Travelers may be reluctant to volunteer information regarding sexual contact abroad, but a complete sexual history is always warranted.

Patients such as volunteers, missionaries, long-term expatriates, and military personnel may present with diseases seen in both travelers and immigrants, presumably reflecting more intense and prolonged exposures.

Clinical Characteristics

Incubation Period

It is important to establish the onset of fever in relation to exposures, because the incubation period of illness can narrow the diagnostic possibilities. Some infections may present long after exposure, such as amebic liver abscess, malaria (especially if due to *Plasmodium vivax*, *P. ovale*, or *P. malariae*), human immunodeficiency virus (HIV), brucellosis, hepatitis B, tuberculosis, visceral leishmaniasis, and human African trypanosomiasis. It is also helpful to note whether the course of illness has been acute or chronic. **Table 20.5** is helpful as a guide, but many of the chronic illnesses listed, such as American and African trypanosomiasis, may also present as acute febrile syndromes during primary infection.

Interval to presentation can serve as a proxy for incubation period. *Falciparum* malaria is most likely to present in the 7- to 14-day post-travel window, whereas malaria due to *P. vivax* may present beyond 42 days post-travel. Dengue seldom presents beyond 10 days post-travel, and chikungunya and rickettsioses rarely beyond 12 days. Similarly, fever due to common agents of traveler's diarrhea or influenza rarely present beyond 1 week post-travel.

Fever Patterns

Fever patterns, although potentially helpful, may not be as characteristic of certain diseases in short-term travelers as they are in immigrants. Fevers of primary malaria rarely exhibit the intermittent pattern of tertian or quartan fevers (every 2 or 3 days, respectively) characteristically experienced by partially immune individuals. "Saddle-back fever," which refers to the phenomenon in which fever lysis is followed within several days by the resumption of high fevers, is found in 60% of cases of dengue fever but can also be seen in relapsing fever resulting from *Borrelia* species or with *P. malariae* (quartan malaria) infection, leptospirosis, and many arboviral infections other than dengue. Continuous fever with temperature/pulse dissociation (relative bradycardia) is often present in enteric (typhoid or paratyphoid) fever, tick typhus, and arboviral infections. Remittent fevers, in which the body temperature fluctuates more than 2°C (3.6°F) but does not completely return to normal, can occur in pulmonary tuberculosis but may also be seen with bacterial sepsis and bacterial abscesses.

Specific Symptoms

Specific symptoms may help establish a diagnosis. Severe myalgia and arthralgia, although characteristic of many febrile illnesses, are extremely severe in arboviral infections such as

TABLE 20.4   Exposures Suggesting Specific Infections

Animal contact
Anthrax
Babesiosis
Brucellosis
Capnocytophaga canimorsus
Hantavirus
Lassa fever
Leptospirosis
Plague
Psittacosis
Q fever
Rabies
Rat-bite fever
Toxoplasmosis
Viral hemorrhagic fevers
All tick-borne diseases

Ticks, fleas, lice, mites
Anaplasmosis
Babesiosis
Colorado tick fever
Crimean-Congo hemorrhagic fever
Ehrlichiosis
Kyasanur Forest disease
Lyme disease
Murine typhus
Omsk hemorrhagic fever
Plague
Q fever
Relapsing fever
Rickettsial spotted fevers
Rickettsialpox
Scrub typhus
Tick-borne encephalitis
Tularemia
Typhus

Transfusions or injections
Babesiosis
Bartonellosis
Chagas disease
Hepatitis B and C
HIV
HTLV-1
Leishmaniasis
Malaria
Q fever
Toxoplasmosis

Raw/uncooked meat/seafood
Cholera
Hepatitis A
Toxoplasmosis
Trichinosis
Vibrio parahaemolyticus, Vibrio vulnificus
Viral gastroenteritis

TABLE 20.4 Exposures Suggesting Specific Infections—cont'd

Sexual contact
Chancroid
Chlamydia (PID)
Gonorrhea (PID and disseminated infection)
Granuloma inguinale
Hepatitis B (and possibly C)
Herpes simplex
HIV
HTLV-1
Lymphogranuloma venereum
Syphilis
Trichomoniasis

Mosquitoes
Bancroftian filariasis
Alphavirus diseases
    Chikungunya
    Eastern equine encephalitis
    Mayaro fever
    O'nyong-nyong
    Ross River
    Sindbis
    Venezuelan equine encephalitis
    Western equine encephalitis
Flavivirus diseases
    Dengue
    Japanese encephalitis
    St. Louis encephalitis
    Yellow fever
    Zika virus
Others
    Bunyavirus diseases
    La Crosse
    Oropouche
    Rift Valley fever
    Tahyna

Fresh water (or unpeeled fruits/vegetables)
Amebiasis
Campylobacter enteritis
Cryptosporidiosis
Cyclosporiasis
Hepatitis A and E
Leptospirosis
Salmonellosis (typhoid fever)
Schistosomiasis
Shigellosis
Viral gastroenteritis

Ingestion of unpasteurized milk
Brucellosis
Listeriosis
Q fever
Salmonellosis
Tuberculosis

HIV, Human immunodeficiency disease; *HTLV-1*, human T-cell lymphotropic virus type 1; *PID*, pelvic inflammatory disease.

TABLE 20.5 Selected Febrile Illnesses of Travelers Classified by Incubation Period and Typical Clinical Course

SHORT INCUBATION (<28 DAYS)		LONG INCUBATION (>28 DAYS)	
Acute Course	Prolonged or Relapsing Course	Acute Course	Prolonged or Relapsing Course
Arbovirus infection	Brucellosis	African trypanosomiasis	African trypanosomiasis
Bacterial dysentery	Epstein-Barr virus	Amebiasis	Amebiasis
Childhood viruses	Q fever	Hepatitis B and C	American trypanosomiasis
Chikungunya			
Dengue	Relapsing fever	Malaria	Brucellosis
Ebola virus disease			
Hepatitis A and E	Schistosomiasis	Rabies	Filariasis
Influenza	Typhoid fever		Leishmaniasis
Leptospirosis			Melioidosis
Malaria			Paragonimiasis
Plague			Schistosomiasis
Rickettsial spotted fevers			Strongyloidiasis
Rubella			Tuberculosis
Rubeola			
Tularemia			
Typhus			
Yellow fever			

Adapted in part from: Salata, R.A., Olds, R.G., 1990. Infectious diseases in travelers and immigrants. In: Warren, K.S., Mahmoud, A.A.F. (Eds.), Tropical and Geographic Medicine, second ed. McGraw-Hill, New York.

chikungunya and dengue. Chills are especially prominent in malaria, bacterial infections or sepsis, and dengue. Spontaneous bleeding suggests the possibility of infection with one of the hemorrhagic viruses (e.g., Lassa fever, yellow fever, dengue hemorrhagic fever) but is also reported with various bacterial and rickettsial diseases (**Table 20.6**). Bleeding may range from easy bruising typical of mild dengue to severe epistaxis, gastrointestinal bleeding, and possible spontaneous central nervous system hemorrhage seen with severe hemorrhagic viral diseases.

Diarrhea associated with fever is typically caused by common bacterial agents of traveler's diarrhea such as *Campylobacter* species, enterohemorrhagic, enteroaggregative, and enteroinvasive *Escherichia coli* strains, *Salmonella* species, *Shigella* species, *Entamoeba histolytica*, and intestinal viruses. Occasionally, febrile diarrhea may present due to other gastrointestinal pathogens such as hookworm, coccidia such as *Cyclospora cayetanensis* or *Cryptosporidium*, and rarely with *Giardia lamblia*. However, many systemic illnesses can present with diarrhea, including malaria.

Respiratory symptoms that suggest viral upper respiratory infections may be manifestations of tuberculosis, bacterial pneumonia, Q fever, melioidosis, or the pulmonary migration phase of helminths such as *Ascaris lumbricoides* and *Strongyloides stercoralis*. Fever with localized respiratory signs and symptoms in a traveler to South Central or Southeast Asia should raise the specter of highly pathogenic avian influenza or severe acute respiratory syndrome

TABLE 20.6   Important Tropical Infections Associated with Spontaneous Bleeding

Infection	Geographic Distribution
Viruses	
Argentine hemorrhagic fever (Junin)	South America
Bolivian hemorrhagic fever (Machupo)	South America
Chikungunya	The Americas (Caribbean, Central and South America), Africa, Asia, Indian subcontinent
Crimean-Congo hemorrhagic fever	Africa, Asia, and Eastern Europe
Dengue	Tropical regions of Africa, South America, Central America, the Caribbean, Asia, and Oceania
Ebola virus disease	Africa
Hantaan virus (hemorrhagic fever with renal syndrome)	Asia, Africa, Oceania, the Americas, Europe
Kyasanur Forest disease	India
Lassa fever	Africa
Marburg virus	Africa
Omsk hemorrhagic fever	Asia (the former USSR)
Rift Valley fever	Africa
Yellow fever	Africa and South and Central America
Bacteria	
Brazilian purpuric fever	South America
Leptospirosis	Widespread
Meningococcal infection	Widespread, particularly sub-Saharan Africa
Melioidosis	Asia, Oceania, Africa, and focal spots in the Americas
Plague	Asia, Africa, Europe, and the Americas
Rocky Mountain spotted fever	North and South America
Typhus	Widespread
Vibrio vulnificus	Widespread in coastal regions

Adapted in part from: Wilson, M.E., 1991. A World Guide to Infections: Diseases, Distribution, Diagnosis. Oxford University Press, New York.

(SARS). Middle East respiratory syndrome coronavirus should be considered when evaluating fever, respiratory symptoms, and recent travel to the Middle East or Korea.

Hepatosplenomegaly along with fever suggests malaria, mononucleosis, hepatic amebiasis, acute schistosomiasis (Katayama fever), visceral leishmaniasis, or enteric fever, among other infectious diseases. Lymphadenopathy evokes mononucleosis, HIV, acute schistosomiasis, plague, typhoid fever, tularemia, and trypanosomiasis, among others (**Table 20.7**). Of course, neoplastic and collagen vascular diseases may also induce lymphadenopathy and fever.

Meningismus, confusion, and other signs of central nervous system dysfunction may be caused by a variety of viral, parasitic, and bacterial agents (**Table 20.8**). Many of these pathogens are restricted to certain ecologic niches, so the patient's geographic itinerary, season of travel, and exposure history are essential. For example, Japanese encephalitis virus is limited to the Far East, is a disease of summer in temperate climates, and is transmitted by mosquitoes. Spinal cord disease associated with fever can result from West Nile virus, schistosomiasis, human T-cell lymphotrophic virus type 1 (HTLV-1) infection, or polio virus infection.

TABLE 20.7   Selected Febrile Illnesses Causing Organomegaly and/or Lymphadenopathy

	Hepatomegaly	Splenomegaly	Generalized Adenopathy	Localized Adenopathy
Viruses				
Cytomegalovirus	+/−	+	+/−	+/−
Dengue	+/−	+/−	+	−
Epstein-Barr virus	+/−	+ +	+ +	+
Hepatitis A and B	+ +	+/−	+/−	−
HIV	+/−	+/−	+ +	+
HTLV-1	+ +	+ +	+ +	+/−
Bacteria				
Anthrax	−	−	−	+
Brucellosis	+	+ +	+	+/−
Ehrlichiosis	+	+	−	−
Endocarditis	−	+	+/−	−
Enteric fever	+ +	+ +	+/−	−
Leptospirosis	+/−	+	+	−
Melioidosis	+/−	+/−	+	+
Plague	+	+	−	+ +
Q fever	+ +	+ +	−	−
Relapsing fever	+ +	+ +	+/−	+/−
Spotted fevers	+	+	+/−	+/−
Tuberculosis	+/−	+/−	+/−	+ +
Tularemia	+/−	+/−	+/−	+ +
Typhus	+/−	+ +	+/−	−
Parasites				
Acute schistosomiasis	+ +	+ +	+ +	+/−
African trypanosomiasis	+/−	+	+ +	+
Amebiasis (hepatic)	+ +	+/−	−	−
Babesiosis	+ +	+ +	+/−	+/−
Fascioliasis	+ +	+/−	−	−
Filariasis	−	−	+	+ +
Malaria	+ +	+	−	−
Toxocariasis visceral larva (migrans)	+ +	+/−	−	−
Toxoplasmosis	+/−	+/−	+	+
Visceral leishmaniasis	+ +	+ +	+	+ +

− No association; + Finding is associated; ++ Finding strongly associated; +/− Finding may or may not be present.
HIV, Human immunodeficiency virus; *HTLV-1*, human T-cell lymphotropic virus type 1.

TABLE 20.8 Important Tropical Infections Causing Meningitis and Encephalitis

Infection	Geographic Distribution
Viruses	
California group encephalitis	The Americas and Asia
Chikungunya	The Americas (Caribbean, Central and South America), Africa, and Asia
Crimean-Congo hemorrhagic fever	Africa, Asia, and Europe
Japanese encephalitis	Asia and Oceania
Kyasanur Forest disease	Asia (India)
Lymphocytic choriomeningitis	Widespread
Murray Valley encephalitis	Oceania (Australia)
Omsk hemorrhagic fever	Europe (former USSR)
Oropouche	South America
Poliomyelitis	Africa and Asia
Rabies	Africa, the Americas, Asia, and Europe
Rift Valley fever	Africa
Tick-borne encephalitis	Asia and Europe
Venezuelan equine encephalitis	The Americas
West Nile fever	Africa, Asia, Europe, and Oceania
Bacteria	
Bartonellosis	South America (Andes)
Brucellosis	Widespread
Leptospirosis	Widespread
Listeriosis	Widespread
Lyme disease	Widespread (especially America and Europe)
Meningococcal infection	Widespread (especially sub-Saharan Africa, northern India, and Nepal)
Rickettsioses	Widespread
Salmonellosis	Widespread
Syphilis	Widespread
Tuberculosis	Widespread
Fungi	
Blastomycosis	Africa, the Americas, Asia, and Europe
Coccidioidomycosis	The Americas
Cryptococcosis	Widespread
Histoplasmosis	Widespread
Paracoccidioidomycosis	Amazonas, Brazil
Sporotrichosis	Widespread
Protozoa	
African trypanosomiasis	Africa, primarily East Africa (game parks)
Malaria	Widespread
Primary amebic meningoencephalitis	Widespread
Toxoplasmosis	Widespread

Continued

TABLE 20.8 Important Tropical Infections Causing Meningitis and Encephalitis—cont'd

Infection	Geographic Distribution
Helminths	
Cysticercosis (*Taenia solium*)	Widespread
Eosinophilic meningitis (*Angiostrongylus cantonensis*)	Asia, Oceania, Africa, and the Americas
Gnathostomiasis	Asia, Oceania, Africa, and the Americas
Paragonimiasis	Africa, Asia, South America
Strongyloidiasis (in immunocompromised hosts)	Widespread
Toxocariasis	Widespread
Trichinosis	Widespread

Adapted in part from: Wilson, M.E., 1991. A World Guide to Infections: Diseases, Distribution, Diagnosis. Oxford University Press, New York.

Cutaneous manifestations of disease are common but seldom specific (**Table 20.9**). The erythema chronicum migrans of Lyme disease and rose spots in typhoid fever are examples of unique, specific rashes. Nonetheless, rash can refine a differential diagnosis considerably. For example, an eschar at the site of inoculation is typical of tick typhus, boutonneuse (Mediterranean spotted) fever, and anthrax. Cutaneous ulcers are seen in leishmaniasis, tropical phagedenic ulcer, Buruli ulcer (*Mycobacterium ulcerans*), cutaneous amebiasis, arthropod bites, syphilis, yaws, tuberculosis, and leprosy. When evaluating a patient who has received previous treatment, it is important to recall that rash can be caused by reactions to drugs, such as sulfa drugs, antimalarials, and other antibiotics. Rickettsial diseases are frequently associated with rash, but the absence of rash may be misleading and does not exclude the possibility of rickettsial disease (see **Table 20.13**). Genital ulcers, such as those seen with syphilis, chancroid, and lymphogranuloma venereum, should be construed as markers of exposure to other sexually transmitted diseases that should be excluded in affected travelers, as well.

APPROACH TO THE TRAVELER WITH FEVER

A thorough but directed evaluation, bearing in mind that most fevers are self-limited, is warranted for the traveler presenting with fever. A careful history covering pre-travel prophylaxis, itinerary, travel style and exposures, apparent incubation period, fever pattern, symptoms, previous treatment, and diagnostic studies is essential. Laboratory tests to consider in the diagnostic evaluation include blood smears for malaria (and *Borrelia*, trypanosomes, *Babesia*, etc.), complete blood count and white cell differential, absolute eosinophil count, serum electrolytes, blood urea nitrogen and creatinine, glucose, bilirubin, hepatic transaminases, urinalysis, chest radiograph, tuberculin skin test, hepatitis serologies, and bacterial cultures of blood, urine, and stool. In many instances, it is prudent to obtain and save an acute serum sample for future comparative serologic studies. Suspected cases of viral hemorrhagic fevers, severe malaria, and enteric fever should be immediately hospitalized. Travel in a rural African environment is a significant risk factor for exposure to viral hemorrhagic fevers, although other hemorrhagic viruses, including those causing dengue fever, Hantaan, yellow fever, and Crimean-Congo hemorrhagic fever, have a more cosmopolitan distribution in widely scattered parts of the world (**Table 20.6**). All cases of suspected viral hemorrhagic fevers should be reported immediately to both the local health department and the Centers for Disease Control and Prevention (CDC).

The clinically stable patient with travel-related fever in whom the initial history, physical examination, and screening laboratory studies, including at least two blood films for malaria

TABLE 20.9   Selected Infections Characteristically Associated with Fever and Cutaneous Signs

Infection	Typical Skin Manifestations/Rash
Viruses	
Dengue	Diffuse scarlatiniform or macular rash; occasional petechiae or ecchymoses
Ebola/Marburg viruses	Maculopapular rash on trunk
Herpes simplex virus	Vesicles
HIV (acute)	Morbilliform rash
Rubella	Maculopapular rash
Rubeola	Maculopapular rash
Varicella	Vesicles or pustules
Viral hemorrhagic fevers	Petechiae, ecchymoses
Yellow fever, hepatitis viruses	Jaundice
Bacteria	
Anthrax	Eschar
Bartonellosis	Angioproliferative papules and nodules
Leptospirosis	Possible pretibial maculopapular rash
Lyme disease	Large, annular erythematous macule(s)
Meningococcal infection	Petechiae and purpura, may involve palms/soles
Rickettsial spotted fevers	Diffuse macular or maculopapular rash, may involve palms/soles; possible petechiae and eschar at primary inoculation site
Scarlet fever	Diffuse maculopapular rash
Scrub typhus	Eschar; diffuse macular or maculopapular rash
Syphilis (secondary)	Papular rash, possibly involving palms/soles
Tularemia	Ulcerated papule at inoculation site
Typhoid fever	Rose-colored papules on trunk ("rose spots")
Typhus	Diffuse macular or maculopapular rash; occasional petechiae
Parasites	
Acute schistosomiasis (Katayama fever)	Urticaria
African trypanosomiasis	Chancre, followed by generalized erythematous rash; possible erythema nodosum
American trypanosomiasis	Erythematous nodule at inoculation site; may be associated with periorbital edema
Leishmaniasis	Ulcers, nodules
Onchocerciasis	Subcutaneous nodule(s), dermatitis
Strongyloidiasis	Cutaneous larva currens (erythematous, serpiginous subcutaneous papules, often perirectal, associated with pruritus)

HIV, Human immunodeficiency virus.

separated by >6 but not more than 24 hours, are unremarkable may be observed. The patient should be instructed to keep a temperature record and return in 2-3 days if fever fails to resolve, or sooner if symptoms worsen. Empiric treatment for enteric fever (and/or rickettsioses) may be considered in patients who continue to have fever >48 hours after all diagnostic work-up has been initiated but in whom specific tests have been noncontributory (see Public Health Agency of Canada, Fever in the Returning Traveller 2011). Because the majority of travel-related febrile illnesses are self-limited viral syndromes, most fevers will resolve spontaneously. If fever persists, however, repeat malarial smears and blood cultures are warranted. Directed serologic studies to detect diseases compatible with the patient's history and physical examination should be considered. Imaging studies (e.g., abdominal computed tomography or ultrasound) and biopsies (e.g., bone marrow, liver, lymph nodes) may be indicated. Hospitalization may be justified to expedite the work-up in certain circumstances. During the evaluation of perplexing cases of apparent travel-related illness, the clinician should bear in mind that non-infectious disorders, such as pulmonary embolism, occult malignancies, systemic lupus erythematosus, and temporal arteritis, may present with fever.

Presumptive empiric therapy directed against a likely pathogen may be justified, especially when adequate diagnostic studies are not readily available or a patient is clinically deteriorating. Examples include intravenous artesunate for suspected severe infection with *P. falciparum*, quinolones or third-generation cephalosporins for suspected enteric fever, doxycycline for suspected rickettsioses, and ribavirin for suspected Lassa fever (**Table 20.2**). Early initiation of appropriate therapy may significantly reduce morbidity and potential mortality from these serious febrile illnesses of travelers.

INFECTIOUS DISEASES IN THE TRAVELER WITH FEVER

Selected infectious diseases that should be considered in the traveler with fever are discussed in this section, with the goal of providing an overview. References to other chapters in this book are given as appropriate; however, the reader is encouraged to consult, when possible, standard textbooks on infectious diseases and tropical medicine and to contact the CDC for current and detailed information on the diagnosis and treatment of exotic diseases. The experts at the CDC can provide 24-hour emergency medical consultation by telephone to healthcare providers dealing with a very ill patient.

Malaria

Fever in a traveler from a malarious area should be evaluated carefully, with multiple blood smears for malaria. Although malaria is discussed in greater detail in Chapter 21, key points are worth repeating here. *P. falciparum* infection can be life-threatening when associated with high parasitemia, blackwater fever, cerebral malaria, or acute respiratory distress syndrome. Chemoprophylaxis is often effective, but only when taken as directed. Of the 231 cases of severe malaria in travelers reported to the CDC in 2012, 75% were due to *P. falciparum*, and 79% of these infections were acquired in sub-Saharan Africa; only 7 of 200 patients in whom information on prophylaxis was known were adherent to their drug regimen. However, drug-resistant *P. falciparum* is now widespread, and even perfect compliance with prophylaxis does not provide absolute protection from malaria infection. The case-fatality rate for *P. falciparum* in US travelers was approximately 0.4% in 2012 (6 deaths among 1687 total cases). Clinical manifestations of *P. vivax* and *P. ovale* infections can develop up to 5 years after exposure. The diagnosis of malaria in immune individuals or individuals who have received prophylaxis or partial treatment may be complicated by low parasitemia. Multiple blood smears in combination with highly sensitive rapid diagnostic tests or, occasionally, nucleic acid amplification tests such as polymerase chain reaction may be helpful in difficult cases (see also Chapters 6 and 21).

Typhoid and Paratyphoid Fever (Enteric Fevers)

Enteric fever is caused by *Salmonella enterica* serovar Typhi (*S. typhi*) or *Salmonella paratyphi*. Persistently rising fever, relative bradycardia, rose spots, and normal leukocyte counts with mild to moderate elevation of hepatic transaminases are all clues to the diagnosis; however, these characteristics are often absent. The organism can be cultured from the blood in >80% of patients during the first week of illness and from bone marrow aspirated from the iliac crest in more than 90% of documented cases, if no antibiotics are administered before obtaining the culture. The organism can be cultured from stool during the incubation period occasionally, and in one-third to two-thirds of patients during the second through fourth weeks of illness.

Neither the oral nor the parenteral vaccine provides complete immunity (Chapter 5). In immunized populations, however, a higher percentage of individuals with enteric fever will have disease caused by *S. paratyphi*, although disease caused by *S. typhi* still occurs. Of the approximate 5700 cases of typhoid fever that occur annually in the United States, up to 75% are travel acquired. Of the 1902 laboratory-confirmed cases of typhoid fever reported by Lynch and colleagues (2009) between 1999 and 2006 in the United States where epidemiologic information was available, foreign travel in the preceding 30 days was reported by 79%, yet only 5% had received typhoid vaccine prior to travel. Seventy-three percent of cases were hospitalized, and 0.2% died. Resistance to antimicrobials has been reported for *S. typhi* isolates in many countries, although fluoroquinolones are usually effective against typhoid fever acquired outside the Indian sub-continent and Southeast Asia (Chapter 31).

Arboviral Diseases

Arboviral diseases are caused by arthropod-borne viruses; most are zoonoses (shared between humans and other vertebrate hosts). More than 400 arboviruses, classified into many families and genera, have been described (**Table 20.10**). Arboviral diseases are present throughout the tropics; however, some arboviruses, such as o'nyong-nyong, Mayaro, Ross River, Oropouche, and Rift Valley fever viruses, are limited in geographic distribution. Diagnosis usually depends on clinical suspicion and serologic confirmation, the latter generally requiring acute and convalescent serum samples.

The arboviral diseases can be divided into four syndromes based on clinical presentation: (1) undifferentiated fever, (2) dengue fever, (3) hemorrhagic fever, and (4) encephalitis. The syndrome of undifferentiated fever (e.g., Oropouche, Mayaro, and sand fly fever) is generally characterized by one or more of the following: fever, headache, myalgia, pharyngitis, coryza, nausea, vomiting, and diarrhea. The dengue fever syndrome (dengue, chikungunya, o'nyong-nyong, Sindbis, West Nile, Ross River viruses) is characterized by fever, rash, arthralgia, and leukopenia. The syndrome of hemorrhagic fevers (Lassa fever, Ebola, Marburg, Crimean-Congo, Argentine, Bolivian, dengue, yellow fever viruses) ranges from mild petechiae to severe purpura and bleeding diathesis. The 2014 West African outbreak of Ebola virus disease (EVD) underscores that prior estimates of the frequency of hemorrhagic manifestations in EVD are likely inflated. In this outbreak of EVD, which has led to >27,000 cases and >11,000 deaths, bleeding and hemorrhagic manifestations have been noted to occur in 5-15% of patients (Chertow et al. 2014; Qin et al. 2015).

Dengue Fever

Dengue is the most widespread arbovirus, distributed throughout the tropics, and frequently encountered in travelers returning from the tropics. Dengue virus is a single-stranded RNA flavivirus transmitted by the day-biting urban mosquito *Aedes aegypti* or the jungle mosquito *Aedes albopictus*. Four serotypes are recognized. Infection with one serotype results in immunity to that particular serotype; however, after a short period of cross-protection, individuals are susceptible to infection with another serotype.

Clinical infection ranges from a mild febrile syndrome to a severe dengue syndrome. Individuals with dengue who recover fully following defervescence are considered to have uncomplicated dengue, while those who deteriorate clinically are classified as having "warning signs," which include any of the following manifestations: abdominal pain, persistent vomiting, fluid accumulation, mucosal bleeding, lethargy, hepatic enlargement, and worsening thrombocytopenia in the setting of hemoconcentration. A minority of patients with warning signs will continue to deteriorate despite fluid resuscitation, and those are

TABLE 20.10 Epidemiology of Important Arboviruses[a]

Family (Genus) Virus	Human Disease	Distribution	Vector
Togaviridae (Alphavirus)			
Mayaro	Fever, arthritis, rash	South America	Mosquito
Ross River	Arthritis, rash, sometimes fever	Australia and South Pacific	Mosquito
Chikungunya	Fever, arthritis, hemorrhagic fever	The Americas, Africa, Asia, and Oceania	Mosquito
Eastern encephalitis	Fever, encephalitis	The Americas	Mosquito
Western encephalitis	Fever, encephalitis	The Americas	Mosquito
Venezuelan encephalitis	Fever, sometimes encephalitis	The Americas	Mosquito
Flaviviridae (Flavivirus)			
Dengue (four types)	Fever, rash, hemorrhagic fever	Worldwide (tropics)	Mosquito
Zika (Human disease)	Fever, rash, Guillan-Barre, microcephaly (during pregnancy) (Distribution)	The Americas (vector)	Mosquito
Yellow fever	Fever, hemorrhagic fever	Tropical Americas and Africa	Mosquito
St. Louis encephalitis	Encephalitis, hepatitis (rare)	The Americas	Mosquito
Japanese encephalitis	Encephalitis	Asia, Pacific	Mosquito
West Nile	Fever, rash, hepatitis, encephalitis	Asia, Europe, Africa, and North America	Mosquito
Kyasanur Forest	Hemorrhagic fever, meningoencephalitis	India	Tick
Omsk hemorrhagic fever	Hemorrhagic fever	Former Soviet Union	Tick
Tick-borne encephalitis	Encephalitis	Europe and Asia	Tick
Bunyaviridae (Bunyavirus)			
La Crosse encephalitis	Encephalitis	North America	Mosquito
Oropouche	Fever	Brazil and Panama	Midge
Bunyaviridae (Phlebovirus)			
Sand fly fever viruses	Fever	Asia, Africa, and tropical Americas	Sand fly, mosquito
Rift Valley fever	Fever, hemorrhagic fever, encephalitis, retinitis	Africa	Mosquito
Bunyaviridae (Nairovirus)			
Crimean-Congo hemorrhagic fever	Hemorrhagic fever	Asia, Europe, and Africa	Tick
Bunyaviridae (Hantavirus)			
Hantaan	Hemorrhagic fever, renal syndrome	Asia	Rodent-borne
Puumala	Hemorrhagic fever, renal syndrome	Europe	Rodent-borne
Sin Nombre	Hantavirus pulmonary syndrome	Western USA	Rodent-borne
Arenaviridae (Arenavirus)			
Junin	Hemorrhagic fever	Argentina	Rodent-borne
Machupo	Hemorrhagic fever	Bolivia	Rodent-borne
Lassa fever	Hemorrhagic fever	West Africa	Rodent-borne

TABLE 20.10 Epidemiology of Important Arboviruses—cont'd			
Family (Genus) Virus	Human Disease	Distribution	Vector
Reoviridae (Orbivirus)			
Colorado tick fever	Fever	Western USA	Tick
Filoviridae (Filovirus)			
Marburg	Hemorrhagic fever	Africa	Unknown
Ebola	Hemorrhagic fever	Africa	Unknown

Adapted from: Shope, R.E., 1992. In: Wyngaarden, J.B., Smith, L.H., Bennett, J.C. (Eds.), Cecil's Textbook of Medicine, nineteenth ed. Saunders, Philadelphia.
ªSome of the viruses listed are not transmitted by arthropods and thus are not arboviruses.

considered to have severe dengue, characterized by severe plasma leakage, severe bleeding, or organ failure (WHO 2009).

The incubation period of dengue is 5-8 days. A viral prodrome of nausea and vomiting is common, followed by high fever for a mean of 5 days; the fever often lyses abruptly. Myalgia and arthralgia are particularly prominent, giving rise to the common name of "breakbone fever." Headache (especially retro-orbital), lymphadenopathy (frequently cervical), and/or rash (scarlatiniform, maculopapular, or petechial; characteristic "islands of white macules on a sea of red") frequently develop. The rash may occur late during the course of illness, and fever may reappear after several days. (*Note*: this "saddleback" fever pattern is present in about 60% of cases.)

Previous infection with one serotype of virus may predispose an individual to more severe disease on infection with another serotype. This immune enhancement of viral pathogenesis is thought to result from immunoglobulin-mediated dengue virus uptake into macrophages, where growth is favored. Thus the hemorrhagic fever/shock syndrome, which is most common in indigenous children, is unlikely to occur in a traveler who has not been previously infected with dengue. Prolonged convalescent periods, characterized by extreme fatigue often persisting for months, have been noted by many travelers who have acquired dengue fever. Dengue vaccine trials in endemic areas show some benefit in children.

Chikungunya

Chikungunya virus infection has been historically noted among travelers from Southeast Asia and Africa. However, in late 2013, the virus emerged for the first time in the Americas, leading to a widespread and ongoing outbreak in the Caribbean and Central and South America affecting at least 44 individual countries, with cases numbering into the hundreds of thousands. This has resulted in high numbers of cases among North American and European travelers to the Caribbean and Central America, in particular. This disease presents in a fashion similar to dengue fever, although incubation and duration of symptoms are typically more prolonged. Myalgia and arthralgia are particularly severe with chikungunya, with function-limiting arthropathy persisting for years in a minority of patients.

Zika

Zika virus was discovered in Uganda in 1947, and human infections were extraordinarily rare until 2015, when an epidemic began to sweep across South and Central America. Most adult patients have a clinical illness very similar to Dengue and Chikungunya, although neurological injury such as Guillain-Barre has been described. Of greatest concern is its association with microcephaly if the patient is pregnant during infection. Women who return from endemic areas with fever should be assessed for this infection, and if infected and pregnant, counseled on strategies for aggressive fetal monitoring or termination options.

Yellow Fever

In the Americas, yellow fever is transmitted by *Haemagogus* mosquitoes in the jungle environment and *A. aegypti* in urban settings. In Africa, transmission to humans occurs via *Aedes* spp. Historically, in both urban and rural environments, only 50–200 cases of yellow fever per year have been reported from the tropical Americas. However, yellow fever is an emerging problem in the Amazon and other jungle regions of Brazil, Colombia, Venezuela, and Peru, with resurgence of the disease in the early 2000s leading to mass vaccination initiatives. Sporadic urban transmission still occurs in large outbreaks in Africa. Although *A. aegypti* is ubiquitous in the Far East, yellow fever virus transmission has never been reported from this region. The reason is unclear, but either the lack of virus importation into the region or possible immune cross-resistance induced by endemic dengue immunity may be responsible. The spectrum of clinical disease ranges from a dengue fever-like illness to a severe hemorrhagic illness associated with hepatic and renal failures. The disease is almost 100% preventable by vaccination with live attenuated 17D-strain vaccine (Chapter 5). Among unvaccinated travelers from the United States and Europe, nine cases of yellow fever occurred between 1970 and 2011, five of which were acquired in sub-Saharan Africa, and four in South America. Eight of these cases were fatal.

Hemorrhagic Syndromes

Viruses causing hemorrhagic syndromes, such as Lassa fever virus, Ebola virus, Marburg virus, and Machupo virus, have been associated with life-threatening infections that can be spread nosocomially. Patients who are suspected of having one of these viruses should be placed in airborne and contact isolation. Laboratory work should be kept to a necessary minimum and the laboratory alerted to the possibility of contagious virus in patient specimens. The CDC and state health department should be contacted immediately.

An arthropod vector has not been identified for many of these viruses, such as Lassa fever, which is transmitted via contact with rodent reservoirs in rural West Africa or with infected humans. Early symptoms include fever, malaise, weakness, and myalgia. A few days later, cough, pharyngitis, and chest and epigastric pain develop. Vomiting and diarrhea occur by about day 5, associated with fever of 39–40°C. By the sixth day, respiratory distress, cardiac instability, hepatic and renal failure, and hemorrhagic phenomena begin to appear. Lassa fever can be diagnosed by either the isolation of virus or the demonstration of a fourfold increase in antibody titer. Early treatment with ribavirin may improve outcome with Lassa fever virus, Hantaan virus, and other hemorrhagic viruses with the exception of Ebola, yellow fever, and dengue viruses. Other viruses of importance are listed in **Table 20.11**. (See also Chapter 28.)

Rickettsial Diseases

Rickettsial diseases are acute, usually self-limited febrile illnesses caused by obligate intracellular Gram-negative bacteria of the order Rickettsiales. Rickettsiae can be divided into the spotted fever group and the typhus fever group. All are transmitted by ticks, fleas, lice, or mites. Rickettsiae are widely distributed throughout the world (**Table 20.12**).

The spectrum of illness ranges widely and includes subclinical infection. Incubation periods for the various diseases vary widely, on the order of 2–30 days (**Table 20.13**). Clinical illness is generally characterized by an abrupt onset of fever, chills, and sweats, frequently associated with rash, headache, conjunctivitis, pharyngitis, epistaxis, myalgias, arthralgias, and hepatosplenomegaly. An eschar often develops at the site of the bite of the mite or tick in scrub typhus, due to *Orientia tsutsugamushi*, and the spotted fever group rickettsioses. Vasculitis underlies the typical pathologic manifestations of rickettsial disease. Complications are rare but include encephalitis, renal failure, and shock.

Most rickettsial disease reported in the United States is acquired domestically (e.g., Rocky Mountain spotted fever). Spotted fever group rickettsioses, including Mediterranean spotted fever/boutonneuse fever and African tick bite fever, appear to be the most common

Continued text to page 293

TABLE 20.11 Epidemiology and Clinical Characteristics of Viral Hemorrhagic Fevers

Disease	Clinical Syndrome	Geographic Distribution	Vector
Yellow fever	Ranges from mild febrile illnesses to severe hepatitis and renal failure (with albuminuria); biphasic course of illness may be noted	Tropical South America and sub-Saharan Africa	*Aedes aegypti* mosquito *Haemagogus* mosquito (urban Americas)
Dengue	Classic dengue: fever, severe myalgia/arthralgia, and morbilliform rash Dengue hemorrhagic fever: shock and DIC	Tropical and subtropical regions of the Americas, Africa, Asia, and Australia	*Aedes aegypti* mosquito
Lassa fever	Fever, severe headache, lumbar pain, chest pain, and thrombocytopenia; possible encephalitis, pneumonitis, and myocarditis	Sub-Saharan Africa	None (high potential for person-to-person transmission)
Argentine hemorrhagic fever (Junin virus)	Insidious onset of fever, myalgia, headache, conjunctivitis, epigastric pain, nausea, and vomiting; possible shock	Argentina (especially Buenos Aires province)	None
Bolivian hemorrhagic fever (Machupo virus)	Similar to Argentine hemorrhagic fever	Bolivia (Department of Beni)	None
Marburg virus	Abrupt onset of fever, headache, conjunctivitis, myalgia, nausea, and vomiting; severe hemorrhagic complications and shock are common	Laboratory outbreaks involved with handling infected monkey tissues/cells	None (high potential for person-to-person transmission)
Ebola virus	Similar to Marburg virus; in West African outbreak, hemorrhagic complications are uncommon; large volume diarrhea common	Large outbreak in West Africa beginning in early 2014; isolated outbreaks in rural sub-Saharan Africa	None (high potential for person-to-person transmission)
Crimean-Congo hemorrhagic fever	Abrupt onset of fever, headache, arthralgia, myalgia, conjunctivitis, and abdominal pain; purpura and ecchymoses are common	Africa, Middle East, and Eastern Europe	*Hyalomma* species (ticks) (potential for nosocomial transmission)
Hemorrhagic fever with renal syndrome (hantavirus)	Abrupt onset of fever, headache, lethargy, abdominal pain associated with oliguria and acute renal failure; petechiae are common	Balkans, former Soviet Union, Korea, and China	None

DIC, Disseminated intravascular coagulopathy.

TABLE 20.12 Epidemiology of Rickettsial Diseases

Disease	Organism	Natural Cycle	Usual Mode of Transmission to Humans	Common Occupational or Environmental Association	Geographic Distribution
Typhus Group					
Murine typhus	*Rickettsia mooseri* (*Rickettsia typhi*)	Fleas	Rodents	Infected flea feces into broken skin or aerosol to mucous membrane	Rat-infected premises (shops, warehouses)	Scattered foci (worldwide grain elevators)
Epidemic typhus	*Rickettsia prowazekii*	Body lice	Humans	Infected feces or crushed lice into broken skin, or aerosol to mucous membranes	Lice-infected human population with louse transfer	Worldwide
Brill-Zinsser disease	*R. prowazekii*	Recrudescence months to years after primary attack of louse-borne typhus				Worldwide
Spotted Fever Group (Selected Examples)					
Rocky Mountain spotted fever	*R. rickettsii*	Ixodid ticks	Ticks/small mammals	Tick bite, mechanical transfer to mucous membranes, ?air-borne	Tick-infested terrain, houses, dogs	Western hemisphere
Ehrlichiosis	*Ehrlichia canis*	Ticks	Dogs	Tick bite	Tick-infested areas	At least 12 states in USA, primarily southern states
African tick bite Fever	*Rickettsia africae*	*Amblyomma* ticks	Ticks	Tick bite	Game hunting; safari	Southern Africa
Boutonneuse fever	*Rickettsia conorii*	Ixodid ticks	Ticks/rodents, dogs	Tick bite	Tick-infested terrain, houses, dogs	Mediterranean littoral, Africa, and Indian subcontinent
Rickettsialpox	*Rickettsia akari*	Mouse mites	Mites/mice	Mouse mite bite	Unique mouse- and mite-infested premises (incinerators)	USA, former Soviet Union, Korea, and Central Africa

Others

Disease	Organism	Vector	Reservoir	Transmission	Exposure	Distribution
Q fever	*Coxiella burnetii*	Ticks	Ticks/mammals	Inhalation of dried air-borne infective material; tick bite	Domestic animals or products, dairies, lambing pens; slaughterhouses	Worldwide
Scrub typhus (tsutsugamushi disease)	*Orientia tsutsugamushi* (multiple serotypes)	Chiggers (harvest mites)	Chiggers/rodents	Chigger bite	Chigger-infested terrain; secondary scrub, grass airfields, golf courses	Asia, Australia, New Guinea, and Pacific Islands
Trench fever	*Bartonella quintana*	Body lice	Humans	Infected feces or crushed louse into broken skin; aerosol to mucous membranes	Lousy human population with louse transfer	Africa, Mexico, South America, and Eastern Europe

Adapted from: Hornick, R.B., 1992. In: Wyngaarden, J.B., Smith, L.H., Bennett, J.C. (Eds.), Cecil Textbook of Medicine, nineteenth ed. Saunders, Philadelphia.

TABLE 20.13 Clinical Features of Important Rickettsial Diseases

Disease	Usual Incubation Period in Days (Range)	Eschar	Onset, Day of Disease	RASH Distribution	RASH Type	Usual Duration of Disease in Days[a] (Range)	Usual Severity[b]	Fever after Chemotherapy (h)
Typhus Group								
Murine typhus	12 (8-16)	None	5-7	Trunk → extremities	Macular, maculopapular	12 (8-16)	Moderate	48-72
Epidemic typhus	12 (10-14)	None	5-7	Trunk → extremities	Macular, maculopapular, petechial	14 (10-18)	Severe	48-72
Brill-Zinsser disease	–	None		Trunk → extremities	Macular	7-11	Relatively mild	48-72
Spotted Fever Group (Selected Examples)								
Rocky Mountain spotted fever	7 (3-12)	None	3-5	Extremities → trunk, face	Macular, maculopapular, petechial	16 (10-20)	Severe	72
Ehrlichiosis	7-21	None	Rare?	Unknown	Petechial	7 (3-19)	Mild	72
Boutonneuse fever	5-7	Often present	3-4	Trunk, extremities, face, palms, soles	Macular, maculopapular, petechial	10 (7-14)	Moderate	–
Rickettsialpox	?9-17	Often present	1-3	Trunk → face, extremities	Papulovesicular	7 (3-11)	Relatively mild	–
Others								
Q fever	10-19	None		None		(2-21)	Relatively mild[c]	48 (sometimes slow)
Scrub typhus (tsutsugamushi disease)	1-12 (9-18)	Often present	4-6	Trunk → extremities	Macular, maculopapular	14 (10-20)	Mild to severe	24-36

Adapted from Hornick, R.B., 1992. In: Wyngaarden, J.B., Smith, L.H., Bennett, J.C. (Eds.), Cecil Textbook of Medicine, nineteenth ed. Saunders, Philadelphia.
[a]Untreated d sease.
[b]Severity can vary greatly.
[c]Occasionally, subacute infections occur (e.g., hepatitis, endocarditis)

rickettsial diseases of travelers, accounting for 231 of 280 cases of rickettsial disease among travelers reported by GeoSentinel between 1996 and 2008 (Jensenius et al. 2009). Typhus fever group rickettsioses are endemic to areas in southern Europe, Africa, and the Middle East, although most cases are also reported in travelers to Africa.

Diagnosis requires clinical suspicion (often mandating empiric antibiotic therapy) and specific serologies. Therapy consists of doxycycline (200 mg/day in divided doses) generally for 3-4 days after defervescence and a minimum of 1 week total therapy. Recent evidence suggests that short courses of macrolide antibiotics, such as azithromycin or clarithromycin, may be acceptable alternatives for the therapy of rickettsioses other than Rocky Mountain spotted fever.

Helminths

Schistosomiasis (Bilharziasis)

Schistosomiasis is caused by a fluke and transmitted by freshwater exposure in endemic regions. Katayama fever, or acute schistosomiasis, develops 2-10 weeks after exposure. This serum sickness-like illness is believed to represent a reaction against antigen–antibody complexes formed as a result of egg deposition. This syndrome is most severe in *Schistosoma japonicum* infections, in which egg production is greatest. Characteristic clinical manifestations include fevers, chills, sweating, headache, cough, lymphadenopathy, hepatosplenomegaly, and eosinophilia. Although death has been reported in *S. japonicum* infections, most patients with Katayama fever experience a self-limited illness that is commonly undiagnosed. Travelers appear to be more likely to develop this syndrome than those raised in endemic areas. Serologic studies are helpful in the diagnosis. Recommended treatment involves administration of praziquantel and corticosteroids (see Chapter 48). Mounting evidence suggests that asymptomatic travelers returning from high-risk areas should be screened (serologically and/or with stool/urine ova and parasites, the latter >6 weeks after exposure) and treated.

Filariasis

The filariasis syndromes associated with fever include onchocerciasis (river blindness), lymphatic filariasis (lymphangitis, often complicated by bacterial superinfection), loiasis, and nocturnal fever with or without pulmonary symptoms resulting from circulating microfilariae. Of these entities, loiasis is most commonly seen in travelers and short-term residents of risk areas (rainforest regions of Central Africa). Eosinophilia is common in patients with filariasis. The diagnosis is usually established by the demonstration of microfilariae in skin snips (onchocerciasis) or in blood. (*Note*: in lymphatic filariasis, the microfilariae circulate nocturnally, while microfilaremia of *Loa loa* peaks in the late afternoon.) Serologic study may be helpful when the disease is suspected (see Chapter 47).

Strongyloidiasis

Strongyloidiasis, usually acquired when larvae in contaminated soil penetrate the skin, rarely causes a febrile illness in travelers. However, a Löffler syndrome, characterized by pulmonary infiltrates with eosinophilia, may occur during the obligate lung migration phase of larvae and may be accompanied by fever. Immunocompromised hosts, particularly due to HTLV-1 or corticosteroids, can develop a life-threatening hyperinfection syndrome, which is frequently complicated by significant disseminated strongyloidiasis outside the gastrointestinal tract (see Chapter 45).

Trichinosis

Trichinosis, usually associated with high-grade eosinophilia, muscle pain, and fever, can be acquired by travelers who ingest undercooked meat (see Chapter 49).

Paragonimiasis

Paragonimiasis is an illness caused by a lung fluke that induces a febrile response either during its migration to the lungs or by its obstruction or destruction of lung parenchyma. Hemoptysis can occur, mimicking pulmonary tuberculosis. The disease is usually acquired by ingestion of raw freshwater crustaceans in Asia, South America, and Africa, though case series are reported in the United States from imported freshwater crab or local crawfish ingestion. Diagnosis can be established by examination of the sputum and stool for ova. Serologic studies are available (see Chapter 48).

Echinococcosis

The ingestion of food or water contaminated by echinococcal eggs from canid feces can cause hydatid cyst disease involving the lungs or liver. Fever is usually absent unless the cyst or cysts become secondarily infected or rupture (see Chapter 46).

Protozoa

Amebiasis

E. histolytica is usually acquired by ingesting cysts in water or food contaminated by human feces but may be transmitted sexually. Both amebic dysentery and amebic liver abscess may cause fever. Amebic liver abscess is associated with right upper quadrant discomfort, hepatomegaly, an elevated right hemidiaphragm, and high serologic reactivity to *E. histolytica* antigens. Often, *E. histolytica* cannot be identified in the stool at the time of presentation of amebic abscess. Treatment is with metronidazole plus another agent to clear luminal cysts, such as iodoquinol (see Chapter 32).

Chagas Disease

Chagas disease (American trypanosomiasis), caused by infection with *Trypanosoma cruzi*, is typically acquired by dwelling in mud or thatched-roof housing, via the feces of the reduviid bug, which defecates on the patient during a silent blood meal. In addition, transmission in Latin America is often congenital or via blood transfusion in endemic countries and occasionally in the United States. It is increasingly recognized as a food-borne illness when cane-sweetened juices are contaminated by crushed reduviid bugs. In typical transmission, after an incubation period of 1-2 weeks, *T. cruzi* causes a febrile illness during the acute stage of infection that persists for 2-4 weeks. The illness is accompanied by local swelling at the site of inoculation of trypanosomes (Romaña sign), lymphadenopathy, hepatosplenomegaly, and influenza-like symptoms. Trypanosomes may be seen during the acute stage of infection in peripheral blood by blood smear or in biopsy specimens obtained from the site of inoculation. Serology studies may be helpful. Treatment during the acute stage of infection with benznidazole or nifurtimox is beneficial in attenuating the progression to chronic Chagas disease. This disease is rare among travelers but is increasingly recognized in non-endemic countries among Latin American immigrants (see Chapter 26).

African Trypanosomiasis

African trypanosomiasis (infection with *Trypanosoma brucei gambiense* or *T. brucei rhodesiense*) cause febrile syndromes due to circulating trypanosomes. West African disease often presents in a subacute or chronic fashion, whereas East African disease is less well adapted to humans and thus has a more fulminant course. Both diseases are transmitted by the bite of the tsetse fly in Africa. Occasionally, a chancre can be seen at the site of inoculation during acute infection. Lymphadenopathy is common, particularly in the posterior cervical chain. Later, the trypanosomes invade the central nervous system, and lumbar puncture must be performed to determine which treatment regimen should be administered. If disease has progressed to the central nervous system, treatment with arsenicals, such as melarsoprol, or difluoromethylornithine is recommended for East and West African trypanosomiasis, respectively. African trypanosomiasis is uncommon among travelers, although clusters have been reported, mainly in travelers returning from East Africa. Both East and West African disease are ultimately fatal without treatment, so recognition and rapid action is essential (see Chapter 27).

Visceral Leishmaniasis

Visceral leishmaniasis, or kala-azar, is characterized by hepatosplenomegaly, severe wasting, and fevers, a syndrome evocative of lymphoma. *Leishmania* spp. are transmitted by the bite of the sand fly. The kala-azar syndrome is usually caused by *Leishmania donovani*. Visceral leishmaniasis is extremely uncommon among travelers. Treatment is with amphotericin B in lipid formulations, pentavalent antimonials, or miltefosine (see Chapter 39).

Toxoplasmosis

Toxoplasmosis, which can cause an acute febrile syndrome, may be acquired by travelers via the consumption of undercooked meat. Transmission may occur in unexpected places, such as France, where infection with *Toxoplasma gondii* is much more common because of the popular ingestion of uncooked meat.

Bacteria

Tuberculosis

Tuberculosis is an uncommon disease among short-term travelers (**Table 20.1**). Travelers at increased risk are those going abroad to perform medical service and those residing abroad for prolonged lengths of time. Occasionally, tuberculosis transmission has been reported among air travelers as the result of relatively poor air turnover on airlines and the presence of a passenger with active pulmonary tuberculosis. In a study of American healthcare workers returning from Botswana, tuberculin skin test conversion occurred in 4.2%, corresponding to a rate of 6.87 per 1000 person-weeks of travel (Szep et al. 2014). Healthcare workers, missionaries, teachers, and others who anticipate close daily contact with resident populations in countries where the incidence of tuberculosis is high should receive the tuberculin skin test before travel to establish a baseline status, and 8-12 weeks following travel (see Chapter 25).

Meningococcal Meningitis

Meningococcal infection occurs sporadically in travelers to endemic areas (sub-Saharan Africa and Nepal) and in epidemics during times of crowding. An example of the latter is the reported high incidence of meningococcal disease and carriage after pilgrimage to Mecca. Purpuric lesions and signs of meningismus are helpful diagnostic clues, but individuals may present with only fever and respiratory symptoms. Diagnosis is established by culture of blood and cerebrospinal fluid, and treatment with parenteral ceftriaxone is usually effective. Close contacts of documented cases should receive prophylaxis with rifampin or ciprofloxacin. Travelers going to areas of known meningococcal transmission should undergo meningococcal vaccination before departure (see Chapter 5).

Leptospirosis

Leptospirosis is acquired by contact with water contaminated by animal urine containing spirochetes. It is common in the tropics and subtropics (Chapter 23). This disease may be contracted by abattoir workers, swimmers, and campers. Large outbreaks have occurred among triathletes in Illinois (98 cases) and competitive swimmers in Borneo (70 cases). Clinical illness ranges from relatively mild disease to fulminant hepatic failure with icterohemorrhagic fever (Weil's disease). Definitive diagnosis is based on either serologic studies or the demonstration of leptospires in specimens of clinical fluids. As with rickettsioses, empiric treatment is often considered.

Brucellosis

Brucellosis is usually transmitted by unpasteurized dairy products but may be encountered in abattoirs. Illness ranges from an indolent febrile syndrome to fulminant endocarditis. Brucellosis is occasionally encountered in the post travel setting, although laboratory acquisition is well documented and remains a risk for medical and laboratory workers who volunteer or work overseas. In their study of >42,000 ill returned travelers entered into the GeoSentinel database between 2007 and 2011, Leder and colleagues (2013) reported 33 cases of acute brucellosis, most of which were acquired in India, the Sudan, and Iraq.

Plague

Plague is reported to be epidemic in humans in certain regions of Vietnam and is endemic in rodent populations in the southwestern United States and other areas of the world. Larger outbreaks can occur, as in India in 1994. Plague causes a clinical syndrome of painful regional lymphadenitis associated with necrotizing pneumonia and septicemia. Prophylactic doxycycline may be given to travelers at risk, since the plague vaccine is not widely available (see Chapter 5).

Melioidosis

Melioidosis, caused by the Gram-negative bacterium *Burkholderia pseudomallei*, produces a tuberculosis-like illness or septicemia. The disease is particularly prevalent in Southeast Asia, where it is especially common in rice-paddy workers. Many Vietnam veterans have serologic evidence of past infection with *B. pseudomallei*. Like tuberculosis, the bacteria may remain dormant for many years before reactivating and causing illness.

Relapsing Fever

Relapsing fever (caused by *Borrelia* species) is a worldwide tick-borne endemic disease, but louse-borne human–human transmission still occurs in highlands of Ethiopia, Sudan, Somalia, Chad, Bolivia, and Peru. Diagnosis depends on the demonstration of extracellular spirochetes by blood smear and Giemsa staining.

Bartonellosis (Oroya Fever)

Bartonellosis, caused by *Bartonella bacilliformis*, is transmitted by sand flies only in Andean river valleys with elevations between 2000 and 8000 ft in Peru, Ecuador, and Colombia. This infection can lead to acute hemolysis (i.e., Oroya fever), in which intraerythrocytic organisms may be detected on pathologic stains (e.g., Giemsa) or in chronic, angioproliferative skin lesions (i.e., verruga peruana, lesions that may be sessile, miliary, nodular, pedunculated, or confluent and may be as large as 1-2 cm). A newly described species, *Bartonella rochalimae*, was reported to cause an Oroya fever-like illness, characterized by anemia, fever, and splenomegaly, in an American traveler to Peru (Eremeeva et al. 2007). The patient had been traveling in an area endemic for *B. bacilliformis*, but to date, no clear vector has been identified. This case highlights the sustained possibility of discovering novel pathogens as international travel becomes increasingly attractive and affordable.

Anthrax

Cutaneous anthrax generally has been associated with exposure to infected animals, contaminated animal hides, and wool. Because *Bacillus anthracis* spores can survive for prolonged periods, contaminated hides or wool remain infectious and may rarely be responsible for disease transmission. Anthrax is sometimes associated with a local eschar, where bacteria proliferate and invade the bloodstream. Travelers purchasing souvenirs or articles of clothing made with contaminated animal hides or wool are a group at theoretical risk for the acquisition of anthrax; hunters are another potential group at risk. In contrast, inhalational anthrax is usually thought to be associated with bioterrorism.

Sexually Transmitted Infections

Gonorrhea, syphilis, chlamydia, lymphogranuloma venereum, herpes simplex virus, HIV, granuloma inguinale, and chancroid are all sexually transmitted diseases that may give rise to fevers (see Chapters 41-44).

Viruses

Respiratory and Enteric Viruses

Common respiratory and enteric viruses are the most common causes of fever in travelers, accounting for over 50% of cases of febrile illness in travelers in most case series.

Hepatitis

Hepatitis viruses are a relatively common cause of fever in travelers (100-200/100,000 travelers); prodromal symptoms associated with fever may precede icterus. Hepatitis A occurs most frequently, but >90% of cases could be prevented by pre-travel immunization with hepatitis A vaccine. Adults over the age of 40 years who acquire hepatitis A are at much greater risk of having a complicated course or dying of their disease than are those who are younger. Hepatitis B and C may occur in healthcare workers, individuals with a history of sexual contact abroad, and patients who receive blood transfusions, although the hepatitis B immunization is also highly effective (see Chapter 22). Hepatitis E has been serologically confirmed in many returned travelers; it undoubtedly occurs more often. In long-term travelers to the developing world, the seroconversion rate for hepatitis E is ~5%.

Human Immunodeficiency Virus (HIV)

Acute HIV infection, resulting from sexual activity, blood transfusion, and intravenous drug use, has been reported among returned travelers (see Chapter 41). In their analysis of GeoSentinel data, Leder and colleagues (2013) reported 84 cases of acute HIV among >42,000 ill returned travelers, making HIV the seventh most common specific cause of fever in this group. Rash and lymphadenopathy combined with appropriate history can be clues to suspect primary infection. Plasma RNA levels are more sensitive than serodiagnostic tests, which may be negative in the early period of infection.

Infectious Mononucleosis

Acute infection with Epstein-Barr virus (EBV) may occur in susceptible travelers, especially in the 15- to 30-year-old age group. Hepatosplenomegaly, lymphadenopathy, mucopurulent pharyngitis, heterophile antibodies, and the presence of atypical lymphocytes on the blood smear are helpful clues. Specific EBV serologies are useful to establish the diagnosis of acute infection. Cytomegalovirus (CMV) infections may cause an infectious mononucleosis-like illness with elevated hepatic transaminases in travelers and may be diagnosed by CMV serologies.

Measles

Rubeola (measles) remains an important cause of morbidity and mortality in developing countries and poses a substantial risk to travelers who have not received adequate immunization. Furthermore, the syndrome of atypical measles may result from exposure to wild virus in individuals who may have received killed virus vaccine (used in the United States before 1963). A large outbreak involving a US theme park in 2014 underscored the risk of measles to unvaccinated individuals and the risk of exported disease via commercial air travel. Complications of measles include progressive pneumonitis (especially in pregnant or immunocompromised patients), pulmonary bacterial superinfection, and encephalitis.

Fungi

Endemic mycoses such as histoplasmosis and coccidioidomycosis are becoming increasingly recognized among international travelers and can present as undifferentiated fever. Among 13 cases of acute pulmonary histoplasmosis in a group of US travelers to Martinique, trekking through a mountain tunnel full of bats emerged as the common epidemiologic risk factor. Participation in construction projects at an orphanage in Tecate, Mexico was similarly associated with a cluster of cases of coccidioidomycosis among US travelers. Penicilliosis can also be acquired by travelers. Endemic mycoses can present as a systemic febrile or flu-like illness, with or without accompanying respiratory, cutaneous, or articular manifestations, and should therefore be considered in the differential diagnosis of post-travel fever.

FURTHER READING

Abramowicz, M. (Ed.), 2013. Drugs for parasitic infections. Med. Lett. 11 (Suppl.), 1.

Ackers, M.L., Puhr, N.D., Tauxe, R.V., et al., 2000. Laboratory-based surveillance of *Salmonella* serotype Typhi infections in the United States: antimicrobial resistance on the rise. JAMA 283, 2668–2673.

Boggild, A., Ghesquiere, W., McCarthy, A., et al., 2011. Fever in the returning international traveller: initial assessment guidelines. Can. Commun. Dis. Rep. 37 (ACS-3), 1–15. Available at: <http://www.phac-aspc.gc.ca/publicat/ccdr-rmtc/11vol37/acs-3/index-eng.php> (accessed July 2, 2015).

Bottieau, E., Clerinx, J., Van den Enden, E., et al., 2006. Etiology and outcome of fever after a stay in the tropics. Arch. Intern. Med. 166, 1642.

Cairns, L., Blythe, D., Kao, A., et al., 2000. Outbreak of coccidioidomycosis in Washington state residents returning from Mexico. Clin. Infect. Dis. 30, 61.

Centers for Disease Control and Prevention, 2001. Update: outbreak of acute febrile illness among athletes participating in Eco-Challenge-Sabah 2000—Borneo, Malaysia, 2000. MMWR 50, 21–24.

Centers for Disease Control and Prevention, 2014. Summary of notifiable diseases—United States, 2013. MMWR 63 (32), 702–715. Available at: <http://www.cdc.gov/mmwr/preview/mmwrhtml/mm6332a6.htm> (accessed July 2, 2015).

Chertow, D.S., Kleine, C., Edwards, J.K., et al., 2014. Ebola virus disease in West Africa: clinical manifestations and management. N. Engl. J. Med. 371 (22), 2054–2057 [E-pub ahead of print, DOI: 10.1056/NEJMp1413084].

El Bashir, H., Coen, P.G., Haworth, E., et al., 2004. Meningococcal W135 carriage; enhanced surveillance amongst east London Muslim pilgrims and their household contacts before and after attending the 2002 Hajj. Travel Med. Infect. Dis. 2, 13–15.

Eremeeva, M.E., Gerns, H.L., Lydy, S.L., et al., 2007. Bacteremia, fever, and splenomegaly caused by a newly recognized Bartonella species. N. Engl. J. Med. 356, 2381.

Freedman, D.O., Weld, L.H., Kozarsky, P.E., et al., 2006. Spectrum of disease and relationship to place of exposure in ill returned travelers. N. Engl. J. Med. 354, 119.

Hill, D.R., 2000. Health problems in a large cohort of Americans traveling to developing countries. J. Travel Med. 7, 259–266.

Huggins, J.W., 1989. Prospects for treatment of viral hemorrhagic fevers with ribavirin, a broad-spectrum antiviral drug. Rev. Infect. Dis. 11, S750–S761.

Janisch, T., Preiser, W., Berger, A., et al., 1997. Emerging viral pathogens in long-term expatriates (I): hepatitis E virus. Trop. Med. Int. Health 2, 885–891.

Jelinek, T., Bisoffi, Z., Bonazzi, L., et al., 2002. Cluster of African trypanosomiasis in travelers to Tanzanian national parks. Emerg. Infect. Dis. 8, 634–635.

Jensenius, M., Davis, X., von Sonnenburg, F., et al., GeoSentinel Surveillance Network, 2009. Multicenter GeoSentinel analysis of rickettsial diseases in international travelers, 1996-2008. Emerg. Infect. Dis. 15 (11), 1791–1798.

Leder, K., Torresi, J., Libman, M., et al., 2013. GeoSentinel surveillance of illness in returned travelers, 2007–2011. Ann Int Med 158, 456–468.

Levy, M.J., Herrera, J.L., DiPalma, J.A., 1998. Immune globulin and vaccine therapy to prevent hepatitis A infection. Am. J. Med. 105, 416–423.

Lewis, M.D., Serichantalergs, O., Pitarangsi, C., et al., 2005. Typhoid fever: a massive, single-point source, multidrug resistant outbreak in Nepal. Clin. Infect. Dis. 40, 554–561.

Liles, W.C., Van Voorhis, W.C., 1999. Fever in travelers to tropical countries. In: Root, R.K., Waldvogel, F., Corey, L., Stamm, W.E. (Eds.), Clinical Infectious Diseases: A Practical Approach. Oxford University Press, New York.

Lynch, M.F., Blanton, E.M., Bulens, S., et al., 2009. Typhoid fever in the United States, 1999–2006. JAMA 302 (8), 859–865.

Meltzer, E., Artom, G., Marra, E., et al., 2006. Schistosomiasis among travelers: new aspects of an old disease. Emerg. Infect. Dis. 12, 1696–1700.

Morgan, J., Bornstein, S.L., Karpati, A.M., et al., 1998. Outbreak of leptospirosis among triathlon participants and community residents in Springfield, Illinois, 1998. Clin. Infect. Dis. 34, 1593.

Panackal, A.A., Hajjeh, R.A., Cetron, M.S., et al., 2002. Fungal infections among returned travelers. Clin. Infect. Dis. 35, 1088.

Public Health Agency of Canada, Committee to Advise on Tropical Medicine and Travel, 2011. Fever in the Returning International Traveller. Available at: <http://www.phac-aspc.gc.ca/publicat/ccdr-rmtc/11vol37/acs-3/index-eng.php>.

Qin, E., Bi, J., Zhao, M., et al., 2015. Clinical features of patients with Ebola virus disease in Sierra Leone. Clin. Infect. Dis. 61, 491–495 [E-pub ahead of print, May 20. pii: civ319].

Rigau-Perez, J.G., Clark, G.G., Gubler, D.J., et al., 1998. Dengue and haemorrhagic fever. Lancet 352, 971.

Ryan, E.T., Wilson, M.E., Kain, K.C., 2002. Illness after international travel. N. Engl. J. Med. 347, 505.

Salata, R.A., Olds, R.G., 1990. Infectious diseases in travelers and immigrants. In: Warren, K.S., Mahmoud, A.A.F. (Eds.), Tropical and Geographic Medicine, second ed. McGraw-Hill, New York.

Salomon, J., Flament Saillour, M., De Truchis, P., et al., 2003. An outbreak of acute pulmonary histoplasmosis in members of a trekking trip in Martinique, French West Indies. J. Travel Med. 10, 87.

Schwartz, E., Shlim, D.R., Eaton, M., et al., 1990. The effect of oral and parenteral typhoid vaccination on the rate of infection with *Salmonella typhi* and *Salmonella paratyphi* A among foreigners in Nepal. Arch. Intern. Med. 150, 349.

Slom, T.J., Cortese, M.M., Gerber, S.I., et al., 2002. An outbreak of eosinophilic meningitis caused by travelers returning from the Caribbean. N. Engl. J. Med. 346, 668.

Stetten, R., Rickenbach, M., Wilhelm, U., et al., 1987. Health problems after travel to developing countries. J. Infect. Dis. 156, 84.

Szep, Z., Kim, R., Ratcliffe, S.J., et al., 2014. Tuberculin skin test conversion rate among short-term health care workers returning from Gaborone, Botswana. Travel Med. Infect. Dis. 12 (4), 396–400.

Wilder-Smith, A., Schwartz, E., 2005. Dengue in travelers. N. Engl. J. Med. 353, 924.

Wilson, M.E., 1991. A World Guide to Infections: Diseases, Distribution, Diagnosis. Oxford University Press, New York.

Wilson, M.E., Weld, L.H., Boggild, A., et al., 2007. Fever in returned travelers: Results from the GeoSentinel Surveillance Network. Clin. Infect. Dis. 44, 1560.

World Health Organization (WHO), 2009. Dengue: Guidelines for Diagnosis, Treatment, Prevention and Control. WHO, Geneva.

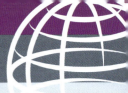

CHAPTER 21

Malaria Diagnosis and Treatment

Kathrine R. Tan and Paul M. Arguin

GENERAL CONSIDERATIONS

Malaria is preventable by taking chemoprophylaxis and using mosquito avoidance measures (Chapter 6). However, healthcare providers should be knowledgeable about the work-up of malaria, as it is not uncommon for a returned traveler to present with fever. When a patient presents with fever, healthcare providers working in malaria-free areas might not consider malaria in the differential diagnosis, especially since this disease can mimic other illnesses, such as influenza or gastroenteritis. However, undiagnosed and untreated malaria can progress rapidly to death. Therefore, healthcare workers must obtain a travel history from patients who present with fever. All febrile patients who have traveled to a malaria-endemic area should be rapidly evaluated for malaria. Patients at risk for malaria most commonly come from one of the following groups:

1. Visitors, immigrants, and refugees from a malaria-endemic area
2. Travelers, regardless of duration of stay (e.g., tourist, business traveler, expatriate), especially first- and second-generation immigrants returning to their countries of origin to visit friends and relatives
3. Military personnel assigned abroad.
   Other groups in which malaria infrequently occurs include:
1. Recipients of blood transfusions or organ or tissue transplant
2. Infants of mothers who have lived or traveled in an endemic area (congenital infections)
3. Injection drug users (parenteral transmission)
4. Residents of non-endemic areas where local transmission might occur from undiagnosed imported infections. For example, Greece and Jamaica, both malaria non-endemic, had outbreaks originating from imported cases of malaria between 2011-2013 and 2006-2011, respectively.

ETIOLOGY

Malaria is a vector-borne protozoan parasite infection spread from person to person in endemic areas by female mosquitoes of the genus *Anopheles*. Four species of malaria regularly cause disease in humans, including *Plasmodium falciparum*, *P. vivax*, *P. ovale*, and *P. malariae*. *P. knowlesi*, a cause of malaria in long-tailed macaques, also naturally infects humans in Southeast Asia, most notably in Malaysia.

PRESENTATION

Epidemiology

In 2013 there were approximately 198 million cases of malaria worldwide, and 500,000 deaths, mostly in children in sub-Saharan Africa. Malaria is endemic in most tropical areas

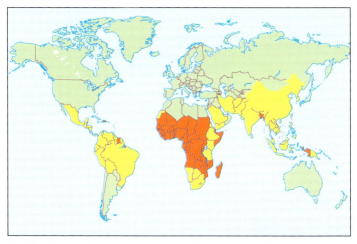

Fig. 21.1 Malaria-endemic countries shown in red (malaria everywhere) and yellow (malaria in select areas) (CDC 2014).

of the world (**Fig. 21.1**). Transmission of malaria can vary within a country and is affected by multiple factors, such as season, altitude, and urbanization. Migration and travel can potentially introduce malaria to previously malaria-free areas where the mosquito vector is present. Drug resistance is an increasing problem. Chloroquine-resistant *P. falciparum* is widespread, and there are very few areas (e.g., Central America west of the Panama Canal, the Dominican Republic, and Haiti) where chloroquine can still effectively treat *falciparum* malaria. Multidrug-resistant *P. falciparum* is present in parts of Southeast Asia, and chloroquine-resistant *P. vivax* is found in parts of Indonesia and Papua New Guinea. Resistance to sulfadoxine-pyrimethamine (Fansidar®) is also widespread.

Malaria endemicity and antimalarial drug resistance can change over time, so healthcare providers should always refer to the most up-to-date information when giving advice to a traveler or when managing malaria. A list of countries and their malaria-related information can be found in "Health Information for International Travel" (the "Yellow Book"), a publication prepared by the Centers for Disease Control and Prevention (CDC) and available online (http://www.cdc.gov/travel/). Reports from the field by way of returned travelers, the news media, and other nonmedical news sources should be confirmed by checking official postings from the CDC (www.cdc.gov/travel or www.CDC.gov/malaria) and World Health Organization (http://www.who.int).

PATHOGENESIS

Natural Life Cycle

After inoculation of the malaria parasites (sporozoites) during feeding by a female anopheline mosquito, the sporozoites invade the liver parenchymal cells within minutes, and then replicate during an asymptomatic incubation period (pre-erythrocytic schizogony) that can last between 1 and 3 weeks but can be as long as a year (*P. vivax*). Relapsing species, *P. vivax* and *P. ovale*, can form hypnozoites in the liver, a dormant stage that can cause relapses weeks to months after the initial infection. Eventually, the hepatic schizonts rupture and parasites (merozoites) are released into the bloodstream, where red blood cells are rapidly infected (erythrocytic stage) (**Fig. 21.2**).

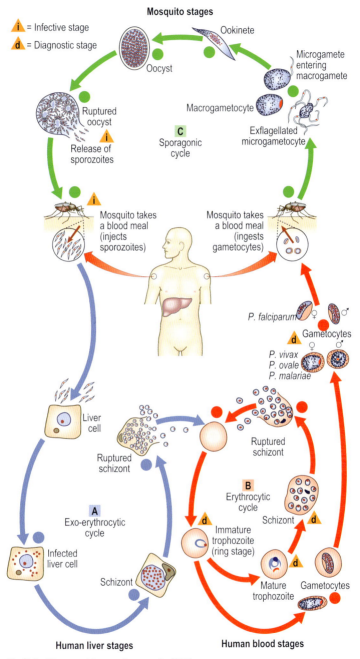

Fig. 21.2   Life cycle of *Plasmodium* parasite (CDC).

1. The merozoites mature in infected red cells, and early stages are called trophozoites, resembling signet rings. The blood-stage infection causes the symptoms and signs of malaria.
2. Most trophozoites undergo asexual division within the red cells to form a schizont, or ball of new merozoites. During this process, the erythrocyte's hemoglobin is consumed. Eventually the cell bursts, liberating new merozoites that invade new red cells. For *P. falciparum*, *P. vivax*, and *P. ovale*, the duration of the asexual life cycle is 48 hours, for *P. malariae* 72 hours, and for *P. knowlesi* 24 hours.
3. After asexual reproduction some merozoites will develop into sexual forms of the parasite called gametocytes. These transmissible stages are ingested by another feeding anopheline mosquito, fuse in the mosquito's midgut to form a zygote, develop in the wall of the gut, and then migrate to the mosquito's salivary gland to complete the cycle.

Pathophysiology

Each of the species has a variable incubation period (the interval between infection and the onset of clinical illness). Incubation periods can be as short as 1 week (rare) or between 2 and 4 weeks (more common), but they can be much longer for vivax or ovale malaria or if the infection is suppressed by partial adherence to chemoprophylaxis. The erythrocytic stage of the infection is associated with spiking fevers and chills, but relapsing fever is not necessarily seen. Fever and illness are caused by the release of proinflammatory cytokines (particularly tumor necrosis factor) and other inflammatory mediators. Cytokines are responsible for many features of severe malaria, but microvascular obstruction is the primary pathologic process. The pathology of severe falciparum malaria is associated with the sequestration of infected red cells in the microvasculature of vital organs. Thus, the pathologies of sepsis and severe malaria are different.

Falciparum malaria may progress rapidly to parasitize a large number of erythrocytes, with severe systemic consequences of multiple organ failure and death unless treated immediately. *P. falciparum* infections are potentially lethal for several reasons:

1. Each blood-stage schizont liberates up to 32 merozoites when it ruptures, potentially infecting many red blood cells quickly.
2. *P. falciparum* causing severe malaria parasitizes circulating red cells of all ages (in contrast to *P. vivax*, which tends to infect young cells only, and *P. malariae*, which has a predilection for older cells).
3. Erythrocytes containing mature forms of *P. falciparum* stick to the endothelium of capillaries and post-capillary venules (cytoadherence). The resulting sequestration results from the interaction between antigenically variant parasite-derived adhesive proteins expressed on the surface of infected erythrocytes and specific receptors on the vascular endothelium. In addition, the deformability of both parasitized and uninfected erythrocytes is markedly reduced in severe malaria. The subsequent interference with microcirculatory flow and regional metabolism is most evident in the brain, resulting in cerebral malaria, but also occurs in the other vital organs. Sequestration accounts for the frequently observed discrepancy between the peripheral parasite count and disease severity and also explains the relative rarity with which mature trophozoites and schizonts are seen in the peripheral blood in falciparum malaria.

Although malaria can be severe with *P. vivax*, *P. ovale*, and *P. malariae* infections, clinical attacks are less likely to be fatal because cytoadherence and sequestration do not occur with these species of malaria. For *P. vivax* and *P. ovale* infections, the hypnozoite, or dormant, stage can cause relapses weeks to months after the initial infection.

Immunity to Malaria

The immune response to malaria infections is incomplete, and frequent repeated attacks are required to induce a degree of protective immunity, which is rapidly lost if the individual leaves the endemic area. Acquired immunity is specific for both the species of malaria and the particular strain(s) causing the infection. The development of immunity to *P. falciparum* is gained at the expense of a high mortality in children living in areas of heavy transmission. For this reason, severe malaria is a disease of childhood in these areas, and adults who have gained protective immunity are less likely to develop severe manifestations, so long as they continue to be exposed via more infected mosquito bites. Without this boosting effect, immunity will wane in time. Thus, in contrast to adult residents of areas of heavy malaria transmission, non-immune travelers—including immigrants—of all ages coming from areas without malaria to malaria-endemic areas are vulnerable to developing severe and potentially fatal infections.

CLINICAL FEATURES

The symptoms and signs of malaria are nonspecific and are most commonly fever, chills, myalgias, and headache. Malaria may present as febrile seizures in children or coma (cerebral malaria). It may be mistaken for infectious hepatitis when jaundice is prominent, for pneumonia when there is respiratory distress, or for enteric infections with fever, vomiting, abdominal pain, and diarrhea. Furthermore, malaria may exist in a patient with other acute travel-related illnesses. Therefore, clinicians should suspect and test for malaria in *all febrile patients* who traveled to a malaria-endemic area.

Malaria is typically classified as either uncomplicated or severe. Indicators for severe malaria are listed in **Table 21.1**. Patients need to have only one of these indicators to have severe malaria; however, patients with severe malaria usually meet multiple criteria.

Hyperparasitemia is defined as more than 5% erythrocytes parasitized. All patients with malaria should have their percent parasitemia calculated at the time of diagnosis, as it is not uncommon for hyperparasitemia to be the only factor that categorizes the patient as having severe malaria requiring parenteral medicine; early initiation of parenteral treatment prior to the development of clinical complications can improve the chances of prompt and complete recovery.

Cerebral malaria can present with either focal or generalized neurologic features, most commonly, altered mental status, seizures (especially in children), or coma. It must be distinguished from other causes of fever and altered consciousness (e.g., bacterial or viral meningoencephalitis).

Acute kidney injury results from acute tubular necrosis. Some patients may develop brisk hemolysis and hemoglobinuric renal failure ("blackwater fever").

Acute respiratory distress syndrome (ARDS), defined as respiratory distress from pulmonary inflammation and characterized by severe hypoxemia with bilateral pulmonary infiltrates on radiograph, is associated with a high mortality. ARDS can occur with all species of

---

TABLE 21.1   Criteria for Severe Malaria

Malaria is severe if one or more of the following is present:
- Acidosis
- Acute respiratory distress syndrome
- Seizures
- Disseminated intravascular congestion
- Hyperparasitemia (>5%)
- Hypoglycemia
- Impaired consciousness
- Jaundice
- Acute kidney injury or macroscopic hemoglobinuria
- Severe anemia (Hb < 7 g/dL)
- Shock

malaria. Respiratory distress in patients with malaria can also be due to metabolic acidosis, iatrogenic volume overload from overly aggressive fluid resuscitation resulting in pulmonary edema, transfusion-related lung injury, and secondary nosocomial pneumonia.

Glucose levels fall in severe malaria infections as a result of increased metabolic demands by the host and parasites, and decreased gluconeogenesis. Hypoglycemia most commonly develops in women in late pregnancy and children with severe malaria, which is hazardous to the viability of the pregnancy. It is usually accompanied by lactic acidosis. Quinine stimulates pancreatic insulin secretion and is an important cause of hypoglycemia.

Severe anemia is defined as hemoglobin levels <7 g/dL. The hematocrit falls rapidly in severe malaria because of the accelerated clearance of both parasitized and unparasitized erythrocytes. The anemia is compounded by bone marrow dyserythropoiesis.

Another poor prognostic indicator is disseminated intravascular coagulation that presents as abnormal bleeding (e.g., petechiae, ecchymosis, bleeding from intravenous lines), thrombocytopenia, and abnormal clotting or coagulation laboratory values. Some degree of thrombocytopenia (at or even below 100,000/μL) is usually seen in all symptomatic malaria cases. Thrombocytopenia alone is not a criterion for severe malaria.

Patients with severe malarial infections are more vulnerable to bacterial infections, such as aspiration pneumonia and spontaneous septicemia with Gram-negative bacteria (particularly nontyphoidal salmonellae), especially in children.

Chronic malaria can manifest in residents of highly endemic areas who, through repeated infections, have developed some degree of immunity, resulting in few to no symptoms despite having parasites in their blood. This asymptomatic parasitemia is a major cause of chronic anemia, particularly in young children. Splenomegaly is also a reflection of repeated malaria attacks in children in endemic areas. Splenic rupture occasionally occurs as a complication of *P. vivax* infection in adults. Hyperreactive malarial splenomegaly (or "tropical splenomegaly syndrome") is sometimes seen in adults in endemic areas and presents as hepatosplenomegaly, anemia, abnormal immunologic findings, and immunosuppression. This appears to reflect an exaggerated immune response to repeated infection. Nephrotic syndrome may develop in children chronically infected with *P. malariae* ("quartan nephropathy").

LABORATORY DIAGNOSIS

The diagnosis of malaria is best made by the identification of malaria parasites on the peripheral blood smear. Preparation of thick and thin smears should be done immediately for any febrile patient living in or returning from a malarious area. Because parasitemia waxes and wanes with the parasite's life cycle, these smears should be performed at least three times, 12-24 hours apart, to achieve acceptable negative predictive value. Although Giemsa stains of the blood smear are preferred for determining speciation of the parasite, the modified Wright's stain used for the routine processing of blood smears in clinical hematology laboratories is adequate. Field's stain may also be used. Both thick and thin smears are first screened at low magnification, then examined using a 100× oil immersion objective for at least 300 fields, because symptoms of malaria can occur at lower parasite densities in nonimmune individuals.

Thick smears are much more sensitive than thin smears, but provide less information regarding the species and infection burden. The thick smear is first examined for presence of parasites. If parasites are present, the thin smear is used to determine the species of parasite, and the percent parasitemia, that is, the percentage of red blood cells infected. To quantify malaria parasites, between 500 and 2000 red blood cells should be examined. Both the species of malaria and the percent parasitemia are key pieces of information when selecting therapeutic options.

The CDC offers training workshops and web-based training on malaria diagnosis for laboratory personnel throughout the United States. DPDx also allows telediagnosis, where outside laboratories can email digital images of their microscopy findings to the CDC and receive same-day feedback from CDC staff (http://www.cdc.gov/dpdx/contact.html).

Rapid Diagnostic Test (RDT)

Immunochromatographic strip assays detect malarial antigens in finger-stick blood samples using test strips or cards impregnated with specific antibodies. These are based either on detection of *P. falciparum* histidine-rich protein 2 (HRP-2) or parasite lactate dehydrogenase isoenzymes or aldolase. Unlike microscopy, which requires a microscope and trained technician, RDTs can be used in places without a skilled microscopist. Only the BinaxNOW® Malaria Test is approved by the US Food and Drug Administration (FDA) for use in the United States. Disadvantages include the cost of the test kits, the inability to determine species of malaria and parasite load, and the potential lack of sensitivity at very low parasitemias. Therefore, use of RDTs should be reserved for situations where quality microscopy is not immediately available and should be followed as soon as possible by microscopy to confirm the results, determine the species, and calculate the parasitemia. Also, HRP-2 may persist in the blood for a number of weeks after an infection has been treated, so use of this test is not recommended to diagnose malaria in a symptomatic patient who has already received a treatment course of antimalarials. However, if a retrospective diagnosis is needed in an asymptomatic patient who treated him- or herself with antimalarials, the persistent positivity of the PfHRP-2 test is helpful.

Polymerase Chain Reaction (PCR)

PCR currently has limited use for the acute management of malaria: it is not widely available, and results are not timely. The advantage of PCR, however, is its ability to detect very low sub-microscopic parasitemias and to identify species; therefore, it can be used following microscopy to confirm the malaria species. All malaria cases diagnosed in the United States should have PCR confirmation of species. This service is available at the CDC free of charge (www.CDC.gov/malaria).

Serology

Measuring malaria antibodies in the blood via indirect fluorescent antibody testing can determine whether infection occurred in the past but will not distinguish between recent or remote infection; thus it is not useful in the acute diagnosis of malaria. Serology may be useful for screening blood donors following diagnosis of transfusion-induced malaria or to confirm the diagnosis retrospectively in a patient who has been treated.

TREATMENT

In choosing which treatment course of antimalarials to give to those with laboratory-confirmed malaria, it is important to distinguish between uncomplicated versus severe malaria, to identify the species of malaria, and to identify where the malaria was acquired to assess the potential for drug resistance. Drug choice may also be affected by availability and licensing of the drug, which varies by country. Travelers who took any malaria prophylaxis should not be treated with the same class of antimalarial drug used for prophylaxis.

Uncomplicated Malaria

Most patients with uncomplicated disease can be treated with oral medications. Parenteral treatment should be used for patients who are vomiting, those with severe disease, or infants under 1 year old. Patients with a diagnosis of uncomplicated *P. falciparum* malaria should not go home unaccompanied, since deterioration can occur after treatment has started. Malaria due to *P. ovale* or *P. vivax*, which can cause relapses, should be treated with two medicines: an antimalarial for the acute infection and primaquine to prevent relapses. Administer the first dose of antimalarial drug(s) as soon as the diagnosis is made, and observe the patient. If vomiting occurs within 30 minutes, readminister the full dose (often after an antiemetic); if it occurs between 30 and 60 minutes, readminister half the dose (repeat the full dose if atovaquone-proguanil). If parenteral therapy must be used, change to oral therapy when the patient is alert and able to swallow. Follow the clinical status of the patient regularly until the individual has improved. Most patients will start to feel better and become afebrile 24-48 hours after starting appropriate therapy. Following the level of parasitemia can be useful to assess patients who are not clinically improving. **Tables 21.2** and **21.3** present the regimens recommended for treatment of uncomplicated malaria.

Antimalarial Drugs for Uncomplicated Malaria

Artemisinin-Based Combination Therapies (ACTs)

Artemisinin (qinghaosu) and its derivatives (artesunate, artemether, dihydroartemisinin) are the most rapidly effective of all antimalarials. They are active against all malaria species. Artemisinin derivatives are used in combination with a drug with a slower rate of elimination to increase efficacy, reduce transmission of the infection, and provide mutual protection from drug resistance. Artemether-lumefantrine (Coartem®, Riamet®) is a highly effective, well-tolerated, fixed combination drug for use in both children and adults. Reliable absorption of this lipophilic drug is dependent on coadministration with food containing fat. Currently, artemether-lumefantrine is the only ACT approved by the FDA for use in the United States. Other ACTs in use in other countries include artesunate-mefloquine, artesunate-amodiaquine, artesunate-sulfadoxine-pyrimethamine, and dihydroartemisinin-piperaquine.

Atovaquone-Proguanil

A fixed dose combination of atovaquone and proguanil (Malarone® and generic) can be used to treat all species of malaria. Atovaquone-proguanil is available as an adult tablet (250 mg/100 mg) and as a pediatric tablet (62.5 mg/25 mg). The medication should be taken with food or drink with fat to enhance absorption. It is very well tolerated, and adverse effects are rare. In the event of vomiting within 60 minutes after dosing, the dose should be repeated. Atovaquone should never be given alone, as resistant mutations arise commonly in approximately one-third of patients receiving the drug.

Chloroquine

Chloroquine-resistant falciparum malaria is present in most areas with falciparum malaria, so this drug should not be used for the treatment of *P. falciparum* infections, with the exception of infections that were acquired in Latin American countries west of the Panama Canal, Haiti, and the Dominican Republic. Chloroquine can be used for nonfalciparum malaria. Chloroquine resistance in *P. vivax* has been reported from parts of Indonesia and Papua New Guinea. In such cases, the guidelines for treating uncomplicated falciparum malaria should be followed and primaquine given in addition.

Mefloquine

Mefloquine (Lariam® and generic) can be used to treat uncomplicated malaria caused by all species. At treatment doses, the risk of side effects from mefloquine increases. Mefloquine-resistant *P. falciparum* parasites are found on the eastern border of Myanmar (Burma) and adjacent parts of China, Laos, and Thailand; the western border of Thailand and adjacent parts of Cambodia and Laos; and southern Vietnam.

Primaquine

Primaquine is the only antimalarial that effectively kills the dormant hypnozoites of *P. vivax* and *P. ovale*. When treating vivax or ovale, primaquine must be given in addition to the course of antimalarials for the acute infection. A severe hemolytic reaction to primaquine can occur in patients with glucose 6-phosphate dehydrogenase (G6PD) deficiency; therefore, prior to receiving primaquine for the first time, all patients must be tested and found to have normal G6PD activity.

Drugs No Longer Recommended

Sulfadoxine-pyrimethamine (SP; Fansidar®): strains of falciparum and vivax malaria resistant to sulfadoxine-pyrimethamine are widespread, therefore SP should not be used for treating acute malaria. However, SP continues to have some niche uses such as when used in the intermittent preventive treatment of malaria in pregnancy in highly endemic areas.

TABLE 21.2 Treatment of Uncomplicated Malaria Due to Presumed Chloroquine-Resistant Infections Including if the Species Has Not Yet Been Identified

Recommended treatments (if patient had been on antimalarials for prophylaxis, DO NOT use same antimalarial)

Artemether-lumefantrine (20/120 mg artemether and lumefantrine)

One dose at hours 0, 8, 24, 36, 48, and 60 according to body weight. Administer with food or drink containing fat.

Body weight (kg)	Tablets per dose
5-14	1
15-24	2
25-34	3
>34	4

Artesunate-amodiaquine (available as 25/67.5 mg, 50/135 mg, or 100/270 mg of artesunate and amodiaquine)

4 mg/kg artesunate and 10 mg base/kg amodiaquine once a day for 3 days

Artesunate-mefloquine (separate tablets of 50 mg artesunate and 250 mg mefloquine)

4 mg/kg artesunate once a day for 3 days and mefloquine 25 mg base/kg split over 2 days (15 mg/kg day 1, 10 mg/kg day 2) or 3 days (8.3 mg/kg daily)

Atovaquone-proguanil (Malarone or generic) (adult tablet: 250/100 mg atovaquone and proguanil; pediatric tablet: 62.5/25 mg atovaquone and proguanil)

Adult dosing: 4 adult tablets as a single daily dose for 3 days

Pediatric dosing:

Body Weight (kg)	Tablets per Dose
5-8	2 pediatric tablets
9-10	3 pediatric tablets
11-20	1 adult tablet
21-30	2 adult tablets
31-40	3 adult tablets
>41	4 adult tablets

Dihydroartemisinin plus piperaquine (40/320 mg dihydroartemisinin and piperaquine)

4 mg/kg dihydroartemisinin and 18 mg/kg piperaquine once daily for 3 days

Quinine + doxycycline

Adults: quinine 650 mg (salt) three times a day for 3 days (7 days for infections from Southeast Asia) and doxycycline 100 mg (base) twice a day for 7 days

Pediatric (for children 8 years and older): quinine 10 mg salt/kg three times a day for 3 days (7 days for infections from Southeast Asia) and doxycycline 2.2 mg base/kg twice a day for 7 days

Quinine + clindamycin

Adults: quinine 650 mg (salt) three times a day for 3 days (7 days for infections from Southeast Asia) and clindamycin 20 mg base/kg per day, divided three times a day for 7 days

Pediatric: quinine 10 mg salt/kg three times a day for 3 days (7 days for infections from Southeast Asia) and clindamycin 20 mg base/kg per day, divided three times a day for 7 days

Quinine + tetracycline

Adults: quinine 650 mg (salt) three times a day for 3 days (7 days for infections from Southeast Asia) and tetracycline 250 mg four times a day for 7 days

Pediatric (for children 8 years and older): quinine 10 mg salt/kg three times a day for 3 days (7 days for infections from Southeast Asia) and tetracycline 25 mg/kg per day divided four times a day for 7 days

---

TABLE 21.3   Treatment of Uncomplicated Malaria Acquired in Areas Without Chloroquine Resistance

Select any option from Table 21.2 or
Chloroquine
    Adults: 1000 mg at time 0, followed by 500 mg at 6, 24, and 48 h
    Pediatric: 16.7 mg/kg at time 0, followed by 8.3 mg/kg at 6, 24, and 48 h
For patients with *P. vivax* or *P. ovale*, in addition to acute treatment as described above, confirm absence of G6PD deficiency in patient, and give
Primaquine
    Adults: 52.6 mg (salt) per day for 14 days
    Pediatric: 0.9 mg salt/kg per day for 14 days

G6PD, Glucose 6-phosphate dehydrogenase.

TABLE 21.4   Treatment of Severe Malaria

Immediate treatment with *one* of the following:
    Artesunate (US clinicians can call the CDC to inquire about acquiring artesunate at 770-488-7100)
        2.4 mg/kg IV at 0, 12, 24, and 48 h
On completion of artesunate, a follow-on antimalarial drug (either atovaquone-proguanil, doxycycline, clindamycin, or mefloquine) must be administered to complete treatment.
    Quinine dihydrochloride
        20 mg salt/kg loading dose IV in 5% dextrose or 0.9% saline over 4 h; then maintenance dose of 10 mg salt/kg (infusion rate should not exceed 5 mg salt/kg/h) 3 times a day.
After at least 24 h of parenteral therapy with quinine, and when patient can tolerate oral medications, give a full oral treatment course with one of the drugs listed in Table 21.2.
    Quinidine gluconate (if parenteral quinidine is not available, or intolerance to quinidine is observed, US clinicians can call the CDC to inquire about acquiring artesunate at 770-488-7100)
        Initial dose of 10 mg salt/kg IV infusion over 1-2 h, followed by maintenance dose of 0.02 mg salt/kg/min for at least 24 h. Once parasite density <1% and patient is able to tolerate oral medications, treatment can be completed with an oral regimen. Quinidine can have cardiotoxic adverse effects, so the electrocardiogram must be monitored continuously, and the infusion slowed or stopped if the QTc interval is prolonged by more than 25%.
IV quinidine should be coupled with doxycycline, clindamycin, or tetracycline, as described in Table 21.2.

Halofantrine (Halfan®). halofantrine is not recommended because it prolongs atrioventricular depolarization and ventricular repolarization and has been associated with sudden cardiac death.

Severe Malaria

Severe falciparum malaria is a serious disease with high mortality that requires admission to the intensive care unit (ICU) and the advice of a specialist. Cerebral malaria has a treated mortality of 15-20%. Concurrent meningitis should be considered for all comatose malaria patients. Intravenous antimalarials (**Table 21.4**) should be given as soon as possible after diagnosis and continued until the parasitemia is less than 1% and the patient is able to tolerate oral medicines. There are several intravenous antimalarial options, including artesunate, quinine, and quinidine; the choice of which to use will ultimately depend on availability. For example, in the United States, currently quinidine gluconate is the only FDA-approved parenteral medicine available for the treatment of severe malaria. Parenteral artesunate has been demonstrated to be superior to quinine; two large randomized multicenter trials in East Asia and Africa showed a reduction in mortality in severe malaria patients treated with artesunate compared with quinine. In the United States, parenteral artesunate is available under an investigational new drug protocol registered with the FDA and may be procured from CDC if the patient meets inclusion criteria, as determined by CDC clinicians. To request intravenous artesunate, US clinicians are encouraged to contact the CDC for consultation (telephone number listed on www.CDC.gov/malaria).

Careful hemodynamic monitoring and attention to fluid balance are critical to ensure adequate cardiac output and urine flow while avoiding overhydration.

Hemodialysis should be instituted if indicated. Renal function typically returns slowly to normal after several days or weeks.

The blood glucose level should be checked regularly, particularly in cerebral malaria patients or pregnant women treated with quinine.

Sudden unexplained deterioration in a patient with severe falciparum malaria can be due to hypoglycemia, ARDS, or supervening bacterial septicemia and will ultimately require supportive management.

After an extensive review of the available evidence, exchange transfusion was not found to have any benefit in the outcome of severe malaria. There have been no randomized controlled clinical trials to assess its efficacy, and there is a low likelihood of such trials ever occurring. Furthermore, the rapidity with which exchange transfusion can reduce parasitemia is comparable to that of artemisinins. Therefore, the use of exchange transfusion is no longer recommended in the management of severe malaria.

The use of steroids or heparin is contraindicated as adjunctive treatment of cerebral and other severe forms of falciparum malaria.

Radical Cure of *P. vivax* or *P. ovale* Malaria

In cases of *P. vivax* or *P. ovale* malaria, when the person is not returning shortly to an endemic malarious area, "radical cure" therapy with 14 days of primaquine phosphate (**Table 21.3**) should be started at the time of the last dose of chloroquine, after G6PD deficiency has been excluded. This is done to kill latent malarial parasites in the liver (hypnozoites) and thus prevent future relapses (Chapter 6). There is little evidence of true *P. vivax* resistance to primaquine. Rather, primaquine failure has been reported in patients with decreased activity of the hepatic isoenzyme cytochrome P450 (CYP) 2D6, an isoenzyme involved in drug metabolism believed to be required for primaquine efficacy.

Prevention of Malaria in Travelers

The best management of malaria is through prevention (Chapter 6), by taking measures such as using mosquito repellants and taking chemoprophylaxis. Although there have been promising developments, a useful vaccine available for large-scale deployment in travelers is still thought to be 5-10 years away.

Travelers who reject the advice to take prophylaxis, who choose a sub-optimal drug regimen (such as chloroquine in an area with chloroquine-resistant *P. falciparum*), or who require a less-than-optimal drug regimen for medical reasons are at increased risk for acquiring malaria and needing prompt treatment while overseas. In addition, some travelers who are taking effective prophylaxis but who will be in remote areas may decide, in consultation with their travel health provider, to bring a reliable supply of a full treatment course of antimalarials. If they are diagnosed with malaria, they will have immediate access to this treatment regimen, which is unlikely to be counterfeit and will not deplete local resources. Although empiric clinical diagnosis and self-treatment are discouraged, in rare instances when access to medical care is not available and the traveler develops a febrile illness consistent with malaria, the reliable medication can be self-administered presumptively. Travelers should be advised that this self-treatment is only a temporary measure and that prompt medical evaluation is imperative.

Two malaria treatment regimens can be prescribed as a reliable supply: atovaquone-proguanil and artemether-lumefantrine. The use of the same or related drugs that have been taken for prophylaxis is not recommended to treat malaria. For example, atovaquone-proguanil may be used as a reliable supply medication by travelers not taking atovaquone-proguanil for prophylaxis.

SPECIAL THERAPEUTIC CONSIDERATIONS

Malaria during Pregnancy

Falciparum malaria in non-immune pregnant women carries a high fetal and maternal mortality. The placenta is a site of preferential sequestration of infected red cells. This reservoir of developing parasites interferes with utero-placental function. In endemic areas, the main adverse effects of malaria in pregnancy are low birth weight and maternal anemia; the primigravida is at greatest risk. There are insufficient data on the safety and efficacy of many antimalarials in pregnancy. Therefore if a woman of childbearing age is diagnosed with malaria, clinicians should always ask if she might be pregnant in order to select the most appropriate antimalarial. Treatment of malarial infections in pregnant women should be started in the hospital, since complications are more likely to arise. The use of primaquine, doxycycline, or tetracycline is contraindicated in pregnancy.

Severe malaria should be treated in the same way as for nonpregnant patients. Hypoglycemia is particularly common in pregnant women receiving quinine. Fetal monitoring is essential (if available), as fetal distress is extremely common in malaria and urgent delivery may be necessary to save the baby.

For uncomplicated disease acquired in areas with chloroquine-resistant *P. falciparum*, quinine sulfate plus clindamycin or mefloquine alone can be used during all trimesters of pregnancy. There are insufficient data and unresolved concerns over the use of artemisinin derivatives in the first trimester. However, for the second and third trimesters, there are published reports of >1000 pregnant women, mainly in the second and third trimesters, who have received an artemisinin derivative and have been effectively treated with no adverse outcome for mother or fetus. An artemisinin-combination drug is recommended for the second and third trimesters by the WHO. In the United States, however, artemether-lumefantrine is not yet approved by the FDA for use during any trimester of pregnancy.

It is recommended that a pregnant returned traveler presenting with an episode of acute vivax or ovale malaria should be given a treatment course of antimalarials (options include chloroquine, quinine plus clindamycin, mefloquine, or ACT where approved by local drug authorities), and then should start weekly chloroquine prophylaxis (500 mg salt) until after delivery. Primaquine therapy for a radical cure should be deferred until after delivery, once G6PD has been excluded in both the woman and her infant if she is breastfeeding.

Malaria in Infancy and Childhood

For newborns of mothers with malaria or history of malaria during pregnancy, congenitally transmitted malaria is rare. In these infants, it is best to be vigilant for fever in the first month of life, to do immediate blood smears if fever occurs, and to give appropriate antimalarials once a malaria diagnosis is established. It is not unusual for newborns to present with a transient parasitemia in the first 7 days of life. If a newborn in a non-endemic area is found to have congenital *P. vivax* or *P. ovale*, no primaquine is needed after the initial antimalarial treatment because they do not have hypnozoites. Hypnozoites are formed only from sporozoites acquired from a mosquito bite (**Fig. 21.2**). In congenital malaria, parasites are acquired at the erythrocytic stage of the life cycle from maternal blood. Newborns of mothers who have some degree of immunity to malaria may receive some temporary protection from maternal antibodies.

Among children, the initial attacks of falciparum malaria are often severe and sometimes fatal. Seizures are common, and sudden death may occur. Children are less likely than adults to develop acute kidney injury, acute respiratory distress, or jaundice, but they are more likely to develop seizures, lactic acidosis, hypoglycemia, and severe anemia. Approximately 10% of children surviving cerebral malaria will have a residual neurological deficit (usually hemiplegia). In 50% of cases this resolves, and in 25% there is partial improvement, but 25% do not recover. More subtle residual deficits may be more common. Children with severe malaria should be admitted to an ICU and treated with parenteral antimalarials (**Table 21.4**). In all comatose children, other causes of concurrent meningitis could be considered. For uncomplicated malaria, although infants <12 months of age are usually able to take oral medications, there is some concern of adequate gut absorption, so parenteral antimalarials are preferred. If oral antimalarials are given, but there is doubt that the dose was retained, or the medication was regurgitated, parenteral treatment may be necessary.

Malaria in Patients with Chronic Diseases

It is recommended that for any patient with chronic conditions or taking medications, healthcare providers should refer to the most up-to-date drug reference for potential contraindications to or drug interactions with antimalarials. For example, patients with human immunodeficiency virus infection may be more susceptible to malaria than non-infected individuals, and there are several interactions between antiretrovirals and antimalarials. Concerns of drug interaction should not delay treatment; treatment should be initiated with the treatment least likely to cause interaction.

General Points

Clinicians should report confirmed malaria cases to their respective public health authorities. The National Malaria Surveillance System collects epidemiological and clinical information on malaria cases diagnosed in the United States. In addition, the CDC is conducting surveillance for emerging antimalarial drug resistance. For all cases of malaria diagnosed in the United States, a sample of the original diagnostic blood sample should be sent to the CDC for both species confirmation by PCR and drug resistance testing. These services are available free of charge (http://www.cdc.gov/malaria/features/ars.html/). Patients traveling to malaria-endemic areas should be advised to seek immediate medical attention if they develop fever in order to avoid a delay in diagnosis and treatment. Healthcare providers who need assistance with the diagnosis or management of malaria may call the CDC Malaria Hotline at 770-488-7788 (Monday-Friday, 8:00 a.m.-4:30 p.m., Eastern Standard Time). A CDC Malaria Branch clinician may be consulted outside those hours at 770-488-7100.

COMMONLY ENCOUNTERED PRACTICAL PROBLEMS

Errors of Diagnosis

A. Malaria was not considered in the differential diagnosis because:
  1. Travel history was not taken in a febrile patient. **Take travel history in all patients presenting with fever.**
  2. Malaria symptoms were ascribed to other more common diseases such as influenza or enteric infections. **Suspect and test for malaria in all febrile patients who have traveled to a malaria-endemic area.**
  3. Infection occurred months after leaving an endemic area. **Relapses of vivax or ovale malaria can present late, so obtain travel history in the past year.**
  4. Patient took malaria chemoprophylaxis. **While rare, it is still possible for the patient to get malaria. Malabsorption of chemoprophylactic drugs may also occur from vomiting, diarrhea, or not consuming foods with fat when taking atovaquone-proguanil.**
B. Blood smears for malaria with same-day results are unavailable because a skilled microscopist or pathologist is not available on site after hours, or smears are sent to an off-site laboratory. **Send patients to the nearest health facility with on-site blood smears for malaria.**

C. A rapid diagnostic test (RDT) is done to diagnose or rule out malaria without a follow-up blood smear. **Immediately follow an RDT with a blood smear to confirm findings, determine species, and quantify parasitemia.**

D. Antibody testing is ordered to diagnose acute malaria infection. **Blood smears, not antibody testing, are used to diagnose acute malaria infection.**

E. False-negative blood smear or RDT:

1. Inexperienced staff processing and reading slides, or administering RDTs. **Skilled staff should be available, and if not, refer patients to the nearest hospital with this capability. US clinicians or laboratories needing immediate assistance can call the CDC for telediagnosis.**

2. For microscopy, failure to examine at least 300 fields. **At least 300 fields should be examined to achieve good sensitivity for even low-level parasitemias.**

3. Very low density parasitemias below the threshold of sensitivity for microscopy or RDT. **At least three negative malaria smears spaced 12-24 hours apart are needed to rule out malaria. If doubt of the diagnosis exists, PCR can be done provided results are available in a timely manner.**

F. False-positive blood smear or RDT.

1. Platelets, dirt, or accumulations of stain are misinterpreted as malaria parasites. **If unsure of blood smear reading, obtain diagnostic assistance immediately from a reference laboratory. US laboratories can ask for assistance from either the state laboratories or the CDC.**

2. PfHRP-2 may persist from a recently cured infection. **Obtain a good history of any recent malaria infection and treatment when RDT is being done.**

G. Misidentification of malaria species. *P. ovale* and *P. vivax* can be difficult to distinguish if microscopist is inexperienced. Unrecognized *P. falciparum* or missed in a "mixed" infection (i.e., *P. falciparum* plus another species) has serious consequences considering its drug resistance. **If unsure about species of malaria, diagnostic assistance should be sought. For US laboratories, all cases of malaria should be PCR confirmed; the CDC can provide assistance with determining malaria species.**

Errors of Management

A. Empiric treatment with antimalarials without laboratory testing. **Always do malaria smears to diagnose malaria prior to treatment and to determine species of malaria and percent parasitemia to help select the appropriate antimalarial course.**

B. Failure to admit patients with *P. falciparum*, anyone with signs of severe malaria, young children, and pregnant women. **These patients should be admitted.**

C. Failure to quantify parasitemia. Patients with parasitemias >5% will require treatment for severe malaria. Also, comparison of pre- and post-treatment parasitemia may help gauge response to treatment.

D. False conclusion that a low parasitemia indicates uncomplicated infection. **Patients with low parasitemia, especially non-immune patients, can present with signs of severe infection.**

E. Not treating asymptomatic parasitemia in a semi-immune individual. **The parasitemia still needs treatment with effective antimalarials.**

Therapeutic Dilemmas (Always Seek Expert Advice)

A. Patient has either severe malaria or uncomplicated malaria with nausea and vomiting, is unable to tolerate oral medications, and intravenous antimalarials are unavailable:

1. For patients with uncomplicated malaria, unable to tolerate oral medications, give antiemetic and acetaminophen suppositories and retry oral antimalarials.

2. In the United States, if intravenous quinidine is unavailable, clinicians can call the CDC at 770-488-7100 to request release of parenteral artesunate.

3. Call nearby facilities for parenteral antimalarials.

B. Patient develops severe hemolytic anemia and "blackwater fever" while receiving parenteral quinine or quinidine:
1. Continue the drugs and transfuse as necessary; if acute kidney injury develops, consider hemodialysis.

C. Patient with severe falciparum malaria, treated with recommended course of antimalarials, has persistent signs of severe malaria despite a 0% parasitemia.
1. Do not extend the antimalarial course, as all parasites have been killed. The clinical sequelae of severe malaria such as ARDS or altered mental status may persist despite completing antimalarials.

D. Microscopic examination of repeat blood slides may suggest poor response to the antimalarial drug regimen (defined as <75% reduction from baseline parasitemia by day three of treatment or persistence of any asexual parasitemia by day 7) *or* the patient returns within a few weeks with another acute episode:
1. Ensure adherence to treatment and consider decreased absorption resulting from acute illness, vomiting, or failure to take artemether-lumefantrine or atovaquone-proguanil with food containing fat.
2. Gametocytes of *P. falciparum* are not eliminated by commonly used drug regimens and therefore may persist on smear despite treatment. These are not harmful to the patient, and no further treatment is required. Gametocytes should not be counted in the parasitemia determination.
3. Consider the possibility of resistance and changing to a different antimalarial, preferably an artemisinin-based combination treatment and seek specialist advice.
4. Relapse with a nonfalciparum species may occur after treatment for falciparum malaria, indicating a misdiagnosed mixed infection. In addition to treating the acute infection, give primaquine.

FURTHER READING

Diagnosis of Malaria
CDC, Malaria Diagnosis (US), available at <http://www.cdc.gov/malaria/diagnosis_treatment/diagnosis.html>.

Treatment of Malaria
CDC, Malaria Treatment (US), available at <http://www.cdc.gov/malaria/diagnosis_treatment/treatment.html>.

Dondorp, A., Nosten, F., Stepniewska, K., et al., South East Asian Quinine Artesunate Malaria Trial (SEAQUAMAT) Group, 2005. Artesunate versus quinine for treatment of severe falciparum malaria: a randomised trial. Lancet 366, 717–725.

Phillips, R.E., Warrell, D.A., White, N.J., et al., 1985. Intravenous quinidine for the treatment of severe malaria: clinical and pharmacokinetic studies. N. Engl. J. Med. 312, 1273–1278.

World Health Organization, 2010. Guidelines for the Treatment of Malaria, second ed. WHO, Geneva. Online. Available at <http://www.who.int/malaria/publications/atoz/9789241547925/en/>.

Management Issues in Severe Malaria
Tan, K.R., Wiegand, R.E., Arguin, P.M., 2013. Exchange transfusion for severe malaria: evidence base and literature review. Clin. Infect. Dis. 57 (7), 923–928.

World Health Organization, 2012. Management of Severe Malaria: A Practical Handbook, third ed. WHO, Geneva. Online. Available at <http://www.who.int/malaria/publications/atoz/9789241548526/en/>.

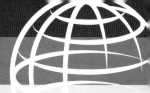

CHAPTER 22

Viral Hepatitis in Travelers and Immigrants

Anne M. Larson and Elaine C. Jong

The various forms of viral hepatitis are a ubiquitous concern for travelers, immigrants, and the healthcare providers responsible for their care (**Table 22.1**). This chapter will cover the five hepatitis viruses that are associated with the majority of human disease: hepatitis A virus (HAV), hepatitis B virus (HBV), hepatitis C virus (HCV), hepatitis D virus (HDV; formerly known as the delta agent), and hepatitis E virus (HEV), formerly known as enterically transmitted non-A, non-B hepatitis (**Table 22.1**). There is evidence to suggest that other types of viral hepatitis also exist, but they have not yet been fully characterized.

Hepatitis A virus is usually transmitted by the fecal-oral route and acquired by ingestion of contaminated food and water. Hepatitis B virus is transmitted through parenteral or mucosal exposure to blood and components, during sexual activities, or from infected mother to unborn child during the birth process. Susceptible travelers originating in areas of low endemicity for HAV and HBV infections going to areas of high endemicity can be immunized against these two vaccine-preventable diseases (**Fig. 22.1**) (Chapter 5). Hepatitis C virus transmission is predominantly through parenteral exposures to blood and components. Sexual transmission is much less common than HBV; however, travelers should be counseled about risk avoidance, as there is as yet no vaccine commercially available. Hepatitis D virus is also transmitted by routes similarly to HBV, but since infection with HBV is the prerequisite for HDV infection, HDV infection is largely prevented by prevention of HBV infection; there is no specific HDV vaccine available. Hepatitis E virus is spread by the fecal-oral route similarly to HAV, and lacking a vaccine against HEV virus (at the time of this publication), travelers need advice about prevention of this infection through selection of safe food and water.

The outcome of an acute viral hepatitis infection depends on the age, co-infections, presence of chronic liver disease, and immune status of the host. With the increasing diversity of international travelers who may have one or more risk factors that will prejudice the outcome of acute hepatitis toward serious sequelae, prevention of travel-acquired hepatitis is of prime importance. Last, in addition to considering the risks of viral hepatitis among departing international travelers, healthcare providers need to be aware of the epidemiology of the various forms of viral hepatitis, the existence of carrier states, and the differential diagnosis of hepatitis in providing care to returning travelers and to newly arrived immigrant populations.

There are many serologic studies available at this time that allow for precise diagnosis and staging of viral hepatitis, together with diagnostic tests of liver function. However, correlation of the test results with the patient's clinical status requires accurate interpretation of test results. Determining the optimal management and treatment for a given patient will often be guided by the consultation of a hepatologist. Complicating the diagnosis of acute liver inflammation, a number of other infections that may be acquired while traveling can

TABLE 22.1   Overview of Hepatitis Viruses

Virus Type	Genetic Material	Incubation Period	Transmission Routes	Risk of Chronicity	Vaccine-Preventable
A	RNA	15-45 days; mean 26 days	Fecal-oral	Absent	Yes
B	DNA	30-180 days; mean 90 days	Sexual, parenteral, blood and components, surgical/odontologic procedure, mother–fetus	High (90% in newborns; 5-10% in adults)	Yes
C	RNA	15-150 days; mean 60 days	Parenteral, blood and components, sexual	High (85%)	No
D	RNA	30-50 days	Sexual, parenteral, blood and components, surgical/odontologic procedure, skin and mucosal wound, mother–fetus	High (79% after superinfection; <5% after co-infection)	No
E	RNA	28-48 days	Fecal-oral	Absent	No

mimic the common symptoms of viral hepatitis, as can adverse effects of a number of drugs and other potential hepatotoxins (**Table 22.2**).

EPIDEMIOLOGY AND ETIOLOGY

Hepatitis A Virus (HAV)

HAV is a 27-nm RNA virus. The transmission of hepatitis A is almost exclusively via the fecal-oral route, although parenteral transmission may occasionally occur, particularly in the setting of intravenous drug use. The virus is found throughout the world, but from the standpoint of the traveler, inadequate sewage facilities and environmental contamination with human excrement in rural tropical areas are most often responsible for hepatitis A transmission (**Fig. 22.1**). Drinking contaminated water and eating fresh fruits and vegetables grown and processed with contaminated water are major routes of infection. Consumption of shellfish grown in contaminated waters is another common etiology of hepatitis A outbreaks, such as the outbreak associated with contaminated clams that caused approximately 300,000 cases of hepatitis A infection in Shanghai in 1988.

Person-to-person transmission can occur through eating food touched by unhygienic food handlers (who failed to wash their hands after defecation) or through close personal contact involving unsanitary conditions, such as found in daycare facilities and institutional domiciles such as prisons and homes for the developmentally disabled. Epidemiologic data have shown that other high-risk populations for HAV infection are men who have sex with men, illegal drug users, and persons with clotting factor disorders. Occupational risk for HAV occurs among those who work with HAV-infected primates or with HAV in research laboratories.

As an indication of the difference in risk in developed versus developing countries, serologic evidence of prior hepatitis A infection was present in 2.3% of young Scandinavian soldiers, in 20-30% of middle-aged middle-class New Yorkers, but in almost 100% of Southeast Asian populations. Epidemiologic evidence shows that the risk of HAV infection

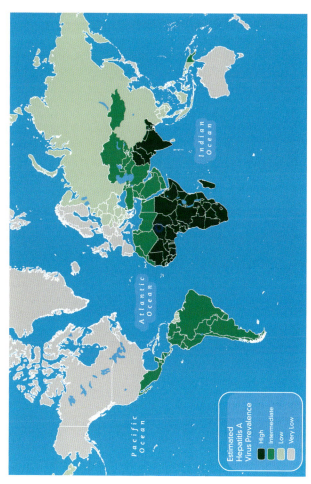

Fig. 22.1 Geographic distribution of hepatitis A prevalence. (From: CDC Health Information for International Travel 2008.)

TABLE 22.2 Historical Clues in Diagnosis of Hepatitis

- Recent travel history
- Ethnic background and birthplace (especially Asian, Oceanic, or North African or close exposure to these individuals)
- Sexual orientation and patterns of contact
- Known exposure to an infectious agent causing hepatitis (including healthcare workers with high-risk exposure)
- Past immunizations against hepatitis
- Past or current medical conditions
  - Previous hepatitis, including type (if known); other liver disease
  - History of, or symptoms suggestive of, biliary tract disease
  - Transfusions or administration of blood products
  - Hemodialysis
  - History of organ transplantation
  - History of recent surgery (benign postoperative jaundice?)
  - History of frequent previous jaundice (Gilbert syndrome?)
  - Current pregnancy (third trimester: consider cholestatic jaundice of pregnancy or acute fatty liver of pregnancy)
- Drug history
  - Illicit drug usage (especially parenteral)
  - Prescription medications (include oral contraceptives)
  - Over-the-counter medications (include vitamins)
- Hepatotoxic exposures
  - Alcohol usage
  - Human immunodeficiency virus infection treated with highly active antiretroviral therapy drugs
  - Occupational exposure
  - Mushroom ingestion

changes as formerly low-resource countries undergo modernization: only 50% of young urban Thais are seropositive, and the massive 1988 hepatitis A outbreak in China indicated that there was a large pool of susceptible young adults who had not previously been infected.

Hepatitis B Virus (HBV)

The agent of HBV is a 42-nm DNA virus. The intact virion, also known as the Dane particle, consists of identifiable sub-viral fragments, including the hepatitis B surface antigen (HBsAg), a core antigen (HBcAg), a DNA polymerase molecule, and the "e" antigen (HBeAg). Circulating HBsAg is the prime marker of active infection. HBeAg is an indicator of high infectivity, except in the setting of the precore mutation, which leads to lack of HBeAg but very high viral levels.

Identifiable groups at risk of contracting HBV include persons receiving contaminated blood products (a low risk in countries where banked blood is screened for HBsAg and other blood-borne pathogens), organ transplant recipients, healthcare workers having frequent contact with blood products, hemodialysis patients, homosexual males with multiple sexual partners, and sexual and household contacts of HBsAg-positive carriers.

The risk of transmission of HBV during travel reflects the prevalence of the disease worldwide (**Fig. 22.2**). In the United States, there is evidence of past HBV infection in 10% of the population, but the HBsAg-positive carrier rate is <2% (1.25 million people). The same figures hold for northern European countries, but areas of North Africa, sub-Saharan Africa, Oceania, and much of East Asia have much higher rates of infection: evidence for previous infection may be present in up to 70-80% of the population, and the underlying carrier rates run from 5 to 15%. An estimated 350 million persons are chronic

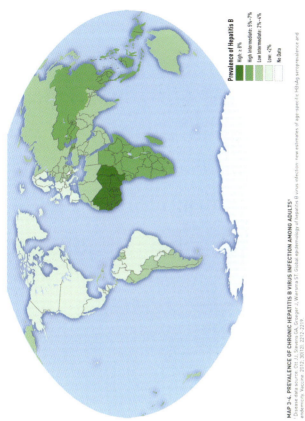

MAP 3-4. PREVALENCE OF CHRONIC HEPATITIS B VIRUS INFECTION AMONG ADULTS[1]

[1] Disease data source: Ott JJ, Stevens GA, Groeger J, Wiersma ST. Global epidemiology of hepatitis B virus infection: new estimates of age-specific HBsAg seroprevalence and endemicity. Vaccine 2012; 30(12): 2212-2219.

Prevalence of Hepatitis B

High ≥ 8%
High Intermediate: 5%–7%
Low Intermediate: 2%–4%
Low: <2%
No Data

Fig. 22.2 Geographic distribution of hepatitis B prevalence. (From: CDC Health Information for International Travel 2008.)

carriers of HBV worldwide. One reason for the high rate of infection and carrier state in highly endemic areas is the phenomenon of peripartum maternal-fetal (vertical) transmission. As many as 30-50% of the women who are HBsAg carriers or who are acutely infected in the third trimester will transmit the infection to their offspring unless specific prophylactic measures are administered to the infant immediately following birth (see below).

Of most concern to the traveler is the risk of exposure through sexual or close personal contact with carriers in the native populations abroad and inadvertent exposure to the virus through contaminated instruments used for personal grooming, for example, haircuts, shaves, manicures, pedicures, tattooing, and waxing. Other travelers at risk include those who seek medical or dental care in countries where hepatitis B is endemic or those who receive unexpected emergency care in sub-optimal situations. The current trend in "medical tourism," that is, travel to foreign countries to obtain surgical procedures at a significantly lower cost than at home, makes the issue of effective practices by blood banks worldwide to screen for blood-borne pathogens (hepatitis B, hepatitis C, human immunodeficiency virus [HIV], West Nile virus, and Chagas disease) a topic of increasing importance.

HBV Infection in Pregnancy

As a general policy, immigrants to the United States from areas where hepatitis B is endemic should be screened for HBsAg, but the screening process becomes extremely important in pregnant women. The influx of refugees from Southeast Asia and other areas where hepatitis B is endemic has made this even more critical (Chapter 3).

The cause for concern is the risk of maternal-fetal transmission. Up to 90% of infants born to HBeAg-positive mothers will themselves become chronic carriers, with the risk of long-term complications and death and also the risk of passing the infection on to their offspring. High-dose (0.5 mL) hepatitis B immune globulin (HBIG) given within 12 hours of birth has been shown to decrease the immediate infection rate by 80%. When the passive immunity granted by HBIG disappears, significant risk of infection via maternal-fetal contact returns, so it is recommended that infants at risk also receive the first of their three hepatitis B vaccinations at birth. This combination of HBIG and HBV vaccine has been shown, in general, to be 90% effective in preventing infection in children born to mothers who are HBV carriers. However, depending on the study, in women with high viral levels the percentage of infants developing HBsAg ranges from 7 to 32%. Antiviral therapy should be considered during the third trimester in women with high-level viremia.

Hepatitis C Virus (HCV)

The HCV was identified in 1989 and proved to be the viral agent causing 96% of cases of what was previously referred to as non-A, non-B hepatitis (NANBH). HCV became the most common cause of transfusion-associated hepatitis in the United States after screening for HBsAg decreased the percentage of post-transfusion hepatitis due to HBV to 10%. Older studies suggested that as many as 3-7% of units of what would now be regarded as high-risk blood products were capable of transmission of NANBH, and rates of infection from 5 to 15% in patients receiving 1-5 units of blood were documented. The risk of post-transfusion hepatitis due to HCV initially decreased when blood was screened for surrogate markers for NANBH (using the liver enzyme alanine aminotransferase [ALT] and the core antibody to hepatitis B); it has now undergone about a 10-fold decrease with routine screening of donor blood for antibody to hepatitis C. Transmission via blood products in the United States is now rare.

Transmission of HCV also occurs with parenteral drug abuse and less often by the mechanisms by which HBV is spread. Although data from studies have been contradictory, there may be a mildly increased incidence of infection in homosexual males and in those with multiple heterosexual partners who are infected; inoculation of body fluids containing virus through mucosal lesions is presumed to be the mechanism of spread. However, this mechanism of viral spread is extremely inefficient. Sexual transmission of HCV between stable monogamous couples is uncommon. The likelihood of transmission to healthcare workers following needle-stick or other parenteral exposure to blood or body fluids is correlated to the viral load of the source patient. Rates of transmission from 1 to 10% have been reported for HCV, in contrast to 5-30% for HBV.

Worldwide, an estimated 180 million people are infected with HCV. In the United States, it is estimated that 1.6% of the population (4.1 million persons) have antibody to hepatitis C virus, and at least 80% are chronically infected. At the time of this publication, HCV is the leading cause of death from liver disease and leading indication for liver transplantation in the United States. Unfortunately, a large proportion of infections with HCV abroad have no clear reason for transmission established; however, medical care, drug use, tattooing, body piercing, and traditional medicine (i.e., ritual scarification, acupuncture) have all been cited as causes. The traveler must be counseled to avoid risk factors for transmission similar to those with HBV. It has been established that some countries have a particularly high prevalence of anti-HCV antibody. Included in this group are certain sub-Saharan African nations, Egypt and parts of the Arabian Peninsula, Thailand, and Japan (**Fig. 22.3**).

Hepatitis D Virus (HDV)

Hepatitis D (formerly the "delta agent") is a defective RNA virus that is dependent on host enzymes and viral enzymes of HBV for its own replication. The HDV RNA is replicated by the host polymerases and requires HBV for its HBsAg coat, which is necessary for HDV assembly. Active hepatitis D is found only in patients who are positive for HBsAg, and anti-hepatitis D antibody has been found only in the sera of active HBsAg carriers or those with serologic evidence of past infection. The overall prevalence of anti-HD in HBsAg carriers is about 8-15% in Western Europe. Hepatitis D is most prevalent in southern Italy and North Africa, but increased rates are also seen in the Middle East and sub-Saharan Africa. Epidemics have also occurred in the Amazon basin, Russia, Greenland, and Mongolia. Risk factors for the transmission of the virus appear to be much the same as for HBV. In the United States, hepatitis D has been found almost exclusively in drug abusers with concomitant hepatitis B infection or in HBV carriers with a history of many transfusions. However, as immigration from endemic countries increases, this population must not be forgotten. The mortality rate in acute HBV infection appears to be greater when hepatitis D co-infection is present, but not as high as when hepatitis D superinfection of a chronic hepatitis B carrier occurs.

Hepatitis E Virus (HEV)

What had previously been called enterically transmitted non-A, non-B hepatitis is now known as hepatitis E. HEV has been demonstrated in stool using immune electron microscopy, and while the virus resembles HAV in terms of both transmission and epidemiology, it is serologically unrelated. Five genotypes have been identified, four of which infect humans, and genotype distribution varies geographically.

HEV is endemic in Southeast and Central Asia (**Fig. 22.4**). It has been the source of several large epidemics in India, Nepal, and Burma, usually in association with flooding or other problems with the water supply. Well-studied outbreaks have occurred in northern and western Africa, the Middle East, and Mexico. With the advent of serologic testing, evidence for frequent sporadic transmission of endemic infection has been documented in a number of countries, including Egypt, Hong Kong, and nations in sub-Saharan Africa.

Classic epidemic HEV infection is secondary to genotypes 1 or 2 HEV, which have no known animal reservoir. Patients who develop acute hepatitis after recent travel to endemic areas are generally infected with these genotypes. Studies have shown that HEV genotypes 3 and 4 are likely to be a zoonosis for which pigs are the most common reservoir. Genotype 4 has also been reported in other reservoirs such as wild boars, chickens, rodents, mongooses, shellfish, and, to a lesser extent, dogs. Based on limited serum surveys of HEV antibodies among high-risk populations in endemic regions, most zoonotic HEV infections appear to be asymptomatic among occupational risk groups where reported seroprevalence was elevated, ranging from 6% among Brazilian pig farmers up to 33% among Italian abattoir

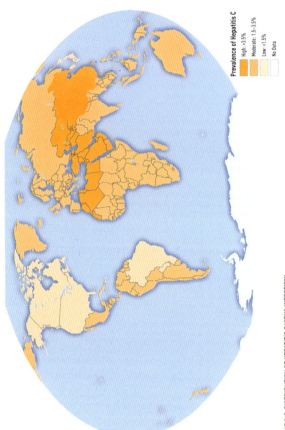

MAP 3-5. DISTRIBUTION OF HEPATITIS C VIRUS INFECTION[1]

[1] Disease data source: Mohd Hanafiah K, Groeger J, Flaxman AD, Wiersma ST. Global Epidemiology of Hepatitis C Virus Infection. New Estimates of Age-Specific Antibody to HCV and Seroprevalence.[2] Hepatology 2013; 57:1333-1342.

Prevalence of Hepatitis C
- High: >3.5%
- Moderate: 1.5-3.5%
- Low: <1.5%
- No Data

Fig. 22.3 Geographic distribution of hepatitis C prevalence. (From: CDC Health Information for International Travel 2008.)

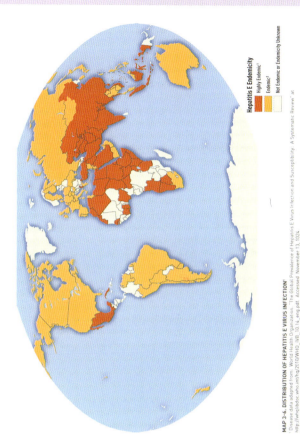

MAP 3-6. DISTRIBUTION OF HEPATITIS E VIRUS INFECTION[1]

[1] Disease data adapted from: World Health Organization. The Global Prevalence of Hepatitis E Virus Infection and Susceptibility. A Systematic Review at http://whqlibdoc.who.int/hq/2010/WHO_IVB_10.14_eng.pdf. Accessed November 13, 1024.

[2] Defined as waterborne or confirmed Hepatitis E virus infection in ≥25% of sporadic non-A, non-B hepatitis

[3] Defined as confirmed Hepatitis E virus infection in <25% of sporadic non-A, non-B hepatitis

Hepatitis E Endemicity

Highly Endemic[1]

Endemic[2]

Not Endemic or Endemicity Unknown

Fig. 22.4   Geographic distribution of hepatitis E prevalence. (From: CDC Health Information for International Travel 2008.)

workers. Symptomatic cases seem to occur in young adults or older children. The very few cases of HEV in the United States have generally been imported by recent travelers from abroad, primarily Mexico and India; secondary transmission has not been documented. However, there have been reports of HEV infection secondary to undercooked deer, pig liver, and shellfish.

In general, hepatitis E is clinically similar to hepatitis A; however, the mortality in some outbreaks has been higher than that seen with hepatitis A, perhaps due to malnutrition and concomitant disease among the victims. A *mortality rate of 10-20% among women late in pregnancy* has been a consistent finding in HEV epidemics, particularly with genotypes 1 and 2. There is no commercially available vaccine against hepatitis E, although one is in development and appears promising. Administration of immune globulin derived from pooled serum banks in non-endemic regions for hepatitis E appears to offer no protection against infection.

CLINICAL SYNDROMES

Uncomplicated infections with the different viral agents have both similarities and differences but can be divided into the prodromal, icteric, and convalescent phases. Some hepatitis infections can result in either acute liver failure or chronic hepatitis, both of which can lead to complications, including death.

Prodrome

The incubation period for hepatitis A is 2-6 weeks, with a mean of 3.7, and the onset of the disease is typically rather rapid. The incubation time for hepatitis E is similar to HAV at 2-8 weeks, with a mean of 40 days. The incubation times for hepatitis B (2-6 months; mean 11.8 weeks) and hepatitis C (6-12 weeks; mean 7.8 weeks) are longer, and the onset is generally more indolent. The incubation periods for hepatitis D are less well defined, but for HDV, it appears to range from 3 to 6 weeks.

Beyond the differing incubation periods, and the rapidity of onset of symptoms, the prodrome in the different types of infections may be remarkably similar. Fatigue, flu-like myalgia, and malaise are often the initial symptoms, followed by gastrointestinal symptoms including anorexia, nausea, and occasional diarrhea. A low-grade fever may also be present. Right upper quadrant tenderness is almost universally found, and hepatomegaly is detectable in many cases.

Arthralgia and an urticarial rash are seen about 10% of the time as part of the prodrome of hepatitis B. They are thought to be due to the formation of hepatitis B antigen–antibody immune complexes. This is seen rarely in HAV infection, although may occur occasionally in hepatitis C.

Patients with hepatitis A are infectious for approximately 2 weeks before the onset of clinical disease, during which time they are shedding viral particles in their stool. Shedding declines with the onset of jaundice, and the patient is non-infectious 1-2 weeks after clinical disease develops. There is no carrier state. By contrast, patients with HBV infection may have low levels of HBsAg detectable within 1-2 weeks after infection and theoretically may be infectious; a smaller infectious inoculum will delay the appearance of HBsAg in serum. The timing for infectivity with HCV is not known.

Icteric Phase

Most cases of all three major types of hepatitis remain subclinical. In the case of hepatitis A, this is because worldwide most infections occur in children, who seldom become very ill; adults are much more likely to become jaundiced. An estimated 10-20% of HBV and 30% of HCV infections result in jaundice. Patients may first notice darkening of the urine, then the appearance of scleral or palatine icterus, and, finally, frank jaundice. Pruritus may become prominent. At this stage, symptoms of hepatitis A begin to improve, and infectivity clears as HAV disappears from the stool. However, symptoms of hepatitis B and hepatitis C may persist after the onset of jaundice, and infectivity remains.

Convalescent Phase

Gradual return to well-being is the rule in all types of hepatitis that do not become fulminant or progress to a chronic carrier state. Some 90% of cases of hepatitis A are characterized by return of liver function tests to normal within 12 weeks; the balance takes somewhat longer, but no carrier state develops. In contrast, the resolution of infection in hepatitis B typically takes 6-20 weeks, and the marker of cure is disappearance of HBsAg and appearance of antibody to it (anti-HBs); 5-10% of adult patients become chronic carriers of HBsAg. Hepatitis C symptoms may resolve quickly or may follow a smoldering course; the latter is highly associated with development of a chronic carrier state.

Acute Liver Failure

The development of acute liver failure (previously called fulminant liver failure) is the most feared complication of acute hepatitis infection. It is an overwhelming infection that results in massive hepatic necrosis, extreme initial elevation of bilirubin, and persistently abnormal bilirubin despite a return of hepatic enzymes to normal. Hepatic encephalopathy and elevated international normalized ratio (INR) develop due to the extreme liver dysfunction.

Acute liver failure (ALF) develops in only a small number of cases of acute hepatitis but is more common in hepatitis B (1-3%) than in hepatitis A (0.5-1.0%). Acute HAV super-infection in persons with chronic HCV may cause a higher rate of ALF. Regardless of viral etiology, the prognosis in cases of infectious ALF is grim: without liver transplantation, the mortality rate can be as high as 60-90%. The mortality rate for hepatitis B ALF is much higher if hepatitis D co-infection is present, and the rate in hepatitis D superinfection of chronic hepatitis B is particularly high.

Chronic Hepatitis

Chronic hepatitis does not occur after hepatitis A but can be seen following HBV, HCV, HDV, or HEV infection. Some 5-10% of people in the United States infected with HBV develop chronic hepatitis. The rate is higher (15-20%) in geographic areas with high endemic rates of disease; the development of chronic hepatitis is more likely following maternal-fetal transmission (90%). The most dreaded complication of chronic HBV is the development of hepatocellular carcinoma, which is 300 times more likely to develop in those with chronic disease compared with the general population. Additionally, those with chronic HBV can progress to cirrhosis, liver failure, and death. Chronic hepatitis develops in approximately 85% of those infected with HCV. Chronic HCV infection can lead to cirrhosis in 30-40% of infected individuals, which is then associated with the development of hepatocellular carcinoma in up to 4% per year. There is some evidence that chronic HCV co-infection may increase the likelihood of hepatocellular carcinoma in HBV carriers. Chronic HEV infection can develop in immunocompromised individuals, such as organ transplant recipients or those infected with HIV, and is associated with rapid development of cirrhosis (within 2-3 years).

Viral Hepatitis Co-Infections

Acute HAV infections in persons with chronic HBV and HCV infections are associated with more severe disease and a higher risk of death. Acute HAV infection in persons infected with HIV may result in a prolonged HAV viremic stage (median duration 53 days vs. 22 days, $p < 0.05$) and potentially more severe disease as well as increased transmissibility.

HBV and HCV co-infection may result in more serious medical complications than HCV alone, in that there is an increased chance of progression to cirrhosis and an increased risk of development of hepatocellular carcinoma.

Among HIV-infected persons, chronic HBV infection occurs in 10-15%, and up to 30% may be co-infected with HCV. An increased risk of death has been reported in HIV/HBV co-infected men. Reports from several countries have shown significantly increased rates of death from end-stage liver disease among HIV-infected persons in the era of highly active antiretroviral therapy (HAART) compared with the pre-HAART era. One hypothesis is that chronic HBV and/or HBC infections can potentiate the inherent hepatotoxicity of the antiretroviral therapy drugs.

DIFFERENTIAL DIAGNOSIS

Before the diagnosis of a specific viral hepatitis can be made, other potential sources of hepatocellular injury must be considered. Particular attention should be paid to diseases endemic to areas from which travelers or immigrants have come, but other less exotic causes of jaundice must be considered (**Table 22.2**).

Viral Diseases

Yellow Fever

Yellow fever should be considered in any jaundiced patient who has been traveling in the endemic areas of South America or West and Central Africa. However, the incubation period of the severe, icteric form of yellow fever is 3-6 days, and the diagnosis can be effectively excluded if the patient departed from an endemic area more than a week previously. Also, the onset is quite abrupt, with marked systemic symptoms, rather than the often more insidious onset typical of viral hepatitis.

Epstein-Barr Virus (EBV)

The syndrome of mononucleosis can include hepatic enzyme abnormalities. Although they are typically low grade, serum enzyme levels as high as several thousand international units (IU) can be seen. Jaundice can also be seen with more severe inflammation.

Cytomegalovirus (CMV)

A syndrome similar to that of mononucleosis can also be seen in this infection. CMV infection generally develops in immunocompromised individuals and is rarely seen in the immunocompetent.

Herpes Simplex

Disseminated infection can result in hepatic necrosis, but this complication is generally seen only in immunocompromised patients.

Coxsackievirus

Severe infections can result in hepatitis.

Nonviral Infections

Typhoid

Diffuse hepatic involvement in typhoid may result in frank jaundice. Acute cholecystitis, with resultant biliary stasis, may also develop in the first stage of typhoid. The same risk factors that predispose a traveler to hepatitis A predispose to typhoid.

Malaria

Hepatomegaly and jaundice occasionally occur, most commonly in severe falciparum malaria.

Liver Abscess

Both bacterial and amebic liver abscess may cause focal hepatomegaly and tenderness. Amebic liver abscess is particularly a risk in travelers to underdeveloped tropical countries.

Q Fever

Hepatomegaly and jaundice may be prominent symptoms. Exposure to cows, goats, or sheep when the animals are giving birth is a major risk factor for the disease, but exposure to the animal hides of these species can also result in transmission.

Secondary Syphilis

Alkaline phosphatase levels will be markedly elevated if liver inflammation is associated with secondary syphilis.

Leptospirosis

Liver dysfunction may occur in the "immune" secondary phase of the disease.

Toxoplasmosis

The infection usually results in only mild liver function abnormalities in immunocompetent individuals.

Helminthic Infestations

Ascariasis

Hepatosplenomegaly may be seen when a patient is first infected, and biliary tract obstruction is a late complication that may occur in immigrants or returning long-time travelers.

Schistosomiasis

Marked systemic illness accompanied by hepatomegaly can be seen in acute illness due to *Schistosoma mansoni* or *Schistosoma japonicum*.

Flukes

A number of other flukes may cause infections that ultimately result in biliary tract obstruction. These include *Clonorchis sinensis*, the *Opisthorchis* species, and *Fasciola hepatica* (which may cause a picture of acute liver disease during the invasive phase).

Toxic Hepatitis

Many toxins, including prescription medications, over-the-counter medications, fat-soluble vitamins and niacin, alcohol, industrial agents, and the toxin of the mushroom *Amanita phalloides*, can cause hepatitis. A detailed drug history should be taken in any jaundiced patient.

Biliary Tract Disease

Cholecystitis or obstructive biliary tract disease should be in the differential if the diagnosis of hepatitis is considered. This can generally be excluded by imaging studies.

Gilbert Syndrome

This benign defect in hepatic glucuronyl transferase activity can cause increased bilirubin in fasting or mildly ill patients. The increase is virtually all unconjugated (indirect) bilirubin.

Pregnancy

In the third trimester of pregnancy, three syndromes can be seen. Cholestatic jaundice of pregnancy (also called intrahepatic cholestasis of pregnancy) is a benign condition without significant hepatic damage. However, acute fatty liver of pregnancy or HELLP syndrome (hemolysis, elevated liver enzymes, low platelet count) can result in marked hepatocellular damage and may have a high mortality rate.

DIAGNOSIS

The diagnosis of hepatitis is generally dependent on the demonstration of abnormal liver enzymes and evidence of liver cell inflammation. Hepatic function, as evidenced by the INR, is generally normal. Screening laboratory tests will usually confirm that hepatitis is present, although liver enzymes may be normal in those with chronic hepatitis.

The serum aminotransferases, alanine aminotransferase (ALT) and aspartate aminotransferase (AST), are the prime markers for hepatocellular injury. They will usually be quite elevated in acute hepatitis, with values as high as several thousand international units (IU). In chronic hepatitis, they may be normal or just mildly elevated until an acute exacerbation of the disease occurs, at which point they may rise dramatically. Decreasing levels of the aminotransferases will generally parallel the resolution of acute liver inflammation, although normalization in the setting of worsening INR following acute liver failure may be an ominous indicator of massive hepatocellular death.

Abnormalities in the serum bilirubin level directly reflect the functional abnormality in hepatitis. The level will generally mirror the degree of hepatic enzyme elevation. An exception to this can occur when massive cell death has occurred. The aminotransferases can be deceptively normal while the bilirubin remains quite high, reflecting the poor functional capability of the little remaining parenchymal tissue. In a mildly ill or otherwise normal patient who is jaundiced, fractionation of bilirubin to determine the proportion that is unconjugated (indirect) may be useful to establish the diagnosis of Gilbert syndrome rather than hepatitis.

Unfortunately, although these general screening tests may be of benefit in detecting that the patient's liver is diseased, they are of little benefit in identifying which type of hepatitis the patient may have. For this, more specific laboratory tests are necessary.

Hepatitis A

For the diagnosis of hepatitis A, there is an assay for antibody to the HAV (anti-HAV). In the acute disease, the anti-HAV will be of immunoglobulin class IgM, whereas within 6 months of resolution of the infection, the anti-HAV will all be IgG. If the IgM fraction is identified in the serum of the acutely jaundiced patient, a presumptive diagnosis of acute hepatitis A is made (**Fig. 22.5**).

The presence of anti-HAV IgG antibody is believed to confer immunity to reinfection, and it will generally be present for life following infection. Persistence of protective antibody levels for >10 years following hepatitis A immunization has been demonstrated; there is no official recommendation at the time of writing for additional vaccine doses after the second dose of the primary series has been received.

Hepatitis B

The diagnosis of hepatitis B infection is much more complex (**Figs. 22.6–22.8**). A number of serologic tests aid in the diagnosis. The results reflect the presence of the viral components or the immune system's response to them during the various stages of the disease. Early in the course of the acute infection, the HBsAg can be detected, often before there are any clinical signs of infection. As long as this is found in the serum, the patient remains

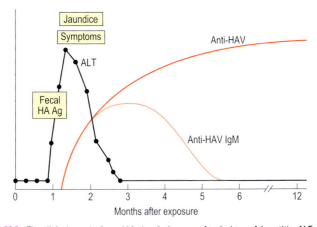

Fig. 22.5 **The clinical, serologic, and biochemical course of typical type A hepatitis. *ALT*, Alanine aminotransferase; *anti-HAV*, antibody to hepatitis A virus; *HA Ag*, hepatitis A antigen; *IgM*, immunoglobulin M.** (Reprinted from: Hoofnagle, J.H., 1981. Perspectives on Viral Hepatitis, Vol. 2, first ed. Abbott Laboratories, Rahway, NJ, p. 4, with permission of publisher.)

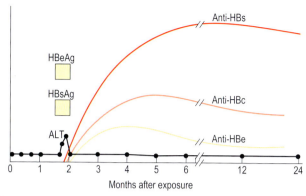

Fig. 22.6 The clinical, serologic, and biochemical course of a subclinical asymptomatic hepatitis B virus infection. *ALT*, Alanine aminotransferase; *anti-HBc*, antibody to hepatitis B core antigen; *anti-HBe*, antibody to HBeAg; *anti-HBs*, antibody to HBsAg; *HBeAg*, hepatitis B "e" antigen; *HBsAg*, hepatitis B surface antigen. (Reprinted from: Hoofnagle, J.H., 1981. Perspectives on Viral Hepatitis, Vol. 2, first ed. Abbott Laboratories, Rahway, NJ, p. 7, with permission of publisher.)

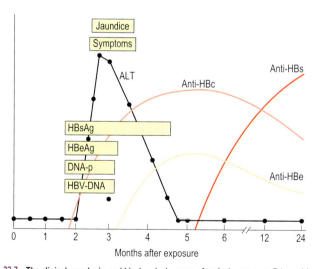

Fig. 22.7 The clinical, serologic, and biochemical course of typical acute type B hepatitis. *ALT*, Alanine aminotransferase; *anti-HBc*, antibody to hepatitis B core antigen; *anti-HBe*, antibody to HBeAg; *anti-HBs*, antibody to HBsAg; *DNA-p*, serum hepatitis B virus DNA polymerase activity; *HBeAg*, hepatitis B "e" antigen; *HBsAg*, hepatitis B surface antigen; *HBV-DNA*, serum hepatitis B virus DNA. (Reprinted from: Hoofnagle, J.H. 1981. Perspectives on Viral Hepatitis, Vol. 2, first ed. Abbott Laboratories, Rahway, NJ, p. 6, with permission of publisher.)

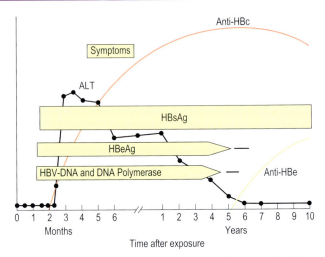

Fig. 22.8 The clinical, serologic, and biochemical course of a chronic type B hepatitis infection. *ALT*, Alanine aminotransferase; *anti-HBc*, antibody to hepatitis B core antigen; *anti-HBe*, antibody to HBeAg; *HBeAg*, hepatitis B "e" antigen; *HBsAg*, hepatitis B surface antigen; *HBV-DNA*, serum hepatitis B virus DNA. (Reprinted from: Hoofnagle, J.H., 1981. Perspectives on Viral Hepatitis, Vol. 2, first ed. Abbott Laboratories, Rahway, NJ, p. 8, with permission of publisher.)

infectious, and if it remains present at least 6 months after the onset of jaundice, the patient is presumed to be chronically infected.

Disappearance of the HBsAg from the blood is followed, after a period of several weeks, by the development of the anti-HBs antibody. This is a marker for resolution of the infection. The patient is not infectious and is considered cured. This is also the only hepatitis B serology that should be positive in the patient who has been successfully vaccinated.

Subsequent to the development of HBsAg, but before anti-HBs appears, antibody to the core of HBV develops (anti-HBc). This generally occurs at about the time of the onset of clinical illness, but it may be the only marker of HBV present if HBsAg has disappeared and anti-HBs has not yet appeared (the "core window"). An assay for IgM and IgG can determine if the anti-HBc present is due to acute or remote infection.

Another marker for hepatitis B infection is the HBeAg, or "e," antigen. This viral component is part of the nucleus and circulates freely during the acute infection. It is indicative of a high degree of infectiousness; presence of HBeAg more than 10 weeks beyond the symptomatic period indicates that the patient will probably develop chronic hepatitis (25-50% of chronic carriers are positive). By contrast, if the patient develops anti-HBe, it is a sign of either resolution of infection or development of an inactive carrier state (**Table 22.3**).

Hepatitis C

The diagnosis of hepatitis C is two-fold. The detection of HCV antibody by the enzyme-linked immunosorbent assay (ELISA) indicates exposure to the disease. This presence of acute or chronic infection is then confirmed by HCV RNA testing.

Hepatitis D

An antibody assay exists for hepatitis D, but it is often only transiently positive at the time of acute infection; it does remain persistently positive in chronic carriers of the infection.

TABLE 22.3 Interpretation of Hepatitis B Serologic Tests

HBsAg	Anti-HBs	Anti-HBc	Serologic Test
			Suggested diagnoses and follow-up
+	–	–	Early hepatitis B infection: probably pre-clinical or early clinical illness.
			HBeAg/anti-HBe testing possibly indicated: If –/– ("e window") or –/+: resolution likely. If +/–: still highly infectious.
			Needs follow-up testing until anti-HBs is positive, i.e., acute infection has resolved.
+	–	+	Diagnostic of either of the following:
			1. Acute HBV infection: has not developed anti-HBs yet. Consider "e" antigen testing as outlined above. Needs follow-up until anti-HBs positive. Anti-HBc IgM distinguishes 1 from 2.
			2. Chronic HBV carrier Consider hepatitis A, hepatitis C, or hepatitis D superinfection as diagnosis if acute hepatitis present. Consider other virus or toxin.
+	+	+	Acute hepatitis B. Atypical pattern; usually HBsAg is gone by the time anti-HBs appears; should resolve, since antibody is present.
–	+	+	Remote hepatitis B infection.
			Recovery is indicated by positive anti-HBs.
			Consider hepatitis A, hepatitis C, other virus, or other cause if acute hepatitis present.
–	–	+	One of the following:
			1. Remote HBV infection: anti-HBs now at undetectable level. If HBeAg is negative, assume remote infection and consider HAV, HCV, other virus, or other cause if acute hepatitis present.
			2. Immediate past HBV infection: the "core window" after HBsAg disappears but before anti-HBs appears. A positive test for HBeAg suggests this diagnosis: while the patient is still infectious (positive HBeAg), the infection is in the process of resolution, since HBsAg has disappeared. Follow-up is needed to be sure anti-HBs becomes positive. The immunoglobulin class of anti-HBc may distinguish 1 from 2.
			3. Low-level carrier state: HBsAg is too low to measure. If acute infection is present, consider HAV, HCV, other virus, or other cause.
–	+	–	Either of the following:
			1. Remote HBV infection: anti-HBc now too low to detect.
			2. Past immunization with hepatitis B vaccine: the vaccine contains low levels of HBsAg only. If acute infection is present, consider HAV, HCV, other virus, or other cause of hepatitis.
–	–	–	No evidence of HBV infection.
			Consider HAV, HCV, other virus, or other cause if hepatitis present.

HAV, hepatitis A virus; *HBcAg*, hepatitis B core antigen; *HBeAg*, hepatitis B "e" antigen; *HBsAg*, hepatitis B surface antigen; *HBV*, hepatitis B virus; *HCV* hepatitis C virus.

An IgM assay will be positive in acute infections and can differentiate acute from chronic disease. Hepatitis D should be considered in cases of acute liver failure or when a patient who is a known hepatitis B carrier suffers an acute exacerbation.

Hepatitis E

During the 3- to 8-week incubation period, HEV RNA can be detected in the serum or stool. By 8 weeks, anti-HEV IgM appears in the serum and persists for months, with IgG developing with resolution of disease. A commercially available HEV IgM ELISA test is available. HEV RNA is considered confirmatory, but is not yet available in the United States at the time of this publication. This can be requested through the National Institutes of Health. Serologic tests for hepatitis E have been used in studies to screen for both prevalence and incidence in countries where this disease is endemic.

Epstein-Barr Virus and Cytomegalovirus

The other viral infections that are most commonly considered in the differential diagnosis of hepatitis, EBV and CMV, can be ruled out by using acute and convalescent antibody titers. The Monospot test may be useful for the diagnosis of mononucleosis due to EBV, but it is frequently negative early in the course of the illness and may remain so.

TREATMENT

There is no specific treatment for acute viral hepatitis other than supportive care. Hospitalization is indicated for those people who are unable to care for themselves or who are unable to eat and hydrate. The other indication for hospitalization is hepatic failure, which requires intensive support and careful laboratory monitoring.

Diet was formerly a matter of great concern in treating hepatitis, but the feeling now is that a general diet with relatively high carbohydrate and low fat content is tolerated best. Activity level is also generally recommended to be as tolerated by the patient: people will usually respond more positively to being as active as possible rather than confined to bed until liver enzyme results approach normal.

Medications in acute hepatitis represent a difficult issue. In general, it is wise to avoid all medications, if possible, but especially any medications that are known to be hepatotoxic. Alcohol, even in modest quantities, should be completely avoided in the immediate period of infection, although it is probably not necessary to proscribe it for 12 months (as some urge) in the absence of evidence of severe liver disease.

The prothrombin time/INR is a functional assay of the liver's ability to synthesize coagulation factors. Vitamin K may be indicated in modest doses if it appears that acute liver infection is interfering with normal factor production. If the INR continues to rise, this is most indicative of acute liver failure, and these patients should be hospitalized.

There are several antiviral therapies currently being used for chronic hepatitis B infection, and patients with either hepatitis Be antigen (HBeAg)-positive or HBeAg-negative chronic hepatitis B are potential candidates for therapy. The drugs include tenofovir, entecavir, interferon α-2b, and peginterferon α-2a. Lamivudine, adefovir, and telbivudine are used less often due to frequent development of significant viral resistance. The goal of treatment is to suppress HBV replication, reduce progression of disease to cirrhosis with decompensation, and decrease the risk of development of hepatocellular carcinoma. Treatment is complicated and several guidelines exist. In general, treatment is indicated in those with HBV DNA levels ≥2000-20,000 IU/mL and ALT levels more than twice the upper limit of normal, and/or liver biopsies showing moderate inflammation/necrosis. Interferon had been used with moderate success in treatment of chronic hepatitis C. There now exist several direct acting antiviral agents for chronic hepatitis C virus infection that carry cure rates of over 90-95%. Treatment of HDV infection is directed at the underlying HBV infection. The greatest experience with treatment of HEV infection is in the solid organ transplant population. Clearance of HEV can be achieved in most cases with pegylated interferon alpha monotherapy, ribavirin monotherapy, or a combination of the two.

PREVENTION

Hepatitis A Vaccine

Travelers who are at risk for hepatitis A may opt for prophylaxis with one of the inactivated hepatitis A virus vaccines currently available. The inactivated vaccines have a rate of sero-conversion of >95% 1 month following immunization, but a booster dose 6-12 months after the initial dose is recommended to ensure long-lasting high levels of immunity (see Chapter 5). To avoid unnecessary immunization, if there is sufficient time before departure, it may be cost-effective to perform HAV antibody screening in travelers who are likely to have been previously infected. Examples of people in whom to consider testing would include those with a history of jaundice, natives or long-term residents of areas where hepatitis A is endemic, or those born before the close of World War II, when sanitary conditions were not as carefully maintained.

Reasonable precautions should be exercised in eating and sanitation habits, regardless of vaccine status. These include drinking hot, carbonated, or canned or bottled beverages; eating hot, well-cooked food and particularly avoiding raw or poorly cooked seafood; and avoiding unpeeled fruits and uncooked vegetables, which may be fertilized with night soil. Hepatitis A virus can be inactivated by heating at 85° C (185° F) for 1 min and partly inactivated at 60° C (140° F) for 60 min under test conditions. There is limited evidence from a food-borne outbreak that microwaving the surface-contaminated cooked food for 30 seconds or more during reheating appears inactivate the virus.

HAV Vaccine in Compromised Hosts

Patients with chronic HBV and HCV respond to hepatitis A immunization with rates of seroconversion comparable to those of healthy adults. Hepatitis A vaccine is less immuno-genic in patients with decompensated cirrhosis (66% seroconversion) compared with those with compensated cirrhosis (98%) at 7 months (1 month after the second dose of vaccine). Seroconversion after two hepatitis A vaccine doses in liver transplant recipients was only in the 0-26% range. Immunogenicity of HAV vaccine in HIV-infected individuals was related to the CD4+ cell count: those with CD4+ >300 had seroconversion rates comparable to healthy controls, whereas individuals with CD4+ <300 had a somewhat decreased response rate.

Immune Globulin

For persons unable to receive hepatitis A vaccine or who have underlying medical condi-tions that are predictive of a suboptimal immune response to vaccine, hepatitis A infection can be prevented through the administration of immune globulin (IG). Recipients receive protection against infection with hepatitis A virus immediately after IG administration from the transfer of pre-formed antibodies contained in the product. Recommendations are that short-term travelers receive 0.02 mL/kg (2 mL) of IG, while those contemplating stays of 3 months or longer should receive 0.06 mL/kg (4-5 mL). In those staying for prolonged periods, additional doses of IG are necessary every 5 months. Studies suggest that protective efficacy in preventing seroconversion is about 85%, and that over 1 year, about 1 in 500 people relying on IG prophylaxis will develop icteric hepatitis.

Hepatitis B

Immunization against hepatitis B is indicated for travelers depending on risk of exposure. This would include healthcare workers, those who anticipate receiving medical care in endemic regions, and those who expect to have sexual or other intimate contact with natives in countries where hepatitis B is endemic. Included in this group are families participating in international adoptions. Long-term travelers (>6 months) to endemic areas should be immunized as well, regardless of anticipated activities. If protection against both hepatitis A and hepatitis B is needed by a traveler, the hepatitis A plus hepatitis B combination vaccine may be used (see Chapter 5).

Household contacts and sexual contacts of HBV carriers should be screened and offered prophylaxis with hepatitis B vaccine when appropriate (Chapters 5 and 19). Persons who are chronically infected with hepatitis B should receive hepatitis A vaccine to avoid more serious pathology.

HBV Vaccine in Compromised Hosts

HBV vaccine is immunogenic in patients with chronic HCV hepatitis, with seroprotection (anti-HBs ≥10 mIU/mL) after three doses comparable to healthy controls. However, several studies have shown uncertain immunogenicity of HBV vaccine administered to individuals with advanced chronic liver disease or post-liver transplant. Among HIV-infected persons, response to HBV vaccine was associated with CD4$^+$ cell counts >200 cells/μL and undetectable HIV-RNA levels, with seroconversion in up to 87.5% following three doses of HBV vaccine reported in subjects with a CD4$^+$ cell count >500/μL. However, among responders, the antibody titers were lower than in HIV-negative controls. In HIV-infected persons with <500/μL CD4$^+$ cells, one study suggested an increased number of HBV vaccine doses could be improved by administering an additional three doses of vaccine on a monthly schedule.

Hepatitis C

No hepatitis C vaccine is commercially available at the time of writing, and its development remains elusive. There are no firm data that indicate IG is protective against hepatitis C if given before exposure. Prevention consists of avoiding high-risk activities and blood products where the virus is known to be endemic. Persons who are chronically infected with hepatitis C will benefit from immunization against both hepatitis A and B, as morbidity and mortality is higher with either co-infection.

Hepatitis D

Immunity to hepatitis D is conferred with immunity to hepatitis B; the vaccine for hepatitis B should be given to those at risk. Prevention for HBV carriers is to avoid risky exposures for HDV.

Hepatitis E

Prevention of HEV consists predominantly of risk avoidance. IG manufactured in the United States and other non-endemic areas does not contain antibodies against HEV, and there is some evidence that IG manufactured where hepatitis E is endemic does not confer good protection, either. Women who are pregnant or who are of childbearing potential should be informed of the heightened risk of acute HEV infection during pregnancy and should consider deferral of travel to HEV-endemic areas as appropriate. A recombinant hepatitis E vaccine (HEV-239) has been developed. Early data have shown that the vaccine is immunogenic (87% efficacy) and provides protection for up to 4.5 years. Safety data suggest that the vaccine is well tolerated. Should this vaccine become widely available, it would be crucial in the prevention and control of hepatitis E virus disease.

FURTHER READING

American Association for the Study of Liver Diseases. Recommendations for Testing, Managing, and Treating Hepatitis C. Available at <http://www.hcvguidelines.org> (accessed April 10, 2015). *Website maintained by the American Association for the Study of Liver Diseases in conjunction with the Infectious Diseases Society of America. Testing and linkage to care figure 1, CDC recommended testing sequence for identifying current HCV infection.*

Centers for Disease Control and Prevention (CDC), Division of Viral Hepatitis Home Page (DVH). Available at <http://www.cdc.gov/hepatitis/> (accessed April 11, 2015). *Website maintained by the CDC DVH that provides up-to-date statistics, surveillance, and guidelines for diagnosis, treatment, and prevention of hepatitis A, hepatitis B, hepatitis C, hepatitis D, and hepatitis E. Content for health professionals and for the public. Considerations for populations at special risk: Asians and Pacific Islanders, those with diabetes, STDs or HIV/AIDS, men who have sex with men, people who inject drugs, and African Americans, as well as specific settings: healthcare settings, hemodialysis, corrections, long-term care.*

Centers for Disease Control, 2012. Yellowbook. Estimated hepatitis A prevalence worldwide. <wwwnc.cdc.gov/travel/pdf/yellowbook-2012-map-03-03-estimated-prevalence-hepatitis-a.pdf> (Accessed February 11, 2016.).

Centers for Disease Control, 1991. Hepatitis B virus: a comprehensive strategy for eliminating transmission in the United States through universal childhood vaccination: Recommendations of the Immunization Practices Advisory Committee (ACIP). MMWR 40, 1–25.
Background and rationale for the introduction of hepatitis B virus vaccine into the program of routine childhood immunizations in the United States.

Costa-Mattioli, M., Allavena, C., Poirier, A.S., et al., 2001. Prolonged hepatitis A in patients infected with human immunodeficiency virus. Clin. Infect. Dis. 32, 297–299.
Immunization against hepatitis A is important among HIV-infected patients.

Halliday, M.L., Kang, L.Y., Zhou, T.K., et al., 1991. An epidemic of hepatitis A attributable to the ingestion of raw clams in Shanghai, China. J. Infect. Dis. 164, 852–859.
Account of a massive hepatitis A epidemic among an urban population in China that overwhelmed the existing local health facilities.

Lange, W.R., Frame, J.D., 1990. High incidence of viral hepatitis among American missionaries in Africa. Am. J. Trop. Med. Hyg. 43, 527–533.
Early report on increased occupational risk associated with international travel.

Laurence, J., 2005. Hepatitis A and B immunizations of individuals infected with human immunodeficiency virus. Am. J. Med. 118, 75S–83S.
Eliciting protective immune responses following administration of hepatitis vaccines to HIV-infected persons is dependent on level of cellular immunity.

Rizzetto, M., Alvian, S.M., 2013. Hepatitis delta: the rediscovery. Clin. Liver Dis. 17, 475–487.
Updated review on hepatitis D viral infections.

Wedemeyer, H., Pischke, S., Manns, M.P., 2012. Pathogenesis and treatment of hepatitis E virus infection. Gastroenterology 142, 1388–1397.
Updated review on hepatitis E viral infections.

CHAPTER 23

Leptospirosis

Vernon E. Ansdell

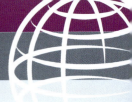

Leptospirosis is the commonest zoonosis worldwide. It occurs in all areas except polar regions and is particularly common in the tropics and subtropics. Typical cases present abruptly with high fever and chills, intense headache, severe myalgias, and conjunctival suffusion. Many cases have a nonspecific presentation, however, and are often misdiagnosed. Adventurous travelers, especially to tropical and subtropical regions, are at increased risk of leptospirosis and should be identified and counseled appropriately prior to departure. The diagnosis of leptospirosis is fraught with problems. A combined approach using culture (blood, urine, cerebrospinal fluid [CSF]) plus serology (acute and convalescent sera) is recommended in order to help make the diagnosis. If available, polymerase chain reaction (PCR) may provide rapid, early diagnosis. Appropriate antibiotic treatment should be started as soon as possible after the diagnosis is suspected.

ETIOLOGY

Leptospirosis is caused by an aerobic, tightly coiled, highly motile spirochete with hooked ends measuring 0.1 μm in diameter and from 6 to 20 μm in length. Because the organism is slender and highly motile, it is capable of passing through membrane filters 0.2 μm in diameter. This may be an important consideration for anyone planning to use water filters to purify their drinking water. The organism survives best in moist, warm conditions (optimal temperature 28-30°C) in a slightly alkaline environment (optimal pH 7.2-7.4). The genus *Leptospira* includes two species: *L. interrogans*, which is pathogenic, and *L. biflexa*, which is saprophytic and nonpathogenic. *L. interrogans* is divided into 23 serogroups and more than 200 serovars, most of which can cause infections in humans. Serovars from common serogroups that cause infection in humans include *australis*, *ballium*, *canicola*, *grippotyphosa*, *hardjo*, *hebdomadis*, *icterohaemorrhagiae*, and *pomona*.

EPIDEMIOLOGY

Leptospirosis occurs worldwide, except in polar regions. Human infection may be epidemic, sporadic, or endemic. Leptospirosis is most common in warm, moist, tropical and subtropical regions, especially areas that have heavy rainfall and neutral or alkaline soil. Infection is often seen in agricultural areas with large numbers of livestock or rodents or in areas with large wildlife populations. It is most common in the rainy season in the tropics and in the summer and fall in temperate climates, probably reflecting the increased opportunity for exposure to contaminated fresh water. Outbreaks of leptospirosis may be a serious threat after severe flooding.

Leptospirosis is a zoonosis with many wild and domestic animal reservoirs, including rats, mice, mongooses, pigs, dogs, and cattle. The cycle of transmission is shown in **Figure 23.1**. Following infection, animals often harbor leptospira in the kidneys. The organism multiplies and may be shed in the urine for months or years. Infected animals are often asymptomatic.

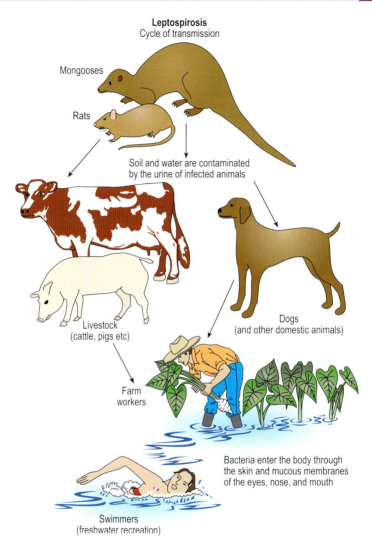

Leptospirosis
Cycle of transmission

Mongooses

Rats

Soil and water are contaminated
by the urine of infected animals

Livestock
(cattle, pigs etc)

Dogs
(and other domestic animals)

Farm
workers

Bacteria enter the body through
the skin and mucous membranes
of the eyes, nose, and mouth

Swimmers
(freshwater recreation)

Fig. 23.1 **Cycle of transmission of leptospirosis from animal to man.** (From the Hawaii Department of Health.)

Leptospira proliferate in fresh water, damp soil, vegetation, and mud. Humans become infected by exposure to infected animal urine either by direct contact or as the result of indirect exposure through contaminated water or moist soil. Indirect contact is the commonest source of infection and may occur via contaminated mud or fresh water in rivers, lakes, and streams. It occurs in a wide variety of occupational (e.g., rice or sugar cane farmers, sewage workers, or miners) and recreational (e.g., rafting, hiking, swimming, fishing, or gardening) situations. Direct contact with contaminated urine and tissues of infected animals may occur in hunters, dairy or cattle farmers, abattoir workers, or veterinarians. Infection is acquired through damaged skin, for example, cuts and abrasions, or via exposed mucous membranes of the nose, mouth, and eyes. Very rarely, infection may be the result of laboratory accidents, animal bites (contaminated with urine), blood transfusions, organ transplants, ingestion of breast milk, sexual intercourse, or congenital transmission.

High antibody prevalence rates have been reported from many tropical and sub-tropical countries. Examples include Belize 37%, Tahiti 30%, Thailand 27%, and Vietnam 23%. Average annual incidence rates in tropical and subtropical countries are also high, for example, Tahiti 20/100,000 and Barbados 123/100,000. In contrast, the average annual incidence rate in the United States is 0.02/100,000. Typically, at least half the cases of leptospirosis diagnosed in the United States are from Hawaii, and average annual incidence rates on the island of Kauai may be as high as 24/100,000. Leptospirosis is commonest on the Hawaiian Islands that have the most rainfall (Kauai and Hawaii Island), especially in the windward (wetter) areas of those islands. Historically an occupational disease of sugar cane workers in Hawaii, leptospirosis has become increasingly recognized as a recreational disease in recent years.

Some serovars appear to be associated with particular animals. Examples include *icterohaemorrhagiae* (rats), *canicola* (dogs), *pomona* (swine), *autumnalis* (rats, raccoons), *hardjo* (cattle), and *bratislava* (swine, badgers).

It has been noted that outbreaks of leptospirosis often occur after periods of heavy rainfall and flooding. It is thought that rain washes the organism from the river banks into surface waters, while, at the same time, flooding results in increased human contact with water and forces infected animals into closer contact with humans. A major outbreak occurred after widespread flooding in Nicaragua in 1995 and was responsible for more than 2000 cases and more than 40 deaths. An outbreak in white-water rafters in Costa Rica in 1996 was also linked to heavy rainfall. In 1998, the largest outbreak in recorded U.S. history involved a group of tri-athletes who had swum in a lake after heavy rainfall in Illinois. A total of more than 60 cases were reported in this outbreak. A further example of the association of leptospirosis with flooding was in late 1998, in the aftermath of Hurricane Mitch, when outbreaks of leptospirosis were reported from various countries in Central America, including Honduras, Guatemala, and Nicaragua. In 2000 an important outbreak of leptospirosis occurred in participants of an "Eco-Challenge" multisport athletic event in Borneo following very heavy rainfall. More recently, outbreaks have been reported after flooding in urban slums of Brazil, India, and Thailand. In addition, many areas of the Philippines have experienced large outbreaks of leptospirosis following recent typhoons, prompting the government to provide antimicrobial prophylaxis with doxycycline to millions of people.

There have been many reports of leptospirosis in travelers, but despite this, the infection continues to be underrecognized in this group. With the increased popularity of recreational and wilderness activities in travelers, there is an increased risk of leptospirosis, particularly in tropical and subtropical regions. Travel medicine specialists should make special efforts to identify and counsel travelers at risk of leptospirosis. This is particularly important in travelers to areas that have experienced recent flooding, because they may be at increased risk of infection. In certain situations, prophylactic antibiotics may be indicated. It is also very important to consider the diagnosis of leptospirosis in a returned traveler who presents with appropriate exposure history and relevant clinical features. Clinicians who see returned travelers need to have a high index of suspicion for leptospirosis, particularly bearing in mind the potentially long incubation period of up to 30 days. Prompt clinical diagnosis is particularly important, because appropriate antibiotic treatment needs to be started early to maximize its benefit.

CLINICAL

The incubation period is usually 7-14 days but may range from 2 to 30 days. Over 90% of cases are relatively mild and self-limited. The remaining cases may be severe, often associated with jaundice and potentially life-threatening, sometimes referred to as Weil syndrome

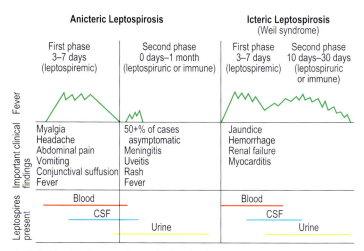

Fig. 23.2 **The clinical course of leptospirosis: anicteric and icteric disease.** *CSF,* **Cerebrospinal fluid. (**Adapted from: Feigin, R.D., Anderson, D.C., 1998. Leptospirosis. In: Feigin, R.D., Cherry, J.D. (Eds.), Textbook of Pediatric Infectious Diseases, fourth ed, vol. 2. Saunders, Philadelphia.**)**

(named after Adolf Weil, who was the first to describe the severe form of leptospirosis in 1892). Totally asymptomatic infections are probably rare.

The illness may be biphasic. The first, or "leptospiremic," phase typically lasts 3-7 days and represents the period when organisms are present in the blood. The second ("leptospiruric"), or immune phase, may be clinically silent or last for up to 1 month or longer. It coincides with the formation of circulating IgM antibodies. In the commoner, milder (anicteric) form of leptospirosis, there may be a clinically apparent, symptom-free interval of 1-3 days between the first and second phases (**Fig. 23.2**).

Anicteric Leptospirosis

Leptospirosis has protean manifestations. The classic presentation is with fever, headache, myalgias, and conjunctional suffusion. Typically, the onset is abrupt with high fever (often >39°C), chills, and a severe frontal headache. Patients may report that this is the worst headache they have ever experienced. Muscle pain and tenderness is common and typically involves the muscles of the calves, thighs, and lower back. Conjunctival suffusion (dilatation of conjunctival vessels without inflammation, not conjunctivitis) is virtually pathognomonic of leptospirosis when observed. It usually appears on the third or fourth day of illness and is probably very common, although it may be mild and easily overlooked if not sought diligently. Large studies have shown a prevalence of anywhere from 8 to 100%. Subconjunctival hemorrhages are often present.

Gastrointestinal symptoms may include abdominal pain, nausea, vomiting, and diarrhea. Pulmonary involvement occurs in 20-70% of cases. Respiratory symptoms may include cough, sometimes with hemoptysis, dyspnea, chest pain, and sore throat. Rashes are present in 10-30% of patients during the first week of illness, but typically last only 1-2 days. They may be erythematous, macular, maculopapular, urticarial, petechial, or purpuric.

There may be a symptom-free period of 1-3 days followed by the second (leptospiruric), or immune phase. This is often clinically inapparent. The hallmark of this phase is aseptic meningitis, and symptoms include headaches, neck stiffness, nausea, vomiting, and photophobia. There may be a low-grade temperature. Rashes may also be present during this phase. Inflammation of the anterior uveal tract has been reported in 2-10% of patients. It presents clinically as iritis, iridocyclitis, or chorioretinitis several weeks or months after the initial illness. It is usually bilateral and may run a prolonged or recurrent course. Rarely, long-term neuropsychiatric changes such as headaches, inability to concentrate, mood swings, depression, and psychosis have been reported following infection.

Severe (Icteric) Leptospirosis (Weil Syndrome)

Approximately 10% of patients with leptospirosis develop a severe, potentially life-threatening form of the disease. The onset of illness is indistinguishable from the milder form of leptospirosis. After 4–9 days, however, there is progression to a severe illness characterized by complications such as jaundice, renal failure, hemorrhage, and cardiopulmonary insufficiency or failure. Jaundice usually appears between the fifth and ninth days of illness and may last for several weeks. It may be marked, but liver failure is rare, because severe hepatocellular damage is very unusual. Tender hepatomegaly is common, and splenomegaly may occur. Renal involvement is common and may be evident within 3–4 days of onset. Several factors may be involved in the pathogenesis of renal insufficiency, including hypovolemia, hypotension, and acute tubular necrosis. Oliguric or non-oliguric renal failure usually occurs during the second week of illness. Peritoneal or hemodialysis may be required, although many cases can be managed without dialysis.

Hemorrhage appears to be the result of severe vasculitis, with endothelial damage resulting in capillary injury. Hemorrhagic manifestations include petechiae, purpura, bleeding gums, epistaxis, hemoptysis, gastrointestinal hemorrhage, and, rarely, subarachnoid or adrenal hemorrhage. Cardiac involvement may result in myocarditis or pericarditis, and there may be arrhythmias such as atrial fibrillation, atrial flutter, and a variety of conduction disturbances. Congestive heart failure may occur, and evidence of myocarditis is often present in fatal cases.

Pulmonary Leptospirosis

Pulmonary involvement may be prominent in severe leptospirosis. It may manifest as pulmonary hemorrhage, pneumonic consolidation, pleural effusions, or adult respiratory distress syndrome. Epidemics of leptospirosis with severe, sometimes fatal, pulmonary hemorrhage have been reported in Korea, China, Brazil, and Nicaragua. No single serovar was isolated in these cases. Typically, jaundice was rare or absent in these cases, distinguishing them from classic Weil syndrome and emphasizing that jaundice is not necessarily present in severe leptospirosis.

Overall mortality for leptospirosis is probably <1%. In severe leptospirosis, however, the mortality rate is about 5–10% and may be even higher in developing countries where facilities for dialysis and intensive care are often not readily available. Mortality tends to be particularly high in cases of pulmonary leptospirosis, in the elderly, or if there is serious underlying disease. Leptospirosis in pregnancy may be responsible for spontaneous abortion, particularly if infection occurs early in pregnancy. Congenital infection is probably rare.

DIFFERENTIAL DIAGNOSIS

Clinical manifestations of leptospirosis are very variable and often nonspecific. Clinicians should have a high index of suspicion to avoid misdiagnosis. There may be diagnostic clues or "red flags" that should alert clinicians to the possibility of leptospirosis (**Box 23.1**). There is often a broad differential diagnosis, particularly in a traveler who has recently returned from the tropics (**Box 23.2**). For example, leptospirosis may present as an unexplained febrile illness, pharyngitis, aseptic meningitis, or hemorrhagic fever, or it may mimic infections such as dengue fever, malaria, viral hepatitis, or typhus.

DIAGNOSIS

Cultures

Cultures should be obtained whenever possible, because they may aid in detecting cases that would be missed by serology alone. Blood and, where appropriate, CSF should be

Box 23.1   Diagnostic Red Flags

- History of contact with fresh water or mud
- History of contact with animals
- History of skin cuts or abrasions
- Abrupt onset of severe headache
- Severe myalgias (calves, thighs, lumbar area)
- Conjunctival suffusion
- Fever and new onset atrial fibrillation
- Jaundice with relatively mild transaminase elevation
- Fever, jaundice, and thrombocytopenia
- Hepatitis and neutrophil leukocytosis
- Fever and elevated creatine kinase levels
- Fever and elevated amylase levels

Box 23.2   Differential Diagnosis

- Influenza
- Streptococcal pharyngitis
- Viral hepatitis
- Aseptic meningitis
- Acute human immunodeficiency virus
- Legionnaires' disease
- Lyme disease
- Brucellosis
- Toxoplasmosis
- Hantaan virus
- Dengue fever
- Malaria
- Typhoid fever
- Rickettsial diseases (e.g., typhus, Q fever)
- Hemorrhagic fevers
- Relapsing fever
- Melioidosis
- Zika virus
- Chikungunya

cultured during the first 7-10 days of illness, prior to the administration of antibiotics. Urine should be cultured during the second week of illness and for up to 30 days after onset (**Fig. 23.2**). Tissue specimens and dialysis fluid can also be cultured in appropriate situations. Cultures should be inoculated as soon as possible using special media, for example, Fletcher semisolid or Tween 80-albumin (EMJH). Blood that cannot be inoculated immediately should be heparinized. If there is any delay in inoculating urine, it should be alkalinized using bovine serum albumin. It is important to emphasize that cultures may take anywhere from 1 to 6 weeks to become positive.

Immunodiagnosis

IgM antibodies appear as early as 4 days after the onset of symptoms but are usually not demonstrable until the second week. They usually peak by the third or fourth week. The appearance of serum antibodies may be suppressed or delayed by antibiotics or corticosteroids. The current reference standard is the microscopic agglutination test (MAT), a very labor- and skill-intensive test available only in specialized reference laboratories worldwide. Paired sera drawn 14-28 days apart should be obtained. Serologic diagnosis is usually based on demonstrating a four-fold rise or single MAT titer of at least 1 in 200. To make the diagnosis of leptospirosis, it is particularly important to obtain convalescent serum, because the acute serum is often negative for antibodies. Even paired sera may fail to detect infection in up to 10% of patients with culture-positive leptospirosis. Unfortunately, serovars present in the tropics may not be represented in the serovar pool, so that sera from patients with leptospirosis from tropical areas may test negative, emphasizing the importance of obtaining cultures whenever possible.

Rapid screening serologic tests that are sometimes used include enzyme-linked immunosorbent assay (ELISA), dot-ELISA, indirect hemagglutination, IgM dipstick, latex agglutination, and indirect fluorescent antibody. These alternative tests tend to have variable sensitivities and specificities depending on the location of the test and the case definition used.

Real-time PCR offers the attractive possibility of rapid, early diagnosis. Fortunately, the test is becoming more readily available, although it is not routinely offered in most settings.

LABORATORY AND RADIOLOGIC FINDINGS

The total white blood cell count is variable but is usually elevated in severe disease. A neutrophil (polymorphonuclear) leukocytosis is common, in contrast to viral hepatitis. A mild to moderate thrombocytopenia (platelet counts 50,000-120,000/mm³) is not uncommon and may occur in up to 50% of cases. Platelet counts of <50,000/mm³ are less common but may be seen in severe disease. Prothrombin time may be prolonged in severe leptospirosis but can be corrected with vitamin K. Erythrocyte sedimentation rate is very commonly elevated and is often >50 mm/h.

Liver function abnormalities include elevated bilirubin (up to 20 mg/dL or higher) but with relatively mild increase in alkaline phosphatase and transaminase levels. Elevated serum amylase has been reported in 47-80% of cases, but only a few of these patients have any evidence of pancreatitis. Creatine kinase levels are elevated in over half the patients during the first week of illness. This may help to differentiate leptospirosis from viral hepatitis.

Urinalysis is abnormal in at least 70% of cases, although the abnormalities may be slight and transient, particularly in mild cases. Abnormalities may include proteinuria, hyaline or granular casts, pyuria, and hematuria.

CSF obtained during the second (immune) phase of illness shows features of an aseptic meningitis. The CSF cell count is usually <500/mm³. Polymorphonuclear leukocytes (neutrophils) predominate early in the illness, but mononuclear cells increase later. CSF protein may be elevated (up to 300 mg/dL), but CSF glucose is usually normal.

Chest radiograph abnormalities have been noted in 23-67% of patients. Abnormalities develop 3-9 days after the onset of illness. Radiographs may be abnormal despite normal clinical examination. Abnormalities include small nodular densities, large confluent areas of consolidation, and diffuse, ill-defined, ground-glass densities. These abnormalities are usually bilateral, nonlobar, and predominantly peripheral.

TREATMENT

Antibiotic treatment should be started as soon as the diagnosis of leptospirosis is suspected, because antimicrobials are most effective if initiated during the first 4 days of illness. Early antibiotic treatment has been shown to reduce the duration and severity of illness. There is evidence of some benefit, however, even if treatment with intravenous penicillin is started relatively late in the course of severe illness. Antibiotics should be continued for 7-10 days. The organism is sensitive to a wide range of antibiotics. Penicillin, ampicillin, amoxicillin, or doxycycline are often recommended. Erythromycin, third-generation cephalosporins such as ceftriaxone and cefotaxime, and some fluoroquinolones also appear to be very effective. The organism may be resistant to chloramphenicol, vancomycin, aminoglycosides, and first-generation cephalosporins.

In the early stages of infection, it is usually impossible to be certain of the diagnosis of leptospirosis. Hence, antibiotic coverage needs to be broad enough to include other possible diagnoses. Supportive care, if necessary in an intensive care unit, is also important, and meticulous attention to fluid and electrolyte balance is essential. Peritoneal or hemodialysis has helped to reduce mortality from leptospirosis, since in the past renal failure was an important cause of death. Jarisch-Herxheimer reactions have been reported following treatment of leptospirosis with penicillin, but they appear to be less common than with other spirochetal infections. Steroids have not yet been proved to be of any benefit.

PREVENTION

Travelers at risk of leptospirosis should be identified and counseled appropriately prior to departure. Recommendations for prevention include avoiding potentially contaminated fresh water, damp soil, or mud whenever possible; wearing protective waterproof clothing; and covering cuts and abrasions with waterproof dressings. Submersion in potentially contaminated fresh water should be avoided, since the organism can enter via the mucous membranes of the eyes, nose, and mouth. Drinking water may be contaminated with leptospires and should be purified by boiling or treating with iodine or chlorine. Filtration may not be adequate, since the organism is slender and highly motile and can pass through membrane filters up to 0.2 μm in diameter.

Travelers to areas that have recently experienced flooding may be at increased risk of infection and should be especially careful. In high-risk situations, they may be candidates for prophylactic antibiotics.

A killed whole-cell vaccine is available for immunization of high-risk humans in China, Japan, Vietnam, Israel, and certain European countries. Safety and efficacy in humans remains uncertain, however. In addition, it is important to emphasize that the vaccines are serovar-specific, and even if an inexpensive, safe, and effective vaccine were available, it would have limited value for travelers. Animal vaccines are effective and widely available but offer only short-term, serovar-specific protection. Previous infection provides protection only against the infecting serovar. Second infections are possible, therefore, in high-risk individuals with recurrent exposure to infection (e.g., rice farmers).

Chemoprophylaxis using doxycycline 200 mg once weekly, beginning prior to the first exposure and ending after the last exposure, was effective in preventing leptospirosis in US military in Panama. Short-term, high-risk travelers may be suitable candidates for chemoprophylaxis. Doxycycline 100 mg, once daily, for prevention of malaria probably also protects against leptospirosis. Travelers at risk of both malaria and leptospirosis may be particularly appropriate candidates for doxycycline chemoprophylaxis rather than alternative antimalarials such as atovaquone plus proguanil (Malarone) or mefloquine.

FURTHER READING

Adler, B., 2015. Leptospira and Leptospirosis. Springer Publishing Company, New York.

Antony, S.J., 1996. Leptospirosis—an emerging pathogen in travel medicine: a review of its clinical manifestations and management. J Travel. Med. 3, 113–118.

CDC, 1997. Outbreak of leptospirosis among white-water rafters—Costa Rica 1996. MMWR 46, 577–579.

Faine, S., 1994. Leptospira and Leptospirosis. CRC Press, Boca Raton, FL.

Farr, R.W., 1995. Leptospirosis. Clin. Infect. Dis. 21, 1–6.

Gaynor, K., Katz, A.R., Park, S.Y., et al., 2007. Leptospirosis on Oahu: an outbreak associated with flooding of a university campus. Am. J. Trop. Med. Hyg. 76 (5), 882–886.

Griffith, M.E., Hospenthal, D.R., Murray, C.K., 2006. Antimicrobial therapy of leptospirosis. Curr. Opin. Infect. Dis. 19, 533–537.

Heron, L.G., Reiss-Levy, E.A., Jacques, T.C., et al., 1997. Leptospirosis presenting as a haemorrhagic fever in a traveler from Africa. Med. J. Aus. 167, 477–479.

Jackson, L.A., Kaufmann, A.F., Adams, W.G., et al., 1993. Outbreak of leptospirosis associated with swimming. Pediatr. Infect. Dis. J. 12, 48–54.

Katz, A.R., Ansdell, V.E., Effler, P.V., et al., 2002. Leptospirosis in Hawaii 1974–1998: epidemiologic analysis of 353 laboratory-confirmed cases. Am. J. Trop. Med. Hyg. 66 (1), 61–70.

Katz, A.R., Ansdell, V.E., Middleton, C.R., et al., 2001. Assessment of the clinical presentation and treatment of 353 cases of laboratory confirmed leptospirosis in Hawaii 1974–1998. Clin. Infec. Dis. 33 (11), 1834–1841.

Lau, C., Smythe, L., Weinstein, P., 2010. Leptospirosis: an emerging disease in travellers. Trav. Med. Inf. Dis. 8, 33–39.

Monsuez, J., Kidouche, R., LeGueno, B., et al., 1997. Leptospirosis presenting as haemorrhagic fever in a visitor to Africa. Lancet 349, 254–255.

O'Neill, K.M., Rickman, L.S., Lazarus, A.A., 1991. Pulmonary manifestations of leptospirosis. Rev. Infect. Dis. 13, 705–709.

Sasaki, D.M., Pang, L., Minette, H.P., et al., 1993. Active surveillance and risk factors for leptospirosis in Hawaii. Am. J. Trop. Med. Hyg. 48, 35–43.

Sejvar, J., Bancroft, E., Winthrop, K., et al., 2003. Leptospirosis in "Eco-challenge" athletes, Malaysian Borneo, 2000. Emerg. Infect. Dis. 9, 702–707.

Takafuji, E.T., Kirkpatrick, J.W., Miller, R.N., et al., 1984. An efficacy trial of doxycycline chemoprophylaxis against leptospirosis. N. Engl. J. Med. 310, 497–500.

Trevejo, R.T., Rigan-Perez, J.G., Ashford, D.A., et al., 1998. Epidemic leptospirosis associated with pulmonary hemorrhage—Nicaragua, 1995. J. Infect. Dis. 178, 1457–1463.

Van Crevel, R., Speelman, P., Grevekamp, C., et al., 1994. Leptospirosis in travelers. Clin. Infect. Dis. 19, 132–134.

Van de Werve, C., Perignon, A., Jaureguiberry, S., et al., 2013. Travel-related leptospirosis : a series of 15 imported cases. J. Travel Med. 20 (4), 228–231.

Watt, G., Padre, L.P., Tauzon, M.L., et al., 1988. Placebo-controlled trial of intravenous penicillin for severe and late leptospirosis. Lancet 1, 433–435.

CHAPTER 24

Lyme Disease

Paul S. Pottinger

In 1977, Steere and co-workers reported on an epidemic of arthritis in the region of Old Lyme, Connecticut. This breakthrough work catalyzed a flurry of studies that soon described *Ixodes* ticks as the vector, identified the spirochete *Borrelia burgdorferi* as the causative infectious pathogen, and characterized the broad clinical manifestations of Lyme disease. Interestingly, several authors had previously described patients in Europe with clinical manifestations similar to patients with Lyme disease, and subsequently European cases were also shown to be caused by infection with *Borrelia* species. Currently, Lyme disease is appreciated as an important vector-borne disease that occurs worldwide and is the most common tick-borne infection in both North America and Europe.

CAUSATIVE ORGANISM

B.burgdorferi is a 0.2×25 μm unicellular spirochete bacteria. In different regions of the world, distinct *B. burgdorferi* species exist, based on specific antigenic differences: (1) *B. burgdorferi* sensu stricto, (2) *B. garinii*, (3) *B. afzelii*, and (4) *B. japonica*. In the United States, all isolates to date have been *B. burgdorferi* sensu stricto. In Europe, however, most isolates have been either *B. garinii* or *B. afzelii*. The distinct antigenic strains may explain some of the differences observed in the predominant clinical manifestations in persons infected with *B. burgdorferi* in the United States versus those infected in Europe. In 2016, a new species provisionaly called *B. mayonii* was described in the blood of six patients from the Midwestern US who presented with atypical and severe Lyme Disease; whether this species will emerge as an important pathogen, and whether it should be diagnosed or treated differently from *B. burgdorferi* infection, remains to be seen.

All strains of *B. burgdorferi* have a central protoplasmic cylinder surrounded by an outer envelope that contains important surface proteins. In 1995, Schwan and colleagues reported that *B. burgdorferi* present in unfed ticks is predominantly covered by outer surface protein (Osp)A, but after the tick feeds for several days on a mammal, OspC replaces OspA. The change from spirochete OspA to OspC coating results from increased expression of the OspC gene in response to the increase in tick temperature that takes place during feeding. This change in surface proteins evidently serves as a prerequisite for the spirochete to migrate from the tick's midgut to the tick's salivary gland. Available data suggest that infection of humans involves *B. burgdorferi* coated with OspC, not OspA. More recent work has described two other heat-sensitive *B. burgdorferi* outer surface proteins, known as decorin-binding proteins A and B (DbpA and DbpB); these are lipoproteins that may act as spirochetal adhesins. Mice immunized with DbpA antigen develop antibodies that block *B. burgdorferi* dissemination from the site of cutaneous inoculation, and antiserum from persistently infected mice had cidal activity against both cultured and plasma-derived *B. burgdorferi*. These findings suggest DbpA antibodies may contribute to control of acute and persistent infection.

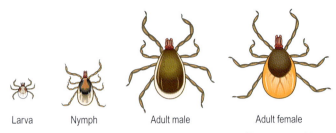

Larva   Nymph   Adult male   Adult female

Fig. 24.1 **Non-engorged *Ixodes* ticks at different life cycle phases.** (To reproduce with permission from University of Rhode Island; TickEncounter Resource Center)

TRANSMISSION

In the United States, *B. burgdorferi* can be potentially transmitted to humans via one of two types of *Ixodes* ticks: *Ixodes scapularis* (formerly known as *Ixodes dammini* and commonly referred to as the deer tick) and *Ixodes pacificus* (commonly referred to as the Western black-legged tick) (**Fig. 24.1**). In the United States, *I. scapularis* ticks are most concentrated in the Northeastern, mid-Atlantic and north-central states, and *I. pacificus* is clustered in West Coast states. In Europe, *Ixodes ricinus* serves as the primary vector, whereas in Asia *Ixodes persulcatus* is the major vector. In the Northeastern and upper north Midwestern United States, the white-footed mouse, *Peromyscus leucopus*, serves as the most common reservoir for *B. burgdorferi*. The white-tailed deer also play a major role, because the adult *I. scapularis* ticks prefer to mate on these animals. In most of the Western United States, the dusky-footed wood rat is the major reservoir for *B. burgdorferi*, but two species of *Ixodes* ticks, *Ixodes neotomae* and *I. pacificus*, are involved in the life cycle of *B. burgdorferi*. In this so-called California bi-cycle, the *I. neotomae* ticks play the role of infecting the wood rat with *B. burgdorferi*, whereas the *I. pacificus* ticks play the role of transmitting *B. burgdorferi* to humans after acquiring *B. burgdorferi* from the wood rat reservoir.

In contrast to many other infections discussed in this book, Lyme disease is *not* typically acquired in the tropics, due to the life cycle of the vector.

The life cycle of these *Ixodes* ticks includes three stages, typically lasting 2 years and requiring a blood meal at each stage in order to mature to the next stage. The cycle begins in the spring when the adult female tick releases her eggs and they hatch as six-legged larvae. During the summer, the larvae take a blood meal, followed by a dormant phase in the fall. In the spring, the ticks molt and enter the second phase of their life cycle as eight-legged nymphal ticks. In the late spring or summer, the nymphal ticks take a blood meal and subsequently molt as eight-legged adults in the fall. The adults then mate and the male dies; the female, however, takes one more blood meal before she lays her eggs and dies. Although ticks at any of these three stages are competent vectors for *B. burgdorferi* transmission to humans, most cases of Lyme disease result from the bite of the 2-3 mm nymphal tick. In the United States, *Ixodes* ticks also serve as the vector for the infectious pathogens that cause babesiosis (*Babesia microti*) and human granulocytic anaplasmosis (*Anaplasma phagocytophilum*), formerly referred to as ehrlichiosis. Thus, a bite from an *I. scapularis* tick may lead to an infection with any one of these agents as a single infection or possibly as a co-infection.

Bites from *Ixodes* ticks are generally painless, and <50% of patients with Lyme disease recall a tick bite. Animal laboratory studies show efficient transmission of *B. burgdorferi* by *I. scapularis* requires a minimum of 36-48 hours of tick attachment, but human cases have apparently occurred after shorter periods of tick attachment. Nevertheless, it does appear that, in general, transmission to humans probably requires at least 8 hours of attachment. The requirement for prolonged attachment correlates with the change in *B. burgdorferi* OspA (non-infectious state) to OspC (infectious state).

EPIDEMIOLOGY

In 1982, following the realization that Lyme disease had emerged as a major vector-borne disease in the United States, the Centers for Disease Control and Prevention (CDC) initiated surveillance for Lyme disease. In 1991 Lyme disease became a reportable disease, with a case defined for surveillance purposes as: (1) physician-diagnosed erythema migrans rash of at least 5 cm or (2) at least one objective late manifestation (i.e., musculoskeletal, cardiovascular, or neurologic) with laboratory evidence of infection with *B. burgdorferi* in a person with possible exposure to infected ticks.

In 2013, CDC reported a total of 27, 203 confirmed cases, yielding a national incidence of 8.6 confirmed cases per 100,000 population. An additional 9,104 probable cases that year would result in a higher case incidence, if included in the calculation. However, Lyme disease happens in a very focal manner: 95% of the cases in 2013 occurred among residents of 14 states where the disease is considered endemic: Connecticut, Delaware, Maine, Maryland, Massachusetts, Minnesota, New Hampshire, New Jersey, New York, Pennsylvania, Rhode Island, Vermont, Virginia, and Wisconsin (**Fig. 24.2**). These highly endemic regions for Lyme disease correlate with the regions that have a high density of *Ixodes* ticks.

From 1982 until the present time, reported cases of Lyme disease have shown a gradual increase, despite the fact that Lyme disease surveillance is subject to both underreporting and overdiagnosis of cases, in addition to probable variation in diagnostic and reporting practices. In August 2013, the CDC shared new, higher estimates of Lyme disease incidence: up to 300,000 cases per year in the United States.

In the United States, most human infections with *B. burgdorferi* occur during the months of May-August, corresponding with the most active feeding period of the *Ixodes* nymphal ticks and maximal human outdoor exposure. The timing of cases in the Western United States is generally several weeks later than in the Eastern United States, mainly because of the later onset of warmer weather. In the 2003-2005 CDC data, 61% of cases were in children aged 5-14, with a male predominance. However, this gender difference diminishes with age, and overall males accounted for 54% of reported cases in that data set.

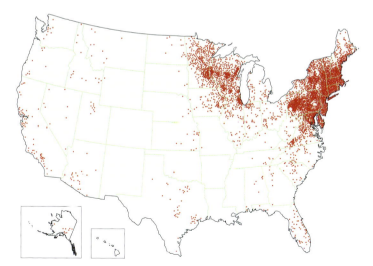

Fig. 24.2 **Reported cases of Lyme disease—United States, 2014. One dot was placed randomly within the county of patient residence for each reported case (not necessarily the location of infection). (Source: CDC.gov/lyme.)**

Several lines of evidence suggest *B. burgdorferi* can be transmitted transplacentally, but adverse birth outcomes related to maternal Lyme disease appear to be rare.

CLINICAL MANIFESTATIONS

From a conceptual standpoint, Lyme disease can be categorized into three different stages: (1) early-localized (onset days to weeks after infection), (2) early-disseminated (days to months), and (3) late (months to years). From a practical perspective, most patients do not pass through all three phases; the manifestations of the stages can overlap; specific clinical manifestations can occur independently; and some patients develop asymptomatic infection. Clinical features of Lyme disease in the United States differ somewhat from those in Europe; erythema migrans and arthritis occur more frequently among patients in the United States, whereas neurologic and chronic skin conditions are more common in European patients.

The most common clinical manifestation of Lyme disease in the United States is the erythematous macular rash known as erythema migrans. This lesion develops in 60-80% of Lyme disease cases, typically appearing at the site of the tick bite an average of 7 days following the bite (range 3-30 days). Patients often also have concomitant mild to moderate constitutional symptoms, including low-grade fever, headache, fatigue, myalgias, and regional lymphadenopathy. The typical appearance of erythema migrans is a round or oval, well-demarcated, erythematous lesion at least 5 cm in diameter (median, 15 cm). The lesion can appear in one of several forms, including a solid lesion, a bull's-eye pattern, or as multiple rings. If untreated, the erythema migrans lesion gradually expands, typically developing partial central clearing and reaching a diameter of >30 cm. Erythema migrans and associated early symptoms typically persist for 3-4 weeks if left untreated. In some instances, patients and medical providers may confuse erythema migrans with an allergic reaction to an insect bite. An insect bite typically is painful, has its onset within 24 hours of the bite, and usually resolves within several days. Erythema migrans, on the other hand, is usually painless, has a delayed onset of typically 7-10 days, and will persist for weeks if not treated.

Although *B. burgdorferi* infection is initially limited to the primary cutaneous site, dissemination from the site of infection to distant sites can occur within days to a few weeks after initial inoculation. Some patients will show evidence of dissemination early in their course by developing multiple, widespread, secondary annular erythema migrans lesions; these secondary lesions are generally smaller than the initial erythema migrans lesion and can vary in number from one lesion to >50. Years after the initial infection, patients may develop a late-stage cutaneous manifestation known as acrodermatitis chronica atrophicans; this chronic scarring skin lesion can resemble scleroderma and is considerably more common among European patients with Lyme disease than among those in the United States.

Months after the initial infection, approximately 60% of patients with Lyme disease in the United States will develop arthralgias or arthritis. The arthritis typically consists of brief attacks of asymmetric, oligoarticular arthritis involving large joints, interspersed with months of remission. Only about 10% of patients with untreated Lyme disease will develop chronic arthritis, and these patients often have the HLA-DR4 haplotype. In addition, patients with HLA-DR4 often have a poor response to antimicrobial therapy. Even with chronic Lyme arthritis, patients generally have resolution of their active flares within 5-6 years, and most do not develop permanent joint damage. The arthralgias tend to also involve large joints, have intermittent recurrences, and usually resolve within 5-6 years.

Overall, about 20% of patients with Lyme disease have some type of neurologic manifestation. Early in the course of Lyme disease, patients may develop unilateral or bilateral facial palsy. Less frequently, patients may present with a lymphocytic meningitis or meningoencephalitis within months of the initial infection. Later in the course (months to years after infection), patients may develop peripheral neuropathy that can manifest as radiculoneuritis, mononeuritis multiplex, or diffuse peripheral neuropathy. The late-appearing chronic neurologic manifestations pose special difficulty, since many of these symptoms are nonspecific and can overlap with many other diseases. The Lyme-associated chronic neurologic manifestations include subacute encephalopathy, axonal polyneuropathy, and, less frequently, leukoencephalopathy. Available studies suggest that sub-acute encephalopathy is the most common of these chronic neurologic manifestations; it is characterized by cognitive deficits and disturbances in mood and sleep. Unfortunately, patients with untreated chronic neurologic Lyme disease may have persistence of their symptoms for several years, even longer than 10 years in some cases. However, this rarely happens in current practice, where antibiotics are often given on suspicion of Lyme disease. There is no evidence that patients who have received an appropriate course of treatment (see below) but who still complain of fatigue or cognitive disability have "chronic Lyme disease." Rather, these patients carry a diagnosis of "post-treatment Lyme disease syndrome," an important distinction that emphasizes the fact that further courses of antibiotics will not be of benefit.

Although cardiac manifestations develop in <10% of patients with Lyme disease, they can have potentially fatal consequences. The most common cardiac abnormality is atrioventricular block, occurring in about 5-8% of patients with Lyme disease, typically weeks to months after the initial infection. Although some patients have required a temporary pacemaker for severe atrioventricular conduction disturbances, these abnormalities generally do not necessitate placing a permanent pacemaker if the patient receives appropriate therapy for Lyme disease. Other less common cardiac manifestations include myocarditis, pericarditis, and pancarditis. Rare reports have described cases of chronic cardiomyopathy caused by *B. burgdorferi*. The prevalence of cardiac abnormalities among persons with Lyme disease who have received antibiotic therapy—typically for erythema migrans—is the same as for persons without a history of Lyme disease.

In addition to the cutaneous, joint, neurologic, and cardiac manifestations, rare reports have described involvement of other body sites, which poses a diagnostic challenge for even the most astute clinician.

DIAGNOSIS

As noted earlier, the CDC has generated a case definition for Lyme disease for surveillance purposes. This case definition, however, is not meant to be a rigid guideline for actual clinical decisions regarding who should or should not receive therapy for Lyme disease. Multiple factors play a role in the clinical decision making regarding the clinical diagnosis of Lyme disease. From a clinical perspective, a diagnosis of Lyme disease should initially be based on compatible clinical findings in a patient with a reasonable probability of previous exposure to *Ixodes* ticks; serologic testing for evidence of *B. burgdorferi* infection can then serve as an adjunct to clinical judgment. Most laboratories use the serum enzyme immunoassay (EIA) as a screening test and the serum Western immunoblot as a confirmatory test.

Recommendations for serologic testing of patients with suspected Lyme disease arose from expert groups that convened at the Second National Conference on Serologic Diagnosis of Lyme Disease in 1994; these expert groups included the CDC, the Association of State and Territorial Public Health Laboratory Directors, the Food and Drug Administration (FDA), and the National Institutes of Health. In general, these groups recommended using a two-step diagnostic process for suspected cases, with initial testing consisting of an EIA or an immunofluorescent antibody test (**Fig. 24.3**). If the initial test is positive or equivocal, further "confirmatory" testing should be performed using a standardized Western immunoblot, because the screening tests have less than optimal specificity. If the Western immunoblot is positive, the patient is considered to have laboratory evidence of Lyme disease. Because adequate antibody responses to *B. burgdorferi* may not be generated in the first several weeks of infection, patients with a negative screening test taken <4 weeks after possible infection should undergo follow-up convalescent repeat testing. If, however, the patient has a negative screening test taken after 4 weeks of infection, they do not have laboratory evidence of Lyme disease and would, in general, not need further testing for Lyme disease.

The same expert panel also generated recommendations that standardized the criteria for a positive Western immunoblot serology test. Specifically, they recommended that the Western immunoblot IgM should be considered positive if at least two of the following bands are present: 21/24 kDa (OspC), 39 kDa (BmpA), and 41 kDa (Fla). The

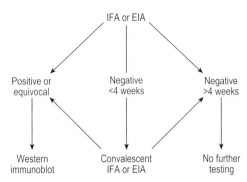

Fig. 24.3 **Recommended approach for serologic testing of patients with suspected Lyme disease.** *EIA*, Enzyme immunoassay; *IFA*, immunofluorescent antibody test. (Source: Centers for Disease Control and Prevention.)

recommended criteria for a positive Western immunoblot IgG are presence of at least five of the following 10 bands: 18 kDa, 21/24 kDa (OspC), 28 kDa, 30 kDa, 39 kDa (BmpA), 41 kDa (Fla), 45 kDa, 58 kDa (not GroEL), 66 kDa, and 93 kDa. Most commercial laboratories that perform *B. burgdorferi* Western immunoblot assays now incorporate these specific diagnostic criteria into their interpretation of the test.

Although standardization of *B. burgdorferi* Western immunoblotting now exists, several major problems still exist with serologic testing for Lyme disease. First, false-negative antibody tests are common during the initial 4-6 weeks of the patient's illness, a time when patients most often present with the initial erythema migrans rash. Second, antimicrobial treatment of early Lyme disease can blunt antibody responses and thus generate a false-negative test. Third, false-positive results can result from other infectious agents and other diseases, including Epstein-Barr virus, oral treponemes, syphilis, relapsing fever, and rheumatoid arthritis. Fourth, test results vary significantly in different laboratories, a problem compounded by the multitude of laboratories that now perform *B. burgdorferi* serologic testing. Other diagnostic tests, such as culture, antigen detection, polymerase chain reaction (PCR), and measurement of cell-mediated immunity to *B. burgdorferi*, are considered investigational and are not recommended for routine clinical purposes. Among these investigational techniques, PCR-based tests show the most promise, especially for patients for early-stage Lyme disease, as well as those with potential false-negative antibody titers. However, this technique is experimental, and clinical decisions should not be based on PCR results from commercial laboratories. Although several investigators have cultured *B. burgdorferi* from clinical specimens, performing cultures requires a special medium (Barbour-Stoenner-Kelly) that is neither rapid nor widely available. Some reference laboratories perform *B. burgdorferi* cerebrospinal fluid antibody titers, but interpretive criteria are not standardized.

Several studies have shown that significant problems exist with the overdiagnosis of Lyme disease. In particular, two studies both found that only about one-quarter of patients referred to their clinic with suspected active Lyme disease actually had active Lyme disease. One of these studies also reported that among persons referred to their clinic who had not responded to antibiotic therapy for Lyme disease, nearly 80% had not responded because the initial diagnosis of Lyme disease was not warranted. Patients may present with a diagnosis of Lyme made by a self-described "Lyme literate doctor," which is a warning sign that their workup and management may have been incomplete or flawed. Healthcare workers can combat this problem in two ways:

(1) *Blood should be tested for Lyme disease only when clinically appropriate.* Unless there is pre-test suspicion for this infection based on epidemiological risk factors and clinical

manifestations, the reliability of the test falls dramatically, and the odds of a positive test reflecting true infection are greatly reduced. A common error is to test for Lyme during the initial work-up of chronic fatigue syndrome. Instead, a stepwise approach should be pursued, as suggested by the CDC (www.CDC.gov/cfs).

(2) *Use an appropriate laboratory.* The importance of sending specimens to a reputable laboratory cannot be overemphasized. Some laboratories have been outlawed in certain states, due to their questionable business and scientific practices. Ensure that the laboratory you use is certified by the FDA and College of American Pathologists and performs other blood work services for your institution; in general, avoid labs that "specialize" exclusively in Lyme diagnostics and exercise skepticism when reviewing results ordered by a patient before seeking formal medical care.

THERAPY

Patients with early Lyme disease, especially erythema migrans, respond well to antimicrobial therapy. In general, with long delays in the initial diagnosis of Lyme disease, patients have poorer responses to antimicrobial therapy. The following treatment recommendations are based on the Infectious Diseases Society of America (IDSA) clinical practice guideline "The Clinical Assessment, Treatment, and Prevention of Lyme Disease, Human Granulocytic Anaplasmosis, and Babesiosis" (**Table 24.1**). The primary goal of treating patients with early-stage Lyme disease is to decrease the duration of the acute manifestations (such as erythema migrans), as well as to diminish the likelihood that later sequelae of Lyme disease will develop. More than 90% of patients with erythema migrans respond to a 10- to 21-day course of oral doxycycline (100 mg twice/day), amoxicillin (500 mg three times/day), or cefuroxime axetil (500 mg twice/day). In general, doxycycline should not be used to treat Lyme disease in pregnant women, lactating women, or children ≤8 years old. Either amoxicillin or cefuroxime axetil could be used instead of doxycycline in these individuals. In children, amoxicillin should be dosed at 50 mg/kg per day in three divided doses (maximum of 500 mg/dose), and cefuroxime axetil dosed at 30 mg/kg per day in two divided doses (maximum of 500 mg/dose). In children ≥8 years of age, doxycycline would be dosed at 4 mg/kg per day in two divided doses (maximum of 100 mg/dose). Because the macrolide antibiotics (azithromycin, clarithromycin, erythromycin) have treatment success rates lower than doxycycline or amoxicillin, they are not recommended as first-line therapy for the treatment of Lyme disease.

Treatment with doxycycline provides an advantage over amoxicillin in geographic areas where patients with Lyme disease may have concomitant human granulocytic anaplasmosis because doxycycline effectively treats both of these tick-borne diseases. Doxycycline is not recommended for the treatment of babesiosis (initial therapy for babesiosis consists of a 7- to 10-day course of either atovaquone plus azithromycin or clindamycin plus quinine).

Initial therapy of Lyme arthritis with oral therapy gives response rates similar to those seen with intravenous regimens. Overall response rates are in the range of 50-60%, but lower among those who previously received intra-articular steroids. In addition, responses are often delayed several months. For patients with recurrent arthritis after treatment with an oral regimen, another course of oral therapy for 28 days or a course of intravenous therapy for 14 days may be considered.

For patients with early-stage neurologic Lyme disease that manifests only as a facial palsy, oral therapy is recommended, whereas those with acute meningitis or radiculopathy should receive parenteral therapy. Recommended treatment for late neurologic Lyme disease consists of parenteral therapy. Overall, about 60% of patients with neurologic involvement show significant improvement in their neurologic manifestations, but, similar to patients with Lyme arthritis, improvement may be delayed for several months after therapy. Treatment for neurological infection with antibiotic courses beyond 28 days has not been shown to help patients in carefully constructed randomized trials, and thus the IDSA recommends against this practice.

TABLE 24.1 Preferred Regimens for the Initial Treatment of Lyme Disease in Adults

Manifestation	Therapy	Route	Dose	Duration in Days (Range)
Erythema migrans	Doxycycline	p.o.	100 mg b.i.d.	14 (10-21)
	Amoxicillin	p.o.	500 mg t.i.d.	14 (14-21)
	Cefuroxime axetil	p.o.	500 mg b.i.d.	14 (14-21)
Arthritis (without neurologic disease)	Doxycycline	p.o.	100 mg b.i.d.	28
	Amoxicillin	p.o.	500 mg t.i.d.	28
	Cefuroxime axetil	i.v.	500 mg b.i.d.	28
Cardiac				
Mild (AV block with PR <0.3 s)	Doxycycline	p.o.	100 mg b.i.d.	14 (14-21)
	Amoxicillin	p.o.	500 mg t.i.d.	14 (14-21)
	Cefuroxime axetil	p.o.	500 mg b.i.d.	14 (14-21)
Serious	Ceftriaxone	i.v.	2 g q.d.	14 (10-28)
Early Neurologic				
Meningitis or radiculopathy	Ceftriaxone	i.v.	2 g i.v. q.d.	14 (10-28)
Cranial nerve palsy	Doxycycline	p.o.	100 mg b.i.d.	14 (14-21)
	Amoxicillin	p.o.	500 mg t.i.d.	14 (14-21)
	Cefuroxime axetil	p.o.	500 mg b.i.d.	14 (14-21)
Late neurologic (central or peripheral nervous system disease)	Ceftriaxone	i.v.		14 (14-28)

AV, Atrioventricular; *b.i.d.*, twice per day; *i.v.*, intravenous; *p.o.*, by mouth; *q.d.*, once per day; *t.i.d.*, three times per day.
(Based on recommendations from: Wormser, G.P., Dattwyler, R.J., Shapiro, E.D., et al., 2006. The clinical assessment, treatment, and prevention of Lyme disease, human granulocytic anaplasmosis, and babesiosis: clinical practice guidelines by the Infectious Diseases Society of America. Clin. Infect. Dis. 43, 1089–1134.)

Patients with mild cardiac disease (asymptomatic and PR interval ≤0.3 s) can be treated with oral therapy. For all other patients with cardiac disease, intravenous therapy should be used. In general, patients with cardiac involvement should be observed closely and may require a temporary pacemaker.

Many patients treated for Lyme disease do not improve after therapy. The complex reasons for poor response may include initial misdiagnosis, concomitant chronic illnesses such as fibromyalgia or depression, slowly resolving Lyme disease, permanent tissue damage caused by *B. burgdorferi*, post-Lyme autoimmune disease, persistent tissue infection with *B. burgdorferi*, and sterile inflammation caused by dead organisms. For those patients who do not respond to antibiotics and have no objective evidence of active Lyme disease, repeated courses of antibiotics have no proven benefit but do carry substantial risk of harm and are not recommended. They do not have "chronic Lyme disease" but rather should be diagnosed with "post-treatment Lyme disease syndrome." This condition is very real, and suffering should be validated; optimum treatment is not certain, but antibiotics are clearly not beneficial here and indeed are often harmful. An excellent resource for patients is the website www.CDC.gov/lyme/postlds.

PREVENTION

The three major strategies involved in preventing Lyme disease include avoiding tick bites, administering prophylactic antibiotics in the event a tick bite occurs, and using a vaccine. The vaccine option is no longer available in the United States.

Tick Bite Prevention

The easiest and first step in preventing Lyme disease and other *Ixodes* species-transmitted pathogens involves decreasing the risk of receiving an *Ixodes* tick bite and minimizing the duration of a bite if it does occur. In general, specific preventive measures consist of staying in the middle of trails when walking through wooded areas, avoiding tall grass and shrubs, wearing light-colored clothing to more easily spot any tick that may crawl onto clothing, wearing long pants tucked into socks, wearing shoes or closed-toed sandals, and wearing an effective tick repellent (Chapter 1). Frequent checks for ticks are recommended, because *B. burgdorferi* is usually not transmitted to humans unless a tick has been attached for at least 8 hours. If an attached tick is found, a pair of tweezers should be used to grasp the tick as close to the skin as possible, and then it should be removed by pulling perpendicular to the skin with slow, steady pressure.

Post-Exposure Antibiotic Prophylaxis

Recommendations on whether to give prophylactic antibiotics to persons following an *Ixodes* tick bite have generated controversy over the years. Clinical practice guidelines from the IDSA guidelines state that "a single dose of doxycycline may be offered to adult patients (200 mg dose) and to children ≥8 years of age (4 mg/kg up to a maximum dose of 200 mg) when all of the following circumstances can be met: (a) the attached tick can be reliably identified as an adult or nymphal *I. scapularis* tick that is estimated to have been attached for ≥36 h on the basis of degree of engorgement of the tick with blood or of certainty about the time of exposure to the tick; (b) prophylaxis can be started within 72 h of the time that the tick was removed; (c) ecologic information indicates that the local rate of infection of these ticks with *B. burgdorferi* is ≥20%; and (d) doxycycline treatment is not contraindicated." The guidelines go on to state that "prophylaxis after *I. pacificus* bites is generally not necessary, because rates of infection with *B. burgdorferi* in these ticks are low in almost the entire region in which the tick is endemic."

These IDSA guidelines regarding the use of prophylactic antibiotics after a tick bite are predominantly based on results from a study conducted in a region in New York hyper-endemic for Lyme disease. The major findings of this study were that a single 200-mg dose of doxycycline was highly effective for post-exposure prophylaxis if given within 72 hours of the *Ixodes* tick bite and that only those bites involving partially or fully engorged ticks led to clinical disease. Whether or not the person receives prophylactic antibiotics, he or she should receive specific information on the signs and symptoms of early Lyme disease and should promptly return for further evaluation if any signs or symptoms develop that are suggestive of Lyme disease.

Lyme Disease Vaccine

Two recombinant *B. burgdorferi* OspA Lyme disease vaccines have been developed and have undergone large-scale evaluation: LYMErix (SmithKline Beecham) and ImuLyme (Pasteur Merieux Connaught). These vaccines have a novel mechanism of action in that they stimulate human antibodies to OspA, and these antibodies neutralize *B. burgdorferi* in the midgut of the *Ixodes* tick, while the tick takes a blood meal. Because *B. burgdorferi* within the tick changes its outer protein covering from OspA to OspC after prolonged feeding, the human OspA antibodies would not likely provide reliable protection if *B. burgdorferi* entered the human bloodstream. The LYMErix vaccine received FDA approval in the United States in 1999 for immunization of persons aged 15-70 years, but the manufacturer discontinued production in early 2002, citing insufficient consumer demand.

FURTHER READING

Bunikis, J., Barbour, A.G., 2002. Laboratory testing for suspected Lyme disease. Med. Clin. North Am. 86, 311–340.

Burgdorfer, W., Barbour, A.G., Hayes, S.F., et al., 1982. Lyme disease: a tick-borne spirochetosis? Science 216, 1317–1319.

Campbell, G.L., Fritz, C.L., Fish, D., et al., 1998. Estimation of the incidence of Lyme disease. Am. J. Epidemiol. 148, 1018–1026.

Cassatt, D.R., Patel, N.K., Ulbrandt, N.D., et al., 1998. DbpA, but not OspA, is expressed by *Borrelia burgdorferi* during spirochetemia and is a target for protective antibodies. Infect Immunol 66, 5379–5387.

Centers for Disease Control and Prevention, 1995. Recommendations for test performance and interpretation from the Second National Conference on Serologic Diagnosis of Lyme Disease. MMWR 44, 590–591.

Centers for Disease Control and Prevention, 2007. Lyme disease—United States, 2003–2005. MMWR 56, 573–576.

Dattwyler, R.J., Luft, B.J., Kunkel, M.J., et al., 1997. Ceftriaxone compared with doxycycline for the treatment of acute disseminated Lyme disease. N. Engl. J. Med. 337, 289–294.

Dennis, D.T., Nekomoto, T.S., Victor, J.C., et al., 1998. Reported distribution of *Ixodes scapularis* and *Ixodes pacificus* (Acari: Ixodidae) in the United States. J. Med. Entomol. 35, 629–638.

Henry, M., Feder, M.D., Jr., Barbara, J.B., et al., 2007. A critical appraisal of "chronic Lyme disease." N. Engl. J. Med. 357, 1422–1430.

Fix, A.D., Strickland, T., Grant, J., 1998. Tick bites and Lyme disease in an endemic setting. Problematic use of serologic testing and prophylactic antibiotic therapy. JAMA 279, 206–210.

Halperin, J.J., 2008. Prolonged Lyme disease treatment: enough is enough. Neurology 70 (13), 986–987.

Klempner, M.S., Hu, L.T., Evans, J., et al., 2001. Two controlled trials of antibiotic treatment in patients with persistent symptoms and a history of Lyme disease. N. Engl. J. Med. 345 (2), 85–92.

Logigian, E.L., Kaplan, R.F., Steere, A.C., 1990. Chronic neurologic manifestations of Lyme disease. N. Engl. J. Med. 323, 1438–1444.

Massarotti, E.M., 2002. Lyme arthritis. Med. Clin. North Am. 86, 297–309.

Nadelman, R.B., Nowakowski, J., Fish, D., et al., 2001. Prophylaxis with single-dose doxycycline for the prevention of Lyme disease after an *Ixodes scapularis* tick bite. N. Engl. J. Med. 345, 79–84.

Piesman, J., Maupin, G.O., Campos, E.G., et al., 1991. Duration of adult female *Ixodes dammini* attachment and transmission of *Borrelia burgdorferi*, with description of a needle aspiration isolation method. J. Infect. Dis. 163, 895–897.

Sangha, O., Phillips, C.B., Fleischmann, K.E., et al., 1998. Lack of cardiac manifestations among persons with previously treated Lyme disease. Ann. Intern. Med. 128, 346–353.

Schwan, T.G., Piesman, J., Golde, W.T., et al., 1995. Induction of an outer surface protein on *Borrelia burgdorferi* during tick feeding. Proc. Natl. Acad. Sci. U.S.A. 92, 2909–2913.

Shapiro, E.D., 2014. Lyme disease. N. Engl. J. Med. 370, 1724–1731.

Sigal, L.H., 1994. Persistent complaints attributed to chronic Lyme disease: possible mechanisms and implications for management. Am. J. Med. 96, 365–374.

Smith, R.P., Schoen, R.T., Rahn, D.W., et al., 2002. Clinical characteristics and treatment outcome of early Lyme disease in patients with microbiologically confirmed erythema migrans. Ann. Intern. Med. 136, 421–428.

Spach, D.H., Liles, W.C., Campbell, G.L., et al., 1993. Tick-borne diseases in the United States. N. Engl. J. Med. 329, 936–947.

Steere, A.C., Malawista, S.E., Snydman, D.R., et al., 1977. Lyme arthritis: an epidemic of oligoarticular arthritis in children and adults in three Connecticut communities. Arthritis Rheum. 20, 7–17.

Steere, A.C., 1989. Lyme disease. N. Engl. J. Med. 321, 586–596.

Steere, A.C., Sikand, V.K., Meurice, F., et al., 1998. Vaccination against Lyme disease with recombinant *Borrelia burgdorferi* outer-surface lipoprotein A with adjuvant. N. Engl. J. Med. 339, 209–215.

Steere, A.C., Taylor, E., McHugh, G.L., et al., 1993. The overdiagnosis of Lyme disease. JAMA 269, 1812–1816.

Tugwell, P., Dennis, D.T., Weinstein, A., et al., 1997. Laboratory evaluation in the diagnosis of Lyme disease. Ann. Intern. Med. 127, 1109–1123.

Wormser, G.P., Dattwyler, R.J., Shapiro, E.D., et al., 2006. The clinical assessment, treatment, and prevention of Lyme disease, human granulocytic anaplasmosis, and babesiosis: clinical practice guidelines by the Infectious Diseases Society of America. Clin. Infect. Dis. 43, 1089–1134.

CHAPTER 25

Tuberculosis in Travelers and Immigrants

Masahiro Narita and Christopher Spitters

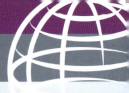

Approximately 2 billion people, one-third of the world's population, are infected with *Mycobacterium tuberculosis*, and the majority of burden is in developing countries. The World Health Organization (WHO) estimates that the annual incidence of active tuberculosis (TB) cases was 9 million worldwide with mortality of 1.5 million in 2013 (WHO, 2014).

In 2013, 65% of reported TB cases in the United States were foreign born; the case rate among the foreign born (15.6 cases per 100,000 persons) was 13 times higher than that of US-born persons (1.2 cases per 100,000). In this chapter, we briefly review the standard approach to evaluate patients for TB and address unique aspects in evaluation and management of TB among travelers and immigrants.

TRANSMISSION AND PATHOGENESIS

TB is caused by bacteria of the *Mycobacterium tuberculosis* complex, which belong to the family Mycobacteriaceae and the order Actinomycetales. Among the species of the *M. tuberculosis* complex, *M. tuberculosis* is the most common in human disease. The *M. tuberculosis* complex also includes *Mycobacterium bovis* (see section on *Mycobacterium bovis* and Nontuberculous Mycobacterial Infection). *M. tuberculosis* is characterized by a waxy component of the cell wall, mycolic acid, which is neutral on Gram stain. The designation of *M. tuberculosis* as the "acid-fast bacillus" derives from its distinctive staining property: resistance to decolorization by acid alcohol after stained with basic fuchsin.

The typical mode of transmission is inhalation and deposition of droplet nuclei containing *M. tuberculosis* on the respiratory bronchiole or alveolus, located beyond the protective mucociliary blanket of the respiratory tree. When droplet nuclei are deposited in the terminal airway passages, bacilli are asymptomatically engulfed by alveolar macrophages. *M. tuberculosis* survives within alveolar macrophages and proliferates intracellularly. Thereafter, bacilli are transported to hilar lymph nodes and then, via thoracic duct, spread systemically to other organs. In the majority of hosts, cell-mediated immunity effectively contains bacilli by formation of granulomas in 2-10 weeks after acquisition of *M. tuberculosis*, and subsequently TB infection becomes latent. Latent TB infection (LTBI) is marked by a positive tuberculin skin test (TST) or a positive interferon-gamma release assay (IGRA). A small proportion of infected individuals show fibrotic or fibronodular lesions in the upper lung fields on chest radiographs (CXRs), presumably as a result of self-limited pulmonary disease that may have been sub-clinical in the past. Persons with these radiologic findings, however, are at greater risk of reactivation and should be encouraged to take treatment for LTBI (see section on Treatment). In addition, a conventional notion was that once someone has LTBI, this person is protected against further acquisition of *M. tuberculosis*. Studies showed that reinfection can occur in high-incidence settings, especially among human immunodeficiency (HIV)-infected individuals (Sonnenberg et al. 2001). Reinfection is uncommon in low-incidence settings, especially among immunocompetent hosts (Jasmer et al. 2004).

TABLE 25.1   Tuberculosis Risk Assessment: Factors Increasing the Risk of LTBI Reactivation

- Recent exposure to an infectious case
- Silicosis
- Diabetes mellitus
- Chronic renal failure/hemodialysis
- Intravenous drug use
- Gastrectomy and jejunoileal bypass
- Tobacco smoking
- Immunocompromising diseases (e.g., HIV infection) or treatment (e.g., corticosteroids, TNF inhibitors, organ transplant) associated with suppression of cell-mediated immunity
- Malnutrition and extremely low body weight

HIV, Human immunodeficiency virus; *LTBI*, latent tuberculosis infection; *TNF*, tumor necrosis factor.

Most cases of active TB arise from reactivation of dormant foci of infection. All the factors that determine the small proportion of individuals whose TB infections will become reactivated are not known. However, certain conditions are known to increase the risk of reactivation. (**Table 25.1**)

When TB is "reactivated" at a later time, pulmonary TB is the most common form, but TB in extrapulmonary sites can be seen (see section on Extrapulmonary Tuberculosis).

Those who have spent substantial time indoors with an infectious TB case may become infected with *M. tuberculosis*. The infection rate among the household contacts of sputum acid-fast bacilli (AFB) smear-positive pulmonary TB cases is around 30-40%. At least 8 hours in a confined indoor space is considered the minimal duration for raising concern about TB transmission.

Persons with LTBI are not infectious and cannot spread TB infection to others. The rate of progression from LTBI to active TB is around 5% within the first 2 years of acquisition and, thereafter, approximately 0.1% per year in immunocompetent adults. Age less than 5 years and immunocompromised status, especially HIV infection, increase the risk of progression to active TB (Horsburgh 2004).

EPIDEMIOLOGY

The global epidemiology of TB has been affected by the acquired immunodeficiency syndrome (AIDS) epidemic. Most of the estimated TB cases in 2013 occurred in Asia (56%) and the African region (29%). Incidence rates vary from high in sub-Saharan Africa and in South and Southeast Asia to fewer than 10/100,000 population in the United States, Canada, and most of Western Europe (**Table 25.2**) (WHO 2014).

CONDITIONS MIMICKING TUBERCULOSIS

In evaluating patients with symptoms of pulmonary TB, clinicians should be reminded that TB may simulate many other diseases. Pneumonia, lung abscess, neoplasm, and fungal and parasitic infections may be mimicked by TB. The patient who originates from or who has traveled to a foreign country presents an additional diagnostic challenge. For example, as coccidioidomycosis is prevalent in persons from northern Mexico, it should be considered in the differential diagnosis of fibrosing, cavitary pulmonary disease in Mexican immigrants. While deep tissue fungal infections are rare in refugees from Southeast Asia, paragonimiasis is often confused with TB. Paragonimiasis is endemic in Asian countries and should be considered, particularly when raw crawfish consumption is reported. The diagnosis is made by identifying the parasite in sputum or in lung biopsy specimens (Chapter 48).

TABLE 25.2   Tuberculosis Incidence Rates in 2013[a]

Region/Nation	Case Rate per 100,000 Population
Sub-Saharan Africa	
South Africa	862
Mozambique	552
Zimbabwe	552
Nigeria	338
Democratic Republic of the Congo	326
Kenya	268
Ethiopia	224
Uganda	166
South and Southeast Asia	
Cambodia	400
Myanmar	373
Philippines	292
Pakistan	275
Bangladesh	224
Afghanistan	189
Indonesia	183
India	171
North America and Western Europe	<10

[a]Globally, 13% of new TB cases in 2013 were HIV co-infected.

MYCOBACTERIUM BOVIS AND NONTUBERCULOUS MYCOBACTERIAL INFECTION

M. bovis and other nontuberculous mycobacterial infections may be seen in immunocompetent patients who have lived or traveled abroad. Generally, *M. bovis* infection is acquired by consumption of unpasteurized milk from infected cows. Human infections with *M. bovis* have been essentially eliminated in developed countries as a result of the pasteurization of milk and TB-control programs for cattle. TB caused by *M. bovis* is almost exclusively recognized in immigrants to the United States from the regions where these two control measures are absent (Barnett and Walker 2008).

Mycobacteria other than *M. tuberculosis*, or nontuberculous mycobacteria (NTM), can cause pulmonary and extrapulmonary diseases. Most cases of cervical adenitis in refugee or immigrant children from African or Asian countries should be presumed to be *M. tuberculosis* disease rather than NTM, whereas cervical adenitis caused by *Mycobacterium avium* complex would be more likely in US-born children.

TUBERCULOSIS IN TOURISTS

Despite the high incidence of TB in many parts of the world, tourists from the United States, Canada, or western European countries to TB-endemic areas do not seem to be at significant risk of exposure when the purpose of their trip is business, tourism, missionary, research, or volunteering (Boggild et al. 2014; Monge-Maillo et al. 2014; Schlagenhauf et al. 2015). Epidemiologic studies have shown that casual contact with an infectious TB case usually does not result in transmission of infection. The important determinants of transmission consist of (1) infectiousness of the index case, (2) environment where TB exposure occurs (e.g., a confined, small space with poor ventilation increases the risk of transmission), and (3) cumulative hours of exposure (e.g., at least 6-8 hours in a confined space even if the index case is highly infectious). TB transmission is typically seen among the family members or within a close social network. Although transmission might occur during long air travel exceeding 8 hours, the public health risk from this is considered very low. Therefore, visitors to TB-endemic areas who follow normal tourist routes for a period of less than 2-3 weeks are unlikely to experience sufficient personal contact with infectious TB cases to acquire TB infection. TB in persons with foreign travel histories is more likely to occur in those who have traveled or lived abroad for several months or years, as is the case with students and expatriates.

Other travel scenarios more relevant to concern for TB transmission include health professionals providing medical aid work in high-risk settings and outbound medical tourists who obtain services in hospitals where TB patients may also be cared for.

TB Risk in Tourists	
Lower Risk	Higher Risk
• Standard tourist routes or business trips • Trips lasting 2-3 weeks	• Visiting friends and relatives for several weeks • Healthcare workers providing medical aid work • Receiving medical services in hospitals where TB patients are also cared for

CLINICAL FEATURES

Pulmonary Tuberculosis

The onset of symptoms and signs of TB is usually gradual, over a period of weeks or months. The first symptoms are often nonspecific, consisting of fatigue, anorexia, weight loss, night sweats, or low-grade fever. Pulmonary symptoms usually include a cough, which slowly progresses over weeks to become more frequent and producing mucoid or mucopurulent sputum. Hemoptysis or chest pain may develop when the pulmonary process is advanced. Dyspnea is uncommon in the absence of pleural or advanced disease.

Extrapulmonary Tuberculosis

Extrapulmonary TB (EPTB) is TB outside the lungs. EPTB includes lymphadenitis (often cervical), pleuritis, meningitis, abdominal TB including peritonitis, skeletal TB such as Pott disease (spine), and genitourinary (renal) TB. Miliary TB results from hematogenous spread of *M. tuberculosis* and affects both pulmonary and extrapulmonary sites. Approximately 10% of all TB cases have both pulmonary and extrapulmonary TB, and an additional 20% have EPTB without pulmonary involvement (CDC 2014). HIV-infected patients, especially with low CD4 counts, have higher rates of EPTB. Children are more likely to have EPTB than adults.

In general, EPTB is more difficult to diagnose than pulmonary TB and often requires invasive procedures to obtain tissue and/or fluid specimens. Besides possible fever and weight loss, the symptoms and signs of EPTB often relate specifically to the affected organ system. Lymphatic TB, which appears to be frequently seen in Asians and Africans, can involve any regional lymph nodes but often affects those of the neck and supraclavicular regions (scrofula). TB of the bones and joints usually causes persistent localized pain and swelling. An exception may be Pott disease of the spine, which can progress insidiously and become advanced with neurologic deficits before diagnosis is made. Meningeal TB typically presents with headache and, if advanced, altered mental status or other neurologic deficits.

Tuberculosis in Children

While only a small fraction of children entering school in the United States have a TST, immigrants of comparable age from TB-endemic countries have a higher rate of TST positivity due to increased prevalence of true LTBI as well as influence of overseas bacillus

Calmette-Guérin (BCG) vaccination. BCG vaccine for infants is routinely used in many countries outside the United States. The primary benefit of the vaccine is prevention of severe forms of TB, particularly TB meningitis, in children. Evaluations of BCG's efficacy on prevention of pulmonary TB have yielded inconsistent results. Regardless of BCG history, small children (aged <5 years) with active TB are generally not transmitters of TB.

Tuberculosis in Persons with HIV Infection

The clinical presentation of TB in persons with HIV infection may be similar to those in HIV-negative patients, particularly if CD4 counts are still relatively preserved (e.g., >200/μL). On the other hand, the symptoms of TB may be indistinguishable from other respiratory diseases, such as *Pneumocystis jiroveci* pneumonia, bacterial pneumonia, and even progressive HIV infection itself. In advanced HIV (e.g., CD4 <200/μL), TB disease is more likely to be extrapulmonary and to involve serous cavities and regional lymph nodes (particularly thoracic and retroperitoneal). A high index of suspicion for the diagnosis must be maintained. Miliary and meningeal TB occurs with increased frequency in persons with HIV infection. These two forms of TB are uniformly lethal if not recognized and treated promptly. Consequently, they must be included in the differential diagnosis when HIV-infected patients experience a severe, abrupt illness with nonspecific signs, neurologic symptoms, or headache. In Africa, a high proportion of patients with "slim disease," the wasting syndrome attributed to AIDS, who come to autopsy are found to have had unsuspected TB.

DIAGNOSIS

Radiographic Findings

Immunocompetent patients with pulmonary TB who have disease sufficient to cause symptoms will virtually always have an abnormal CXR. Pulmonary opacities are usually seen in the apical and/or posterior segments of the upper lobes or in the superior segments of the lower lobes. HIV-infected patients with pulmonary TB are associated with a wide variety of radiographic abnormalities, including hilar, paratracheal, or mediastinal adenopathy; lobar consolidation; patchy pneumonitis; and diffuse miliary infiltration. Cavitation is infrequent, and CXRs can be even normal in advanced HIV infection with very low CD4 counts (e.g., <200/μL).

Hilar and mediastinal adenopathies are not commonly seen with pulmonary TB in immunocompetent adults. When these findings are noted, another diagnosis, such as lymphoma, should be considered. In children, however, active primary TB commonly includes hilar or mediastinal adenopathy or both. The adenopathy on the radiograph is usually unilateral and in approximately half the cases is associated with parenchymal opacities.

Tuberculin Skin Testing

The TST using purified protein derivative (PPD) is a time-honored diagnostic aid in the evaluation of a patient with suspected TB infection, but its limitations must be understood. TST measures T-cell response to TB antigens and thus has limited sensitivity in those with impaired T-cell function. Furthermore, the test is unable to differentiate LTBI from active TB disease. However, when used appropriately, TST can yield valuable epidemiologic information and identify individuals who may be at high risk for progression to active TB disease.

It is recommended to use different cutoff points between a positive and negative test depending on either the risk of TB infection or the risk of progression to TB disease (**Table 25.3**) (CDC 2000b). The lowest cutoff point, a diameter of induration of 5 mm, should apply to those at highest risk of disease progression (e.g., HIV-infected patients, solid organ transplant recipients) and close contacts of an infectious TB case. The highest cutoff point, a diameter of induration of 15 mm, should apply to those who lack all identified risk factors.

TABLE 25.3   Criteria for Tuberculin Positivity by Risk Group[a]

≥5 mm Induration	≥10 mm Induration	≥15 mm Induration
HIV infection	Recent immigrants (<5 years of arrival) from high-prevalence countries	Persons without risk factors listed in previous two columns.
Recent close contacts of a patient with infectious TB	Injection drug users	
Persons whose chest radiograph shows fibrotic lesions likely to represent untreated yet healed tuberculosis	Residents and employees of high-risk settings: prisons and jails, nursing homes and long-term care facilities, hospitals, homeless shelters	
Patients with organ transplants and other immunosuppressed patients (receiving the equivalent of 15 mg/day of prednisone for ≥1 month)	Persons with medical conditions reported to increase risk of tuberculosis once infection has occurred, e.g., silicosis, gastrectomy, jejunoileal bypass, chronic renal failure, diabetes mellitus, immunosuppressive therapy, and some hematologic disorders and malignancies, and weight loss >10% of ideal body weight	
Persons receiving treatment with TNF-α antagonist therapy	Mycobacteriology laboratory personnel	
	Children <4 years or older children exposed to adults at high risk.	

[a]Test performed by intradermal injection of 0.1 mL of PPD-S, containing 5 TU, usually into forearm, with reading at 48-72 h. Induration is measured across the forearm, ignoring any erythema.
HIV, Human immunodeficiency virus; *TNF-α*, tumor necrosis factor alpha.
From CDC 2000b.

Interferon-γ Release Assays

Recently, IGRAs have been developed as an alternative to TST (CDC 2010). Two FDA-approved tests, QuantiFERON-Gold (Qiagen, Venlo, Netherlands) and T-SPOT.*TB* (Oxford Immunotec, Marlborough, MA) are available in the United States. These tests measure the ex vivo production of interferon-gamma from T cells that are stimulated with the TB-specific antigens (peptides called ESAT-6 and CFP-10). ESAT-6 and CFP-10 are not present in BCG nor most of the commonly encountered nontuberculous mycobacteria (with the exception of *M. kansasii*, *M. szulgai*, and *M. marinum*). Conversely, TST uses whole extracts of TB (i.e., PPD) as a stimulant, and positive results may represent cross-reactivity to BCG and nontuberculous mycobacteria that share some of the antigens present in PPD. Therefore, the specificity of IGRA is higher (>90%) than TST, especially among BCG-vaccinated populations (Pai et al. 2008). The sensitivity of IGRAs to detect TB infection is similar to that of TST, but T-SPOT.*TB* appears to have slightly higher sensitivity.

There are a few concerns about the use of IGRAs. While high cost and limited availability were problematic in the initial roll-out of IGRAs, most clinical settings are now served by a clinical or reference laboratory that can provide the test at a reasonable price. Except for children <5 years of age, the CDC recommends that IGRAs can be used in all other settings where TST is currently utilized.

AFB Smear and Culture

The recovery of *M. tuberculosis* organisms in culture from clinical specimens is essential for the definitive diagnosis of TB and drug susceptibility testing. A patient suspected of having active TB disease based on epidemiologic information, signs, symptoms, and compatible abnormalities on radiographs should have the appropriate specimens submitted for AFB smear and culture. Most patients with pulmonary TB are able to produce specimens of sputum that yield *M. tuberculosis* on culture. Respiratory specimens should be examined microscopically for the presence of AFB (smear). The sensitivity of AFB microscopy is only 50-60% in pulmonary TB cases, but it is inexpensive, has short turn-around time (within a day), and correlates with infectiousness of the case.

Although sputum smears are positive for AFB among patients with pulmonary TB who have advanced symptoms and extensive radiographic abnormalities and for virtually all those with cavitary pulmonary TB, negative AFB smears should *not* lead the clinician away from the diagnosis of TB, especially when epidemiologic information and radiographic findings are consistent with active TB. At least one-third of patients with pulmonary TB who produce positive sputum cultures have negative sputum smears.

Invasive procedures, such as bronchoscopy and lung biopsy, are usually not necessary to establish the diagnosis of pulmonary TB but may be performed to rule out other etiologies such as malignancy. Children with hilar and mediastinal lymphadenopathy typically have negative sputum smears, and a positive culture may not be required for the diagnosis in appropriate settings (e.g., household exposure and clinical response to empirical TB treatment). Because of similarity in the onsets, symptoms, and radiographic appearances of several AIDS-associated respiratory diseases, bronchoscopy may be necessary to obtain additional specimens in HIV-infected patients to arrive at the correct diagnosis and to begin appropriate therapy as rapidly as possible.

Compared with most bacteria, *M. tuberculosis* multiplies very slowly, dividing every 18-24 hours. Using the most modern method of culture, the isolation and identification of the causative organism require 2-6 weeks.

When EPTB is suspected on clinical grounds, it is usually necessary to obtain tissue or other body fluids from the affected sites to establish the diagnosis. Whenever possible, both tissue and fluid obtained from either open or closed biopsy should be submitted for AFB smear and culture. The yield on culture will be improved by submission of multiple specimens. This is particularly true with pleural and lymphatic TB, in which culture of tissue gives a greater yield than culture of aspirated fluid.

Nucleic Acid Amplification Testing

To distinguish among the more than 100 mycobacterial species, laboratories have traditionally used biochemical methods. More recently, nucleic acid amplification testing (NAAT) has been increasingly used for species identification, since it is more timely and specific (e.g., GeneXpert, Cepheid). Amplification techniques can be applied to specimens before the organism grows in culture to determine whether *M. tuberculosis* is present. At least one specimen submitted for AFB smear and culture should also be submitted for NAAT as part of the initial evaluation for active TB. In some laboratories, NAAT is also being used to identify common mutations conferring drug resistance before culture-based drug susceptibility testing results become available.

TREATMENT OF ACTIVE TUBERCULOSIS

The goals of TB treatment are (1) to cure illness caused by TB in a patient and (2) to interrupt transmission of TB in a community. With available chemotherapeutic agents, both goals are readily achievable if drug susceptible. The treatment of TB generally requires at least 6 months, and thus adherence to the treatment is challenging.

The four most commonly used antituberculous drugs—isoniazid, rifampin, ethambutol, and pyrazinamide—are described in **Table 25.4**. Second-line agents may be used in case

TABLE 25.4 Chemotherapeutic Agents Commonly Used to Treat Tuberculosis

Drug	Daily Dose	Side Effects	Interactions	Remarks
Isoniazid	5-10 mg/kg up to 300 mg p.o.	Hepatitis, peripheral neuritis, rash, dizziness	Potentiation of phenytoin, Antabuse	Inexpensive
Rifampin	10-15 mg/kg up to 600 mg p.o.	Hyperbilirubinemia, fever, purpura	Inhibition of many drugs: oral contraceptives, warfarin, methadone, many antiretrovirals (e.g., protease inhibitors), azole antifungal agents, sulfonylurea hypoglycemics, some statins, calcium channel blockers, and immunosuppressive agents (e.g., corticosteroids, cyclosporine)	Colors urine and other body secretions orange
Ethambutol	15-25 mg/kg p.o.	Optic neuritis (rare at 15 mg/kg), rash		Use with caution in patients with renal disease
Pyrazinamide	20-25 mg/kg up to 2 g p.o.	Hyperuricemia, rash, hepatitis		When used for the first 2 months with isoniazid and rifampin, can shorten total duration of therapy to 6 months

p.o., By mouth.

of drug-resistant TB or intolerance to first-line agents. They include fluoroquinolones, streptomycin, capreomycin, amikacin, ethionamide, cycloserine, para-aminosalicylic acid, linezolid, and bedaquiline. The second-line agents are better used under the guidance of experts in this field, as these are less potent against *M. tuberculosis* (with the exception of fluoroquinolones and injectables) and are difficult to administer because of frequent and/or serious side effects.

To prevent development of acquired drug resistance, it is critical to treat active TB with at least two drugs known to be potent against the infecting organism. Susceptibility testing of *M. tuberculosis* isolates is an essential component of optimum management of a case of active TB. Throughout the United States, susceptibility testing of TB is available free of cost through local or state health departments.

The initial empiric treatment regimen should consist of four drugs for the first 2 months: isoniazid, rifampin, pyrazinamide, and ethambutol. This regimen gives excellent results in pulmonary, extrapulmonary, and primary TB. The regimen should be adjusted after the results of sensitivity testing on the patient's isolate are known.

A number of factors influence the decision regarding the total duration of therapy. For patients who have a negative sputum culture at 2 months, have a fully susceptible organism, and do not have cavitation on their CXR, therapy can be completed in 6 months (2 months of initiation phase [four first-line drugs] and 4 months of continuation phase [isoniazid and rifampin]). Patients with cavitation on CXR whose sputum cultures remain positive at 2 months have high relapse rates if they are treated for only 6 months. As a result, 9 months of therapy is recommended in this setting. The patient with persistently positive sputum cultures despite initial four-drug therapy should be suspected of non-adherence, having a drug-resistant strain, or malabsorption of TB medications.

Most HIV-infected TB patients respond well to routine TB treatment. Nevertheless, some authorities recommend extending the TB treatment for 3 additional months (a total of 9 months), because of the possibility of relapse resulting from impaired immunity in HIV-infected patients. The authors recommend that treatment of TB in HIV-infected patients be individualized and that the patient be monitored closely throughout the course of treatment to ensure that the response is satisfactory.

Drug-Resistant TB

Whereas the prevalence of resistance to any of the four first-line antituberculous drugs in **Table 25.4** is <10% among active cases of TB in those born in the United States, resistance is more common in *M. tuberculosis* isolates from other parts of the world. For example, the prevalence of isoniazid resistance among TB patients who immigrated from Southeast Asian is 10-15%; among Filipino immigrants, it is 15-25%.

Emergence of increasingly resistant strains of *M. tuberculosis* has been reported and necessitates complex treatment options. Multidrug-resistant (MDR) TB is resistant to at least both isoniazid and rifampin. More recently, MDR TB strains with additional resistance to key second-line medications (i.e., fluoroquinolones and injectables), known as extensively drug-resistant (XDR) TB, have been reported. Challenges of treatment of MDR TB include the need to use more expensive, less effective second-line drugs, frequent serious side effects, and the risk of increased mortality from less effective treatment.

Globally, 3.5% of new and 20.5% of previously treated TB cases were estimated to have been MDR TB in 2013. This translates into an estimated 480,000 people having developed MDR TB in 2013. WHO has recommended the use of Xpert MTB/RIF, the first automated molecular test that both confirms the presence of *M. tuberculosis* and detects mutation suggestive of rifampin-resistance. Because most rifampin-resistant isolates are also isoniazid-resistant, detection of a rifampin-resistance mutation indicates MDR TB. While Xpert MTB/RIF is very useful in developing countries with high incidence of TB and MDR TB, its use and results in developed countries with low incidence of MDR TB should be carefully interpreted (Sohn et al. 2014).

When applying available information on drug resistance to the management of the individual TB patient, several important principles of treatment should be emphasized:

- When there is a reasonable possibility that a TB patient acquired the infection in a country with high drug-resistance rates, drug susceptibility testing is absolutely essential.
- Before the results of susceptibility testing become available (usually 3-6 weeks from the time of specimen collection), treatment regimens must include at least two drugs to which the infecting organism is likely to be susceptible. A treatment regimen using the four recommended first-line drugs (i.e., isoniazid, rifampin, pyrazinamide, and ethambutol) is recommended for TB patients in the United States, regardless of national origin, and it should be adequate in >98% of patients.
- When susceptibility test results indicate that the organism is susceptible to isoniazid and rifampin, ethambutol can be discontinued. Pyrazinamide may be withdrawn after 2 months, and the total length of treatment should be 6-9 months. If the organism is resistant to isoniazid, the other three agents of the original regimen (rifampin, pyrazinamide, and ethambutol) should be continued for 6-9 months. In patients with isoniazid-resistant TB, the response to therapy must be monitored carefully.
- When susceptibility test results indicate resistance to isoniazid and rifampin or extensive drug resistance, consultation with a TB expert is recommended.

The predominant risk factor for MDR TB in the United States is foreign birth. Therefore, clinicians who are involved in the healthcare of immigrants, refugees, and travelers at high risk of TB infection must be aware of global trends of MDR TB. In addition, treatment of MDR TB is exceedingly difficult and has significant public health implications. Care of such patients should be coordinated by a local health department.

Treatment Precautions

Three of the first-line TB drugs are safe for use in pregnancy: isoniazid, rifampin, and ethambutol. The safety of pyrazinamide during pregnancy has not been verified. Streptomycin and other injectables may be nephrotoxic and should be used carefully in persons with renal disease. In addition, ethambutol is excreted via the kidneys, and thus the dosing should be adjusted when used in patients with renal disease; serum drug levels may be necessary to determine appropriate dosing. As isoniazid, rifampin, and pyrazinamide can be hepatotoxic, they should be used cautiously by patients with underlying liver disease or persons at risk of hepatitis (e.g., excessive alcohol use).

With the advancement of antiretroviral therapy for patients with HIV infection, treatment of TB in persons with HIV infection has become complex. For example, rifampin—the key drug that determines the effectiveness of TB treatment—may not be readily used along with some antiretrovirals because rifampin accelerates the metabolism of those agents and lessens their antiretroviral effect. Conversely some antiretrovirals affect drug levels of rifampin substantially. Given the increasing complexity of TB treatment of HIV-infected patients, it is ideal for a clinician with expertise in managing both HIV infection and TB to supervise the HIV and TB treatment in such patients. At a minimum, it is crucial to emphasize communication and coordination between HIV and TB care providers.

Adherence to TB Treatment

Because of the long duration of the drug therapy that is required to cure a case of active TB, patient adherence (i.e., the ability of patients to take their medications and complete the treatment as advised) is a major issue. When treatment is based on susceptibility testing, as described earlier, failure to eradicate the infection is commonly due to non-adherence, even in patients with HIV infection.

Many non-adherent patients are discovered when they fail to return for follow-up clinic visits. While adherence should be monitored in all TB patients, it must be emphasized particularly among patients with mental illness, substance abuse, or homelessness. When the patient comes from an ethnic culture that stigmatizes TB or when the understanding of medical advice is difficult due to a language barrier, non-adherence may occur.

Non-adherence with anti-TB medications undermines both the personal and public health goals of TB treatment. Non-adherent patients should be reported to the local health department for appropriate evaluation and management. Most public health TB control programs in the United States require directly observed therapy (DOT), if not for all cases, then at least for pulmonary cases. DOT is a practice of observing patients swallow their medications. Because of the key role of drug therapy in terminating the spread of TB and in preventing development of drug resistance during TB treatment, DOT is the standard of care especially for infectious TB cases in the United States.

PREVENTION

Although medical practice has traditionally focused on curing human disease, there has been a wide interest in disease prevention and health maintenance. In this context, clinicians who provide medical care to foreign-born patients have both the opportunity and the responsibility to practice preventive medicine with respect to TB in that population.

Review of the pathogenesis of TB reveals that there are two targets for prevention of TB: (1) prevention of acquiring TB infection in uninfected persons and (2) prevention of progression from latent TB infection to active TB disease in those who already have latent TB infection. The primary way to prevent the acquisition of latent TB infection is to eliminate the excretion of tubercle bacilli from infectious patients. This is achieved, as noted previously, by administering effective chemotherapy to persons with pulmonary TB.

A second means of preventing TB is vaccination with BCG, a live vaccine made from an attenuated strain of *M. bovis*. BCG has been used for decades for the prevention of severe forms of TB in infants and children in many parts of the world. However, because of uncertainty regarding its efficacy and its interference with interpretation of the TST, it was never chosen for use in TB control programs in the United States (see Chapter 5).

The second line of approach to prevention of TB—preventing disease in those with latent TB infection—has a place in modern medical practice. A number of studies by the US Public Health Service in the 1950s and 1960s showed that administration of isoniazid 300 mg/day, for 9 months, had a 50-80% efficacy rate in preventing TB disease in persons with latent TB infection. The protective effect of isoniazid preventive therapy is believed to be lifelong if the patient is immunocompetent. In addition to isoniazid, two other regimens for LTBI are used: rifampin self-administered daily for 4 months and isoniazid-and-rifapentine directly observed once weekly for 12 weeks (WHO 2015).

Treatment should be offered in the following situations:

1. The patient may have been recently infected with *M. tuberculosis*. Recent infection is likely in close contacts of an infectious case of TB and in young children with diagnosis of LTBI.
2. The patient has one (or more) of the following medical conditions that raise the risk of progression from latent TB infection to active TB: HIV infection; treatment with immunosuppressive medications such as corticosteroids or TNF inhibitors; diabetes mellitus; certain malignancies; conditions associated with low weight, such as malnutrition, gastrectomy, and intestinal bypass surgery; and fibrotic pulmonary lesions consistent with untreated yet healed pulmonary TB.
3. The patient is under 50-60 years of age and has an estimated cumulative lifetime risk of reactivation that exceeds the risk of significant adverse effects from LTBI therapy.

One tool for patient-centered decision making is to first calculate lifetime risk of developing active TB (e.g., www.tstin3d.com). Then, clinicians inform the patient of a balance between benefits and risks of LTBI treatment options. Shared decision making may increase the engagement of the patients and thus potentially increase adherence with LTBI treatment.

Patients receiving LTBI treatment should be evaluated monthly during treatment and given prescriptions for 1-month supplies of medicine at each follow-up appointment. Personal interviews for adherence and side effects should be performed at these monthly intervals. The most important side effect of isoniazid is hepatotoxicity. Although potentially fatal, the frequency of this side effect appears to be low. Every patient who starts LTBI treatment should be educated about the symptoms of hepatotoxicity and instructed to stop treatment immediately if such symptoms develop. Patients capable of following these instructions do not require laboratory monitoring of liver-related enzymes during LTBI treatment. However, it is recommended to conduct baseline and periodic monitoring of liver function tests in patients with co-existing chronic liver disease or who are at increased risk of drug-induced hepatitis (e.g., excessive alcohol use, hepatitis B or C infection, concurrent use of other hepatotoxic drugs, and pregnancy). A 2-month regimen of rifampin-pyrazinamide was previously recommended as an alternative to isonicotinic acid hydrazide for treating latent TB. However, significant rates of serious hepatotoxicity were observed with this combination, and it is no longer recommended.

TB RISK ASSESSMENT

Figure 25.1 illustrates each step of TB risk assessment when a clinician evaluates a person for TB infection. The first two steps are to assess significant TB exposure and potential TB acquisition. At minimum, we consider TB exposure significant when someone spends more than 8 hours in a confined indoor space with someone who has infectious TB. When a person has an immature or impaired immune system (e.g., an infant or someone with HIV infection), rapid progression to active TB disease must be ruled out after significant TB exposure. Otherwise, risk of reactivation TB and an opportunity for prevention (i.e., treatment of latent TB infection) should be addressed. In rare circumstances, those with latent TB infection or a history of cured TB may be reinfected with a different strain of *M. tuberculosis* after substantial TB exposure. Diagnosis of reinfection and prevention of post reinfection disease has not been established yet.

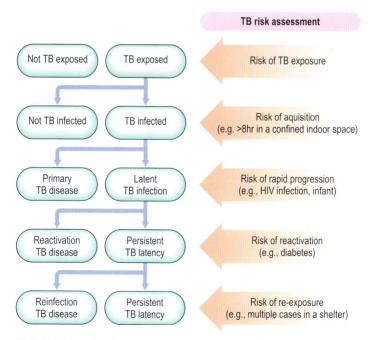

Fig. 25.1 **Tuberculosis risk assessment.**

EVALUATION OF IMMIGRANTS FOR TB

Evaluation of immigrants from TB-endemic countries is crucial for TB control in the United States. There are two steps. First, to exclude active TB disease and to evaluate for LTBI; second, to treat appropriately. Those who apply for permanent resident status ("a green card") have to undergo CXR. If abnormal, sputum examination for AFB smear and culture is completed prior to emigration. Refugees are also screened in this way, but those with student, work, or tourist visas generally do not undergo health screening, including TB screening. While treatment of active TB is mandatory, treatment of LTBI is not required for immigration purposes.

EVALUATION OF TRAVELERS WHO VISIT TB-ENDEMIC COUNTRIES

Pre-Travel

While sensitivity of TST and IGRA to detect TB infection is reasonably high (~80%), positive predictive values of TST and IGRA in a population with low prevalence of TB infection are concerning (**Table 25.5**). Both tests, especially IGRA, appear to have limited reproducibility when used in a low-LTBI prevalence group. This raises concerns because of consequences of positive TST or IGRA (e.g., CXR, possible treatment for LTBI especially after conversion). Knowledge of positive predictive values in BCG-vaccinated and nonvaccinated populations with various likelihoods of TB infection should help a clinician whether LTBI testing is beneficial or not (**Table 25.5**). At this point, the authors do not recommend testing a US-born traveler for LTBI prior to a trip to TB-endemic countries

TABLE 25.5   Positive Predictive Values of Latent Tuberculosis Infection Testing[a]

Non-BCG Vaccinated	TST	QFT-G	
	Sensitivity 77%	Sensitivity 78%	
LTBI Prevalence	Specificity 97%	Specificity 99%	
1%	20%	44%	
3%	44%	70%	
5%	57%	80%	
10%	74%	90%	
BCG Vaccinated			
	TST	QFT Gold	TSpot
	Sensitivity 77%	Sensitivity 78%	Sensitivity 90%
LTBI Prevalence	Specificity 59%	Specificity 96%	Specificity 93%
5%	9%	51%	40%
10%	17%	68%	59%
20%	32%	83%	76%
30%	45%	89%	85%

[a]Based on the sensitivities and specificities published in a systematic review.
BCG, Bacillus Calmette-Guérin; LTBI, latent tuberculosis infection; QFT-G, QuantiFERON-TB Gold test; TST, tuberculin skin test.

when the purpose of the travel is business, tourism, missionary, research, or volunteer work in nonhealthcare settings. If foreign-born persons plan to visit their families and friends in TB-endemic countries, the information on prior TST or IGRA is helpful. If a negative result had been documented, we recommend considering pre- and post-travel LTBI testing especially if the duration of the trip is longer than a few weeks. Detailed interview of anticipated activities in TB-endemic countries (e.g., being a healthcare volunteer in a TB hospital) can be used to help determine the need for pre- and post-travel LTBI testing. The following recommendations may be given to travelers:

- Avoid places where people at high risk for TB congregate (e.g., hospitals, jails, prisons, homeless shelters)
- Use mitigating measures (e.g., augmentation of airflow or ventilation, N-95 mask) if high-risk exposure cannot be avoided
- Consider pre- and post-travel testing for LTBI if high-risk TB exposure is unavoidable or if the stay in a TB-endemic country is over 3 months. Be mindful of poor positive predictive value of TST and IGRA when the likelihood of acquisition of TB infection is remote.

Some experts suggest a single dose of BCG as a pre-travel preventive measure when healthcare and humanitarian workers have high risk of exposure to MDR or XDR TB, especially in settings where the TB infection control measures are not fully implemented (Seaworth et al. 2014).

Post-Travel

Urgent evaluation is indicated if the traveler has signs or symptoms consistent with active TB disease. Otherwise, a test for TB infection (TST or IGRA) should be obtained 8-10 weeks after return to the United States for high-risk travelers. If the stay exceeds 3 months, repeat testing for TB infection overseas (i.e., prior to return) may be appropriate.

REFERENCES AND FURTHER READING

Barnett, E.D., Walker, P.F., 2008. Role of immigrants and migrants in emerging infectious diseases. Med. Clin. North Am. 92 (6), 1447–1458, xi–xii.

Boggild, A.K., Geduld, J., Libman, M., et al., 2014. Travel-acquired infections and illnesses in Canadians: surveillance report from CanTravNet surveillance data, 2009–2011. Open Medicine: A Peer-Reviewed, independent, Open-Access Journal. 8 (1), e20–e32.

CDC, 2000a. Diagnostic standards and classification of tuberculosis in adults and children. Am. J. Respir. Crit. Care Med. 161, 1376–1395.

CDC, 2000b. Targeted tuberculin testing and treatment of latent tuberculosis infection. MMWR Recomm. Rep. 49, 1–51.

CDC, 2003. Treatment of tuberculosis. MMWR Recomm. Rep. 52, 1–77.

CDC, 2010. Updated guidelines for using interferon gamma release assays to detect Mycobacterium tuberculosis infection—United States, 2010. MMWR Recomm. Rep. 59, 1–25.

CDC, 2014. Reported Tuberculosis in the United States, 2013.

Horsburgh, C.R., Jr., 2004. Priorities for the treatment of latent tuberculosis infection in the United States. N. Engl. J. Med. 350 (20), 2060–2067.

Jasmer, R.M., Bozeman, L., Schwartzman, K., et al., 2004. Recurrent tuberculosis in the United States and Canada: relapse or reinfection? Am. J. Respir. Crit. Care Med. 170 (12), 1360–1366.

Monge-Maillo, B., Norman, F.F., Perez-Molina, J.A., et al., 2014. Travelers visiting friends and relatives (VFR) and imported infectious disease: travelers, immigrants or both? A comparative analysis. Travel Med. Infect. Dis. 12 (1), 88–94.

Pai, M., Zwerling, A., Menzies, D., 2008. Systematic review: T-cell-based assays for the diagnosis of latent tuberculosis infection: an update. Ann. Intern. Med. 149 (3), 177–184.

Schlagenhauf, P., Weld, L., Goorhuis, A., et al., 2015. Travel-associated infection presenting in Europe (2008-12): an analysis of EuroTravNet longitudinal, surveillance data, and evaluation of the effect of the pre-travel consultation. Lancet Infect. Dis. 15 (1), 55–64.

Seaworth, B.J., Armitige, L.Y., Aronson, N.E., et al., 2014. Multidrug-resistant tuberculosis. Recommendations for reducing risk during travel for healthcare and humanitarian work. Ann. Am. Thorac. Soc. 11 (3), 286–295.

Sohn, H., Aero, A.D., Menzies, D., et al., 2014. Xpert MTB/RIF testing in a low tuberculosis incidence, high-resource setting: limitations in accuracy and clinical impact. Clin. Infect. Dis. 58 (7), 970–976.

Sonnenberg, P., Murray, J., Glynn, J.R., et al., 2001. HIV-1 and recurrence, relapse, and reinfection of tuberculosis after cure: a cohort study in South African mineworkers. Lancet 358 (9294), 1687–1693.

WHO, 2014. WHO Global TB Report 2015: <http://www.who.int/tb/publications/global_report/en/>.

WHO, 2015. Guidelines on the management of latent tuberculosis infection <http://www.who.int/tb/publications/ltbi_document_page/en/>.

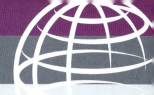

CHAPTER 26

Chagas Disease

Frederick S. Buckner, Anne C. Moore, and Martin S. Cetron

Chagas disease, first described in 1909 by Carlos Chagas, is endemic throughout Central and South America. An estimated 8 million people are infected with *Trypanosoma cruzi*, the etiologic agent of this disease. *T. cruzi*, a protozoan of the order Kinetoplastida, has a complex lifecycle passing between insects and mammals. Blood-sucking triatomine bugs serve as the principal transmission vector by depositing *T. cruzi*-infected feces onto the skin. The parasite is then inoculated into dermal breaks or mucosal surfaces by inadvertent rubbing or scratching. Most transmission occurs in rural areas of Latin America, where poor housing conditions promote contact with the insect vector. *T. cruzi* can also be transmitted by transfusion of blood from chronically infected donors, by organ transplantation, from mother to fetus, in laboratory accidents, and by contaminated food or drink. Infection is lifelong if not treated.

Progress in reducing vector- and blood-borne transmission in endemic areas and migration within endemic countries and to non-endemic countries are changing the epidemiology of Chagas disease. It is becoming an increasingly global problem. Based on limited data from seroprevalence studies among blood donors and other populations, an estimated 300,000 people residing in the United States are infected with *T. cruzi*. Most are unaware of their infection and remain undiagnosed.

EPIDEMIOLOGY

Parasite Distribution versus Disease Distribution

T. cruzi infection of vertebrate hosts and insect vectors occurs widely throughout the Americas from 42° North latitude to 46° South latitude. This encompasses much of the United States and extends through Mexico and Central America to most of South America. The risk of vector-borne transmission to humans is low in the United States, probably because of better housing conditions and less efficient vectors; however, autochthonous transmission is increasingly recognized in the southern United States. Transmission to humans by vector occurs mainly in endemic areas in Mexico, Central America (Belize, Costa Rica, El Salvador, Honduras, Guatemala, Nicaragua, Panama), and South America (Argentina, Bolivia, Brazil, Colombia, Ecuador, Guyana, Suriname, French Guiana, Paraguay, Peru, Venezuela). Interestingly, the Amazon region with mainly sylvatic triatomine species is an area with relatively low prevalence of Chagas disease in humans. Successful vector control programs in the "Southern Cone" of South America have substantially reduced transmission by reduviid bugs. Uruguay, Chile, and parts of Brazil have been certified free of vector-borne transmission. Despite these successes, Chagas disease represents a serious health problem in 17 countries in Latin America, with 20% of the population living in endemic areas. The prevalence of infection in Latin America is estimated to be ~8 million seropositive individuals; 100 million are estimated to be at risk for acquiring the infection.

Due to emigration of seropositive individuals, Chagas disease is increasingly found in countries without vectorial transmission (**Fig. 26.1**).

Vectors

T. cruzi is transmitted to mammalian species by insects of the family Reduviidae, subfamily Triatominae (**Fig. 26.2**). More than 100 triatomine species exist, each with its own feeding pattern, vertebrate host preference, and geographic/ecologic distribution. In the sylvatic cycle, the bugs prefer forested areas, but they become domesticated as a result of conversion of natural habitat to domestic uses. Most bug species prefer tropical climates with a

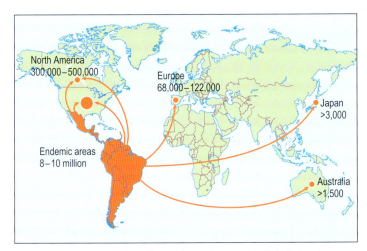

Fig. 26.1 Worldwide distribution of Chagas disease. Cases outside the Latin Americas are mainly due to seropositive individuals who have moved to these locations. (From: Barcelona Institute for Global Health. Available at <http://www.infochagas.org/en/en-que-paises-hay-chagas>.)

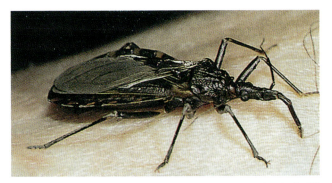

Fig. 26.2 *Triatoma infestans* feeding on a human arm. One of many species of reduviid bugs capable of transmitting *Trypanosoma cruzi*. (With permission from: Wallace, P., Pasvol, G., 2007. Atlas of Tropical Medicine and Parasitology, sixth ed. Elsevier, Mosby, image #1TF231.)

TABLE 26.1 Popular Regional Names for Triatomine Bugs

Name	Countries Where Used
Barbeiros, bicudos, chupanca, fincao, percevejo da parede	Brazil
Vinchucas	Argentina, Uruguay, Bolivia, Chile
Chirimacha or *chinchon*	Peru
Chupasangre	Ecuador
Chinche or *chincha*	Mexico, Colombia, Venezuela, Central America
Chinchona, chince picuda, or *pik*	Mexico
Chinchorro or *chinchorra*	Ecuador, Guatemala
Timbuck or *chincha-guasu*	Paraguay
Telepate	Guatemala, El Salvador
Bush chinch	Belize
Pito	Colombia
Cone nose bugs, kissing bugs, assassin bugs, Arizona tigers	USA

From: Garcia-Zapata, M.T.A., Marsden, P.D., 1986. Chagas' disease. Clin. Trop. Med. Commun. Dis. 1, 558.

temperature range from 24 to 30°C and relative humidity from 60 to 70%. Climatic factors account for increased transmission during the warmer months.

Triatoma infestans, Triatoma dimidiata, Panstrongylus megistus, and *Rhodnius prolixus* are important vectors in human transmission. Colloquial names for the reduviid are commonly used (**Table 26.1**). In northeast Brazil, for example, they are known to locals as *barbeiros* or *bicudos*. The word *barbeiro* comes from the Portuguese word for "barber," used because the bugs like to bite the exposed chin and neck. In Argentina, Uruguay, Bolivia, and Chile they are referred to as *vinchucas*. In English, one hears the terms *bed bugs* or *kissing bugs*, which refer to the insect's preference for feeding at night and about the face of sleeping children. Adult bugs are about 2.5 cm in length. They should not be confused with bed bugs of the Cimicid family (adults are 4-5 mm) found around the world.

Reservoir Hosts

T. cruzi is found in a broad range of species of sylvan mammals including monkeys, sloths, rodents, marsupials, rabbits, bats, and various carnivores. Birds, amphibians, and reptiles are naturally resistant. Humans can become infected by entering into the sylvatic transmission cycle of *T. cruzi*, but transmission primarily occurs because the reduviid vectors move into the domestic environment and infect peridomiciliary, then domestic animals. In endemic areas, the seroprevalence among domestic animals is high; studies in South America have shown the following rates: 80% in dogs, 60% in cats, 19% in sheep, and 9% in goats. Guinea pigs and rabbits are often domesticated and have been shown to have a seroprevalence of 60% and 12%, respectively. Among rodents, up to 90% of mice and 60% of rats have been shown to be infected. In most cases, animals acquire their infection directly from insect bites, but in others the acquisition of infection appears to be via the food chain (e.g., cats eating infected mice).

Transmission by Vector

Transmission by insect vector occurs in both sylvan and domestic cycles. It is the interface of these cycles, brought about by infected peridomiciliary animals such as rodents and, particularly, opossums, that leads to high rates of infection of more domestic animals, such as dogs, and eventually of humans. Chagas disease tends to occur in low socioeconomic settings because of the primitive type of housing the triatomine bugs prefer. They tend first to colonize outbuildings and move into houses built with walls of sticks and mud and covered with thatched roofs. Cracks in the walls and roofs provide the insects with a daytime hiding place and ready nighttime access to domestic animal and human hosts to obtain blood meals.

In some animals, acquisition of the parasite is via the food chain. Human outbreaks following ingestion of food or drink contaminated with infected insects or their feces have been documented and often associated with fatal cases.

TRANSMISSION RELATED TO TRANSFUSIONS AND ORGAN TRANSPLANTS

Although most people chronically infected with *T. cruzi* are asymptomatic, low levels of parasites are present in blood and other tissues. Blood transfusion is considered the second most common mode of transmission. Between 12 and 48% of recipients of blood from a *T. cruzi*-seropositive donor become infected, depending on the volume and type of blood product transfused and the level of donor parasitemia.

Many Latin American countries have made considerable progress in improving blood safety in the past two decades. In 10 of the 17 endemic countries, >99% of donated blood is screened by at least one assay for *T. cruzi* antibodies. However, a substantial risk of blood-borne *T. cruzi* infection is still present in countries with low screening coverage (e.g., Costa Rica, Panama) or in countries with relatively good, but incomplete, coverage and a high prevalence of infection (e.g., Bolivia).

Increased Latin American immigration to the United States has generated concerns about the presence of *T. cruzi* in the US blood supply. Based on seroprevalence data, the overall risk is estimated at 1 in 27,500 donations, although it varies with location and may be as high as 1 in 3000 in areas with large Latino populations. At least eight cases of transfusion-associated transmission have been reported in the United States and Canada. These were mainly detected in immune-suppressed patients who developed serious infection, but it is likely that many additional cases have occurred but were unrecognized, because acute *T. cruzi* infection in immunocompetent patients is usually a mild illness. The Food and Drug Administration approved a screening assay for *T. cruzi* antibodies in blood donations, and in early 2007, screening was implemented by blood collection agencies accounting for ~70% of the blood supply. As a result, clinicians in the United States are likely to encounter an increasing number of patients with suspected or confirmed Chagas disease. For more information from the Centers for Disease Control, see http://www.cdc.gov/parasites/chagas/resources/A_Test%20Positive_Chagas_Flyer_508.pdf.

Transmission of Chagas disease can also occur through solid organ or bone marrow transplantation from chronically infected donors. In the United States, at least five cases of infection associated with solid organ transplantation have been reported. Newly acquired *T. cruzi* is of special concern in transplant recipients because of their limited ability to control the infection. It is now recommended that donors who have resided in endemic areas be screened for Chagas disease.

CONGENITAL TRANSMISSION

Congenital transmission is a more serious problem than previously realized, especially in highly endemic areas of Bolivia, Chile, and Brazil, where prevalence among offspring from seropositive pregnant mothers ranges from 1 to 8%. Congenital *T. cruzi* infection may be responsible for prematurity and low birth weight, although most infected newborns are asymptomatic.

It is known that parasitemia is common among infected neonates; hepatosplenomegaly, meningoencephalitis, hemorrhagic disorders, and disseminated cutaneous lesions are also well described.

Transmission by breast feeding deserves mention because of the conflicting information previously available. Despite sporadic anecdotal reports implicating breast milk, the most recent systematic studies from Bahia (Brazil), Cordoba (Argentina), and Santa Cruz (Bolivia) do not support transmission of *T. cruzi* via colostrum. Current World Health Organization

(WHO) policy explicitly states "there is no reason to restrict breast-feeding by *T. cruzi*–infected mothers."

CLINICAL FEATURES

Infection in humans is characterized by two principal phases: acute and chronic.

Acute Disease

Along with fever, patients experience local swelling at the inoculation site; this is referred to as a chagoma. If the conjunctiva or eyelid is the portal of entry, one may develop the classic unilateral periophthalmic cellulitis and palpebral edema referred to as Romaña sign (**Fig. 26.3**). This is a reliable diagnostic indicator seen in 90% of recognized acute cases acquired through the eye. Flu-like symptoms such as malaise, fever, rash, anorexia, diarrhea, and vomiting are common but nonspecific.

Acute Chagas disease often passes undetected. It is diagnosed in only 1-2% of all cases, but electrocardiographic (EKG) or radiographic evidence of acute myocarditis is found in as many as 30% of acute cases if it is sought. Fulminant systemic symptoms requiring hospitalization occur only occasionally during acute Chagas disease but include generalized lymphadenopathy, hepatosplenomegaly, severe myocarditis, and meningoencephalitis. Disease of sufficient severity to require hospitalization carries a 5-10% mortality rate. The younger the patient at the time of acquisition, the more severe the acute syndrome,

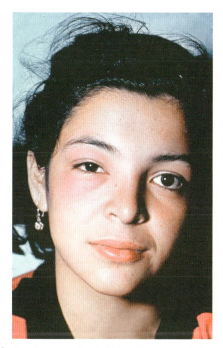

Fig. 26.3   **Romaña sign. A symptom of acute Chagas disease characterized by unilateral conjunctivitis and periorbital swelling due to rubbing infected reduviid bug feces into the eye.** (With permission from: Wallace, P., Pasvol, G., 2007. Atlas of Tropical Medicine and Parasitology, sixth ed. Elsevier, Mosby, image #1TF235.)

especially if the patient is ≤2 years old. After the initial infection, widespread dissemination of *T. cruzi* occurs; this is followed by lifelong infection. Incubation periods of 20-60 days have been observed in transfusion recipients. In most instances, acute symptoms resolve within 4-8 weeks. The host then enters the chronic phase of infection.

Chronic Disease

Most chronically infected individuals are asymptomatic and will remain asymptomatic for their lives. These patients have so-called indeterminate infection characterized by a positive serology, normal electrocardiogram and chest radiograph, and the absence of gastrointestinal symptoms. Despite a lack of symptoms, persons with chronic infection have a low level of circulating parasites. Parasitemia can be detected in ~50% of patients using polymerase chain reaction or the technique of xenodiagnosis (i.e., allowing laboratory-reared reduviids to feed on subjects' blood and monitoring the reduviids for *T. cruzi* infection). Conversion from asymptomatic to symptomatic disease occurs at a rate of ~2% per year. By the fourth decade of life, 20-30% of chronically infected individuals have progressed to symptomatic disease.

Symptomatic chronic Chagas disease is characterized by cardiac, gastrointestinal, and neurologic disorders. Cardiac problems include conduction system disturbances (high-degree heart block or arrhythmias), progressive dilated cardiomyopathy with congestive heart failure, and thromboembolic events. The most common digestive syndromes include mega-esophagus, with symptoms similar to idiopathic achalasia, and megacolon, which causes bloating, constipation, and abdominal pain. Co-existence of cardiac and gastrointestinal symptoms can occur in the same patients. Neurologic symptoms of the central, peripheral, and autonomic nervous systems have been described in chronic Chagas disease, but these are rare and not well studied.

Theories of the pathogenesis of Chagas disease have evolved in recent decades. Due to the paucity of parasites observed by microscopy in affected tissues, it was long believed that autoimmune mechanisms drove the pathological response. This view contributed to the perceived lack of value in providing etiologic treatment for *T. cruzi* infection. However, in recent decades more sensitive laboratory methods such as polymerase chain reaction (PCR) convincingly demonstrate that *T. cruzi* are in fact present in involved tissues. These parasites are thought to drive the inflammatory response responsible for tissue damage. Consequently, antiparasitic treatment is now viewed to be important in managing patients, particularly before end-stage organ disease has manifested. As will be discussed below, ideal anti-*T. cruzi* chemotherapeutics have unfortunately not been developed.

Table 26.2 summarizes the salient clinical features of each of the three principal manifestations of chronic infection ("indeterminate," cardiac, and gastrointestinal).

Host factors alone may not entirely explain the striking regional differences in disease manifestations that occur throughout Latin America. Areas in northern Brazil have cardiac disease two to three times more commonly than intestinal disease, whereas in Argentina, Chile, and some parts of Bolivia, gastrointestinal megasyndromes predominate. These geographic differences may be due in part to differences among strains of the parasite rather than to host factors.

Chronic *T. cruzi* Infection in Immunosuppressed Patients

T. cruzi-infected patients who become immunocompromised may experience a reactivation of the infection, characterized by high levels of parasitemia and by increased intracellular parasite replication. The incidence is unknown, but reactivation occurs more often with the use of highly immunosuppressive regimens. It also occurs in a subset of patients co-infected with human immunodeficiency virus (HIV). Clinical features of reactivated Chagas disease depend on the underlying type of immunosuppression (i.e., the manifestations in transplant patients differ from those in patients with acquired immunodeficiency syndrome). In bone marrow or solid organ transplant recipients, subcutaneous nodules containing large numbers of parasites, inflammatory panniculitis, and myocarditis are frequent manifestations of

TABLE 26.2 Clinical Features of Chronic Chagas Disease

- Indeterminate[a]
  - Applies to 50-80% of chronically infected people
  - Begins 8 weeks post-infection and lasts decades, if not for life
  - Serologic tests for *T. cruzi* are positive
  - Sensitive methods of parasite detection (e.g., PCR or xenodiagnosis) demonstrate low levels of circulating *T. cruzi*
  - Physical examination, EKG, and chest radiograph studies are normal
  - Patients are asymptomatic and capable of normal activity
  - As many as one-third of this population may have minor abnormal findings in echocardiographic or autonomic testing
  - Patients are often unaware of infection and serve as reservoirs
- Cardiac[b]
  - Most frequent symptoms are palpitations, dizziness, syncope, dyspnea, edema, and chest pain
  - Arrhythmias of many varieties are a hallmark of chronic chagasic heart disease
  - Multifocal PVCs are commonly seen early in the course
  - Sick sinus syndrome and sinoatrial block also occur frequently
  - Right bundle branch block with left anterior hemiblock is the classic and most common conduction abnormality
  - Complete heart block requiring mechanical pacing is not uncommon
  - Sudden death is not rare and is usually due to ventricular fibrillation
  - Cardiomegaly is common and causes regurgitant systolic murmurs
  - Congestive heart failure is due to chronic inflammatory changes in the myocardium, not coronary artery disease
  - Apical left ventricular aneurysms are seen frequently at autopsy; they predispose patients to arterial embolization
  - Pancarditis is seen on histopathology
- Gastrointestinal syndromes[c]
  - Most commonly affected segments are the esophagus and rectosigmoid colon
  - Pathologic inflammatory lesions are found in Auerbach plexus, which is responsible for the autonomic coordination of peristalsis
  - Esophageal dysmotility may result in progressive dilation of the lumen
  - Patients experience variable degrees of dysphagia and regurgitation
  - In the extreme form of esophageal disease, radiographic evaluation shows megaesophagus, contraction abnormalities, and distal esophageal stricture
  - Colonic dysmotility is manifest initially by constipation
  - Progressive obstipation leads to dilated megacolon, fecaloma, and severe abdominal pain
  - Volvulus may occur

[a]Disease state is labeled indeterminate because it is unclear when, or if, patients will develop symptomatic Chagas disease.
[b]Consider chagasic heart disease in a young patient from an endemic area (or who has a history of blood transfusion) who presents with unexplained cardiomyopathy, EKG abnormalities, or arterial emboli.
[c]Consider Chagas disease in any patient from an endemic area who presents with megaesophagus or megacolon.
EKG, Electrocardiogram; *PCR,* polymerase chain reaction; *PVC,* premature ventricular contraction.

reactivation, and central nervous system involvement is uncommon. However, in patients co-infected with HIV who have low CD4[+] lymphocyte counts, the clinical picture most often includes meningoencephalitis and space-occupying central nervous system lesions that can resemble those of toxoplasmosis. Reactivation in HIV-infected patients can also cause acute myocarditis.

DIAGNOSIS

The vast majority of diagnoses for Chagas disease are made during the chronic phase in patients with appropriate epidemiological risk factors. Serology is the most import tool for establishing chronic infection. During acute infection or in immune-compromised patients with reactivation, direct parasite detection methods become important.

Serologic Detection Methods

Antibodies appear during the acute phase and generally persist for life. The most widely used serological tests are immunofluorescent antibody detection (IFA), hemagglutination, and enzyme-linked immunoassay (ELISA). Antigens from epimastigote lysates or recombinant proteins are used for detecting *T. cruzi* antibodies (usually IgG antibodies, except when using IFA, which can distinguish between IgG and IgM). Sensitivity for these tests in reliable laboratories with standardized reagents and careful quality-control practices is on the order of 98%. False-positive results can occur with sera from patients with leishmaniasis (a co-endemic infection in many areas of Latin America) or *Trypanosoma rangeli*, an animal trypanosome nonpathogenic to humans. Because of variable test specificity, most authorities recommend performing at least two different types of serologic tests based on different antigens (e.g., whole parasite lysate and recombinant antigens) or principles (e.g., IFA and ELISA) per patient.

The Parasitic Diseases Division of the Centers for Disease Control and Prevention (CDC) (404-718-4745; email chagas@cdc.gov) is available for consultation regarding the diagnosis and therapy of Chagas disease.

Parasite Detection Methods

During the acute phase, one may culture *T. cruzi* from the blood or see circulating trypomastigote forms on direct examination of the blood. Although they can be seen on Giemsa-stained specimens either by thin or thick smear (sensitivity 60-70%), superior methods of detection are microscopic examination of peripheral blood buffy coat wet preparations, culture, or PCR, all of which have a detection rate of 90-100% in the acute phase.

Blood Cultures

Centrifugation blood culture in liver infusion tryptase or brain–heart infusion medium can detect parasites in about 30% of chronically infected patients. Cultures can be repeated serially to increase yield, although time to positivity can take weeks.

Polymerase Chain Reaction

Detection of *T. cruzi* DNA in blood can now be achieved using PCR. DNA is extracted after whole blood lysis by using various techniques; unique *T. cruzi* gene fragments are then amplified in a thermocycler. PCR-based methods have a high sensitivity when used for diagnosis of acute infection or for monitoring reactivated disease. However, the performance of PCR for patients with chronic Chagas disease is variable, and it is used primarily as a research tool.

EVALUATION AND TREATMENT

Evaluation

Patients newly diagnosed with chronic Chagas disease should have a complete medical history recorded, physical examination, and a resting 12-lead electrocardiogram with a 30-second lead II rhythm strip. If the initial evaluation is normal, it should be repeated annually. Patients with symptoms or signs suggestive of Chagas heart disease should receive a complete cardiac evaluation, including 2D echocardiogram, 24-hour ambulatory EKG monitoring, and exercise testing. Barium studies should be performed for patients with gastrointestinal symptoms.

Antitrypanosomal Agents

Antitrypanosomal treatment is strongly recommended for all cases of acute, congenital, and reactivation infection, as well as for all children with infection and patients up to 18 years of age with chronic disease. Antitrypanosomal drugs should generally be offered to adults aged 19-50 without advanced heart disease; it is optional for those >50 years of age, because the benefit has not been proven in this group. Nonrandomized clinical trials in patients with chronic Chagas disease show slowed progression of cardiac disease in patients receiving etiological therapy. However, the drugs are usually not provided to patients with advanced symptoms of Chagas disease (cardiac or gastrointestinal) due to poor tolerability and ineffectiveness. The current drugs (benznidazole and nifurtimox) are contraindicated in pregnancy, although strong consideration should be given to treatment of reproductive-age women, because this may reduce the risk of congenital transmission. The drugs are also contraindicated in patients with severe renal or hepatic dysfunction. Treatment should also be considered for patients who have not been previously treated and who anticipate future immunosuppression. Antitrypanosomal therapy of reactivated disease in immunosuppressed patients results in improvement of symptoms and a decrease in the intensity of parasitemia. The need for secondary prophylaxis in these patients has not been established.

Two antiparasitic drugs, benznidazole (Rochagan) and nifurtimox (Lampit) have proven efficacy in Chagas disease. Unfortunately, these trypanocidal agents carry the risk of serious toxicity and should be used only if clearly indicated. Benznidazole is usually regarded as the first-line agent, because it is slightly better tolerated than nifurtimox. Neither drug is currently licensed in the United States; however, both drugs are available from the CDC for use under investigational protocols (see http://www.cdc.gov/parasites/chagas/health_professionals/tx.html).

Table 26.3 provides a summary of these medications and precautions associated with their use. Alternative therapy with posaconazole, itraconazole, or allopurinol has not been shown to be efficacious in humans.

Proving parasitological cure after treatment is a challenge due to the localization of parasites in tissues and difficulty detecting low levels of circulating parasites. Negative seroconversion using conventional assays may take years to occur after successful treatment. The

TABLE 26.3	Chemotherapy for Acute Chagas Disease	
Drug	**Dosage**	**Adverse Effects**

Benznidazole (preferred due to shorter duration and fewer side effects)	Adults
	  5-7 mg/kg per day p.o. divided b.i.d. × 60 days
	Children
	  5-10 mg/kg per day p.o. divided b.i.d. × 60 days
		1. Photosensitive rash: 30%
		2. Peripheral neuropathy: 30%
		3. Anorexia and weight loss
		4. Hematologic abnormalities (bone marrow suppression): rare

Nifurtimox	Adults
	  8-10 mg/kg per day p.o. divided t.i.d. or q.i.d. × 90 days
	Children
	  (11-16 years): 12.5-15 mg/kg per day p.o. divided t.i.d. or q.i.d. × 90 days
	  ≤10 years: 15-20 mg/kg per day p.o. divided t.i.d. or q.i.d. × 90-120 days
		1. Anorexia and weight loss: 50%
		2. Polyneuropathy
		3. Tremors and excitation
		4. Insomnia
		5. Nausea/vomiting
		6. Myalgia

b.i.d., Twice per day; *p.o.*, by mouth; *q.i.d.*, four times per day; *t.i.d.*, three times per day.

interval between treatment and negative seroconversion appears to be related to the duration of infection (up to 5 years for acute infection, up to 10 years for <10 years' duration of infection, and up to 20 years in patients with duration >10 years). PCR-based techniques are useful for monitoring for treatment failure after therapy of acute disease but are of limited utility for patients treated for chronic *T. cruzi* infection.

Symptomatic Treatment

Therapeutic approaches are dictated by the type and severity of end-organ damage. Patients with Chagas heart disease may benefit from the use of angiotensin-converting enzyme inhibitors, amiodarone, pacemaker placement, or intracardiac defibrillator implantation. Patients who undergo heart transplantation for Chagas disease have survival rates equal to or greater than patients transplanted for idiopathic dilated cardiomyopathy. Megaesophagus can be managed by non-invasive dilation or by surgical intervention to remove strictured regions. Megacolon should be surgically treated by resection of the dilated segment before fecaloma or vascular complications occur. Recurrences of gastrointestinal megasyndromes that require multiple surgeries are known to occur.

PROGNOSIS

The overall prognosis of patients with chronic Chagas disease is fairly good: 70% or more will remain in the seropositive but asymptomatic indeterminate phase, and the survival of these individuals is the same as the general population. Symptomatic chronic Chagas disease carries a variable prognosis depending on severity of end-organ damage. Ventricular conduction defects (typically right bundle branch block or left anterior fascicular block) are early manifestations of Chagas heart disease that develop years before the onset of symptoms and are associated with increased mortality risk. Predictors of increased mortality risk among patients with symptomatic disease include congestive heart failure (NYHA class III or IV), cardiomegaly, ventricular systolic dysfunction on echocardiography, nonsustained ventricular tachycardia on 24-hour ambulatory monitoring, low QRS voltage, and male sex. Patients in the highest risk group for these factors have only about a 15% 10-year survival rate. Digestive syndromes are better tolerated and tend to progress slowly over decades. It is difficult to know the morbidity and mortality directly attributable to Chagas disease, but overall life expectancy in endemic areas is estimated to be 9 years less than in non-endemic areas.

PREVENTION

For Persons Living in Endemic Areas

Prevention strategies in endemic areas are a major priority of the WHO, the Pan American Health Organization, and the health ministries of many Latin American countries. In the absence of vaccines and fully effective therapies, control focuses on surveillance and vector control. Several approaches to control are used: (1) blood bank screening to eliminate transfusion-related transmission, (2) insecticide spraying to eradicate domiciliated triatomine bugs, and (3) housing improvements to minimize contact between the insect vector and human hosts.

For Persons Traveling to Endemic Areas

For the traveler to Latin America, protecting oneself against *T. cruzi* infection is largely a matter of educational awareness; there are no prophylactic medications or vaccines available. Travelers should be encouraged to become familiar with pictures of the triatomine bug before departure. However, the typical traveler is at low risk for infection. It is estimated that risk of infection by one encounter with a reduviid bug is only 1 in 1000. In 25 years of CDC surveillance, there have been no cases of acute Chagas disease in US travelers to endemic areas. Preventive measures include the following:

1. Be aware of the risk of transmission in each of the endemic areas.
2. Be familiar with the regional names and appearance of triatomine (reduviid) bugs.

3. Avoid overnight stays in poor-quality housing constructed of adobe brick, mud, or thatch. The insects typically infest cracks and roofing and feed at night.
4. If overnight stays in high-risk areas are unavoidable, spraying infested dwellings with residual-action insecticide and sleeping under an insecticide-treated bed net may offer some protection.
5. Be aware that blood products may not always be screened routinely for Chagas disease.
6. Seek medical attention as early as possible if signs or symptoms of acute Chagas disease occur. Antitrypanosomal therapy is most effective in the early stages of Chagas infection.

The findings and conclusions in this chapter are those of the authors and do not necessarily represent the views of the Centers for Disease Control and Prevention.

REFERENCES AND FURTHER READING

Bern, C., 2011. Antitrypanosomal therapy for chronic Chagas' disease. N. Engl. J. Med. 364, 2527–2534.

Bern, C., Montgomery, S., 2009. An estimate of the burden of Chagas disease in the United States. Clin. Infect. Dis. 49, e52–e54.

Chagas, C., 1909. Nova tripanozomiaze humana. Estudos sobre a morfolojia e o ciclo evolutivo de *Schizotrypanum cruzi* ajente etiolojico de nova entidade morbida do homen. Mem. Inst. Oswaldo Cruz 1, 159.

Coura, J.R., 2014. The main scenarios of Chagas disease transmission. The vectors, blood and oral transmissions—a comprehensive review. Mem. Inst. Oswaldo Cruz [ePub ahead of print].

de Andrade, A.L., Zicker, F., de Oliveira, R.M., et al., 1996. Randomised trial of efficacy of benznidazole in treatment of early *Trypanosoma cruzi* infection. Lancet 348, 1407–1413.

de Oliveira, R.B., Troncon, L.E., Dantas, R.O., et al., 1998. Gastrointestinal manifestations of Chagas' disease. Am. J. Gastroenterol. 93, 884–889.

Marin-Neto, J.A., Rassi, A., Jr., Avezum, A., Jr., et al., 2009. The BENEFIT trial: testing the hypothesis that trypanocidal therapy is beneficial for patients with chronic Chagas heart disease. Mem. Inst. Oswaldo Cruz 104 (Suppl. 1), 319–324.

Rassi, A., Jr., Rassi, A., Rassi, S.G., 2007. Predictors of mortality in chronic Chagas disease: a systematic review of observational studies. Circulation 115, 1101–1108.

Rassi, A., Jr., Rassi, A., Little, W.C., et al., 2006. Development and validation of a risk score for predicting death in Chagas' heart disease. N. Engl. J. Med. 355, 799–808.

Rassi, A., Jr., Rassi, A., Marin-Neto, J.A., 2010. Chagas disease. Lancet 375, 1388–1402.

Sartori, A.M., Ibrahim, K.Y., Nunes Westphalen, E.V., et al., 2007. Manifestations of Chagas disease (American trypanosomiasis) in patients with HIV/AIDS. Ann. Trop. Med. Parasitol. 101, 31–50.

Sosa Estani, S., Segura, E.L., Ruiz, A.M., et al., 1998. Efficacy of chemotherapy with benznidazole in children in the indeterminate phase of Chagas' disease. Am. J. Trop. Med. Hyg. 59, 526–529.

Torrico, F., Alonso-Vega, C., Suarez, E., et al., 2004. Maternal *Trypanosoma cruzi* infection, pregnancy outcome, morbidity, and mortality of congenitally infected and non-infected newborns in Bolivia. Am. J. Trop. Med. Hyg. 70, 201–209.

Villar, J.C., Perez, J.G., Cortes, O.L., et al., 2014. Trypanocidal drugs for chronic asymptomatic *Trypanosoma cruzi* infection. Cochrane Database Syst. Rev. (5), CD003463.

Viotti, R., Vigliano, C., Lococo, B., et al., 2006. Long-term cardiac outcomes of treating chronic Chagas disease with benznidazole versus no treatment: a nonrandomized trial. Ann. Intern. Med. 144, 724–734.

WHO Expert Committee, 2002. Control of Chagas Disease. WHO technical report series number 905. World Health Organization, Brasilia, Brazil.

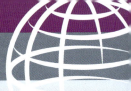

CHAPTER 27

Human African Trypanosomiasis (Sleeping Sickness)

Anna McDonald and Neil R.H. Stone

Human African trypanosomiasis (HAT), or African sleeping sickness, is a parasitic infection caused by the flagellated protozoa of the *Trypanosoma brucei* complex, which is spread by the tsetse fly. Sleeping sickness occurs in more than 30 countries in Africa, putting 60 million people at risk of infection. HAT ranks third among the world's most important parasitic diseases, behind malaria and schistosomiasis, in calculated disability-adjusted life years (DALYs) lost (Kennedy 2008), and as a result it remains on the World Health Organization (WHO) list of neglected tropical diseases. The most affected countries include the Democratic Republic of the Congo (DRC), which accounts for more than 70% of cases; South Sudan; Angola; the Central African Republic (CAR); Uganda; Tanzania; Malawi; and Zambia (Barrett et al, 2003; Krishna and Stitch, 2012). The past several years have shown progress toward the elimination of HAT, though this disease remains a public health threat in many areas of Africa, especially those that are plagued by poverty, conflict, and lack of effective governmental control.

EPIDEMIOLOGY

In 1995, the WHO's Expert Committee on Trypanosomiasis estimated that there were approximately 300,000 new cases of HAT in Africa each year and that less than 10% of these cases were appropriately diagnosed and treated (WHO, Human African Trypanosomiasis). The number of new cases reported annually has decreased significantly in recent years, with 2009 marking the first time in more than 50 years that less than 10,000 new cases were reported. A further decrease was seen in 2010, with the WHO reporting only 7,139 cases that year. Although there has been a general decrease in disease prevalence, disease transmission is characterized by focal epidemics during periods of political unrest, war, and famine—largely due to decreased surveillance and treatment (Kennedy 2008).

Transmission of HAT requires the presence of a competent vector, the tsetse fly (*Glossina* species). These insects are found in warm, shaded areas in a geographic region between 14° North and 19° South of the equator in Africa (Kennedy 2004). They inhabit an area that covers approximately one-third of Africa's landmass and is roughly the size of the United States (Kennedy 2008). The average lifespan of a tsetse fly is between 1 and 6 months, and once a fly is infected, it remains so for life (Kennedy 2004). Although an infected tsetse fly remains a vector for disease transmission for the duration of its lifecycle, the trypanosome undergoes complete transformation in only about 10% of infected flies (Berriman et al. 2005).

While exclusively endemic to the African continent, there are approximately 50 cases of HAT per year diagnosed outside Africa, mostly in travelers returning from visits to East African game reserves (Kennedy 2008).

PATHOGEN/LIFECYCLE

There are two forms of HAT, both of which are transmitted by the bite of the tsetse fly. The disease caused by the species *Trypanosoma brucei rhodesiense* occurs mostly in Southern and Eastern Africa (and therefore is often referred to as "East African sleeping sickness") and causes a more rapidly progressive disease, while infection with *Trypanosoma brucei gambiense* occurs mostly in West and Central Africa ("West African sleeping sickness") and leads to a more chronic form of disease. In either case, the infected tsetse fly bites its host, thereby injecting metacyclic trypomastigotes into the skin (Kennedy 2004). The trypomastigotes then transform into bloodstream trypomastigotes, allowing them to travel throughout the body, where they multiply by binary fission (CDC, Parasites—African Trypanosomiasis). To complete the lifecycle, the host must then be bitten by another tsetse fly. During the second ingestion, the trypomastigotes move to the midgut of the fly where they transform and, after approximately 3 weeks, migrate to the salivary gland of the tsetse fly. In the salivary gland, they undergo a final transformation into the infective form, which allows them to be transmitted to another host with the next meal (**Fig. 27.1**).

The genome of *T. brucei* was fully sequenced in 2005. It contains approximately 9000 genes, with 10% of these coding for variable surface glycoproteins. The lifecycle of *T. brucei* involves near continuous modulation of these proteins, which allows the parasite to rapidly switch expression of surface proteins to constantly evade host immune responses, a process known as antigenic shift (Kennedy 2008). As a result, there are typical waves of parasitemia that occur with each antigenic shift, and then subside as the immune system begins to develop a response.

CLINICAL MANIFESTATIONS

Trypanosome infection involves both an early, or hemolymphatic, stage and a late stage in which there is central nervous system (CNS) involvement. In *T.b. gambiense* infection, this is a slowly progressive process marked by indolent symptoms that persist for months to years. In *T.b. rhodesiense*, there is a more rapid progression, often associated with early onset of CNS involvement (Barrett et al. 2003) (**Table 27.1**).

In either form of disease, a trypanosomal chancre may be the herald of infection and typically appears about 5-15 days after a tsetse fly bite. These are well-circumscribed, painful, indurated lesions at the site of the bite and are more common with *T.b. rhodesiense* than *T.b. gambiense* infections (**Fig. 27.2**).

For 1-3 weeks after the initial bite, the trypanosome parasites spread through the bloodstream and lymph nodes in the hemolymphatic stage of infection. It is during this stage that trypomastigotes can be seen on blood smear.

Early symptoms of disease are nonspecific and include fevers, malaise, headaches, and arthralgias. Symptoms may coincide with waves of parasitemia as the trypanosomes undergo antigenic variation, thus evading host immune response. Conversely, symptoms may temporarily subside as the immune system begins to develop a response. This leads to nonspecific polyclonal B cell activation with large production of IgM and resultant enlargement of the spleen and lymph nodes (Kennedy 2004). Diffuse lymphadenopathy, hepatomegaly, and, more commonly, splenomegaly, are often present. Lymphadenitis can occur anywhere, but in the *T.b. gambiense* form it is classically seen in posterior cervical nodes, with painless enlargement of these mobile nodes referred to as Winterbottom sign (Barrett et al. 2003). This phase can last up to 3 years in the *T.b. gambiense* form, whereas *T.b. rhodesiense* is more rapidly progressive and can lead to death within weeks or months (Malvy and Chappuis 2011). Other nonspecific symptoms that are recognized include pruritus, rash, weight loss, and facial swelling (Barrett et al. 2003).

Because the trypomastigotes can pass through blood vessel walls, they easily spread into connective tissue and can enter the cerebrospinal fluid (CSF) (Kennedy, 2004). Progression to the second stage of infection (the "late" or encephalitic stage) occurs when parasites cross the blood–brain barrier. This may happen within weeks in *T.b. rhodesiense* infection or

LIFE CYCLE

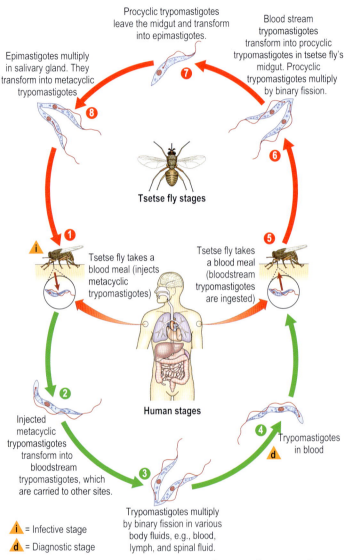

Procyclic trypomastigotes leave the midgut and transform into epimastigotes.

Blood stream trypomastigotes transform into procyclic trypomastigotes in tsetse fly's midgut. Procyclic trypomastigotes multiply by binary fission.

Epimastigotes multiply in salivary gland. They transform into metacyclic trypomastigotes

Tsetse fly stages

Tsetse fly takes a blood meal (injects metacyclic trypomastigotes)

Tsetse fly takes a blood meal (bloodstream trypomastigotes are ingested)

Human stages

Injected metacyclic trypomastigotes transform into bloodstream trypomastigotes, which are carried to other sites.

Trypomastigotes in blood

Trypomastigotes multiply by binary fission in various body fluids, e.g., blood, lymph, and spinal fluid.

i = Infective stage

d = Diagnostic stage

Fig. 27.1 **Lifecycle and transmission of trypanosomiasis.** (From: http://www.cdc.gov/parasites/sleepingsickness/biology.html.)

TABLE 27.1   Routes of Trypanosome Infection

	T.b. rhodesiense	T.b. gambiense
Location	East Africa	West and Central Africa
Reservoir	Animals: wild game, cattle	Humans (domestic pigs)
Progression	Weeks to months	Months to years

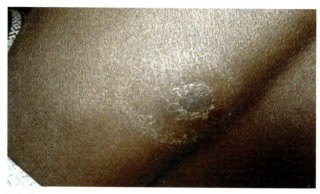

Fig. 27.2   Trypanosomal chancre on the back of a patient with human African trypanosomiasis, Uganda 2013. (Courtesy of N. Stone.)

months in *T.b. gambiense* infection. This stage is defined by increased white blood cells (WBCs) in the CSF.

Clinically, stage II disease manifests as a progressive, diffuse meningoencephalitis, which can have a broad range of features, including headaches, poor concentration, difficulty completing tasks, psychosis, personality change, tremor, and/or ataxia. One of the hallmarks of late disease is alteration in the normal circadian rhythm, with reversal of the sleep–wake cycle, hence the name "sleeping sickness." Convulsions may occur as the disease progresses, especially in children, though meningismus and focal neurologic signs are often absent (Barrett et al. 2003). As the disease progresses, there is clinical deterioration until coma or stupor results. Wasting and cachexia are common. Stage 2 disease is universally fatal without treatment.

TESTING AND DIAGNOSIS

Because clinical features are nonspecific, diagnosis depends on appropriate laboratory testing. Numerous nonspecific laboratory findings are associated with HAT infection. Common findings include anemia, leukocytosis, and thrombocytopenia, likely due to splenic sequestration (Barrett et al. 2003). Hypergammaglobulinemia with polyclonal IgM is characteristic. Other common findings include elevated erythrocyte sedimentation rate and C-reactive protein, and hypoalbuminemia.

There is neither antigen nor antibody testing for *T.b. rhodesiense*. Antibody testing is available for *T.b. gambiense* but is not sufficient for definitive diagnosis. The most frequently used detection method is the card agglutination test for *T.b. gambiense* (CATT), which relies on the agglutination of trypanosomes and antibodies and has a sensitivity of 94-98% (Truc et al. 2002). This test is not available in the United States but is often used in large-scale screening programs in endemic areas. All patients with a positive CATT require further evaluation.

Definitive diagnosis requires detection of parasites in blood, CSF, or lymph node aspirates. Microscopic detection of parasites is relatively straightforward and more widely available than serologic testing. Diagnosis is often made incidentally, with trypanosomes being visualized on a smear done to look for malaria parasites, as HAT is often clinically suspected to be malaria in early stages. Because *T.b. rhodesiense* disease is often associated with a high parasite load, parasites are usually seen on microscopy. When available, examination of the buffy coat from centrifuged specimens can increase sensitivity if parasite counts are low and organisms are not easily seen (CDC, Parasites—African Trypanosomiasis). *T.b. gambiense* is more difficult to detect and has been traditionally tested via biopsy of suspicious enlarged posterior lymph nodes when present. Serologic testing for *T.b. gambiense* may be useful in screening programs but requires confirmation for definitive diagnosis (see below). If initial testing is negative and clinical suspicion remains high, repeat smears should be collected on subsequent days, as parasitemia fluctuates during the course of disease due to antigenic shift and immune response (**Fig. 27.3**).

CSF testing is essential in anyone with suspected diagnosis of HAT both to confirm and to stage the disease. Typical CSF findings include pleocytosis, elevated protein, and increased opening pressure (Barrett et al. 2003). A rare but pathognomonic finding is the presence of eosinophilic plasma cells with high levels of IgM, or so-called morula cells of Mott (Lejon and Buscher 2005). It may also be possible to visualize trypanosomes in the CSF. Antitrypanosomal antibody testing has been developed for CSF analysis, but these tests lack sensitivity and it is generally felt that a WBC count >5-6 or high levels of IgM in the CSF are the most sensitive markers for CNS involvement (Lejon and Buscher 2005).

Both antigen detection via enzyme-linked immunosorbent assay testing and polymerase chain reaction-based testing methods have been developed but are not yet commercially available. Other clinical tests, such as magnetic resonance imaging and electroencephalography, may show nonspecific abnormalities but are not yet widely available in endemic areas at this time.

TREATMENT

Treatment for HAT is based on the type and stage of infection. CSF analysis should always be performed, even in the absence of CNS symptoms, in order to stage the infection. All

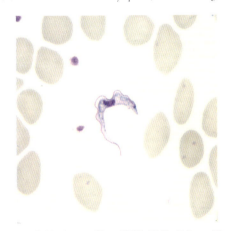

Fig. 27.3 **Trypanosome in blood smear.** (From: CDC Public Health Image Library/Blaine Matheson ID 11820.)

TABLE 27.2   Treatment of Trypanosomiasis

	Stage 1 (Hemolymphatic stage)	Stage 2 (CNS involvement)
T.b. gambiense	Pentamidine	Nifurtimox plus Eflornithine combination therapy
T.b. rhodesiense	Suramin	Melarsoprol

CNS, Central nervous system.

of the drugs used to treat HAT are toxic, and appropriate therapeutic monitoring is indicated. As such, any patient diagnosed with HAT should consult with an expert and ideally transferred to a specialist center with experience in treating this rare and potentially life-threatening infection. Patients will often require admission to an intensive care setting, particularly those presenting with stage 2 disease (i.e., CNS involvement).

Antitrypanosomal drugs are generally not routinely available. In the United States, melarsoprol, eflornithine, and suramin are available from the CDC, which can also provide specialist treatment advice (telephone 404-718-4745; email parasites@cdc.gov). Pentamidine is more widely available.

It is crucial to determine both the stage of infection and the species of trypanosomes causing infection (*T.b. gambiense* or *T.b. rhodesiense*), as this has significant consequences for the selection of treatment, as summarized in **Table 27.2**. A careful travel history and knowledge of the geographical distribution of each subspecies is therefore essential, as this is usually sufficient to make an initial treatment decision while awaiting laboratory confirmation. Awaiting laboratory sub-speciation should not delay the initiation of treatment, especially when the travel history is suggestive of East African (*T.b. rhodesiense*) trypanosomiasis, which tends to run a more aggressive clinical course.

As a neglected tropical disease, there is a paucity of clinical trial data to guide treatment strategies, although there have been recent advances in this respect. Randomized trial data is now available for second stage *T.b. gambiense* infection; however, particularly in the case of stage 2 *T.b. rhodesiense* trypanosomiasis, the optimal therapy often remains at the level of expert opinion on a case-by-case basis. **Treatment regimens vary considerably depending on local and national guidelines. The doses given in this chapter are given as a guide only—each case should be discussed with an expert in managing the disease.**

Treatment of *T.b. gambiense* Trypanosomiasis

Stage 1

Pentamidine

Dose 4 mg/kg/day IV or IM for 7-10 days

Pentamidine has poor CNS penetration and limited activity against *T.b. rhodesiense*, therefore its indication is confined to early-stage *T.b. gambiense* infection; it has been used in this capacity since the 1940s. It is generally well tolerated, but side effects are common. The intravenous route is associated with hypotension and is irritating to veins; therefore, central venous access may be required. A slow infusion, over 2 hours, can reduce the risk of hypotension. Other significant adverse reactions include hypo- and hyperglycemia, electrolyte disturbance (particularly hyperkalemia), and cardiac dysrhythmias including QT interval prolongation. Nephrotoxicity can occur with prolonged use, as can leukopenia and thrombocytopenia. Liver enzymes may also be elevated. Careful blood glucose, blood count, and blood chemistry monitoring is therefore required.

Intramuscular administration is painful and can lead to sterile abscess, although is less likely to cause hypotension and is widely administered this way in resource-limited settings.

Stage 2

Nifurtimox/Eflornithine Combination Therapy (NECT)

In a landmark clinical trial by Priotto et al. (2009), which evaluated a cohort of 103 adults with stage 2 *T.b. gambiense* trypanosomiasis in the DRC, researchers demonstrated non-inferiority of a combination of eflornithine of 200 mg/kg intravenously every 12 hours for 7 days plus nifurtimox (15 mg/kg/day orally every 8 hours for 10 days) as compared with a 14-day course of eflornithine at a dose of 400 mg/kg/day intravenously in four divided doses for 14 days. It was a remarkable achievement to perform a randomized trial in such a challenging setting, and its results have changed practice. NECT is less toxic and less costly than 14 days of IV eflornithine, and as such it has since been placed on the WHO list of essential medicines. NECT is therefore now the recommended treatment regimen for stage 2 West African HAT.

Nifurtimox

15 mg/kg/d orally in three divided doses for 10 days (given in combination with eflornithine)

Significant side effects are primarily gastrointestinal, with anorexia, weight loss, nausea, and vomiting commonly experienced. Neurological side effects include dizziness, headaches, insomnia, myalgia, and paresthesias. Occasionally, leukopenia can occur, warranting CBC monitoring.

Eflornithine

200 mg/kg IV every 12 hours for 7 days (given in combination with nifurtimox)

Numerous side effects have been observed with parenteral eflornithine, including dizziness, headache, arthralgias, cardiac arrhythmias, pruritus, nausea, vomiting, abdominal pain, and neutropenia.

Staggering the doses of nifurtimox and eflornithine is recommended, as concurrent administration of the two potentially toxic medications is associated with more severe side effects.

Treatment of *T.b. rhodesiense* Trypanosomiasis

Stage 1

Suramin

1 g IV on days 1, 3, 7, 14, and 21 (*Note*: local and national guidelines may vary on precise dosing intervals)

Suramin has been in clinical use for nearly a century, having been discovered in 1916. It is given intravenously at a dose of 1 g on days 1, 3, 7, 14, and 21. There is a small risk of an anaphylactic reaction, therefore a test dose of 100 mg is recommended prior to initiating full dose therapy. Nephrotoxicity, myelosuppression, and peripheral neuropathy have been reported but are uncommon side effects. It is generally well tolerated; however, it does not cross the blood–brain barrier and therefore is not effective in stage 2 trypanosomiasis—highlighting the critical importance of CSF testing for appropriate staging prior to initiation of treatment.

Pretreatment with suramin prior to lumbar puncture is performed in some centers, because there is a theoretical risk that performing a lumbar puncture can mechanically introduce trypanosomes from the bloodstream into the central nervous system. This must be weighed against a delay in staging the infection. Pre-treatment with suramin is also believed to reduce the risk of a severe reaction to melarsoprol if it is required, by reducing the parasitic load prior to its administration. However, there is no firm evidence supporting this approach.

Stage 2

Melarsoprol

2.2 mg/kg IV daily for 10 days

Melarsoprol, an arsenic derivative, is the only currently available treatment for stage 2 *T.b. rhodesiense* trypanosomiasis. It is highly trypanocidal but is also toxic to the patient. Until recently, a complex treatment schedule of three dose cycles followed by a rest period of 5-7 days was used, requiring lengthy hospitalization. Thankfully, recent evidence suggests that a shortened and condensed protocol is as effective and no more toxic; therefore, it is now given at a dose of 2.2 mg/kg daily for 10 days (Priotto et al. 2009). Common side effects include irritation at the injection site, abdominal pain, vomiting, diarrhea, myocarditis, and peripheral neuropathy. The most feared complication is an encephalopathic reaction. This has been reported in up to 10% of cases and carries a mortality of 50% for those who experience it. There is some evidence that corticosteroids reduce the risk of this devastating complication; therefore, daily prednisone during melarsoprol therapy is often given. The significant toxicity of this drug raises two important issues in the treatment of sleeping sickness: first, the importance of staging and speciating HAT in order to be sure of the need to commit the patient to such a toxic therapy and, second, the desperate need for development of new drugs. At present, melarsoprol remains the only treatment option for stage 2 *T.b. rhodesiense* trypanosomiasis, which is universally fatal if left untreated.

NEW DRUGS

There is renewed impetus in drug discovery for trypanosomiasis. At the time of writing this chapter, an oral nitroimidazole agent, fexinidazole, is being investigated in clinical trials in the DRC and CAR for stage 2 *T.b. gambiense* trypanosomiasis. This is an oral agent and has activity against both species of trypanosomes in vitro, and the results of this study are eagerly awaited.

PREVENTION

Travelers to areas where sleeping sickness is endemic should be counseled regarding the nature of the disease and its transmission. In a Western setting, those at risk are most often travelers planning to visit game reserves in eastern and southern Africa or aid workers planning to spend prolonged periods of time in remote settings in West or Central Africa. It should be emphasized that the disease is very rare in travelers; however, the severity of HAT warrants awareness, and providers should take time to counsel travelers on appropriate exposure prevention measures. At present, the only effective prevention is avoidance of tsetse fly bites. No vaccine against HAT exists, in part because of the challenges associated with antigenic variation. Given the toxicity of trypanocidal drugs and the relative rarity of the disease in travelers, prophylactic chemotherapy cannot be recommended.

Wearing ankle- and wrist-length clothes with neutral colors that blend into the environment (khaki or beige) is recommended because tsetse flies are attracted to vivid dark colors, particularly dark blue. The CDC recommends that travelers wear medium-weight fabric, as tsetse flies can bite through lightweight clothing (Moore 2015). DEET is relatively ineffective in repelling tsetse flies but may be of some benefit. Because tsetse flies are day biters, sleeping under a bed net has little impact on reducing tsetse fly bites. Travelers should be reassured, however, that even in the event of tsetse fly bites, the vast majority will not result in infection with trypanosomes. They should be aware of the symptoms and be encouraged to seek healthcare advice in the event of developing symptoms or signs, such as a chancre at the bite site.

REFERENCES AND FURTHER READING

Barrett, M.P., Burchmore, R.J., Stich, A., et al., 2003. The trypanosomiases. Lancet 362, 1469–1480.

Berriman, M., Ghedin, E., Hertz-Fowler, C., et al., 2005. The genome of the African trypanosome: *Trypanosoma brucei*. Science 309, 416–422.

CDC (Centers for Disease Control and Prevention). Parasites—African Trypanosomiasis. Available at <http://www.cdc.gov/parasites/sleepingsickness/> (accessed May 27, 2015).

Franco, J., Simarro, P., Diarra, A., et al., 2014. Epidemiology of human African trypanosomiasis. Clin. Epidemiol. 6, 257–275.

Kennedy, P.G., 2004. Human African trypanosomiasis of the CNS: current issues and challenges. J. Clin. Invest. 113, 496–504.

Kennedy, P.G., 2008. The continuing problem of human African trypanosomiasis (sleeping sickness). Ann. Neurol. 64, 116–126.

Krishna, S., Stitch, A., 2012. Human African trypanosomiasis. In: Magill, A.J., Maguire, J.H., Ryan, E.T., et al. (Eds.), Hunter's Tropical Medicine and Emerging Infections, ninth ed. Elsevier.

Kuepfer, I., et al., 2012. Safety and efficacy of the 10-day melarsoprol schedule for the treatment of second stage *rhodesiense* sleeping sickness. PLoS. Negl. Trop. Dis. 6 (8), e1695.

Lejon, V., Buscher, P., 2005. Review article: cerebrospinal fluid in human African trypanosomiasis: a key to diagnosis, therapeutic decision and post-treatment follow-up. Trop. Med. Int. Health 10, 395–403.

Magill, A.J., et al. (Eds.), 2013. Hunter's Tropical Medicine and Emerging Infections, ninth ed. Saunders/Elsevier, London, New York.

Malvy, D., Chappuis, F., 2011. Sleeping sickness. Clin. Microbiol. Infect. 17, 986–995.

Moore, A. Trypanosomiasis, African (Sleeping Sickness). CDC Yellow Book. Available at <http://wwwnc.cdc.gov/travel/yellowbook/2014/chapter-3-infectious-diseases-related-to-travel/trypanosomiasis-african-sleeping-sickness> (accessed May 27, 2015).

Priotto, G., et al., 2009. Nifurtimox-eflornithine combination therapy for second-stage African *Trypanosoma brucei gambiense* trypanosomiasis: a multicentre, randomised, phase III, non-inferiority trial. Lancet 374 (9683), 56–64.

Truc, P., Lejon, V., Magnus, E., et al., 2002. Evaluation of the micro-CATT, CATT/*Trypanosoma brucei gambiense*, and LATEX/*T b gambiense* methods for serodiagnosis and surveillance of human African trypanosomiasis in West and Central Africa. Bull World Health Organ. 80, 882–886.

World Health Organization. Human African Trypanosomiasis. Available at <http://www.who.int/trypanosomiasis_african/en/> (accessed May 27, 2015).

CHAPTER 28

Ebola Virus Disease and Hemorrhagic Fevers

Christopher A. Sanford, Timothy E. West, and Shevin T. Jacob

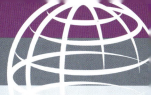

HEMORRHAGIC FEVERS

Overview and Transmission

Hemorrhagic fevers are caused by infection with single-stranded, small RNA viruses in the Arenaviridae, Filoviridae, Bunyaviridae, or Flaviviridae families (**Table 28.1**). The clinical picture is usually one of hemodynamic instability and coagulation abnormalities leading to bleeding.

The viruses are primarily zoonotic, existing in mammalian reservoirs. Humans may become infected by interaction with the reservoir or via an arthropod vector. While human-to-human transmission may occur with certain viruses and contribute to epidemics (with the exception of dengue), humans are not considered reservoirs. Therefore, infection primarily occurs in geographic locales that support the reservoir or the vector. However, all inhabited continents and climates host these viruses (**Table 28.1**). In light of the recent epidemic of Ebola virus disease (EVD), special attention is given to this infection below. Yellow fever and dengue are discussed in other chapters.

Clinical Manifestations

The many different viruses that cause viral hemorrhagic fever (VHF) can result in a variety of clinical presentations. Early disease or mild infection can be nonspecific and potentially confused with respiratory viruses, hepatitis, gastroenteritis, primary human immunodeficiency virus, malaria, sleeping sickness, bacterial sepsis, or other infections. A variety of types of rash may be seen. In Lassa fever, the pharynx may be erythematous or exudative. Bleeding may not be overt and may be delayed; however, more severe disease may be characterized by bleeding, capillary leak, or shock. Laboratory findings may be variable but are often suggestive of disseminated intravascular coagulopathy. In severe disease, there may be pronounced electrolyte and acid-base disturbances.

Diagnosis

A high level of clinical suspicion for VHF in individuals who may have been exposed to reservoirs or vectors of infection is required. Confirmation of infection generally requires detection of viral antigen or RNA. These tests are performed in specialized laboratories; commercial kits for diagnosis are not currently available. Serology may be useful in the convalescent phase of illness. It is important to exclude other causes of infection.

Treatment

While there is substantial variation in the pathogenicity of the viruses, care of the patient with VHF is primarily supportive. Diligent organ support including correction of hypovolemia and electrolyte abnormalities, management of hemorrhage and coagulation derangements, mechanical ventilation, and renal replacement therapy has the potential to markedly

391

TABLE 28.1 Hemorrhagic Fever Viruses in Humans

Family	Virus	Disease	Main Reservoir or Vector	Geographic Distribution of Disease
Arenaviridae	Lassa	Lassa fever	Rodent (multimammate rat, or *Mastomys natalensis*)	West Africa
	Lujo	Lujo hemorrhagic fever	Unknown; presumed rodent	Zambia
	Junin	Argentine hemorrhagic fever	Rodent (corn mouse, or *Calomys musculinus*)	Argentine Pampas
	Machupo	Bolivian hemorrhagic fever	Rodent (large vesper mouse, or *Calomys callosus*)	Beni Department, Bolivia
	Guanarito	Venezuelan hemorrhagic fever	Rodent (cane mouse, or *Zygodontomys brevicauda*)	Portuguesa State, Venezuela
	Sabiá	Brazilian hemorrhagic fever	Unknown; presumed rodent	Rural area near São Paulo, Brazil?
	Chapare	Chapare hemorrhagic fever	Unknown; presumed rodent	Cochabamba, Bolivia
Filoviridae	Ebola	Ebola hemorrhagic fever	Unknown; fruit and insectivorous bat species have been implicated	Sub-Saharan Africa
	Marburg	Marburg hemorrhagic fever	Fruit bat (Egyptian fruit bat, or *Rousettus aegyptiacus*; perhaps others)	Sub-Saharan Africa

Family	Viruses	Disease	Reservoir/Vector	Distribution
Bunyaviridae	Hantaan, Seoul, Puumala, Dobrava-Belgrade, others	Hemorrhagic fever with renal syndrome	Rodent (Hantaan: striped field mouse, or *Apodemus agrarius*; Seoul: Norway rat, or *Rattus norvegicus*; Puumala: bank vole, or *Clethrionomys glareolus*; Dobrava-Belgrade: yellow-necked field mouse, or *Apodemus flavicollis*)	Hantaan: northeast Asia Seoul: urban areas worldwide Puumala and Dobrava-Belgrade: Europe
	Sin Nombre, Andes, Laguna Negra, others	Hantavirus pulmonary syndrome	Rodent (Sin Nombre: deer mouse, or *Peromyscus maniculatus*; Andes: long-tailed rat, or *Oligoryzomys longicaudatus*; Laguna Negra: vesper mouse, or *Calomys laucha*)	Sin Nombre: North America, Andes Laguna Negra: southern South America
	Rift Valley fever	Rift Valley fever	Domestic livestock/mosquito (*Aedes* and others)	Sub-Saharan Africa, Saudi Arabia, Yemen
	Congo-Crimean hemorrhagic fever	Congo-Crimean hemorrhagic fever	Wild and domestic vertebrates/tick (primarily *Hyalomma* species)	Africa, Balkans, southern Russia, Middle East, India, Pakistan, Afghanistan, western China
Flaviviridae	Yellow fever	Yellow fever	Monkey/mosquito (*Aedes aegypti*; other *Aedes* and *Haemagogus* spp.)	Sub-Saharan Africa, South America up to Panama
	Dengue	Dengue hemorrhagic fever	Human/mosquito (*A. aegypti* and *Aedes albopictus*)	Tropics and subtropics worldwide
	Kyasanur Forest disease	Kyasanur Forest disease	Vertebrate (rodents, bats, birds, monkeys, others)/tick (*Haemaphysalis* species and others)	Southern India; Yunnan Province, China; Saudi Arabia
	Omsk hemorrhagic fever	Omsk hemorrhagic fever	Rodent/tick (primarily *Dermacentor* and *Ixodes* species)	Western Siberia

Adapted from Bausch, D.G., 2011. Viral hemorrhagic fevers. In: Goldman's Cecil Medicine, twenty-fourth ed. Saunders Elsevier, Philadelphia, pp. 2147–2155.

reduce death rates. For specific infections, including Lassa fever, hemorrhagic fever with renal syndrome, South American hemorrhagic fevers, and Crimean-Congo hemorrhagic fever, ribavirin, a purine nucleoside, may be considered, but robust data regarding its efficacy are lacking. Post-exposure vaccination, passive immunotherapy, and novel immunomodulatory agents are largely experimental but may carry some benefit. Suspected or confirmed co-infection should also be treated.

EBOLA VIRUS DISEASE

Overview and Transmission

Ebolavirus was discovered in 1976 near the Ebola River in what was then Zaire (now Democratic Republic of Congo). Ebola is one of three known filoviruses; the other genera within the family Filoviridae are *Marburgvirus* and, more recently discovered, *Cuevavirus*. Five species of the genus *Ebolavirus* have been identified: *Sudan ebolavirus*, *Zaire ebolavirus*, Tai Forest (Ivory Coast) *ebolavirus*, *Reston ebolavirus*, and *Bundibugyo ebolavirus*. *Bundibugyo*, *Zaire*, and *Sudan* have caused large outbreaks in Africa. *Z. ebolavirus* is the cause of the epidemic that began in West Africa in December 2013. *R. ebolavirus* is not pathologic in humans.

While transmission from a zoonotic reservoir is suspected, no definitive link between animal species and transmission of Ebola to human beings has been made. Some evidence suggests fruit bats, family Pteropodidae, as the natural reservoir, but other studies including recent work from the West African Ebola outbreak implicate an insectivorous bat species, *Mops condylurus*. Ultimately, the primary mode of transmission of Ebola virus into humans remains unknown.

In humans, the majority of *Ebolavirus* transmission is via contact with bodily fluids of symptomatic patients. It is not known to be transmitted by eating food (with the exception of handling bush meat), by drinking water, or via the bites of mosquitoes or other insects. *Ebolavirus* RNA has been identified in the blood, breast milk, semen, vaginal fluid, placental/amniotic fluid, skin/sweat, saliva, eyes, urine, and feces of infected individuals. Detection of viral RNA, however, does not indicate infectiousness, whereas viral isolation through culture is more suggestive. Of the bodily fluids and sites where viral RNA has been detected, blood, breast milk, saliva, aqueous fluid, urine, and semen have yielded cultured virus. Regarding human-to-human transmission of Ebola virus from sexual fluids or other routes (e.g., airborne), limited data exist, and epidemiologic patterns reported during outbreaks have not supported these types of transmission playing a major role in outbreak transmission dynamics.

Epidemics begin when the human index case either has contact with a reservoir species or when transmission of an infection to a person by a blood-borne mechanism occurs during activities such as preparing the meat of wild animals (also called bushmeat), which have become exposed and infected with Ebola virus.

Amplification of human-to-human transmission in the community has been linked to burial practices common to indigenous groups throughout Africa, in which family and community members prepare the dead body. A study on deceased Ebola-infected macaques found that viable virus could be recovered for at least 7 days after death. Also, transmission of Ebola virus by health workers not suspecting EVD in a symptomatic patient for whom they provided care has been an important cause of both community and nosocomial amplification of the outbreak.

In the first 9 months of the West African outbreak, an average incubation period of 11.4 days was observed. Symptom onset after exposure is under 21 days in 95% of patients (which is the recommended follow-up period for contacts).

Given that Ebola is a zoonosis, its eradication is unlikely.

Epidemiology and Outbreaks

Prior to the West African outbreak that began in late 2013, the largest outbreak of Ebola was in Uganda in 2000, with 425 cases. In that epidemic the case fatality rate was 53%.

Between 1967, when Marburg virus was first identified, and 2011, there were 30 outbreaks of either Ebola or Marburg hemorrhagic fever, totaling almost 2500 cases.

Almost all outbreaks of Ebola prior to 2014 were rural. Two urban outbreaks did occur, in Kikwit, Zaire, population 400,000, in 1995, and in Gulu, Uganda, population 100,000, in 2001; each caused about 250 deaths.

One group at markedly elevated risk for infection with Ebola is healthcare workers. As of early May 2015, more than 850 healthcare workers have been infected with Ebola in current epidemic, of whom almost 60% have died.

The largest outbreak of Ebola began in December 2013 in the Guéckédou and Macenta districts of Guinea. The outbreak, however, was not identified as Ebola until the spring of 2014. By that time, cases had also been reported across the border in neighboring Liberia. Unconfirmed cases were also reported around that time in neighboring Sierra Leone, but the first officially diagnosed case of EVD was not reported until May 2014. On August 8, 2014, the World Health Organization (WHO) declared the epidemic to be a "public health emergency of international concern." As of May 10, 2015, the West African EVD outbreak has resulted in almost 27,000 cases reported in Guinea, Liberia, Sierra Leone, Mali, Nigeria, Senegal, Spain, United Kingdom, and United States. The overall reported case fatality rate is 41.4% and varies considerably depending on the country and across sites within countries.

As of May 2015, there have been 11 cases of Ebola in the United States: seven were evacuated to the United States from West African countries, and four were first diagnosed in the United States (two of which were contracted in the United States). Two (18%) of these 11 patients died.

Clinical Manifestations

In general, patients with Ebola have a somewhat predictable clinical course (Chertow et al. 2014). During the first couple days of infection, patients present with a mild fever, decreased appetite, and headache. During this time, patients are ambulatory and generally able to drink and eat. Over the next 2-3 days, fever increases (as high as 40° C), headache continues with onset of arthralgias and myalgias, and mild gastrointestinal symptoms arise, including anorexia, nausea, onset of diarrhea (two to three bowel movements daily), epigastric pain, and occasionally hiccups. During these first 3-4 days of illness, patients may still be ambulating; clinicians should monitor for the onset of asthenia and lassitude.

For patients whose illness progresses beyond this stage, a severe gastroenteritis phase ensues with increased diarrhea (reported up to 10 L daily in some cases) and vomiting; hematemesis and bloody diarrhea can be seen in a minority of cases. During this phase, manifestation of signs of systemic involvement and shock can be seen, including tachycardia and hypotension, conjunctival injection, chest pain, dysphagia, decreasing urine output, and little to no ambulation. In addition, a subset of patients experience an encephalopathic/encephalitic phenotype with delirium (both hypoactive and hyperactive), manifested by confusion, impaired cognition, agitation, and, less commonly, seizures. It is uncertain whether these central nervous system sequelae are secondary to direct cytopathic injury from the Ebola virus, electrolyte disarray, or a combination of both.

The gastrointestinal phase lasts for approximately 5 days, after which a convalescent or terminal phase ensues. During this phase, fever and gastrointestinal symptoms subside, generally corresponding with a decrease in Ebola viral load. Many patients recover during this period. Some patients, however, will have suffered from end-organ damage with oliguria/anuria and progression to coma. While primary hypoxia is uncommon, end-stage cases may also manifest tachypnea and respiratory distress likely to represent respiratory compensation for metabolic acidosis developed as a result of shock and acute kidney injury. Patients in this terminal phase may require higher levels of supportive care (e.g., mechanical ventilation and hemodialysis) without which many of these patients will succumb to their illness.

On physical exam, rash is reported in 25-52% of clinical reports; it is often nonpruritic, erythematous, and maculopapular and may be difficult to discern in dark-skinned individuals.

Other exam findings may include hyperemic conjunctivae, pharyngeal erythema, enlarged lymph nodes, and tender hepatomegaly with the edge of the liver palpable below the ribcage.

Other conditions to consider in patients presenting with nonspecific symptoms concerning for Ebola include bacterial sepsis, other hemorrhagic fevers (such as Crimean-Congo hemorrhagic fever, Lassa fever, Marburg hemorrhagic fever, and dengue hemorrhagic fever), dysentery, malaria, typhoid fever, hepatitis, cholera, rickettsioses, and leptospirosis.

The majority of EVD patients have been cared for in sub-Saharan Africa where collection of clinical laboratory data is rare. Nonetheless, some insight has been gained through minimal data from various outbreaks and newer clinical data from EVD patients who have been evacuated to higher resource settings. A common feature of patients with EVD is leukopenia at time of presentation, with a reduced number of lymphocytes and an increased proportion of granulocytes. As the illness progresses, the total white cell count can rise above normal, with an increase in immature granulocytes and the appearance of atypical lymphocytes. Thrombocytopenia is often present at during the patient's clinical course and can decline to very low levels in more severe cases.

Metabolic derangement is also common with the excessive gastrointestinal losses. Renal function is often normal at time of presentation, but acute kidney injury is common with oliguria and anuria occurring in severe cases. Related electrolyte abnormalities include hypo- and hypernatremia due to fluid and sodium losses and fluid shifts from diarrhea and vomiting. Hypokalemia is also common from potassium loss in diarrhea, but hyperkalemia can also occur, especially in patients with severe acute kidney injury.

Liver enzymes are often abnormal with a disproportionate elevation in aspartate aminotransferase (AST) over alanine aminotransferase. Creatinine kinase can also be elevated, consistent with mild rhabdomyolysis and perhaps suggesting a dual liver and muscle source for the elevated AST level. When tested, partial thromboplastin time is more commonly prolonged than prothrombin time, and bilirubin levels are usually within normal limits. Though described as being a pathogenic feature in some nonhuman primate models, disseminated intravascular coagulation has not been reported commonly in human cases of EVD, likely because of lack of tests to measure for it.

Patients who die of Ebola more commonly progress from prostration and obtundation to hypotension and shock to coma. Some deaths, however, occur suddenly, perhaps resulting from dysrhythmias in the setting of electrolyte derangements. Most deaths occur between days 7 and 12 of illness, with a median survival of 9 days from symptom onset to death. The mean time from admission to hospital to death in the current West African epidemic is 4.2 days.

Independent risk factors for mortality reported from different cohorts include elevated Ebola viral load at the time of admission, increased age (>40 years), and end-organ damage, particularly involving the liver and kidneys. Other factors observed to be associated with a high mortality include age <2 years, pregnancy, and hemorrhage. Historically, case fatality rates have ranged from 25 to 90%. In the first 9 months of the 2014 West African outbreak, a case fatality rate (CFR) of 71% was observed with a decline to around 55% later in the epidemic. The reason for the decreased CFR is unclear but likely attributable to increased availability of safe facilities and decreased time to seeking care by patients and their families in the community.

At approximately day 10 of illness, about 40% of patients begin to improve. Patients who live to day 13 of illness have a higher likelihood of surviving. Current recommendations for discharge criteria include ≥3 days without fever or any significant symptoms (e.g., diarrhea, vomiting, bleeding), significant improvement in clinical condition, ability to perform activities of daily living, and a negative blood polymerase chain reaction (PCR) test for Ebola virus on the third day of being asymptomatic. If the PCR test remains positive despite lack of symptoms, current recommendations are to repeat PCR in 48 hours and counsel patients that the PCR test can take several days to become undetectable despite resolution of symptoms.

In survivors, convalescence is prolonged, lasting weeks to months. Common signs and symptoms reported during convalescence include asthenia, weight loss, headache, dysesthesias, migratory arthralgias, sloughing of skin, and loss of scalp hair. Survivors have also reported blurred or partial loss of vision, dizziness, headache, insomnia, and myalgia.

Diagnosis

The CDC defines a "person under investigation" for Ebola as someone with both (1) a history of exposure (travel to a country with widespread Ebola transmission or contact with a person with confirmed Ebola) within the past 21 days and (2) signs and symptoms potentially consistent with Ebola (fever, either subjective or ≥100.4° F [38° C], or headache, weakness, muscle pain, vomiting, diarrhea, abdominal pain, or hemorrhage). Similarly, the WHO identifies a suspect case as one of the following: any person (1) having had contact with a clinical case and presenting with an acute fever (>100.4° F [38° C]); (2) having had contact with a clinical case and presenting with three or more of the following symptoms: headache, generalized or articular pain, intense fatigue, nausea or vomiting, loss of appetite, diarrhea, abdominal pain, difficulty in swallowing, difficulty in breathing, hiccups, miscarriage; (3) presenting with acute fever and three or more of the above-mentioned symptoms; (4) with unexplained bleeding or miscarriage; and (5) who has an unexplained death. Across outbreaks, the case definition may require refinement depending on epidemiologic data specific to a particular outbreak. To improve the performance of existing case definitions for identification of suspect cases during the West African outbreak, clinical data from one Ebola Treatment Unit in Liberia were used to develop a clinical prediction score that could help determine whether a person has EVD. The Ebola Prediction Score comprised six independent predictors (having a sick contact, diarrhea, loss of appetite, muscle pain, difficulty swallowing, and absence of abdominal pain).

Establishing a diagnosis of Ebola ultimately requires isolation of Ebola virus, viral antigen capture, or virus-specific antibody from a bodily fluid sample. In settings where diagnostic capacity exists, the most commonly utilized test for diagnosing Ebola is real-time reverse transcription PCR (RT-PCR). Persons with Ebola are not known to be viremic during the incubation period; however, virus has been detected in blood samples on the day of symptom onset. A negative PCR test obtained on a patient who has had symptoms of <72 hours' duration may represent a false negative test. Tests obtained before 72 hours of symptoms should be repeated at or after 72 hours after onset of symptoms if there is ongoing clinical suspicion of EVD. Diagnosis of Ebola in deceased patients can be made using PCR testing of blood (often collected by cardiac puncture) or a sample collected by oral swab. If appropriate biosafety facilities are available, immunohistochemistry testing and virus culture can also be utilized.

Ebola is usually undetectable in the blood by the end of the second week. In survivors, however, infectious virus may persist in some immune privileged anatomic sites, including the testes and eyes. Later in the course of the disease (around day 10) or after recovery, evidence of current or past Ebola infection can be detected by virus-specific immunoglobulin (IgM and IgG antibodies). Most fatal cases fail to mount an antibody response. Hence, detecting virus-specific immunoglobulin in serum is a favorable finding. Virus-specific IgG has been detected in survivors as long as 11 years after infection.

Recent development of an antigen-based rapid diagnostic test for Ebola has been a promising addition to the arsenal of EVD diagnostics in light of its good performance characteristics (92% sensitivity, 85% specificity) and rapid turn-around time of 15 minutes. Further validation is required, however, before it formally can be used as a diagnostic in an outbreak.

Treatment

Despite the use in high-resource settings of investigational therapies (see below), the mainstays of treatment in both high- and low-resource settings are aggressive fluid replacement, electrolyte repletion, antiemetics, antimicrobials to treat co-infections, analgesia and antipyretics, nutrition, and targeted organ support. In the United States, the lower fatality rate of 18% seen in the first 11 cases suggests that even critically ill patients with end-organ damage can survive with aggressive treatment that, when necessary, may include mechanical ventilation and hemodialysis.

During an outbreak such as the West African Ebola outbreak, triaging patients by severity of illness enables health workers to appropriately manage and treat high volumes of patients. For example, Chertow et al. (2014) recommend the following three triage categories:

1. Clinically hypovolemic, not in shock, and able to provide self-care
2. Clinically hypovolemic, not in shock, not able to provide self-care
3. In shock with evidence of organ failure whose outcome would not be altered by available medical intervention.

For those patients falling in the first category, priority should be placed on encouragement of oral rehydration salts and nutrition complemented by symptomatic treatment such as oral analgesics, antinausea, and antiemetic medications.

A proportion of patients from group 1 will inevitably progress to group 2, and other patients may be presenting to the treatment unit at this level of severity. Health workers should be trained to identify early those patients who are beginning to deteriorate by monitoring for increased gastrointestinal losses, decreased ability for self-care, lethargy, and lassitude. Once identified as entering into group 2, these patients should immediately receive short-term intravenous therapy aimed to match gastrointestinal losses and electrolyte replacement, if capacity for electrolyte monitoring is available. Importantly, being able to establish intravenous access, deliver adequate volume of fluids, and safely manage needles and devices requires appropriate staff and triage planning to ensure that the sickest patients receive the necessary care. In addition, broad-spectrum antibiotics are often administered for prophylaxis against pathogenic translocation of intestinal bacteria in severely ill patients and for empiric treatment of non-Ebola diarrhea and pneumonia (especially in children).

In addition to supportive care, a number of investigational therapeutics have been developed or repurposed for treatment of EVD. During the West African Ebola outbreak, a number of these therapeutics were used under compassionate use, particularly in patients who were repatriated to either the United States or United Kingdom. These therapeutics include (1) ZMapp (and a related drug called ZMab), a combination of three different monoclonal antibodies that bind to the protein of the Ebola virus; (2) brincidofovir, a lipid-conjugated version of cidofovir, an oral nucleotide analog with broad-spectrum in vitro antiviral activity; (3) favipiravir, a broad-spectrum antiviral compound with activity against RNA viruses; and (4) TKM-Ebola, a combination of small interfering RNAs targeting several proteins in the RNA virus. Additionally, convalescent whole blood and plasma transfusions from patients who have recovered from Ebola have been administered. Though the efficacy of these treatments is unknown, trials to evaluate ZMapp, TKM-Ebola, and convalescent plasma are currently under way in Sierra Leone and Guinea.

Ribavirin has not shown anti-*Ebolavirus* activity in vitro and does not protect *Ebolavirus*-infected primates. Other agents that have been studied for the treatment or prevention of EVD include nucleoside analog inhibitors of S-adenosylhomocysteine hydrolase, interferon beta, horse- or goat-derived immune globulins, human-derived convalescent immune globulin preparations, recombinant human interferon alpha-2, recombinant human monoclonal antibody against the envelope glycoprotein (GP) of Ebola virus, DNA vaccines expressing either envelope GP or nucleocapsid protein genes of Ebola virus, protein C, and recombinant inhibitor of factor VIIa/tissue factor.

Public Health Measures

Historically, the cornerstone of control in low-resource regions has been isolation of the ill. While this strategy, in and of itself, may have been effective in small rural outbreaks, it has little to offer to infected people and their families.

Because Ebola is transmitted by contact with bodily fluids of symptomatic patients, transmission can be interrupted by a combination of early diagnosis, contact tracing, patient isolation, infection control, and safe burial practices. As has been demonstrated in the West African outbreak, however, the quality of clinical management of EVD patients while in treatment units, active communication with family members, and increased numbers of discharged patients plays a critical role in the success of efforts that target interrupting outbreak transmission. In effect, if the community is not convinced that an Ebola treatment unit is providing quality care, they are likely to avoid that treatment unit, which results in infectious patients remaining longer in the community.

When clinicians encounter patients with a history of exposure to Ebola and symptoms that are potentially consistent with EVD, they should first notify local public health authorities. In the United States, this would be county public health departments.

The CDC has designated US hospitals into three categories: those without special capacity to care for patients with suspected or proven EVD, those where patients with suspected EVD can be safely assessed and cared for while the infection is ruled out (usually within 72 hours), and those where comprehensive care of confirmed EVD patients can be safely provided. Every front-line healthcare worker should be confident that he or she can safely move patients with suspected EVD to the next higher level of care. Regardless of the level of care of a particular center, only trained employees should be permitted to care for these patients. Personal protective measures include diligent, rigorous, observed use of contact precautions via full barrier protection and flawless hand hygiene after care duties. These patients can produce prodigious volumes of infectious diarrhea and other body fluids, which must be handled with utmost care.

Given the relative immunosuppression of pregnancy, and epidemiologic data suggesting that pregnant women have a more severe than usual course when they become infected with Ebola, it is recommended that pregnant women not care for patients with Ebola.

The CDC recommends that women with Ebola and female survivors of Ebola not nurse their infants. Also, male survivors of EVD are recommended to either abstain from sexual activity or use condoms after recovery. The duration of these measures has not yet been delineated.

Vaccines

During the West Africa Ebola outbreak, at least two vaccines for Ebola have been under investigation in clinical trials. One (NIAID/ GSK Ebola vaccine) is a recombinant chimpanzee cold virus used as a vector to deliver segments of genetic material from Zaire Ebola virus (cAd3-ZEBOV). The other (VSV-EBOV Merck vaccine) is a genetically engineered version of vesicular stomatitis virus (VSV) in which the outer protein is replaced with a gene segment from the outer protein of Zaire Ebola virus. In March 2015, preliminary results from a phase II trial involving more than 600 participants in Liberia showed that both cAd3-ZEBOV and VSV-EBOV were safe. In addition, between October 2014 and June 2015, 120 Swiss adult participants receiving either high-dose cAd3-ZEBOV, low-dose cAd3-ZEBOV, or placebo were enrolled in a phase 1/2a randomized, double-blind, placebo-controlled trial which demonstrated that the vaccine was well tolerated and could elicit a robust immune response lasting 6 months after vaccination. Between April and July 2015, a phase III cluster-randomized trial utilizing a ring vaccination strategy to test safety and efficacy of VSV EBOV in contacts of newly infected EVD cases took place in southwestern Guinea: when a new case was identified, close contacts were randomized to receive VSV-EBOV either immediately or 3 weeks later. Interim analyses suggested a significantly lower incidence of EVD in participants who received early VSV-EBOV vaccination compared to participants who received delayed vaccination, and randomization was discontinued so that all participants could receive this vaccine immediately. No one who received the vaccine has yet developed clinical EVD beyond a defined incubation period. While guidelines for widespread deployment of the vaccine have not been established, under investigational protocols, VSV-EBOV has been administered for post-exposure prophylaxis in some repatriated patients who were exposed to Ebola virus while caring for EVD patients in West Africa. In addition, since October 2015, VSV-EBOV vaccination has been administered to contacts from the UK and Sierra Leone who had been exposed to EVD survivors with recrudescent infection; no secondary infections have been reported in these vaccinated contacts.

FURTHER READING

Bausch, D.G., 2011. Viral hemorrhagic fevers. In: Goldman's Cecil Medicine, twenty-fourth ed. Saunders Elsevier, Philadelphia, pp. 2147–2155.

CDC, 2014. Clinical Inquiries Regarding Ebola Virus Disease Received by CDC—United States, July 9–November 15, 2014. MMWR 63 (Early Release), 1–5.

CDC, 2014. Interim U.S. Guidance for Monitoring and Movement of Persons with Potential Ebola Virus Exposure. Updated December 24. Available at <http://www.cdc.gov/vhf/ebola/exposure/monitoring-and-movement-of-persons-with-exposure.html> (accessed February 16, 2015).

CDC, 2014. Support Services for Survivors of Ebola Virus Disease—Sierra Leone, 2014. MMWR 63 (50), 1205–1206.

CDC, 2015. Ebola (Ebola Virus Disease)—Diagnosis. Available at <http://www.cdc.gov/vhf/ebola/diagnosis/> (accessed February 20, 2015).

CDC, 2015. 2014 Ebola Outbreak in West Africa—Case Counts. Available at <http://www.cdc.gov/vhf/ebola/outbreaks/2014-west-africa/case-counts.html>.

CDC, 2016. CDC Health Information for International Travel. Oxford University Press, New York.

Chertow, D.S., Kleine, C.K., Edwards, J.K., et al., 2014. Ebola virus disease in West Africa—clinical manifestations and management. N. Engl. J. Med. 371, 2054–2057.

Epstein, H., 2014. Ebola in Liberia: an epidemic of rumors. New York Review of Books, 91 95.

Henao-Restrepo, A.M., Longini, I.M., Egger, M., et al., 2015. Efficacy and effectiveness of an rVSV-vectored vaccine expressing Ebola surface glycoprotein: interim results from the Guinea ring vaccination cluster-randomised trial. Lancet 386 (9996), 857–866. Online, July 31.

International Committee on Taxonomy of Viruses. Available at <http://ictvonline.org/virusTaxonomy.asp?version=2012> (accessed February 16, 2015).

Ippolito, G, et al., 2012. Viral hemorrhagic fevers: advancing the level of treatment. BMC Med. 10, 31.

King, J.W., Ebola virus infection. Medscape. Available at <http://emedicine.medscape.com/article/216288-overview> (accessed February 16, 2015).

Kortepeter, M.G., Bausch, D.G., Bray, M., 2011. Basic clinical and laboratory features of filoviral hemorrhagic fever. J. Infect. Dis. 204 (Suppl. 3), S810–S816. doi:10.1093/infdis/jir299.

Knust, B., Rollin, P.E., Infectious Diseases Related to Travel: Viral hemorrhagic fevers. CDC 2016 "Yellow Book" Chapter 3. Available at <http://wwwnc.cdc.gov/travel/yellowbook/2016/infectious-diseases-related-to-travel/viral-hemorrhagic-fevers>.

Lyon, G.M., et al., 2014. Clinical care of two patients with Ebola virus disease in the United States. N. Engl. J. Med. 371, 2402–2409.

Meltzer, E., 2012. Arboviruses and viral hemorrhagic fevers (VHF). Infect. Dis. Clin. N. Am. 26, 479–496.

Prescott, J., et al., 2015. Post-mortem stability of Ebola virus. Emerg. Infect. Dis. doi:10.3201/eid2105.150041. Available at <http://wwwnc.cdc.gov/eid/article/21/5/15-0041_article>.

Towner, J.S., Rollin, P.E., Bausch, D.G., et al., 2004. Rapid diagnosis of Ebola hemorrhagic fever by reverse transcription-PCR in an outbreak setting and assessment of patient viral load as a predictor of outcome. J. Virol. 78 (8), 4330–4341.

West, T.E., von Saint André-von Arnim, A., 2014. Clinical presentation and management of severe Ebola virus disease. Ann. Am. Thorac. Soc. 11 (9), 1341–1350.

WHO, 2015. WHO Fact Sheet: Ebola Virus Disease. Available at <http://www.who.int/mediacentre/factsheets/fs103/en/> (accessed December 11, 2014).

WHO Ebola Response Team, 2014. Ebola Disease in West Africa—The First 9 Months of the Epidemic and Forward Projections. N. Engl. J. Med. 371, 1481–1495.

CHAPTER 29

Antibiotic-Resistant Bacteria in Returning Travelers

Paul S. Pottinger

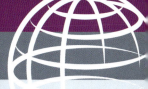

International travel often brings us into contact with multidrug-resistant (MDR) organisms (MRDOs), especially bacteria. These germs may or may not colonize or infect the traveler, but when they do, they present challenges to the clinician. This chapter will focus on strategies to prevent, diagnose, and treat MRDO infections in international travelers.

OVERVIEW OF ANTIBIOTIC RESISTANCE

Long before the human era, microbes competed for ecological niches in the environment. Thus, ancient bacteria developed the ability to resist the assault of naturally occurring antibacterial substances, especially those made by fungi and other soil-dwelling organisms. By harnessing these substances (and by developing new antibiotics) for clinical use, we have dramatically accelerated this evolutionary process. The more we expose bacteria to these medications, the sooner we select resistant phenotypes. Nobel Laureate Alexander Fleming warned long ago that this process was inevitable and that medical professionals have an ethical responsibility to use antibiotics in a responsible fashion. Less than a century later, his concerns have proven prophetic. Antibiotic resistance to at least one class of drugs has been documented in almost all bacteria studied, including Gram-positive bacteria (e.g., methicillin-resistant *Staphylococcus aureus*, vancomycin-resistant *Enterococcus*, and drug-resistant *Streptococcus pneumoniae*), and Gram-negative bacteria (e.g., extended-spectrum beta-lactamase–producing *Escherichia coli*, MDR *Pseudomonas aeruginosa*, and carbapenem-resistant *Enterobacteriaceae*). Some mechanisms of resistance are specific to a particular species, but in many cases the genetic determinants of resistance lie on mobile elements, such as plasmids and integrons, which can move between species. Thus, in some regions of the world there seem to be ideal conditions for the creation and spread of resistant microbes, in which antibiotic use is uncontrolled and sanitation is insufficient. There is no single, reliable, international surveillance system for detecting and reporting antimicrobial resistance. The World Health Organization oversees a consortium of regional laboratories around the globe, but their funding streams and staffing are often insufficient to generate timely data, especially in sub-Saharan Africa. High-quality data are essential for our understanding of this phenomenon, and they are sorely lacking—this situation needs to change right away. However, the trend is clear: many bacterial infections are becoming tougher to treat worldwide, including in the tropics.

There is no hope of eradicating pathogenic bacteria from the face of the earth with antibiotics—resistance is inevitable. The global question is whether we can reduce, delay, and anticipate the emergence of resistance in a way that helps humans live side-by-side with bacteria in a sustainable way. Our understanding of the human microbiome—the universe of microorganisms on and inside us—is still incomplete. But we do know that more than 90% of the cells on us and in us are microorganisms, so by the numbers we are more "them" than "us." The notion of human dominance over the microscopic world is naïve, and a more nuanced view of our position in the world is called for. For medical providers dealing with MDRO infections in their individual patients, these questions have very urgent clinical meaning.

PREVENTION OF MDRO INFECTION: PUBLIC HEALTH

Reducing the threat of MDROs on an international scale will require coming to terms with several key factors that are currently out of control.

- *Meager drug pipeline.* New antibiotics may help turn the tide, but the current pace of progress is discouraging. Industry has precious few financial incentives to develop novel agents, because the process is time-consuming and expensive. And with resistance on the rise, there is concern that new agents will have limited effective lives—and, thus, limited profit potential. A new "public-private partnership" model may be called for, in which government incents industrial activity via financial rewards beyond traditional drug sales. Viewing these drugs as national assets, rather than simple profitable commodities, may yield meaningful change.

- *Ineffective infection control.* Limiting the spread of infection between patients is common sense, with an importance easily grasped by physicians. However, there are other crucial reasons to limit the transmission of pathogens: bacteria are sometimes able to swap genetic information with each other, across species. Many genetic determinants of antibiotic resistance are contained within mobile elements such as plasmids and integrons. When infected patients are cared for in clinics or hospitals, these genes may be transferred efficiently if hygiene protocols are breached. Even more alarming is the frequency with which this may happen in the built environment when sanitation practices are insufficient, and human effluent mixes together and then enters the water supply without proper treatment. Fortunately, simple interventions, such as hand hygiene by healthcare workers and the installation and use of proper pit latrines or flush toilets in austere settings, can have a huge impact.

- *Agricultural use of antibiotics.* The more selective pressure we assert on the microbiome, the more we accelerate the evolution of MDROs. According to the Food and Drug Administration (FDA), over 80% of antibiotics in the United States—more than 13 million kilograms annually—are given to livestock to promote growth or prevent infection. This practice has been associated with the development of MDR Gram-negative rods, such as fluoroquinolone-resistant *Campylobacter* species, which can be transmitted to humans via unsafe meat handling processes. These massive quantities of antibiotics may also enter the water supply, and then the human host, leading to unpredictable alterations in the gastrointestinal microbiome. Other nations have banned this practice, without suffering detrimental increases in the cost of producing poultry or beef. Whether the United States will reduce this practice from a regulatory perspective or whether market demands will lead to change remains to be seen.

- *Injudicious use of antibiotics in human medicine.* Although the use of antibiotics in humans is less than in animals in most industrialized nations, medical providers around the world bear a huge portion of the blame for our current predicament. Multiple expert reviews of large patient cohorts reveal a stubborn truth that has not changed appreciably over the decades: in general, 50% of antibiotic prescriptions are inappropriate (in terms of indication, spectrum, dose, or duration). The wise use of antibiotics is called "antimicrobial stewardship." All clinicians have important roles to play as good antimicrobial stewards. Resources are listed in the Further Reading section of this chapter. Fundamentals are included in **Table 29.1**.

PREVENTION OF MDRO INFECTION: THE TRAVELING PATIENT

MDRO infections are part of the reality of traveling abroad, and this topic should be included in pre-travel counseling. Core points to discuss with patients before leaving include the following:

- *Protect yourself without becoming a "germophobe."* Most of the toughest-to-treat MDROs acquired overseas are Gram-negative rods, from the family *Enterobacteriaceae.* In other

TABLE 29.1   Principles of Effective Antimicrobial Stewardship

- **Maintain Meticulous Infection Control.** Minimize the risk of passing resistance genes to bystander bacteria by keeping drug-resistant pathogens away from other patients—and yourselves. Clean hands before and after every encounter, obey other special precaution protocols, and maintain a clean examination area or hospital room.

- **Establish a Firm Diagnosis.** Is the patient truly infected with a bacterial pathogen? Some diseases mimic infection but do not respond to antibiotics. If bacterial infection is present, culture data are extraordinarily helpful, because they will reveal not only the pathogen but also its susceptibility profile. Ideally, cultures should be obtained before antimicrobials are started. But for patients who have a severe infection, delays in starting treatment may have grave consequences; start antibiotics immediately and send specimens for culture as soon as possible.

- **Say NO to Antibiotics for Viral Rhinosinusitis.** The common cold is due to viral infection approximately 95% of the time. Encourage patients to "get smart" about antibiotics, treat their symptoms, and emphasize the importance of maintaining the effectiveness of these medications if they should eventually require them.

- **Deescalate When Possible.** If broad-spectrum empiric treatment was initiated for severe infection, be willing to trust the results of positive cultures and focus treatment. More expensive, newer drugs may not be superior to tried and true therapies.

- **Shorter May Be Better.** Using the briefest duration of therapy possible may reduce selective pressure on bystander, normal flora. Subtherapeutic doses or intermittent, haphazard dosing are enormous mistakes, but treating at a full dose for a short period may have benefits for resistance—so long as the underlying infection has been adequately treated.

- **Collaborate with Experts.** Specialists in the field of infectious diseases medicine are always eager to collaborate with other physicians, both to generate protocols and to care for specific patients. Consult these specialists when patients are severely ill, when they fail to improve as expected, when the resistance profile is unexpectedly severe, or when treatment involves multiple or toxic drugs.

---

words, human fecal bacteria. Prevention of gastrointestinal illness is an excellent way to prevent gut colonization with these MRDOs. Hands should be cleaned before and after eating, and after using the lavatory, with soap, water, and a clean towel—or a hand rub containing at least 60% alcohol if this is not possible. Food should be chosen wisely, because of concern for contamination with human coliform bacteria introduced during preparation and storage. The mantra "Peel it, boil it, cook it, or forget it" is a fine start, but this may be difficult for patients to accomplish. The principles of smart eating and drinking habits are reviewed in depth in Chapters 7 and 8. Wearing a surgical mask when in public has a very small chance of preventing bacterial MDRO infections and is not usually recommended for this purpose.

- *Get all appropriate immunizations, including seasonal influenza.* Some bacterial MDRO infections may be directly prevented by immunizations (e.g., typhoid fever and pertussis). But the prevention of viral infections can also reduce the risk of MDRO bacterial infection, principally by reducing the likelihood of developing a febrile illness that might lead to healthcare interactions and inappropriate antibiotic use. Add this to the list of the many reasons why travelers should receive all appropriate vaccinations before leaving.

- *Avoid "medical tourism."* As the cost of surgical procedures seems to continue to rise in industrialized nations, some patients seek more affordable care overseas, particularly in Mexico, India, and China. Certainly, there are centers of excellence in these nations and elsewhere around the globe. Furthermore, post-procedural infections still happen in North America with unacceptable frequency. However, numerous case reports substantiate the concern that infection control and quality assurance overseas are often provided at a level below that achieved in Europe and North America. Patients may fail to grasp the impact—personal and financial—of healthcare infections acquired overseas. These can be dangerous, debilitating, disfiguring infections, and the cost of aftercare alone may meet or exceed the savings envisioned. Thus, in general, planning trips for medical procedures should be discouraged. Seeking care for an acute medical problem while overseas is quite different, and patients should not be discouraged from seeing a healthcare provider if the need arises.

- *Use antibiotics wisely.* As described above, antimicrobial stewardship can have major impacts on public health; it can also benefit individual patients. Every prescription for antibiotics written pre-departure should come with clear guidance on when to initiate self-treatment during the trip. Patients who take antibiotics for uncomplicated secretory diarrhea put themselves at risk for *C. difficile* infection, prolongation of symptoms due to altered microbiota ("antibiotic-associated diarrhea"), and development of de novo antibiotic resistance within their own native bacteria. For this reason—among others— antibiotics should not be taken as "routine prophylaxis" but rather reserved for the unusual occurrence of high-risk infections, such as dysentery, except in exceptional cases as described in Chapter 8.

- *Quit smoking.* Most smokers acknowledge that their addiction is hazardous to their health, and are interested in quitting. Here is another motivator: respiratory infections are more frequent among smokers, and thus they are more susceptible to MRDOs; they also require antibiotics more often, which in turn puts them at even higher risk of creating new MDROs in their own bodies.

- *Practice safe sex.* Certain bacterial sexually transmitted diseases (STDs), such as gonorrhea, are becoming more and more drug resistant over time and may require higher doses, longer courses, and parenteral routes of therapy (see Chapter 42). Pre-travel safe sex counseling should pay dividends in terms of preventing acquisition of MDRO STDs.

- *Probiotics are probably safe but of unproven benefit.* The "health-savvy" patient may seek your advice on probiotics. The concept is attractive: use friendly microbes to keep the bad ones at bay. Published studies to date vary in terms of design—different settings, different interventions, and different outcome measures. Recent meta-analyses suggest a trend toward benefit in the treatment arms, but rarely a large enough benefit to achieve statistical significance. Given the complexity of our gastrointestinal microbiomes, it is small wonder that taking megadoses of one or a few microbes fails to reliably set things to right, including prevention of traveler's diarrhea. Further complicating the issue is a lack of ingredient standardization or regulatory oversight by the FDA for these products, which are classified as dietary supplements rather than medications. On the other hand, probiotics are unlikely to harm the patient—unless he or she has a suppressed immune system, in which case the probiotic microbes can become invasive, leading to colitis or bloodstream infection. In summary, patients should be told that the jury is still out, but for those with a healthy immune system it is reasonable to add once- or twice-daily probiotic supplements to their diets while abroad, although this is not a substitute for any of the other interventions outlined above.

RECOGNITION AND MANAGEMENT SUGGESTIONS FOR MDRO INFECTIONS

Because most bacteria have the potential to become MDROs, and because they can infect virtually any part of the body, a comprehensive discussion of the clinical presentation and management of these infections is beyond the scope of this chapter. However, advice regarding the most common MDRO syndromes in returning travelers includes discussions about the following:

- *Silent colonization.* Conceptually, when a germ comes into contact with a human being, one of four things happens: the two simply ignore each other; the germ kills the host; the host kills the germ; or an agreement is reached—a state referred to as "colonization." In colonization, bacteria inhabit an ecological niche within the patient, such as body hair follicles, the anterior nares, the oropharynx, the lower gastrointestinal tract, or the genitourinary tract. By definition, colonizers are clinically silent and cause no signs or symptoms of disease. However, colonizers can become pathogens in a moment, if given the opportunity by the host. This could happen with waning humoral immunity (as during chemotherapy), impaired cellular immunity (as in untreated human immunodeficiency [HIV] infection), anatomical injury (as in surgical wound infections), or alteration of the competitors within an ecological niche (as in antibiotic-associated diarrhea). Surveillance data are lacking, but clinical experience suggests that many patients who acquire MRDOs while overseas have asymptomatic colonization of the gastrointestinal tract. By itself, this is harmless; however, if these germs are allowed to flourish under the selective pressure of antibiotics, or if they migrate to other anatomic sites, then infection may develop. MDRO colonization may last for days, years, or anything in between. Patients who have traveled overseas for any considerable period of time, especially those who received health care during the trip, are at elevated risk for gastrointestinal MDRO colonization for at least the first 6 months after return. However, this is an arbitrary number, and there are many cases in which patients have demonstrated sustained colonization years after their exposure. This may have implications for infection control in the hospital or clinic. Currently there is no national consensus on whether to look for asymptomatic MDRO colonization, for example, via a rectal swab or fecal culture, in part because of the challenges this poses in the laboratory, and because it is not entirely clear what to do with that information. It may be simpler to assume these patients are colonized, and thus to treat them using contact precautions (diligent hand hygiene, gowns, and gloves). However, it is reasonable to consider surveillance cultures as part of a comprehensive infection control strategy if your clinic or center encounters these organisms frequently.

- *Gastrointestinal infection.* The gastrointestinal tract is a leading reservoir for MDRO colonization, although invasive infection is relatively uncommon. As described in Chapters 21 and 30, enteric fever due to *Salmonella enterica* serovars *typhi* and *paratyphi* are leading causes of fever among travelers returning from the tropics. In the past, fluoroquinolones such as ciprofloxacin and levofloxacin were reliable treatment options for these infections; currently, the majority of isolates acquired in Southeast Asia, in particular South Asia, are partially or fully resistant to fluoroquinolones. Third-generation cephalosporins such as ceftriaxone are more reliable empiric choices and can be used in uncomplicated disease, but unfortunately resistance to this class is also on the rise. Someone who is septic with suspected salmonella infection acquired in India should be admitted and treated empirically with a carbapenem such as ertapenem, until antibiotic susceptibility testing confirms a narrower-spectrum agent can be used. Similarly, enterotoxigenic *E. coli* (ETEC), which was once predictably susceptible to fluoroquinolones, is increasingly resistant—again particularly in Southeast Asia—and alternative drugs such as azithromycin are more reliable today. Other MDR Enterobacteriaceae, including carbapenem-resistant species, may require toxic agents such as aminoglycosides for treatment. Fortunately, symptomatic infection of the gut is uncommonly caused by carbapenem-resistant Enterobacteriaceae, presumably because these bacteria infrequently carry extra virulence genes. Drug resistance and increased virulence are not necessarily found together.

- *Urinary tract infection (UTI).* MDR Gram-negative rods, especially from the Enterobacteriaceae group, which includes *E. coli*, may be detected in the urine of returning travelers, particularly women. Presumably, this is because gastrointestinal colonization is a common source of MDROs in travelers (see above), and proximity of the urethral meatus to the anal aperture facilitates bacterial entrance into the urinary tract (just as happens with all UTIs). Because treatment can be challenging, it is essential to distinguish between true UTI and asymptomatic bacteriuria (ABU). If a patient does not have signs or symptoms of UTI such as urinary urgency or frequency, hematuria, pyuria, suprapubic tenderness, or an abnormal urinalysis, or if her urine was tested for reasons that are unclear, then by definition she has ABU, which should *not* be treated with antibiotics. On the other hand, if clinical suspicion for true UTI is high, then treatment is appropriate. Guidelines of the Infectious Diseases Society of America suggest that uncomplicated UTI be treated empirically, without sending a urine culture unless symptoms persist or recur. However, patients who have recently been overseas may not fit into this category of "uncomplicated," and our practice is to send a clean-catch midstream urine specimen for urinanalysis and reflexively for culture if the urinanalysis is abnormal at the first presentation for these patients. Culture data will take time, however, so an empiric prescription will be necessary. Ideally, these patients should receive one dose of fosfomycin 3 gm PO, because resistance to this drug is less common than to the alternative first-line treatments (trimethoprim-sulfamethoxazole 1 dose PO BID for 3 days or nitrofurantoin 100 mg PO BID for 5 days). Alternative oral treatments are even less likely to succeed against MDR Enterobacteriaceae, such as ciprofloxacin or cefpodoxime.

After culture and resistance data are available, empiric treatment can be changed if the patient has failed to improve. In many cases, no oral treatment will have a favorable in vitro resistance profile. This is an appropriate situation in which to consult a specialist in infectious diseases, who may have access to experimental oral treatments or who can assist with parenteral treatment if indicated. In many cases, an intravenous course of a carbapenem, such as ertapenem 1 gm IV daily for 5 days, may be required.

Some patients will develop recurrent UTI symptoms, which can be stubborn and frustrating for everyone. An emerging strategy that may hold promise involves resetting the microbiome of the vagina. *E. coli* does not belong in the vagina in substantial amounts, and most UTIs in otherwise healthy women are caused by *E. coli* ascending the urethra from the introitus. A leading hypothesis is that the vagina is usually protected from high-level *E. coli* colonization because of its low pH, which is provided by the activity of human lactobacilli, including *Lactobacillus crispatus* and *Lactobacillus iners*, among other species. These healthy bacteria may be wiped out inadvertently by antibiotic courses given for other reasons, such as rhinosinusitis. Sadly, most commercially available lactobacillus supplements contain bovine species such as *Lactobacillus rhamnosus*, which do not lower vaginal pH appropriately. Fortunately, clinical trials of human lactobacilli in vaginal suppositories have shown a protective effect, and there is hope that FDA registry trials will result in approval of this product in the near future. If so, it would be appropriate to offer this technique to patients with recurrent UTI (regardless of their bacterial resistance profile). This is also yet another reason to prescribe antibiotics prudently, to prevent altering the vaginal microbiome in the first place. Patients who ask for antibiotics for inappropriate indications may respond to this teaching by their physician.

- *Skin and soft tissue infections.* In developed nations, the origin of skin and soft tissue infections is relatively predictable: cellulitis without purulence is usually caused by streptococcal species (including Group A beta-hemolytic *Streptococcus pyogenes*), whereas purulent infections such as "boils," furuncles, carbuncles, and abscesses are usually caused by *Staphylococcus aureus* (both methicillin-susceptible *S. aureus* and methicillin-resistant *S. aureus*). In a returning traveler, this pattern remains accurate (see Chapter 36). However, other pathogens should be considered as well, depending on host factors and environmental exposures. Providers must obtain a careful, detailed history in order to avoid missing drug-resistant bacterial infections. For example, the risk of MDR Gram-negative skin infections is greatly increased among patients who have undergone surgical procedures overseas or who sustained a wound exposed to fresh water. Such wounds may have become infected by environmental organisms such as *Acinetobacter*, *Pseudomonas*, *Aeromonas*, *Burkholderia*, and rapidly growing mycobacteria, which can be profoundly resistant to most, if not all, antibiotics. Thus, an interdisciplinary approach is required for these patients: there should be a low threshold to admit severely infected patients to the hospital (with full and aggressive contact precautions). There should be tissue and blood specimens should be submitted for culture and sensitivity testing, and consultation should be sought from specialists in both infectious diseases (because toxic medications may be necessary, such as aminoglycosides, polymyxins, or tigecycline) and surgery (because in some cases rapid debridement or even amputation may be life-saving).

- *Respiratory infections.* Infections of the lung and respiratory tract among returning travelers are second only to gastrointestinal infections. The great majority are either presumed or proven to be caused by viruses (e.g., *influenza*, *parainfluenza*, *rhinovirus*, or *coronavirus*).

These infections may be "garden variety" or novel forms acquired during travel, such as highly pathogenic avian influenza (HPAI) or Middle East respiratory corona virus. Furthermore, these viral processes may mask, mimic, or predispose patients to drug-resistant bacterial infections. For example, *S. aureus* or *Haemophilus pneumoniae* infections may follow influenza infection. So-called atypical bacterial pneumonia due to *Legionella* or *Chlamydia* may have a clinical and radiographic appearance that looks very much like viral pneumonia. These infections require early detection and antibiotic coverage in order to prevent substantial risk of morbidity and mortality. All physicians know well the principle of "Occam's razor," in which the single answer with the fewest uncertainties should be selected. This is usually a wise approach in infectious diseases medicine; however, because there are so many microbes that threaten people in austere settings, multiple infections may present simultaneously or in close sequence. Thus, caution should be advised in the ill traveler returning from the tropics, where "Occam's razor may grow rusty in the humid atmosphere," so to speak.

FURTHER READING

Center for Disease Dynamics, Economics and Policy. <www.CDDEP.org>.
Website maintained by the CDDEP, an independent, not-for-profit organization dedicated to collection and dissemination of information regarding antimicrobial resistance.

Centers for Disease Control and Prevention. <www.cdc.gov/GetSmart>.
User-friendly website maintained by the CDC, including patient-oriented information on the importance of wise antibiotic use.

Dellit, T.H., Owens, R.C., McGowan, J.E., Jr., et al., 2007. Infectious Diseases Society of America and the Society for Healthcare Epidemiology of America guidelines for developing an institutional program to enhance antimicrobial stewardship. Clin. Infect. Dis. 44 (2), 159–177. PMID: 17173212.
State-of-the-art guidelines on how to set up an antimicrobial stewardship program from the Infectious Diseases Society of America.

Shepherd, A.K., Pottinger, P.S., 2013. Management of urinary tract infections in the era of increasing antimicrobial resistance. Med. Clin. North Am. 97 (4), 737–757. PMID: 23809723.
Practical advice for medical providers regarding strategies for dealing with urinary tract infections due to MDROs.

World Health Organization. <www.who.int/drugresistance>.
Clearinghouse of information regarding the global burden and epidemiology of antibiotic resistance, maintained by the WHO.

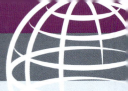

CHAPTER 30

The Role of Point-of-Care Testing in Travel Medicine

Robert Martin, Lucy A. Perrone, and Michael Noble

Health threats to travelers from infectious disease are common, with estimates of up to 75% of travelers becoming ill at some time during their travel. The World Health Organization (WHO) cites an extensive list (http://www.who.int/ith/diseases/en) of potential infectious agents, dependent on the countries visited. Because international travel can expose individuals to serious health risks, it is important that travelers have a medical consultation before traveling to consider appropriate medications for common symptoms such as upper respiratory illnesses and gastrointestinal disturbances, as well as to assure an awareness of health threats in the countries being visited.

For the returning traveler with illness, an accurate travel history is critical for development of a differential diagnosis. The process of developing a diagnosis often requires a number of laboratory tests. The availability and use of point of care (POC) tests for many suspected infectious agents may assist clinicians in more rapid diagnosis and treatment than conventional laboratory-based tests, but there are currently few such tests available that would benefit a healthcare provider attending to a returning traveler. An international survey of the use of POC tests in primary care turns up a long list of tests currently in use globally. However, not all of these POC tests are approved for use in the United States. **Table 30.1** lists some of the tests currently approved by the Food and Drug Administration (FDA) for use by healthcare providers in the United States.

In addition to being a diagnostic aid for acute infections, POC tests are also used for the purpose of monitoring, such as blood glucose control or anticoagulant therapy. For those anticipating international travel, there are a number of issues that must be considered to assure testing accuracy.

It is widely accepted that POC testing has the potential to improve access for the diagnosis and treatment of disease. POC testing is often mentioned as among the solutions in environments where "traditional" laboratory testing is not available. However, there are a number of factors that influence the true impact of POC testing, such as capital costs (equipment), maintaining an inventory in an environment of infrequent use, ease of use, associated instructions, training, and quality assurance of testing. In addition, accredited laboratories and laboratory professionals have the responsibility of documenting training, assuring appropriate quality control, and reporting test results. For nonlaboratory healthcare workers, there may be a lack of awareness of the importance of these elements in providing overall quality of testing. When these key quality issues are addressed, POC tests that have been rigorously evaluated can be important tools in rapid diagnosis of some infectious diseases.

DEFINITION AND USE OF POINT OF CARE TESTS

POC tests are generally defined as diagnostic tests used near the patient that provide results in a time frame that allows diagnostic results to inform clinical decision making while the

TABLE 30.1   Partial List and FDA Classification of Point of Care Tests Currently Available in the United States (i.e., FDA-Approved)

Analyte	TEST COMPLEXITY	
	Waived	Moderate
Bacteria		
Group A Strep	X	
Helicobacter pylori (urease and antibody)	X	
Lyme disease (antibody)		X
Salmonella (culture and detection of toxin in broth)		X
Chlamydia (nucleic acid)		X
Neisseria *gonorrhoeae*		X
Viruses		
Influenza A and B (virus)	X	
Respiratory syncytial virus (virus)	X	
Adenovirus (virus)	X	
HIV (antibody)	X	
Hepatitis C (antibody)	X	
Infectious mononucleosis (antibody)	X	
Hematology		
Hemoglobin	X	
Hematocrit	X	
Erythrocyte sedimentation rate	X	
Prothrombin time	X	
White cell count		X
Chemistry		
Glucose	X	
Glycosylated hemoglobin	X	
Cholesterol, HDL cholesterol, and triglyceride	X	
Troponin		X
Blood gases		X
C-reactive protein		X
Fecal occult blood	X	
Urine test strips	X	
Parasitology		
Trichomonas	X	

FDA, US Food and Drug Administration; *HDL,* high-density lipoprotein; *HIV,* human immunodeficiency virus.

patient is present. In the United States, regulations also play a role in determining which tests can be performed in that environment.

Use and Regulation of Point-of-Care Tests in the United States

The regulation of laboratory testing in the United States is administered by the FDA and is based on complexity of performance, including specimen preparation. The complexity model assigns a category of moderate or high complexity category based on the guidelines in the Clinical Laboratory Improvement Amendments of 1988 (CLIA 88). These moderate and highly complex tests are most often performed in a traditional laboratory setting. Some rapid tests (e.g., Remel XPECT Giardia/Cryptosporidium lateral flow assay) fall into the category of moderate complexity, meaning that they are subject to inspection and that technicians must perform proficiency testing and quality control and meet personnel requirements. POC tests in the moderate complexity category (e.g., blood gases, electrolytes) are often performed in a healthcare environment in which the laboratory supports these requirements. A third category, and the category most often associated with POC testing, is known as "waived tests." Waived tests are defined as "simple laboratory examinations and procedures that have an insignificant risk of an erroneous result." Clearly, this definition is problematic if applied to tests such as human immunodeficiency virus (HIV), hepatitis C virus (HCV), and others that can have significant consequences if results are erroneous. In addition, a single positive result for those tests that require confirmation (e.g., HIV) should never be provided to the patient without confirmation; therefore, personnel performing such POC tests much be trained and have appropriate oversight to prevent such occurrences. In 1988 when the CLIA regulations were written, there were only eight analytes; as of February 2016 there were currently more than 125 analytes and hundreds of test systems available.

Importantly, waived tests, even though they may be regarded as "simple," require knowledge, competence, and an understanding of basic testing procedures. If reagents have expired or are used in either insufficient or excessive volume or the testing times are either prolonged or abbreviated, the results of testing may be difficult to interpret. For example, the interpretation of many tests is based on the accumulation of a specific color reaction after 1-2 minutes of reaction. If reaction times are not monitored closely and tests are allowed to sit for an extra 2-3 minutes or more, the extra time can greatly enhance the accumulation of color, resulting in false positive results.

In the United States it is important to distinguish which POC tests are in the moderate complexity or "waived" category, because that categorization determines the personnel, training, and quality assurance for performing the test. A list of waived analytes is available at http://www.accessdata.fda.gov/scripts/cdrh/cfdocs/cfClia/analyteswaived.cfm and a list of waived test systems is available at http://www.accessdata.fda.gov/scripts/cdrh/cfdocs/cfClia/testswaived.cfm.

For travel clinics in the United States in which there is no laboratory oversight (e.g., no requirements for training, quality assurance, or proficiency testing), there are a limited number of tests in the waived category for infectious diseases. Tests cleared by the FDA as "waived tests" include those for HIV, HCV, influenza, respiratory syncytial virus, Epstein-Barr virus, Group A *Streptococcus*, adenovirus, *Helicobacter pylori*, trichomonas, and presence of Gram-negative bacteria in vaginal specimens (bacterial vaginitis).

An example of a rapid diagnostic test (RDT) that is considered a POC in international settings is the malaria antigen detection assay. While their use in malaria-endemic areas has proven a major step forward in providing rapid treatment, in the United States only one test system (BinaxNOW® Malaria) for malaria has been approved by the FDA. It is categorized as moderately complex and must meet the requirements listed above for performance of moderately complex testing.

Use and Regulation for Point-of-Care Tests in Resource-Limited Settings

Many of the countries that present the highest risk to international travelers lack regulatory standards regarding production or importation of test kits. A WHO report addressing regulation of in vitro diagnostics established that many POC tests sold in limited-resource countries perform poorly due to the lack of regulatory oversight or enforcement. Because many of these low-quality POC tests are inexpensive, countries where there are no quality standards often use cost as the single factor in the decision to purchase and use a test kit.

POC tests in resource-limited settings have been valuable in addressing the HIV epidemic, in providing rapid diagnosis of malaria infections, and, more recently, in transfusion medicine (rapid syphilis test). However, studies describing the value of these tests emphasize that the effectiveness of POC tests is dependent on test quality and conditions of use.

In international settings where there is no oversight of performance or of manufacturing of tests, there are insufficient data to determine common parameters such as sensitivity and specificity, and no studies in populations of intended use to provide data on predictive value. Therefore, test results from these settings should be viewed with caution and repeated if necessary.

Good Laboratory Practices for Point-of-Care Testing

Commonly used tests at POC in the United States include those for glucose, blood gas analysis/electrolytes, activated clotting time, urine dipsticks, occult blood, hemoglobin, and rapid tests for Group A *Streptococcus*. As noted above, the requirement for performing these tests is dependent on the FDA categorization. For the purposes of most travel clinics, these tests will be of limited use for the returning traveler in the United States.

However, regardless of the test being performed, good laboratory practice dictates that performance of any test includes the use of quality control material and that the test be performed by trained personnel who are periodically evaluated on their ability to perform the testing. For example, a survey of general practitioners in the Netherlands found that there is not always attention to quality control measures such as checking storage conditions, performing calibration and maintenance, or performing acceptable hygienic practices such as hand washing prior to collecting a blood sample. In 2005 the Centers for Disease Control and Prevention (CDC) and the Centers for Medicare and Medicaid Services (CMS) published "Good Laboratory Practices for Waived Settings," a guide that provides a list of important considerations before introducing waived testing.

THE TRAVELER USING POINT-OF-CARE TESTS

Patients involved in their own healthcare and using monitoring devices to determine glucose levels or to monitor coagulation times need to be advised of potential problems with equipment and reagents as well as potential problems in maintaining appropriate storage for medications. There are some obvious issues such as assuring monitoring devices will have sufficient power (extra batteries) or assuring the ability to connect to systems with voltage other than the standard 120 V available in the United States. Depending on the country and location within the country, availability of continuous electrical power is a common problem.

In addition to these more obvious issues, a letter from a physician that lists a traveler's diagnoses and the supplies used, including syringes or infusion pumps, may be useful when traveling through airports. All supplies should be transported in carry-on luggage. Assuring a sufficient supply of materials and reagents (some supplies may not be available in resource-limited settings) and the ability to control temperatures of storage while traveling is critical. For example, excessive heat may influence not only the quality of medications, but also the quality of reagents and control materials, and even the ability of the monitoring device to perform properly. For example, the CoaguChek XS meter can be used at temperatures between 2 and 30°C and humidity to 85%. While suitable for the United States and other temperate climates, acceptable operating temperatures and humidity levels are often exceeded in many tropical travel destinations.

For patients monitoring anticoagulant medicine efficacy and their international normalized ratio, it is important they discuss testing options with their physician. To continue to monitor while traveling and modifying dosages based on test results requires the patient to be evaluated and, if a candidate for self-treatment, trained appropriately on the use of the monitoring device and on administration of medication.

ALTERNATIVE SETTINGS AND EMERGENCY USE OF POINT-OF-CARE TESTS

The use of POC tests in alternative settings such as for immigration purposes, adventure travel, on board ships, or during disaster relief (earthquakes, tsunamis, etc.) will require taking into consideration the same issues as noted earlier—that is, accepted good laboratory practices for performance of testing that includes training and assurance of adequacy of test instructions, maintaining records and logbooks of results, and quality control; these issues are often overlooked in environments where waived tests are performed.

A survey by the CDC and CMS found that among clinician offices in the United States performing waived testing, even the simple requirement of assuring the availability of test directions was not being met among 12% of those surveyed, and 21% did not routinely check to assure there were no changes in instructions when new test kits were received.

While there are no routine inspections of physician office laboratories in the United States and no requirement for training of personnel on the testing menu, there is an expectation that good laboratory practices are followed. The absence of basic accepted laboratory practices among survey participants should heighten awareness around decisions to implement POC testing in alternative sites.

Use of Point-of-Care Testing to Address New or Emerging Disease Outbreaks

During outbreaks of new or emerging diseases (the HIV epidemic, the Ebola epidemic, widespread malaria epidemics, etc.), there is a clear need to react quickly to respond to public health emergencies and to assure that test methods assure accurate results. When such a need is established, government and international organizations have modified policies to assure rapid approval of test systems or, in the case of malaria RDTs, the evaluation of test systems.

For example, the WHO has developed an Emergency Use Assessment and Listing procedure to evaluate and make available diagnostic test kits during public health emergencies. The FDA also makes allowances for expedited review when the Secretary of Health declares a public health emergency. The following are several examples of how these policies affected the introduction of new test systems.

HIV

As the HIV epidemic progressed, and as antiretroviral therapy became available, there was a clear need to assure that testing was provided where the patient was being seen to help assure prompt treatment. While the HIV rapid test was initially approved by the FDA as a moderately complex test, that designation presented barriers to the use of the test in alternative settings such as voluntary counseling and testing clinics. In the United States the HIV rapid test was declared a waived test in 2004 with the provision that training and quality assurance was a requirement for use. In the United States, most HIV testing has been implemented through local health departments where there has been provision of training and implementation of quality assurance measures. Algorithms for the determination of HIV infection have been developed and include the use of multiple tests to confirm initial test results.

Malaria

Morbidity and mortality associated with malaria, particularly among children, is greatest in resource-limited countries, and often there is little mechanism for determining the quality of test kits. Recognizing the need to provide information on quality of test system to resource-limited countries, in 2014 the WHO, CDC, and the Foundation for Innovative New Diagnostics published a summary of product testing of RDTs for malaria. The report cites the full evaluation of 206 products from 34 manufacturers for the detection of *Plasmodium falciparum* and *Plasmodium vivax* over a 5-year period. Performance varied widely at low parasite density for all products, but all had a high rate of detection in samples with high parasite density. The report also noted test performance variation among different lots (indicating variation in quality of antibody). In this example of malaria POC tests, it is clearly important that test selection, training, and quality assurance are components of any program anticipating the use of such tests in their clinics.

While not commonly considered as a POC test, microscopy for malaria has many characteristics in common with POC tests. Microscopic analysis can readily be performed in a variety of community and field settings and, if performed by a competent analyst with a functional microscope, can provide diagnostic information in a few minutes. It is important to note that RDTs do not replace microscopy. The use of RDTs must be carefully evaluated to assure consideration of local algorithms that make clear actions to be taken based on RDT results.

The WHO provides similar information to resource-limited countries addressing the quality of HIV test systems as well. The publication of this work enables a resource-limited country to make an informed decision about what will work best in their settings.

Ebola

As the 2014 Ebola epidemic grew, the need for a rapid and accurate test became clear. The WHO performed an emergency use assessment and made a rapid test kit available to Ebola-affected countries (the ReEBOV™ antigen rapid test kit, Corgenix, Broomfield, CO). While the sensitivity and specificity of the test is only 92% and 85%, respectively, when the population being tested is in an endemic area and patients being tested have signs and symptoms, the predictive value of a positive test is high. A positive test is considered presumptive detection of Ebola Zaire virus disease, and where possible, results should be repeated with a new blood sample using nucleic acid testing. On the other hand, in low-prevalence regions, particularly when testing patients with minimal or few symptoms, the risk of false-positive results may greatly outnumber true-positive results.

While POC testing is often a key component of measures used in addressing disease outbreaks and other public health emergencies, it is important to have appropriate oversight that will assure that rapidly developed test systems provide accurate results. Results of testing are among the factors that help determine where to focus scarce resources when mounting a successful public health response.

THE FUTURE OF POINT-OF-CARE TESTS

As technology enables the development of new and simpler formats for a variety of tests, including molecular and genetic assays more commonly offered in traditional laboratory settings, the sites where testing can be offered will expand. Hospital clinics, physician offices, cruise ships, pharmacies, and health fairs are examples where such testing is now being offered.

US manufacturers are currently working on a number of POC tests including those for infectious disease, markers for stroke and sepsis, and tests such as complete blood count and white blood cell count. While it is desirable for more tests to be available where the patient is being seen, POC tests generally cost more than the same test performed in the laboratory. An important issue will be whether or not use of POC testing improves patient outcomes.

POC tests are most useful where the turnaround time is critical, when the training and quality assurance required is minimal, and when the method has been rigorously investigated for the population for intended use.

These examples of the use of POC tests make clear that a number of issues must be considered before implementation of use. For example, understanding what the test is measuring (e.g., antigens vs. nucleic acids) and assuring awareness of the impact of sensitivity, specificity, and disease prevalence in the population being tested both have a bearing on the predictive values of a test. In addition, training, availability of quality control, and oversight of quality assurance activities are critical elements essential to assure accuracy of testing.

FURTHER READING

Bhagat, M., Kanhere, S., et al., 2014. Concurrent malaria and dengue fever: a need for rapid diagnostic methods. J. Family Med. Prim. Care 3 (4), 446–448.

Bissonnette, L., Bergeron, M.G., 2010. Diagnosing infections: current and anticipated technologies for point-of-care diagnostic and home-based testing. Clin. Microbiol. Infect. 16, 1044–1053.

Bottieau, E., 2013. Point-of-care testing: filling the diagnostic gaps in tropical medicine? Clin. Microbiol. Infect. 19, 397–398.

Carter, J., 2014. Point of care tests at sea. J. Travel Med. 21, 4–5.

Carter, M.J., Emary, K.R., et al., 2015. Rapid diagnostic tests for dengue virus infection in febrile Cambodian children: diagnostic accuracy and incorporation into diagnostic algorithms. PLoS Negl. Trop. Dis. 9 (2), e0003424.

Cea, L.M., Espinilla, V.F., del Prado, G.R., 2015. Developing countries: health round-trip. J. Infect. Dev. Ctries. 9 (1), 20–28.

Centers for Disease Control. Clinical Laboratory Improvement Amendments (CLIA). Available at <https://www.cdc.gov/clia/Resources/TestComplexities.aspx>.

Herbert, R., Ashraf, A.N., Yate, T.A., et al., 2012. Nurse-delivered universal point-of-care testing for HIV in an open-access returning traveller clinic. HIV Med. 13 (8), 499–504.

Howerton, D., et al., 2005. Survey findings from testing sites holding a certificate of waiver under CLIA 88 and recommendations for promoting quality testing. Morb. Mortal. Wkly. Rep. 54 (RR13), 1–25.

Howick, J., Cals, W.L., Jones, C., et al., 2015. Current and future use of point-of-care tests in primary care: an international survey in Australia, Belgium, The Netherlands, the UK and the USA. BMJ Open 4, e005611.

Kost, G.K., Tran, N.K., Tuntideelert, M., et al., 2006. Optimizing rapid response diagnosis in disasters. Am. J. Clin. Pathol. 126, 513–520.

Maltha, J., Gillet, P., Jacobs, J., 2013. Malaria rapid diagnostic tests in travel medicine. Clin. Microbiol. Infect. 19, 408–415.

Mbanya, D., 2013. Use of quality rapid diagnostic testing for safe blood transfusion in resource-limited countries. Clin. Microbiol. Inf. 19, 416–421.

National Coalition of STD Directors. Rapid Syphilis Test Approved for Use Outside Traditional Laboratory Settings Is a "Game Changer" for STD Testing. Press Release. December 15, 2014.

Pai, M., Ghiai, M., Pai, N.P., 2015. Point-of-care diagnostic testing in global health: what is the point? Microbe 10 (3), 103–108.

Peeling, R.W., Mabey, D., 2010. Point-of-care tests for diagnosing infections in the developing world. Clin. Microbiol. Infect. 16, 1062–1069.

Pruett, C.R., Vermeulen, M., Zacharias, P., et al., 2015. The use of rapid diagnostic tests for transfusion infectious screening in Africa: a literature review. Transfus. Med. Rev. 29, 35–44.

WHO. Malaria Rapid Diagnostic Test Performance: Summary Results of WHO Product Testing of Malaria RDTs: Round 1–5 (2008–2013).

CHAPTER 31

Approach to Diarrhea in Returned Travelers

Micah M. Bhatti and Mark Enzler

Gastrointestinal infections are the most common illnesses in travelers, occurring in 34% of all travelers, typically those traveling from high-income countries to low and middle-income countries. Traveler's diarrhea (TD) is defined as three or more unformed stools per day and at least one additional gastrointestinal symptom, such as nausea, vomiting, and abdominal pain, and possibly systemic findings including fever and malaise. The majority of TD is commonly attributed to enterotoxigenic strains of *Escherichia coli* (ETEC) and occurs within the first 2 weeks of travel with a mean duration of 4-5 days. Since most patients travel for at least 1 week, a medical provider will seldom see a case of new-onset diarrhea in a returned traveler. Instead, the majority of cases of travel-acquired diarrhea seen by the medical establishment will be protracted or recurrent. Approximately 10% of patients with TD will experience symptoms for more than 1 week, and in 5-10%, symptoms will last for 2 weeks or longer. This chapter will focus on the evaluation of TD that is likely to present to the healthcare system.

EXPOSURE HISTORY AND RISK FACTORS

Many factors influence the acquisition of TD, including geographic location, type of travel, and host factors. Of these factors, travel destination and duration are the most important determinants of attack rate. Highest risk of TD is associated with travel for more than 2 weeks to South and Southeast Asia, sub-Saharan Africa, the Middle East, and Latin America. Gathering information regarding the patient's travel arrangements is important in determining if the patient is suffering from TD and may narrow the list of potential pathogens. While ETEC and enteroaggregative *E. coli* (EAEC) are the most common causes of TD, especially in Africa and Latin America, the invasive pathogens *Campylobacter*, *Vibrio*, and *Salmonella* are just as common in South and Southeast Asia. High rates of TD have been associated with those visiting family and relatives, trekkers and campers, and travelers on adventure tours or cruise ships.

Information about consumption of street food and local water sources increases the risk of TD but is unhelpful in ascertaining the TD etiology. A history of shellfish or seafood consumption may be useful, as they are common sources of *Vibrio*. In addition, hepatitis A virus and noroviruses may be acquired through contaminated shellfish. Acute hepatitis A viral infection is associated with an average of 30 days of missed work and 1% mortality in adults.

Direct contact with animals should raise the suspicion for *Campylobacter*, shiga toxin–producing *E. coli* (STEC), and *Giardia* infections. Treatment with antibiotics for TD adds the risk of antibiotic-associated diarrhea caused by *Clostridium difficile*. If antibiotics were administered and an initial response obtained, the recurrence of symptoms may represent recrudescence of resistant bacteria, reinfection with similar or different pathogens, or a post-infectious process. Reviewing the patient's vaccination history is also important; those 415 vaccinated against rotavirus and hepatitis A would be protected against infections caused by these agents. However, given the relatively low efficacy of typhoid fever vaccine (50-80% for both the oral and injectable forms), this diagnosis should remain in the differential diagnosis for returned travelers with signs and symptoms consistent with this.

Host factors can also play a role in the risk of TD, including age, reduced gastric acidity, blood type group O, and other genetic factors. Infants and toddlers can acquire infection though oral contact with nonfood items. Recent studies have suggested that individuals who produce higher amounts of the inflammatory mediators interleukin 8 AA, lactoferrin, and interleukin 10 may be more susceptible to TD. Polymorphisms in the CD14 receptor and osteoprotegerin have also been associated with increased susceptibility to TD. Immunocompromised individuals are at risk for prolonged illness with typical agents and infection with atypical organisms such as microsporidia.

Finally, the likelihood of the patient transmitting infectious diarrhea to other contacts must be explored. Food handlers and institutional caregivers with any type of diarrhea, including TD, should be evaluated regardless of the length of symptoms and their employment deferred until symptoms resolve to avoid a potential outbreak.

CLINICAL PRESENTATION AND EVALUATION

The severity of the illness dictates the level of evaluation required of an ill patient with diarrhea. The first consideration to be made is the need for hospitalization. The combination of orthostatic hemodynamic changes and an inability to maintain oral rehydration necessitates intravenous rehydration and possible hospitalization. If significant systemic toxicity is present, stool and blood cultures should be obtained along with initiation of empiric parenteral antibiotics.

That being said, the average case of TD is not severe (averaging 4.6 stools/day), and symptoms are often those of nausea and cramping abdominal pain. The presence of high fever and/or blood or pus in stool suggest an invasive pathogen such as *Salmonella*, *Shigella*, *Campylobacter*, STEC, or *Entamoeba histolytica* and decrease the likelihood of non-invasive pathogens such as ETEC, norovirus, *Giardia*, and *Vibrio* spp., which tend to cause profuse watery diarrhea and abdominal cramps, without fever or bloody stools. Blood may not be present in all patients infected with invasive organisms, and concurrent infection with more than one enteric pathogen may occur. Persistent watery diarrhea for longer than 14 days, without fever, suggests giardiasis as well as other parasitic infections such as *Cryptosporidium*, microsporidia, and *Cyclospora*.

The physical examination does not usually aid in determining the etiology of travel-acquired diarrhea, although it is useful to assess the general condition of the patient and to exclude other conditions that may present with diarrhea. In TD, the abdomen is typically not tender to palpation, and bowel tones are hyperactive. Focal abdominal tenderness dictates expanding the differential diagnosis to include appendicitis, biliary disease, peptic ulcer disease, pancreatitis, diverticulitis, small bowel perforation and inflammatory bowel disease (IBD). Hepatic tenderness in a traveler with diarrhea could be suggestive of acute viral hepatitis or amebic liver abscess. Unrecognized chronic human immunodeficiency virus infection may present with gastrointestinal complaints. Occult or gross blood in the stool indicates the presence of an invasive organism. If only non-invasive pathogens are identified in stool samples, a non-infectious cause for gastrointestinal bleeding should be considered, including IBD and malignancy.

Physicians seeing travelers with chronic gastrointestinal complaints need to maintain an index of suspicion for previously unrecognized gastrointestinal disease, particularly IBD and irritable bowel syndrome (IBS). Infections with *Salmonella*, *Shigella*, or *Campylobacter* may trigger or exacerbate IBD. Ulcerative colitis or Crohn disease should be suspected in patients with bloody diarrhea, accompanied by systemic signs such as weight loss, oral or perianal lesions, and extraintestinal manifestations including arthropathies or ophthalmologic symptoms. IBD becomes more likely when symptoms have persisted more than 2 months without a microbiologic diagnosis. IBS is one of the most common post-infectious diarrhea processes

TABLE 31.1   Potential Etiologies of Diarrhea in Returned Travelers Suggested by Clinical Presentations

Clinical Presentation	Microorganisms to Consider as Etiologies

Non-inflammatory diarrhea
  Acute watery diarrhea
  Absence of fever
  No blood or fecal WBCs
	Enterotoxigenic *Escherichia coli*
	Enteroaggregative *E. coli*
	Vibrio cholera
	Aeromonas
	Noroviruses and other enteric viruses
	Giardia
	Cryptosporidium
	Cyclospora

Inflammatory diarrhea
  Grossly bloody stool
  Fever present and other systemic symptoms
  Fecal WBCs present
	Salmonella
	Campylobacter
	Shigella
	Shiga-toxin producing *E. coli* (*E. coli* O157:H7)
	Vibrio parahaemolyticus
	Yersinia enterocolitica
	Plesiomonas shigelloides
	Entamoeba histolytica

Persistent diarrhea (lasting ≥14 days)	*Cyclospora* *Cryptosporidium* *Entamoeba histolytica* *Giardia* Microsporidia (immunocompromised)

WBCs, White blood cells.

in returning travelers and may be associated with intermittent cramping pain, bloating, and gas. If IBD or IBS is a consideration, further evaluation should be performed in consultation with a gastroenterologist.

DIAGNOSTIC STUDIES

The decision to perform laboratory studies in the traveler with diarrhea should be based on the duration of symptoms, severity of the illness, and type of diarrhea present: inflammatory (blood or white blood cells present) versus non-inflammatory (primarily watery), as outlined in **Table 31.1**. The traveler seeking medical attention who has had fewer than 5 days of diarrhea does not require investigations unless there is significant fever, abdominal pain, dehydration, blood or mucus is present in the stool, or if the patient is immunocompromised. Before ordering stool studies, it is important to be aware of the capabilities and protocols of the clinical microbiology laboratory at your institution, including testing options, recommended stool sample volume, and preferred stool specimen transport method. **Table 31.2** lists the common causes of TD, associated symptoms, and diagnostic testing.

It is important to educate patients on proper collection of stool samples for laboratory testing, as submission of improperly collected specimens will compromise testing results. The stool specimen should be caught directly in a standard pint-sized specimen container or in a larger clean, dry container. Fecal specimens contaminated with urine or toilet paper or retrieved from the toilet bowl are not satisfactory. It is ideal for stool specimens to arrive in the laboratory within 1-2 hours post collection to ensure reliability of microscopy and culture results. If this is not feasible, specimens for bacterial culture should be placed in an

TABLE 31.2 Etiologic Agents of Diarrhea in Returned Travelers

Etiology	Incubation Period	Signs and Symptoms	Duration of Illnesses	Associated Exposure	Laboratory Testing
Aeromonas	Unknown	Abdominal cramps, watery diarrhea	2-10 days	Contaminated meats and water	Routine stool culture
Campylobacter jejuni	2-5 days	Fever, cramps, vomiting, diarrhea (possibly bloody)	2-10 days	Undercooked poultry, unpasteurized milk, contaminated water	Routine stool culture; requires special media and incubation conditions
Clostridium difficile	5 days to 5 weeks	Fever, abdominal cramps, diarrhea	4 days to weeks	Colonization and prior antimicrobials	Immunoassays or NAT for toxins A and B
Shiga-toxin producing *E. coli*	1-8 days	Abdominal pain, vomiting, severe, often bloody, diarrhea	5-10 days	Undercooked beef, unpasteurized milk, contaminated water and produce	Stool culture Immunoassays or NAT for Shiga toxin
Enterotoxigenic *E. coli*	1-3 days	Abdominal cramps, watery diarrhea	3-7 days	Contaminated water or food	Routine stool culture not useful. Multiplex NAT Specific testing by state or public health laboratories
Plesiomonas shigelloides	24-28 h	Abdominal pain and cramping, watery diarrhea	5-14 days	Contaminated seafood and water	Routine stool culture
Salmonella enteritidis	1-3 days	Fever, abdominal cramps, vomiting, diarrhea	4-7 days	Eggs, poultry, milk, raw fruits and vegetables	Routine stool culture
Shigella spp.	24-48 h	Fever, abdominal cramps, and diarrhea	4-7 days	Contaminated food or water. Also spread person to person	Routine stool cultures

Vibrio cholerae	24-72 h	Severe dehydration due to profuse watery diarrhea and vomiting	3-7 days	Contaminated water, fish, shellfish, street-vended food	Stool culture with specific request for isolation. Antigen immunoassay
Vibrio parahaemolyticus	2-48 h	Watery diarrhea, abdominal cramps, nausea, vomiting	2-5 days	Undercooked or raw seafood	Stool culture with specific request for isolation
Vibrio vulnificus	1-7 days	Vomiting, diarrhea, abdominal pain	2-8 days	Undercooked or raw seafood	Stool cultures; request specific testing
Yersinia enterocolitica	24-48 h	Fever, abdominal pain, vomiting, bloody diarrhea (mimics appendicitis)	1-3 weeks	Undercooked pork, milk, water	Stool culture with specific request for isolation
Norovirus	12-48 h	Fever, myalgia, abdominal cramping, nausea, vomiting, diarrhea	12-60 h	Shellfish, contaminated water, contact with infected individuals	Not routinely available. Immunoassay and NAT by public health labs
Rotavirus	24-72 h	Fever, nausea, vomiting, watery diarrhea	4-10 days	Contact with infected individuals	Immunoassay

Adapted from Center for Disease Control. Diagnosis and management of foodborne illnesses: a primer for physicians and other healthcare providers. *MMWR*. 2004;53(RR-4):1–33. *NAT*, Nucleic acid testing.

appropriate transport medium, such as Cary-Blair. When collecting stools to be examined for parasites, patients should be instructed to collect only one stool sample per day and at least three samples within a 10-day period if the first specimen is negative. It is recommended that stool specimens for ova and parasite examination be sent to the laboratory in a fixative. Preservative kits usually contain two different fixatives: formalin to preserve helminths and coccidian parasites and polyvinyl alcohol for staining to visualize protozoa. Single vial preservatives are now available, such as the alcohol-based Ecofix™ (Meridian Bioscience, Cincinnati, OH), which can be utilized for both the examination of helminths and staining for intestinal protozoa. It is important to note that the transport media used for bacterial cultures are not suitable for parasite examination and that fixed specimens cannot be used for bacterial culture. Thus, if bacterial culture and parasite examination are desired, separate fecal specimens are required, each in the appropriate transport container.

The determination of white blood cells (WBC) in the stool can be helpful in the evaluation of patients with diarrhea. The presence of WBC suggests an inflammatory process in the gastrointestinal tract, possibly due to an invasive infection. The detection of fecal leukocytes in stool samples can be achieved by microscopic examination of a stool smear stained with methylene blue or by using a commercially available enzyme immunoassay (EIA) for lactoferrin. The sensitivity/specificity of fecal leukocytes by microscopy or lactoferrin for predicting inflammatory diarrhea are 73%/84%, and 92%/79%, respectively.

TD studies have shown that the most commonly identified bacterial pathogens are ETEC, *Salmonella*, *Shigella*, and *Campylobacter*, which account for 45-50% of cases. Because bacteria are the most commonly reported cause of TD, stool culture has traditionally served as the backbone for a TD diagnostic work-up. While stool cultures are a commonly ordered test, they are *not* performed the same way at every hospital laboratory. Stool cultures are designed to optimize the recovery of *Salmonella*, *Shigella*, *Campylobacter*, and STEC, including *E. coli* O157:H7. Some laboratories will also isolate *Aeromonas*, *Plesiomonas*, *Yersinia*, and/or *Vibrio* from stool, whereas others will do so only on special request. In view of this, it is crucial to know how your laboratory performs stool cultures to ensure that the enteric pathogens being considered will be recovered. It is important to note that the most common cause of TD, ETEC, is difficult to isolate in stool culture, as there is no reliable way to discriminate between ETEC and endogenous *E. coli* by culture alone. Nucleic acid testing (NAT) platforms are available that will detect ETEC in stool samples as a single target or as part of a multiplex panel along with *Salmonella*, *Shigella*, and *Campylobacter*. Many laboratories will include an antigen-based assay or NAT to detect Shiga toxin in all stool cultures to aid in detecting STEC. However, STEC is an uncommon cause of TD, although it has been seen in outbreaks such as the one in Germany and France in 2011. Another illness to consider in patients with TD is *Clostridium difficile* colitis, based on history of antibiotics use or previous *C. difficile* infections. Detection of *C. difficile* from stool specimens is achieved by detecting toxins A and B using commercially available EIA or NAT methodologies. In addition to feces, cultures of blood, bone marrow, and/or urine samples should be performed in patients with symptoms consistent with disseminated *Salmonella*. Two negative stool cultures from specimens collected on separate days, rules out the majority of bacterial pathogens in patients with diarrhea.

Identification of bacteria and yeast using matrix-assisted laser desorption ionization time of flight mass spectroscopy (MALDI-TOF MS) has become increasingly available in clinical laboratories throughout the world including the United States. Currently, there are two commercially available systems: VITEK® MS (BioMérieux Inc.) and the MALDI Biotyper CA System (Bruker Daltonics Inc.). Each system includes a mass spectrometer, software, and database including a list of microorganisms that are cleared for identification. MALDI-TOF MS based bacterial identification takes minutes to perform and is significantly cheaper to operate than nucleic acid based identification methods such as 16S rRNA sequencing and multiplex panels, leading to a de-emphasis of biochemical-based bacterial identification. However, despite the robust nature of this technology, it cannot reliable differentiate E.

coli from Shigella spp as these are highly related organisms at the molecular level. Thus, there may always be a need for biochemical identification in certain situations.

One major advantage of isolating stool bacterial pathogens is the ability to perform antimicrobial susceptibility testing. This is particularly important in travelers returning from parts of the world known to harbor multidrug-resistant (MDR) bacterial pathogens. MDR Salmonella have become more common in Asia and sub-Saharan Africa. Campylobacter resistance to fluoroquinolones has become a concern in Southeast Asia, with resistance rates up to 80%. Additionally, Enterobacteriaceae producing extended spectrum beta-lactamases and, more recently, carbapenem-resistant Enterobacteriaceae are becoming more prevalent in many parts of the world.

Parasitic infections are estimated to be responsible for 5-10% of TD cases. The index of suspicion for an enteric parasite should increase in travelers with diarrhea lasting longer than 1 week. Microscopic examination of stool for ova and parasites indicating infection is performed by examination of a stool specimen on two glass slides prepared using two different methods. One slide is prepared using concentrated, preserved stool and examined with or without the addition of iodine, looking for helminths and their eggs, or ova. The second slide is of preserved stool stained with trichrome, which facilitates identification of intestinal flagellates and amebic parasites. Microsporidia, Cryptosporidium, Cystoisospora, and Cyclospora are best visualized using special stains other than trichrome. If these organisms are suspected, the laboratory must be notified so the appropriate stains are included. Reliable detection of parasites by microscopy requires examination of multiple (at least three) fecal specimens, since parasites may be excreted intermittently and infections with multiple parasites may not be detected with one or two specimens. Strongyloides may require up to seven stool examinations and the use of special methods such as the Baermann technique or agar plate culture.

As an adjunct to microscopic stool examination, many laboratories utilize EIAs or fluorescent antibody tests for the detection of Giardia and Cryptosporidium antigens in stool because they are more sensitive than microscopic examination and are easier to perform. Stool antigen testing typically requires only one specimen to be diagnostic and effectively rules out infection with two negative results from separate specimens collected on different days. The sensitivity and specificity of Giardia EIAs are greater than 95%, while the performance of the Cryptosporidium EIAs are more variable, with sensitivity and specificity ranging from 80 to 99%.

It is estimated that 5-15% of cases of TD are due to viral infections, the majority of which are norovirus and rotavirus. Diagnostic work-up in these patients is unnecessary, since viral infections are self-limited and there are no directed therapies that will shorten the duration of illness or decrease viral shedding. Immunocompromised individuals are a patient group in whom diagnostic work-up may be beneficial, because determining the etiology of the diarrhea would limit further diagnostic work-up. In travelers in whom viral diagnostic work-up is warranted, stool can be assessed for rotavirus using commercially available EIAs; some laboratories offer NAT for norovirus and rotavirus. Hepatitis A is another viral cause of diarrhea that would be important to consider in unvaccinated individuals and is diagnosed using serology.

The causes of protracted diarrhea and ongoing gastrointestinal complaints will usually reveal themselves after clinical examination and laboratory studies outlined in this section. However, in approximately 30% of cases of traveler's diarrhea, no pathogen can be identified despite multiple, thorough laboratory evaluations. In these instances, consultation with a gastroenterologist is recommended to assist with further diagnostic evaluation. A complete blood count should be obtained to assess for signs of systemic inflammation, suggested by a high WBC and/or eosinophilia, and to assess for anemia from ongoing gastrointestinal blood loss or malabsorption. If tropical sprue or other malabsorption syndromes are being considered, testing for lactose tolerance and D-xylose absorption may be considered. If deemed appropriate, a gastroenterologist can perform a colonoscopic examination to inspect the mucosa and obtain biopsies to assess for Crohn disease, ulcerative colitis, schistosomiasis, and amebiasis.

Currently, there are three FDA-cleared, multiplex NAT panels available for the detection of enteric pathogens from stool specimens: xTag® GI Pathogen Panel (Luminex Corporation, Toronto, Canada), the FilmArray™ GI panel (BioFire, Inc., Salt Lake City, UT), and Verigene® Enteric Pathogens (EP) Test (Nanosphere, Inc., Northbrook, IL). All three panels detect bacterial pathogens commonly isolated in stool culture (*Campylobacter* spp., *Salmonella* spp., *Shigella* spp., *Vibrio* spp., and *Yersinia enterocolitica*) and the enteric viral pathogens Norovirus and Rotavirus. The xTag® and FilmArray™ GI panels can also detect the protozoan parasites *Cryptosporidium* spp., *Entamoeba histolytica*, and *Giardia lamblia*. These assays yield results within hours and require less hands-on time than the laborious, conventional methods for identification of bacteria and parasites. However, these assays may be cost prohibitive for some laboratories and patient populations and none of the currently available multiplex NAT assays can detect helminths. While molecular assays offer improved sensitivity over culture, use of these assays remains controversial due to concerns regarding specificity, clinical correlation and lack of an isolate for antimicrobial susceptibility testing and subtyping analysis to support identification during outbreak investigations. It is important to maintain an open dialog with the clinical microbiology laboratory to ensure that the tests being ordered are the appropriate tests for the patient.

INFECTIOUS DIARRHEA SYNDROMES

The goal of this section is to highlight the important features of bacterial diarrhea syndromes caused by pathogens that may cause protracted symptoms and are more likely to be encountered by a healthcare professional evaluating a patient with TD. The invasive bacterial pathogens *Salmonella*, *Shigella*, and *Campylobacter* are more common in patients with prolonged diarrhea and will be the focus of this section. In addition, several bacterial pathogens that are rare but important causes of TD and those that are emerging organisms of interest, including viral agents, will be discussed. Parasitic infections are discussed in Chapter 32 and will not be addressed in this section. Antibiotic resistance trends will be mentioned, but specific antibiotic treatment options are discussed in Chapter 8.

SALMONELLA

Salmonella are ubiquitous Gram-negative bacteria that cause a range of disease in humans. The nomenclature of *Salmonella* is quite confusing, as there are several subspecies and serotypes (also referred to as serovars). Of the 2500 known serotypes, only about 100 are known to cause human disease and are in the genus *Salmonella*, species *enterica*, subspecies *enterica* (or subspecies I). The other species of *Salmonella* and other subspecies within *S. enterica* rarely infect humans. Included in the *S. enterica* subspecies *enterica* are the serotypes Typhi and Paratyphi, which cause typhoid and paratyphoid fever, respectively. The remaining serotypes are referred to as nontyphoidal and primarily cause intestinal infections. The most common serotypes in the United States are Enteritidis, Typhimurium, Newport, and Javiana, but other serotypes may present in travelers returning from other countries. It is important to note that nontyphoidal *Salmonella* strains can cause extraintestinal infections (e.g., bacteremia, meningitis, and osteomyelitis), particularly in children under 2 years of age, the elderly, and immunocompromised individuals including patients with sickle cell disease.

Salmonella infections are usually acquired through ingestion of contaminated food or water. Eating raw, unpeeled fruits and vegetables, undercooked meat, and unpasteurized dairy products is particularly risky. Infections can also be transmitted by direct contact with infected animals or their excreta. Oysters and shellfish grown in contaminated waters can transmit *Salmonella*. Meals can be contaminated during preparation through unsanitary kitchen practices or infected food handlers. Infections are dependent on the size of the inoculum, the vehicle of transmission, and the susceptibility of the host. An oral inoculum of 10^6 bacteria or greater, ingestion of contaminated foods high in protein and fat, and impaired host status tend to promote infection.

The clinical presentation of *Salmonella* enterocolitis can range from a mild to severe diarrheal illness with cramps, nausea, vomiting, and fever. The incubation period is usually

1-3 days. The acute illness usually lasts for 1-2 weeks, although *Salmonella* are shed in the feces for 4-6 weeks in untreated persons and for up to several months in patients treated with antibiotics. *Salmonella* enterocolitis can result in a bacteremia that can lead to focal infections outside the gastrointestinal tract. Sepsis and even death can occur in patients with pre-existing comorbidities.

Stool specimens from patients suffering from *Salmonella* enterocolitis are usually positive for fecal leukocytes. Clinical microbiology laboratories can isolate *Salmonella* spp. from stool cultures and occasionally blood. If a biopsy or sterile fluid specimen (e.g., synovial or spinal fluid) is sent to the microbiology laboratory with concern for *Salmonella* infection, it is important to alert the laboratory to ensure appropriate cultures are set up. Once an isolate is identified as *Salmonella* by biochemical or molecular analysis, confirmation is performed using *Salmonella*-specific antisera directed at the O antigen. Full serotyping is beyond the scope of most clinical laboratories but can be performed by public health laboratories as part of epidemiologic surveillance.

In general, antibiotic treatment is not indicated for patients with uncomplicated *Salmonella* enterocolitis but may be considered for those who are severely ill or at risk for severe infections, such as neonates, the elderly, and immunocompromised individuals. However, antibiotic treatment may prolong infectious carriage of *Salmonella*. Treatment should be guided by antibiotic sensitivity testing, since drug resistance to multiple antibiotics is prevalent among some *Salmonella* strains.

SHIGELLA

Shigellosis is an acute gastrointestinal infection caused by one of four *Shigella* subgroups that have been historically treated as species: *S. dysenteriae* (subgroup A), *S. flexneri* (subgroup B), *S. boydii* (subgroup C), and *S. sonnei* (subgroup D). This subgroup classification is based on the type of O antigen present on the bacteria. Shigellosis in the United States and other developed countries is primarily caused by *S. sonnei* (subgroup D). In the developing world, the majority of endemic *Shigella* dysentery is due to *S. flexneri* (subgroup B); this is the species most commonly identified in travelers with shigellosis. *S. dysenteriae* serotype 1 is associated with severe disease and high rates of mortality.

Shigella is a strictly human pathogen, can remain viable on inanimate objects for weeks, and can cause infections with an inoculum of just 200 bacteria. Shigellosis outbreaks have been associated with conditions favoring human fecal-oral transmission, such as poor sanitation, inadequate water supplies, and crowded living conditions. Shigellosis is commonly seen among travelers returning from developing areas of the world and among people living or working in refugee camps and institutional settings, such as daycare centers, prisons, and facilities for the developmentally disabled.

Clinical illness ranges from severe inflammatory diarrhea with systemic toxicity, commonly called bacterial dysentery, to mild, nonspecific diarrhea. The incubation period of shigellosis is usually 24-48 hours, with a presentation characterized by fever, abdominal cramps, and watery diarrhea. The illness may progress to a more serious condition with the passage of blood, mucus, and pus, accompanied by left lower quadrant pain and tenesmus. *Shigella* invade the mucosa and submucosa of the colon during this stage of the disease. The duration of symptoms is usually 1 week or less, although *Shigella* may persist in the stools for 1-3 months after cessation of clinical symptoms.

The presence of fecal leukocytes supports the diagnosis of an inflammatory infection but is not specific for shigellosis. Isolation of *Shigella* spp. can be achieved through routine stool culture media. Specific antisera to the O antigen are available for subgroup classifications, and isolates may be sent to public health laboratories for further serotyping analysis. Most laboratories employ a nonculture assay for the detection of Shiga toxin 1 (Stx1) and 2 (Stx2) to enhance the detection of STEC. The toxin produced by *S. dysenteriae* serotype 1 is highly homologous to Stx1 and would be detected by these assays as well.

Treatment of shigellosis is warranted, as it shortens disease and terminates bacterial carriage, and should be based on antimicrobial susceptibilities. Rates of antibiotic resistance are higher in isolates from developing countries. This is particularly true for *S. dysenteriae* 1 isolates acquired during international travel to parts of Africa and Asia where most strains are multidrug resistant. Post-infection complications are rare but can occur in patients with shigellosis. The most notorious complication is hemolytic-uremic syndrome (HUS). While this is associated with Shiga toxin exposure, it is more commonly due to STEC infection rather than shigellosis. Reactive arthritis is another complication that may follow *Shigella* infection, particularly with *S. flexneri*, and does not appear to be associated with antibiotic treatment.

Campylobacter

Campylobacter jejuni is a short, comma-shaped, Gram-negative rod that is a common cause of diarrhea worldwide and may exceed *Salmonella* and *Shigella* as an etiologic agent of acute infectious diarrhea. Of the 22 species within the genus *Campylobacter*, the two responsible for the majority of gastrointestinal disease are *C. jejuni* and *Campylobacter coli*, with *C. jejuni* responsible for about 85% of infections. *Campylobacter fetus* subsp. *fetus* infection is much less common but may cause serious systemic infections in human hosts with impaired immunity. Extraintestinal *Campylobacter* infections can occur but are primarily reported in neonates, the elderly, and immune-compromised individuals.

Campylobacter species are found worldwide and are primarily zoonotic, inhabiting the intestinal tracts of livestock and domesticated pets but rarely causing disease in these animals. The organisms are shed in animal feces, and humans can become infected by close contact with animals. The consumption of poorly cooked meat or dairy products contaminated with animal feces is the most common source of campylobacteriosis.

After an incubation period of 2-4 days, patients develop cramping abdominal pain, fever, and watery diarrhea typically lasting less than 1 week, although recurrent attacks in untreated individuals have been noted. In some cases, colitis symptoms predominate with bloody stools and lower abdominal pain that can mimic appendicitis. Rarely, colonic ulcerations and systemic infections may occur. *C. fetus* subsp. *fetus* is more frequently associated with systemic infections, with diarrhea occurring in only one-third of patients. Infants and immunocompromised patients appear to be more susceptible to the complications of fulminant sepsis, endocarditis, and meningitis caused by this organism.

The diagnosis of campylobacteriosis is made by isolation of the organism from stool, blood, or other tissues. Isolation of *Campylobacter* from clinical specimens requires special growth conditions that are created using unique, commercially available media and incubation under microaerophilic conditions at 42° C. These growth conditions assist in selecting for the thermo-tolerant *C. jejuni* and *C. coli* from other stool flora. However, such conditions may be not optimal for the recovery of other *Campylobacter* species, such as *C. fetus*. Standard stool culture procedures incorporate the appropriate growth conditions for *C. jejuni* and *C. coli*. However, routine work-up for blood, urine, and other specimens do not. Therefore, if the clinician suspects extraintestinal manifestations of *Campylobacter*, the laboratory must be notified so that appropriate culturing conditions are included.

Severe or prolonged gastrointestinal *Campylobacter* infection should be treated with antibiotics, especially in pregnant women or immunosuppressed patients. Fluoroquinolone-resistant *Campylobacter* has become widespread in many parts of the world, particularly in Asia. It is important to be aware of the autoimmune complications such as Guillain-Barré syndrome (GBS) that may occur following *Campylobacter* infection. GBS is an acute, paralytic disease of the peripheral nervous system that is seen in approximately 0.1% of *Campylobacter* infections. GBS has been associated primarily with *C. jejuni*, which expresses lipooligosaccharides that mimic human gangliosides, resulting in autoantibodies that react with epitopes in the peripheral nerves. The onset of GBS usually occurs within 2-21 days of the diarrheal illness. Reactive arthritis affects 2-4% of patients post-infection and is characterized by joint pain and swelling, commonly in the knees, that last for several weeks to a year. Symptoms typically begin days to weeks following intestinal illness; in about 5% of cases the arthritis can be chronic or relapsing.

VIBRIO

The vibrios are Gram-negative bacilli that are widely distributed in marine and estuarine environments, with *Vibrio cholerae* also found in bodies of fresh water. Of the many *Vibrio* species, gastrointestinal infections primarily occur with *V. cholerae* and *Vibrio parahaemolyticus*. While *V. cholerae* is the only species that causes endemic, epidemic, and pandemic cholera, only a small subset of *V. cholerae* strains carry the requisite genes to cause cholera. Serotyping studies have identified more than 200 different O groups within the species *V. cholerae*, with almost all cholera-causing strains belonging to O group 1 or 139. The majority of non-O1/non-O139 *V. cholera* strains are nonpathogenic, or cause mild illness, although some of these strains have been implicated in outbreaks of cholera-like illness. *Vibrio parahaemolyticus* infections are most commonly transmitted by contaminated food. The pathogenicity of *V. parahaemolyticus* has been correlated with production of one of two thermostable direct hemolysins, Vp-TDH and Vp-TRH. Less commonly, gastroenteritis can also be caused by *Vibrio mimicus*, *Vibrio fluvialis*, *Vibrio vulnificus*, and the related organism, *Grimontia hollisae*.

Cholera is primarily seen in severely resource-limited settings where there is inadequate access to potable water. Tourists from developed countries rarely acquire cholera because they are not typically exposed to these environments and have access to potable water. In contrast, *V. parahaemolyticus* is a common cause of acute gastroenteritis in areas where raw, undercooked, or improperly stored and handled seafood is consumed. *V. parahaemolyticus* outbreaks have been reported in Japan and Asia and on cruise ships. Sushi, pre-cooked shellfish, and raw oysters have been implicated in outbreak reports. A relatively large inoculum (10^{10} organisms or more) is necessary to establish an infection in normal human hosts because *Vibrio* is exquisitely sensitive to gastric acid. In patients with decreased gastric acidity, the infectious inoculum is lower ($\leq 10^6$ organisms). *V. vulnificus* gastroenteritis risks include the ingestion of shellfish, especially raw oysters. In addition to vomiting and diarrhea, *V. vulnificus* can become an invasive pathogen, leading to septicemia and intractable septic shock. Pre-existing hepatic disease was present in over 75% of *V. vulnificus* septicemic patients in one report. Therefore, patients with hepatic disease should avoid eating raw oysters.

The incubation period for *Vibrio*-associated diseases ranges from less than 1 day to several days. Patients with cholera present with severe, voluminous watery ("rice-water") diarrhea, abdominal cramps, nausea, and vomiting. *V. parahaemolyticus* usually causes a self-limited, 72-hour, cholera-like gastroenteritis but some strains can penetrate the lamina propria, resulting in dysentery that resembles shigellosis.

A definitive diagnosis of *Vibrio* infection is based on isolation of the organism from clinical samples, which also allows the determination of antibiotic susceptibility. The isolation of *Vibrio* from stool is accomplished using selective salt-containing media that is *not* part of the standard stool culture protocol in most microbiology laboratories. Therefore, if *Vibrio* infection is in the differential, this needs to be communicated to the laboratory. Once cultured, *Vibrio* species can be determined by biochemical tests; serogroup and serotyping can be performed with specific antibodies by public health laboratories. There is a rapid diagnostic test for *V. cholerae* that has been used as part of cholera outbreak investigations (Crystal VC™ Span Diagnostics, Surat, India).

The cornerstone of clinical management for severe gastroenteritis due to *Vibrio* infection is the aggressive replacement of fluid and electrolytes lost in the diarrheal stools. Antibiotic treatment may shorten the duration of *Vibrio* infections by eradicating organisms in the stool, although symptoms may persist because of toxins already bound to the mucosal surface.

OTHER NOTABLE BACTERIAL PATHOGENS

Yersinia enterocolitica is a zoonotic enteric pathogen that is increasingly recognized as a cause of human bacterial enteritis. This pathogen appears to be ubiquitous in nature, with acquisition by ingestion of contaminated food or water. These organisms are able to multiply at room temperature and survive at low temperatures (4° C) for many months under a variety of environmental conditions. Infection requires ingestion of a relatively large inoculum (10^9

bacteria) followed by invasion and involvement of the mesenteric lymph nodes. Patients can present with cramping abdominal pain, fever, and diarrhea, which may last from 1 to 3 weeks. Occasionally, pain localized in the right lower quadrant caused by ileitis and mesenteric lymphadenitis may be severe enough to mimic appendicitis. The laboratory should be notified of a possible *Yersinia* infection to ensure the use of selective media that may not be included in routine stool cultures. *Yersinia* may be present in the stool for weeks after symptoms resolve. Usefulness of antimicrobial therapy in enterocolitis and lymphadenitis caused by *Y. enterocolitica* is uncertain but may be warranted in severe cases and guided by antibiotic susceptibility testing. Post-infectious complications consist of autoimmune disorders, including arthritis, erythema nodosum, Reiter syndrome, and ankylosing spondylitis, which may be more likely to develop in patients with the HLA-B27 histocompatibility tissue type.

Plesiomonas shigelloides is a Gram-negative bacillus found in aquatic environments that has been primarily associated with sporadic cases and outbreaks of diarrheal disease. Risk factors for *P. shigelloides* gastroenteritis include travel to tropical regions, consumption of raw or undercooked shellfish or contaminated water, and exposure to reptiles and tropical fish. *Plesiomonas* enteritis typically presents as a watery diarrhea but may manifest as a dysenteric syndrome. The organism readily grows in the laboratory on standard media, and its presence is usually screened for as part of standard stool culturing. Most infections are characterized by self-limiting diarrhea with blood or mucus, abdominal cramps, vomiting, and fever and do not require antibiotic therapy. Antimicrobial therapy may be warranted with prolonged infections and infections associated with severe illness.

Aeromonas spp. are ubiquitous in freshwater aquatic habitats, and concentrations peak when water temperatures rise during the summer months. While *Aeromonas* spp. are not considered part of the normal gastrointestinal flora, their role as enteropathogens is somewhat contested. Consumption of contaminated meats or water is the most common source of infection. *Aeromonas*-associated diarrhea most commonly presents as an acute watery diarrhea but may be associated with a more invasive disease resembling dysentery or enterocolitis. *Aeromonas* spp. will grow in media used in routine stool culture, but its presence may be overlooked because its growth in culture is difficult to distinguish from endogenous flora. Therefore, it is important to alert the laboratory to screen for this agent in patients suffering from TD. Most infections with *Aeromonas* spp. are self-limiting and require only supportive care. Cases of HUS have been associated with *Aeromonas* diarrheal illness thought to be secondary to the organism expressing Shiga toxin.

Colitis caused by *C. difficile* is not expected to be a primary pathogenic process in travel-acquired infectious diarrhea. However, *C. difficile* diarrheal illness should be considered in cases of diarrhea persisting after travel in patients who recently received of antimicrobials. Clinical features of *C. difficile* colitis include persistent and profuse watery diarrhea, sometimes containing blood and mucus. Systemic toxicity with fever and malaise may be present in severe cases. Diagnosis is made by detecting the presence of *C. difficile* toxins A or B in stools by immunoassay or NAT. Isolation of the organism by culture is rarely performed. Treatment consists of discontinuing the causative antimicrobial and starting either oral vancomycin or metronidazole.

EMERGING BACTERIAL PATHOGENS

Enteroaggregative *E. coli* (EAEC) is another pathotype of *E. coli* that appears to be playing an emerging role in TD. It possesses the ability to aggressively attach to intestinal mucosal epithelial cells and mediate inflammation through a variety of adhesins and toxins. As EAEC is similar to ETEC, accurate identification of EAEC in stool cultures is challenging. The introduction of NAT methods has the potential to improve the diagnosis of these pathogens.

Arcobacter spp. are *Campylobacter*-like organisms that have been isolated from the feces of animals with enteritis. *Arcobacter butzleri* has been reported as a cause of TD in travelers to Mexico, Guatemala, and India and is likely transmitted through the ingestion of contaminated food or water. *Arcobacter* may be an underestimated etiologic agent of TD since its presence in stool cultures is rarely sought, but it can be recovered using the same media to isolate *Campylobacter* incubated under microaerophilic conditions at 37° C rather than 42° C.

Bacteroides spp. are a major component of the normal human fecal flora. Enterotoxigenic *Bacteroides fragilis* (ETBF) have been identified as a cause of acute watery diarrhea and colonic inflammation. In a recent study, ETBF was identified via NAT in the stool of 13% of patients with TD returning from India. The ability to discriminate ETBF from normal anaerobic intestinal flora requires NAT. More study is required to better understand the role of ETBF as a cause of diarrheal illness in those who travel abroad.

VIRAL AGENTS

Norovirus is the leading cause of food-borne infection and the cause of half of all gastroenteritis outbreaks worldwide. This virus may persist in the environment for prolonged periods and is highly contagious, with an infectious dose of only 20 viral particles. Its ability to cause explosive outbreaks in closed communities has been reported in all-inclusive resorts and on cruise ships. A single genotype of norovirus (genogroup II, genotype 4) has been the predominant norovirus strain that has been associated with gastroenteritis outbreaks in many countries. Norovirus may be transmitted by ingestion of contaminated water and foods such as salads, clams, and oysters and from contact with contaminated fomites. Gastroenteritis caused by norovirus is characterized by watery diarrhea, abdominal cramps, and vomiting; fever is rarely present. The disease is self-limited, and the gastrointestinal symptoms last from 1 to 4 days. Antigen detection immunoassays and nucleic acid tests can be used to confirm the clinical diagnosis. Treatment consists of replenishing fluids and electrolytes.

Rotavirus has been implicated as an important cause of TD among adults and children, especially among those visiting Central America and the Caribbean. Transmission is fecal-oral and is typically through direct contact with infected individuals such as caregivers caring for ill children. Symptoms begin with fever and vomiting for 2-3 days followed by profuse nonbloody, non-inflammatory diarrhea. The incidence of rotavirus has decreased secondary to the advent of effective vaccines combined with massive vaccination campaigns throughout the developing world, particularly in Latin America. Nevertheless, unvaccinated travelers to underdeveloped regions remain at risk. Rotaviral antigen can be detected in stool using commercially available immunoassays or by NAT; treatment is achieved through supportive care.

FURTHER READING

Anderson, F.J., Weber, S.G., 2004. Rotavirus infection in adults. Lancet Infect. Dis. 4 (2), 91–99.

Binnicker, M.J., 2015. Multiplex molecular panels for the diagnosis of gastrointestinal infection: performance, result interpretation and cost-effectiveness. J. Clin. Microbiol. pii: JCM.02103-15. [Epub ahead of print]; PMID: 26311866.

de la Cabada Bauche, J., Dupont, H.L., 2011. New developments in traveler's diarrhea. Gastroenterol. Hepatol. (NY) 7 (2), 88–95.

Estrada-Garcia, T., Navarro-Garcia, F., 2012. Enteroaggregative *Escherichia coli* pathotype: a genetically heterogeneous emerging foodborne enteropathogen. FEMS Immunol. Med. Microbiol. 66 (3), 281–298.

Gomi, H., Jiang, Z.D., Adachi, J.A., et al., 2001. In vitro antimicrobial susceptibility testing of bacterial enteropathogens causing traveler's diarrhea in four geographic regions. Antimicrob. Agents Chemother. 45 (1), 212–216.

Hill, D.R., Beeching, N.J., 2010. Travelers' diarrhea. Curr. Opin. Infect. Dis. 23 (5), 481–487.

Humphries, R.M., Linscott, A.J., 2015. Laboratory diagnosis of bacterial gastroenteritis. Clin. Microbiol. Rev. 28 (1), 3–31.

Jiang, Z.D., Dupont, H.L., Brown, E.L., et al., 2010. Microbial etiology of travelers' diarrhea in Mexico, Guatemala, and India: importance of enterotoxigenic *Bacteroides fragilis* and *Arcobacter* species. J. Clin. Microbiol. 48 (4), 1417–1419.

Patel, R., 2015. MALDI-TOF MS for the diagnosis of infectious diseases. Clin. Chem. 61 (1), 100–111.

Ross, A.G., Olds, G.R., Cripps, A.W., et al., 2013. Enteropathogens and chronic illness in returning travelers. N. Engl. J. Med. 368 (19), 1817–1825.

Steffen, R., Hill, D.R., DuPont, H.L., 2015. Traveler's diarrhea: a clinical review. JAMA 313 (1), 71–80.

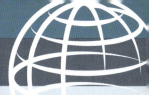

CHAPTER 32

Amebiasis, Giardiasis, and Other Intestinal Protozoan Infections

Abinash Virk

Entamoeba histolytica and *Giardia lamblia* are the most common protozoan pathogens of the human intestinal tract worldwide. In the United States, infections caused by *Giardia* and *Cryptosporidium* are most prevalent. *Giardia* and *E. histolytica* infection rates are significantly higher in developing countries. Despite this, neither protozoan is a common cause of disease in travelers. *Giardia* accounts for 1-4% of traveler's diarrhea, and *E. histolytica* for <1%. However, the prolonged illness and potential for serious complications in both diseases make it important to expeditiously diagnose and treat.

ENTAMOEBA HISTOLYTICA

Pathogenesis

E. histolytica is the only commonly recognized human intestinal pathogen in the subphylum Sarcodina, whose members are distinguished by the use of pseudopods for locomotion. *E. histolytica* exists in two forms: the cyst (infective form) or the ameboid trophozoite (invasive form). The cysts are round, 10-15 μm in size, and have four nuclei and a refractile wall. The trophozoites are larger (10 and 50 μm) and motile with a pleomorphic shape. Infection is usually acquired by ingestion of cysts present in fecally contaminated food or water or by direct person-to-person contact. Transmission can also occur by sexual exposure (either through oral-anal-genital contact or by direct inoculation of traumatized tissue) or from contaminated enema equipment.

The trophozoites are very labile and easily destroyed by gastric acid. Unlike the trophozoites, the cysts can survive for weeks in moist surroundings and are resistant to gastric acid and the low concentrations of chlorine commonly used in commercial water purification.

Intestinal Amebiasis

The initial site of amebic infection is the cecum and colon after *E. histolytica* excysts in the small bowel. Attachment of trophozoites to the colonic mucosa is followed by mucosal invasion, leading to both superficial and deep colonic ulcerations. Host cell lysis and proteolysis of the extracellular matrix by the amebae results in ulceration and tissue invasion. Virulent strains of *E. histolytica* possess lectins and adhesins for adherence, cytotoxins, proteolytic enzymes, and transmembrane ion channel proteins (porins). Strains from different geographic areas vary widely in their relative virulence. Certain isoenzyme patterns appear to serve as markers for strain virulence. A rapid assay for virulence would have great clinical significance, as clinically avirulent strains such as *E. dispar*, *E. moshkovskii*, or *E. bangladeshi*, while morphologically indistinguishable from virulent strains, do not require treatment. For instance, currently approximately 12% of the world population is estimated to have both *E. histolytica* and *E. dispar*; however, only 1% are estimated to have pathogenic *E. histolytica*. Presence of other bacteria in the colon, extremes of age, immunocompromised state, pregnancy, and malnutrition influence the virulence of the amebae.

Extraintestinal Amebiasis

Once local invasion is established in the colon, the amebae can gain access to the portal venous system to establish metastatic sites of infection. Symptomatic invasive amebiasis occurs in approximately 10% of patients with asymptomatic *E. histolytica* fecal carriage state. The most common location is the liver, but amebic abscesses of the lungs, brain, and, rarely, other organs do occur. These metastatic abscesses contain necrotic debris but few leukocytes or trophozoites. Trophozoites are most easily identified in the peripheral tissue. In addition to hematogenous dissemination, local spread of infection from the colon can result in cutaneous amebiasis or in paracolonic inflammatory masses referred to as amebomas.

Immunity

Infected individuals develop both humoral and cell-mediated immune responses to *E. histolytica*. The specific immunoglobulin response is helpful in diagnosis in non-endemic areas (see later discussions), but its importance in vivo is unknown. Cell-mediated responses are important in controlling the disease, particularly in invasive amebiasis, but only partial protection from reinfection is achieved after recovery from the primary episode. Host response determines the severity and relapses of disease. Acquired resistance to infection is thought to be linked to intestinal IgA against the carbohydrate-recognition domain of the *E. histolytica* galactose *N*-acetyl-d-galactosamine lectin. Host HLA class II-restricted immune responses also play a role in protection against *E. histolytica* infection. Recovery from amebiasis does not confer immunity to reinfection.

Epidemiology

Humans and some nonhuman primates are the only natural reservoirs. Therefore, the persistence of endemic disease in a population is dependent on crowding and poor standards of hygiene for water purification, food preparation, and waste disposal.

Amebiasis is a significant health problem in the developing world. Within the United States, risk groups include institutionalized individuals, promiscuous men who have sex with men (sexual transmission in which case trophozoites may be infective as well), recent immigrants, and travelers to high prevalence countries.

Travel to any developing country poses a risk of acquiring amebiasis, but travel to Mexico or to remote rural areas of Asia (e.g., trekking in Nepal) appears to bear the highest risk. The risk of amebiasis among travelers was 0.3% in one study.

Clinical Features

Intestinal Amebiasis

E. histolytica infection is most often asymptomatic. Asymptomatic cyst excretion can be self-limited or persist for years. Symptoms, when present, range from mild diarrhea to severe dysentery. Typically, there is gradual onset of colicky lower abdominal pain and diarrhea. Mucus, tenesmus, fever, and abdominal pain usually accompany diarrhea. Stools are often bloody and may be associated with signs of hypovolemia in severe cases. Spontaneous resolution after 1-4 weeks, sometimes with persistent asymptomatic cyst excretion, is the usual outcome. Persistent disease is not uncommon. Chronic disease may manifest cyclical relapses and remissions mimicking inflammatory bowel disease. Chronic amebic colitis results in anorexia, weight loss, and intermittent abdominal pain.

Several serious complications can develop in about 5% of patients with invasive intestinal amebiasis. Intra-abdominal complications include peritonitis secondary to perforation of a colonic abscess, intestinal hemorrhage from erosion of an abscess into an artery, or toxic megacolon from fulminant amebic colitis. The prognosis is poor in these situations, since the colon is often diffusely necrotic, rendering surgery difficult. Complications are more common in infants, pregnant women, and patients with alcohol abuse or diabetes or receiving corticosteroids. Amebomas are inflammatory mass lesions most common in the cecum, ascending colon, and descending colon; usually solitary, they can be radiologically indistinguishable from colonic neoplasms or intestinal tuberculosis. Involvement of the cecum can result in amebic appendicitis.

Extraintestinal Amebiasis

The liver is the most common site of extraintestinal amebic disease. Amebic liver abscesses (ALA) can present with the dysenteric phase of the illness or several years later. ALA are predominantly solitary (83%) and located in the right lobe (75%) of the liver. Right lobe predilection results from streaming of portal vein blood flow. ALA develops in 3-9% of cases of intestinal amebiasis. However, only 14% of patients with ALA will have active intestinal disease at the time of diagnosis, and majority will have neither active intestinal disease nor a history of dysentery. Incidence peaks in the 20- to 50-year-old age group with a male/female case ratio of 3:1.

The duration of symptoms before presentation is <2 weeks in the majority of cases. Virtually all patients present with right upper quadrant pain. Right lower chest pain, which may be pleuritic, is present in 25%. Other symptoms include upper abdominal swelling, weight loss, malaise, anorexia, pruritus, and cough (10-50%). Diaphragmatic irritation can result in referred pain to the right shoulder. High fever with chills and profuse night sweats may be present. Examination reveals tender hepatomegaly, sometimes with point tenderness. About half of the patients may have abnormal right lung auscultatory findings (rales or dullness). Jaundice is rare.

Primary amebic abscesses of the lung or brain are indistinguishable from pyogenic abscesses. Finally, extraintestinal disease can also result from rupture of a hepatic amebic abscess into the peritoneum, pleural cavity, or pericardium.

Diagnosis

Intestinal Amebiasis

Examination of the stool

Traditionally, intestinal amebiasis was diagnosed by the identification of trophozoites or cysts in fresh feces. However, owing to the more prevalent nonpathogenic, morphologically identical, but genetically distinct *E. dispar* in stool, *E. histolytica* is diagnosed using *E. histolytica*-specific tests. *E. histolytica* trophozoites survive only 2-5 hours at 37°C and 6-16 hours at 25°C, so prompt examination of specimens or refrigeration (survival 48-96 hours) is essential. In active infections, both cysts and trophozoites can be found on microscopic examination of the stool. The finding of ingested red blood cells (hematophagocytosis) is diagnostic of *E. histolytica* infection. More often, however, the number of organisms is small and excretion is sporadic, resulting in a yield of only 33-50% from the examination of a single specimen. Despite invasive disease, fecal leukocytes are not found because of the lytic activity of the amebae. Fecal blood (microscopic or gross) is seen in approximately 70% of patients.

Differentiation from nonpathogenic ameba species or fecal leukocytes can be difficult, and both false-positive and false-negative laboratory errors are common. Therefore, in addition to clinical and epidemiologic correlation, a specific *E. histolytica* test is advised for definitive diagnosis. Specific tests are available to detect and differentiate *E. histolytica* and *E. dispar*. Stool *E. histolytica*-specific antigen has a sensitivity of 87% and specificity of >90% compared with culture. Stool in vitro culture methods are not selective for *E. histolytica*. Isoenzyme analysis is specific but takes about 1-2 weeks. Molecular methods such as polymerase chain reaction (PCR) are also available and effective to identify *E. histolytica*.

Colonoscopy

Colonoscopy is preferred over sigmoidoscopy because amebic colitis lesions can be present in the ascending colon or cecum and be missed on a sigmoidoscopy. Endoscopy may be normal or reveal only nonspecific edema and inflammation of the mucosa. Characteristic ulcers are present only 25% of the time, but scrapings or brushings from the rectal mucosa or the edge of an ulcer frequently are positive for trophozoites (samples must be obtained with a glass pipette or metal implements, since the amebae adhere to cotton fibers). Endoscopic brushings or biopsy from the edge of the ulcer are more sensitive for the diagnosis of amebic colitis than fecal examination.

Radiographic studies

No pathognomonic pattern is present on radiographic studies. Barium studies in particular should be avoided, since barium interferes with stool examination for protozoa.

Blood tests

Several serologic tests are available for the diagnosis of amebiasis. Antibody detection is most useful in patients with extraintestinal disease (i.e., ALA). Of these the most widely used is the enzyme immunoassay (EIA), which has replaced indirect hemagglutination. The EIA detects antibody specific for *E. histolytica* in approximately 95% of patients with extraintestinal amebiasis, 70% of patients with active intestinal infection, and 10% of asymptomatic cyst carriers. Anti-ameba antibodies can remain elevated for years after the initial infection, hence should be evaluated carefully in persons from endemic countries. Serologic tests are particularly useful in excluding amebiasis as the etiology of chronic inflammatory bowel disease before initiating steroid therapy, especially in persons from non-endemic countries.

Extraintestinal Amebiasis (Especially Liver Abscesses)

Blood tests

Most patients with ALA will have a moderate degree of leukocytosis with neutrophilia. Transaminases may be slightly elevated in acute ALA with normal alkaline phosphatase. However, these are elevated in only 20% of patients with chronic ALA.

Radiographic studies

Chest radiography is abnormal in the majority of cases. Elevation of the right hemidiaphragm and right lung base atelectasis are the most common abnormalities. Pleural fluid may be present, despite absence of frank rupture of the abscess into the pleural space. Ultrasonography and computed tomography are equally sensitive in detection of ALA.

Special diagnostic considerations

None of the aforementioned tests will reliably differentiate ALA from pyogenic liver abscesses or from neoplastic masses with central necrosis. Serologic tests for anti-amebic antibodies are positive in 91-98% of patients with ALA, making these tests highly useful in persons from non-endemic areas. In one study of detection of circulating *E. histolytica* Gal/GalNAc lectin in the serum, the TechLab *E. histolytica* II test (TechLab, Blacksburg, VA) had a sensitivity of 96% to diagnose ALA and was helpful in follow-up care after treatment. In endemic areas, a therapeutic trial of metronidazole or a diagnostic aspiration of the lesion may be necessary to establish the diagnosis. Fluid from an amebic abscess is characteristically thin, brownish, and odorless, but amebae may be difficult to detect without a biopsy of the edge of the abscess. In biopsy specimens, detection of the trophozoites is diagnostic. PCR may be more rapid and sensitive where available. If possible, aspiration or surgery should be avoided because of the risk of complications, including secondary infection of the abscess cavity, and because of the excellent therapeutic outcome obtained with chemotherapy alone.

Diagnosis of amebic abscesses of other organs or of amebic peritonitis generally requires serologic evidence of amebiasis and consistent findings in aspirated fluid from the abscess or peritoneum.

Treatment

Treatment regimens for the various *E. histolytica* clinical syndromes are listed in **Table 32.1**. Common side effects associated with these antimicrobial agents are shown in **Table 32.2**. All patients with active intestinal or extraintestinal infection, especially those at high risk for severe complications (immunocompromised or individuals at either extreme of age), should be treated with a tissue agent followed by a luminal agent. Management of an asymptomatic individual who passes cysts is more controversial. Differentiating between *E. dispar* and *E. histolytica* helps clarify management options, as nonpathogenic *E. dispar* does not need treatment. Treatment is recommended for high-risk cyst carriers with either *E. histolytica*/*E. dispar* complex (where differentiation is not possible) or *E. histolytica* alone in the stool. Asymptomatic *E. histolytica* colonization can be treated with a luminal agent alone. In areas

TABLE 32.1 Treatment Regimens for *Entamoeba histolytica* Infections

Drug	Adult Dose	Pediatric Dose	Duration
Asymptomatic cyst passers			
Iodoquinol	650 mg t.i.d.	30-40 mg/kg per day in three doses	20 days
Diloxanide furoate	500 mg t.i.d.	20 mg/kg per day in three doses	10 days
Paromomycin	25-30 mg/kg per day in three doses. Can be used in pregnant women	25-30 mg/kg per day in three doses	7 days
Invasive colitis			
Metronidazole[a]	750 mg t.i.d.	35-50 mg/kg per day in three doses	10 days
	2.4 g q.d.		2-3 days
Tinidazole[a]	2 g orally q.d.	Children >3 years of age: 50 mg/kg per day[b] (up to 2 g a day)	3 days
Dehydroemetine[a]	1-1.5 mg/kg per day i.m. in two doses		5 days
Amebic liver abscess			
Metronidazole[a]	750 mg t.i.d.	35-50 mg/kg per day in three doses	10 days
Tinidazole[a]	2 g orally q.d.	Children >3 years of age: 50 mg/kg per day[b] (up to 2 g a day)	3-5 days
Dehydroemetine[a]	1-1.5 mg/kg per day i.m.	1-1.5 mg/kg per day i.m. in two doses	5 days
Chloroquine base	600 mg q.d. × 2 days, then 300 mg q.d. (may be added to other regimens)		14-21 days

[a]A luminal agent (paromomycin, diloxanide, or iodoquinol) should follow treatment with metronidazole, tinidazole, or dehydroemetine.
[b]Tinidazole tablets (available as 250 mg or 500 mg) can be crushed and mixed with cherry syrup.
i.m., intramuscularly; *q.d.*, one per day; *t.i.d.*, three times per day.

where the risk of reinfection is high, treatment of asymptomatic individuals may not be cost effective. Test-of-cure stool examinations after completion of therapy are important, as all of the recommended regimens have significant failure rates.

Intestinal Amebiasis

Metronidazole is the mainstay of therapy because of its availability and low toxicity. Unfortunately, it fails to eradicate luminal infection in 10-15% of cases because of its excellent absorption from the lumen into the tissues. Tinidazole, a structural analog of metronidazole, is effective for the treatment of intestinal amebiasis. It is also not indicated for the treatment of asymptomatic cyst passage. In four small randomized clinical trials of intestinal amebiasis, tinidazole was equally or more efficacious (one study) than metronidazole, with fewer side effects. Nitazoxanide, a thiazolide antiparasitic drug, has in vitro activity against *E. histolytica/dispar*. In clinical trials, parasitologic cure rates range from 69 to 96%. It is not yet approved by the US Food and Drug Administration (FDA) for the treatment of intestinal amebiasis. Following treatment with metronidazole or tinidazole for invasive amebiasis, all patients should receive a luminal amebicide to eliminate cysts from the colon. The following

TABLE 32.2 Side Effects Associated with Medications Used in the Treatment of Intestinal Protozoal Infections

Drug	Common	Uncommon
Metronidazole	Nausea, vomiting, bloating, metallic taste	Dizziness, vertigo, ataxia, stomatitis, peripheral neuropathy, Antabuse effect
Tinidazole	Nausea, vomiting, bloating, metallic taste	Rash, serum-sickness, peripheral neuropathy
Nitazoxanide	Abdominal pain, diarrhea, headache and nausea	
Diloxanide furoate	Flatulence	Nausea, vomiting, diarrhea, urticaria
Iodoquinol	Rash, acne, enlarged thyroid, nausea, diarrhea, cramps	Optic atrophy
Paromomycin	Nausea, vomiting, diarrhea	Eighth nerve damage, nephrotoxicity
Dehydroemetine	Nausea, vomiting, diarrhea, cardiac arrhythmias, precordial pain, muscle weakness (patients must be hospitalized and electrocardiographic changes monitored)	Dizziness, weakness, heart failure, hypotension
Quinacrine	Vomiting, diarrhea, dizziness, headache, abdominal cramps	Toxic psychosis, hepatic necrosis, blood dyscrasias
Furazolidone	Nausea, vomiting	Allergic reactions, polyneuritis, fever, hemolytic anemia

medications are primarily active against luminal stage of the protozoa. In the United States, the most common luminal amebicide is paromomycin. Diloxanide furoate is available in the United States only through the Centers for Disease Control and Prevention (CDC). Iodoquinol, although approved by the FDA, is difficult to obtain and has the potential for optic neuritis. Paromomycin and tetracycline have activity against luminal disease but have not been tested in rigorous controlled treatment trials with adequate follow-up monitoring. Documentation of cure should be undertaken after treatment. There is a 10% relapse rate if treated with a tissue agent but not followed by a luminal agent.

None of the drugs used in the treatment of amebiasis has been shown to be safe for use during pregnancy. The indications for treatment must be weighed against the potential risk to the fetus in each case.

Extraintestinal Amebiasis

Metronidazole or tinidazole, with or without a luminal amebicide, is the treatment of choice for all forms of extraintestinal amebiasis. Tinidazole is equally as efficacious as metronidazole (seven randomized studies with a total of 133 patients) or more efficacious than metronidazole (one study, 18 patients) for the treatment of ALA. The cure rates range from 86 to 93%. Dehydroemetine (available through the CDC) is extremely toxic and rarely indicated. Emetine is even more toxic and should be avoided.

In a series of ALA treated with metronidazole and followed by hepatic ultrasonography, resolution ranged from 2 to 20 months. After healing, the hepatic sonograph pattern was normal. Routine follow-up ultrasounds are not recommended, since the abscess cavity is likely to remain for months to years after appropriate therapy.

Antimicrobial therapy alone is successful in the majority of cases of amebic abscesses. The prognosis is excellent unless the patient is gravely ill at the initiation of treatment.

Needle aspiration or drainage may be useful in selected cases for symptomatic relief, left-lobe abscess, impending rupture, or abscess that does not respond to conservative medical therapy. Surgery should be reserved for emergent situations, such as impending rupture of ALA into the pericardium or peritoneum.

Prevention

The basic means for eradication of endemic amebiasis is to eliminate fecal contamination of food and water by improving waste disposal systems and water purification. For travelers, avoidance of uncooked, unpeeled fruits and vegetables and untreated drinking water is recommended. Adequate water treatment consists of boiling, filtration, or treatment with high concentrations of iodide. Chlorine is much less effective (see Chapter 7). Prophylactic chemotherapy is not recommended. One agent available for this purpose in some countries, iodochlorhydroxyquin (Entero-Vioform), has been associated with irreversible optic neuritis. In populations at risk of sexually transmitted amebiasis, altering sexual practices to avoid fecal-oral spread may reduce the risk of transmission of amebiasis and other enteric pathogens. Additionally, efforts should be made to decrease the transmission from a cyst-passer to family members or contacts. Contacts and family members of the index case of *E. histolytica* infection should be screened.

GIARDIA LAMBLIA

Pathogenesis

G. lamblia (also called *G. duodenalis* or *G. intestinalis*) is the human species and is acquired by ingestion of a very low inoculum (as few as 10-100) cysts in contaminated food or water. Cysts can survive up to 3 months in water at $4°C$. The free-living trophozoite form is less infectious, since it is more labile in the environment and is easily killed by gastric acid. Excystation occurs in the duodenum and proximal jejunum, the regions predominantly involved in the infection. The incubation period is 3-25 days (median 7-10 days), after which the cysts can be detected in the stool.

The pathogenesis is poorly understood. Trophozoites have a prominent "sucking disk" on their ventral surface, but whether this structure is involved in adherence to the intestinal brush border is unknown. The severity of symptoms does not correlate with the extent of morphologic damage to the epithelial cells (usually limited to disruption of the brush border) or the number of organisms. Organisms have occasionally been noted to penetrate the wall of the gut to the submucosa, but invasiveness does not appear to play a role in pathogenesis. No enterotoxins have been associated with *Giardia*.

The host immune system plays an important role in giardiasis, as illustrated by the predisposition to chronic giardiasis observed in patients with malnutrition, IgA deficiency, agammaglobulinemia, and common variable immunodeficiency. Humoral immune system is important for recovery from the initial infection and protection from reinfection. Cellular immunity also plays a role, as shown in animal models. *Giardia* infection confers partial protection of variable duration.

Epidemiology

Giardiasis occurs as an endemic disease and in large, water-borne outbreaks. In developing countries, where prevalence is 7-10%, it is primarily a disease of children. *G. lamblia* is the most commonly diagnosed intestinal parasite in public health laboratories in the United States. In the United States, major water-borne outbreaks have been reported from many states. *G. lamblia* that infects humans has cross-species pathogenicity for other mammals, and vice-versa. Water-dwelling animals, such as beavers and muskrats, have been implicated as the source of the *Giardia* contamination in some of the outbreaks.

Direct person-to-person spread is also important in the transmission of giardiasis. An infected person may shed 1-10 billion cysts daily in their feces. Shedding may last for several months. High shedding and small infective inoculum contribute to high attack rates in developing countries and daycare centers. At-risk groups include men who have sex with men, institutionalized persons, refugees or immigrants from developing countries, or travelers to those countries. Overall risk of *Giardia* among immigrants is 1180 per 100,000, with the highest risk associated with immigration from Afghanistan and Iraq.

All travelers are at some risk of acquiring *Giardia*, even when traveling in the United States or other industrialized countries. A Swedish study of imported giardiasis showed that the overall risk for acquiring *Giardia* during travel is 5.3/100,000, with the highest risk of acquisition related to travel to the Indian subcontinent (628 per 100,000) and East and West Africa. The largest proportion of imported giardiasis was seen among immigrants visiting friends and family in the country of their origin. Overall, however, it accounts for only a small percentage of cases of traveler's diarrhea. Hikers drinking untreated surface water have the greatest risk for acquisition of giardiasis.

Among the nontraveling patients in the United States, giardiasis is more common among children between 0 and 5 years old and among adults between 31 and 40 years old. There is a seasonal variation, with more cases during late summer and early fall, coinciding with increased water-related outdoor activities. There appears to be geographic variation as well, with higher number of cases reported from the northern states. Annually about 20,000 cases are reported in the United States.

Clinical Features

The acute phase of giardiasis is highly variable in severity, but typically there is sudden onset of diarrhea 7-21 days after ingestion of the cysts. The moderate to large volume of foul-smelling, loose stools accompanied by distention, flatulence, and midepigastric cramps helps to distinguish giardiasis from other infectious diarrheas. Bacterial pathogens of the small bowel, such as enterotoxigenic *Escherichia coli*, tend to cause a more watery diarrhea with less bloating and flatulence. Infectious colitis secondary to amebiasis or *Shigella* infection typically has smaller stool volume, more severe and diffuse cramps, and less abdominal bloating than seen with giardiasis. Dysentery is highly unusual with giardiasis and should prompt an evaluation for other pathogens. Other symptoms with acute giardiasis can include nausea, anorexia, vomiting, low-grade fever, and headache. The acute phase usually lasts 7-14 days but can then evolve into a chronic infection.

Chronic giardiasis symptoms may be persistent or relapsing and include loose, bulky, foul-smelling stools; distention; foul flatus; constipation; and substernal burning. Malabsorption can occur and lead to significant weight loss. Malabsorption results from trophozoites forming a physical barrier between the intestinal epithelial cells and the lumen of the intestine, interrupting the absorption of nutrients from the lumen. Spontaneous resolution is the rule, but occasionally infections can persist for years. Chronic infection most often occurs in patients with hypogammaglobulinemia or agammaglobulinemia. Some individuals become chronic, asymptomatic cyst-passers and become an important reservoir for spread to others. In developing countries, chronic giardiasis in children is associated with malnutrition and resultant growth and cognitive impairment.

Diagnosis

Giardiasis should be suspected in any patient with a diarrheal illness persisting >1 week or malabsorption. Epidemiologic data may be suggestive but do not exclude the diagnosis, since giardiasis is endemic in the United States and sporadic cases occur. Both the cyst and the trophozoite forms can be seen in diarrheal stool, but trophozoites are rare in formed stool. A minimum of three specimens should be examined, since cyst passage is erratic and the numbers may be small. The yield from a single specimen is 50-75% but increases to 90-95% with three or more specimens collected every other day during a 5-day period. *Giardia* antigen detection by enzyme-linked immunosorbent assay and direct fluorescent antibody (DFA) in stool specimens are the preferred diagnostic tests and more sensitive than standard morphologic identification of this parasite in stool specimens. Some of these antigen detection assays are available as combined *Cryptosporidium*/*Giardia* detection kits. The sensitivity and specificity approach 100% compared with microscopy. Newer stool PCR tests, where available, are more sensitive and specific for diagnosis.

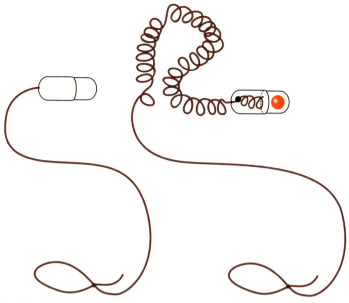

Fig. 32.1 **The string test capsule.**

If suspicion of giardiasis remains high and multiple stool specimens are negative, options include a therapeutic trial with antimicrobial agents or proceeding to the string test (Entero-Test, Hedeco, Palo Alto, CA); upper endoscopy for aspiration of duodenal fluid or biopsy may be helpful. The string test consists of a gelatin capsule containing a string (**Fig. 32.1**). One end of the string is held outside the patient, and the capsule is swallowed. The capsule is weighted with a small metal sphere and is passed into the duodenum, unwinding string from a hole in the proximal end. The gelatin capsule dissolves, leaving the distal end of the string free in the duodenum. After 4 hours it is withdrawn, and the material adhering to the bile-stained end is scraped off and examined for trophozoites (**Fig. 32.2**).

Small-bowel biopsy is most helpful in the evaluation of chronic giardiasis and associated malabsorption. It has little, if any, role in the diagnosis of acute giardiasis. The histopathologic examination of the small bowel in giardiasis is usually normal but may show some nonspecific blunting of the villi. Touch preparations of the biopsy specimen are necessary to see the trophozoites, which inhabit the mucoid layer overlying the epithelial cells.

Routine blood chemistry and hematologic values are normal, and specific serodiagnostic assays for antibodies to *Giardia* are still experimental. Radiographic procedures are unhelpful. Barium studies should be avoided, as barium interferes with detection of Giardia.

Treatment

The agents and appropriate dosage regimens used in the treatment of giardiasis are listed in **Table 32.3**. Common or severe side effects reported with these agents are shown in **Table 32.2**.

Metronidazole or tinidazole is the standard therapy for giardiasis. Metronidazole dosing of 250 mg three times a day for 5 days in uncomplicated giardiasis is associated with a higher failure rate; therefore, a minimum dose of 500 mg three times a day for 5-7 days appears appropriate. Short-course therapy with metronidazole has been tried, but the failure

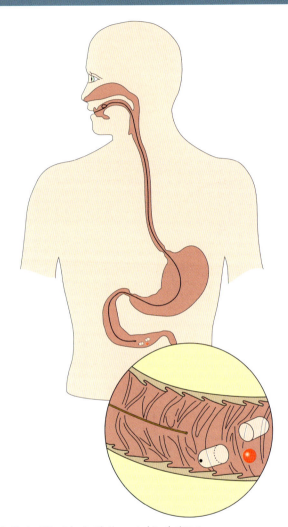

Fig. 32.2 **Route of the string test in the gastrointestinal tract.**

rates have been high with both the 2.0 g single-dose regimen (40-50% treatment failure) and the two-dose (2.0-2.4 g q.d. × 2 days) regimen (20-25% failure rate). A regimen of 2.4 g/day for 3 days has a 91% success rate but is associated with higher gastrointestinal toxicity.

Tinidazole, a second generation nitroimidazole antiprotozoal agent, is FDA approved for the treatment of giardiasis. Tinidazole has in vitro and clinical activity against metronidazole-resistant strains of *Giardia*. A Cochrane Database Systematic Review showed that treatment with a single dose of tinidazole results in higher clinical cure (92% cure rate with a single 2.0-g dose) with fewer adverse effects than metronidazole.

TABLE 32.3   Treatment Regimens for Giardiasis

Drug	Adult Dose (Nonpregnant)	Pediatric Dose	Duration
Metronidazole	500 mg t.i.d.	5-7 mg/kg t.i.d.	5-10 days
Tinidazole	2 g orally	Children >3 years of age: 50 mg/kg per day[a] (up to 2 g a day)	Single dose
Nitazoxanide	>12 years of age: 500 mg tablet or 25-mL suspension twice daily with food	Children 1–3 years of age: 100 mg (5 mL) twice daily with food Children 4–11 years of age: 200 mg (10 mL) twice daily with food	3 days
Quinacrine HCl	100 mg t.i.d. p.c.	2 mg/kg t.i.d. p.c. (max. 300 mg/day)	5 days
Furazolidone	100 mg q.i.d.	1.25 mg/kg q.i.d.	7-10 days

[a]Tinidazole tablets (available as 250 mg or 500 mg) can be crushed and mixed with cherry syrup.
p.c., after meals; *q.i.d.*, four times per day; *t.i.d.*, three times per day.

In 2002, the FDA approved nitazoxanide for the treatment of giardiasis for persons ≥1 year of age. Nitazoxanide interferes with the pyruvate–ferredoxin oxidoreductase enzyme-dependent electron transfer reaction in *Giardia* or *Cryptosporidium*. Its metabolite, tizoxanide, is eight times more active than metronidazole against *Giardia* in metronidazole-susceptible strains and twice as active as metronidazole-resistant strains. In clinical trials, the parasitologic response rate with nitazoxanide varied from 64 to 94%.

Quinacrine, the official drug of choice for treatment of giardiasis, is associated with frequent severe gastrointestinal side effects that limit patient compliance. Few controlled studies have been performed comparing quinacrine with metronidazole. Although these studies had suboptimal follow-up for detection of late relapses, the data suggest that there is little difference in cure rates between these two agents, both being successful in approximately 90% of cases. In the United States, quinacrine can be acquired from a few compounding pharmacies on an individual basis.

Special Therapeutic Considerations

Children

Prior to the approval of tinidazole and nitazoxanide, the treatment of children was difficult owing to the lack of liquid preparations of quinacrine or metronidazole. However, treatment options for children have improved: tinidazole is approved for children >3 years of age (tablets can be crushed and mixed with cherry syrup); nitazoxanide is approved for children >1 year of age and is available as a suspension. Another drug, furazolidone, is FDA approved for treatment of giardiasis but with limited availability. It is less active against *Giardia* (cure rates of 70-80%).

Treatment Failures

Treatment success is generally better in acute giardiasis than in subacute or chronic cases. Drug resistance is not believed to be a major factor in treatment failures, and a second course of the same agent is as likely to be successful as switching to a second drug. Recurrent infections may be related to IgA deficiency and warrant further investigation. Metronidazole-resistant strains have been described. Options for treatment of drug-resistant giardiasis include using a different drug such as nitazoxanide or using a combination of medications with different mechanisms of action, such as metronidazole and albendazole or paromomycin. Tinidazole may still be effective, but since it shares a similar mechanism of action it may not be effective. Additional options include using a higher dose, longer course, or combination of medications.

Pregnant Women

None of the drugs used in the treatment of giardiasis is approved for use in pregnancy. Unless severe or disabling symptoms are present, treatment should be deferred until after delivery. CDC recommends use of paromomycin, a non-absorbable aminoglycoside, in the treatment of giardiasis in pregnant women.

Chronic Gastrointestinal Symptoms

Some individuals, possibly as many as 5%, develop a poorly characterized symptom complex of persistent bloating, flatulence, and upper abdominal cramps after apparently successful therapy for giardiasis. Patients with this "post-giardiasis syndrome" do not have detectable persistent infections as assessed by stool examination and small-bowel aspiration and biopsy, and the giardiasis-like symptoms often persist despite repeated courses of therapy. Destruction of mucosal disaccharidases may play some role, but the symptoms may persist after recovery of the mucosal epithelium. Symptoms resolve slowly over 3-24 months. It is important to avoid repeated courses of antimicrobial agents in this disease if no evidence of ongoing infection is present. In refractory cases or in patients with chronic symptoms with evidence of active infection, a 14-day combination of metronidazole 750 mg, three times a day, and quinacrine 100 mg, three times a day, may be more effective.

Prevention

Contaminated water is the primary mode of transmission for *Giardia*. Boiling (30 s is sufficient at sea level; longer periods may be necessary at high elevations) and filtration are both adequate purification techniques (see Chapter 7). Inactivation by chlorination or by iodine treatment is less effective because these methods are affected by the pH, temperature, and cloudiness of the water, thereby decreasing the reliability of the purification method. The traveler should also avoid uncooked foods that may have been washed with tap water or untreated surface water. Hikers in mountainous regions should regard all surface water as potentially contaminated. Antimicrobial prophylaxis is not advised. Patients should also be advised to avoid fecal exposure and the potential of transmission during sex.

Outbreaks arising from daycare centers may be difficult to eradicate. The efficacy of epidemiologic screening or treatment of daycare staff and family members of infected children is unproven. Even the necessity for screening and treating asymptomatic children attending the daycare centers is unknown, although it would seem reasonable to screen and treat infants in diapers because of the greater potential for fecal-oral spread within and from this population.

OTHER PROTOZOA

Cryptosporidiosis

Protozoa of the genus *Cryptosporidium* are widely distributed among mammalian species, but only *Cryptosporidium parvum* and *C. hominis* are significant human pathogens. Infection, acquired by ingestion of cysts, primarily involves the small intestine, with highest concentration in the jejunum. Water or food contaminated with even a small inoculum (as low as 30 cysts) can cause an infection. Oocysts are highly resistant to chlorine or other common disinfectants.

In immunocompetent hosts, cryptosporidiosis is a self-limited illness that resolves spontaneously in 7-21 days. It is indistinguishable from giardiasis. Children less than 5 years of age are also more susceptible to symptomatic cryptosporidiosis. Immunocompromised hosts, especially patients with human immunodeficiency virus infection (HIV)/acquired immunodeficiency syndrome (AIDS), with cryptosporidiosis develop a prolonged intractable watery diarrhea associated with anorexia and weight loss. Among HIV/AIDS patients, it can also cause infection of the bile duct, gallbladder, pancreas, liver, or lung. Cell-mediated and humoral immunity seem to play a role in pathogenesis.

Cryptosporidium may cause as much as 5-7% of pediatric diarrhea in developing countries but is implicated in only 0.3-1.0% of outpatient diarrheal cases in the United States. The prevalence of cryptosporidiosis among HIV/AIDS patients ranges from 14% in developed countries to 24% in developing countries. Risk factors for cryptosporidiosis include travel to developing countries, use of swimming pools or water recreation parks, animal contact (zoo, farms, etc), daycare exposure, and contact with ill persons, especially children.

Stool *Cryptosporidium* antigen detection by EIA or DFA is the test of choice for detection of *Cryptosporidium* cysts and is more sensitive than modified acid-fast stain testing. Modified acid-fast stains of direct or concentrated stool are labor intensive and require more skill. Small-bowel biopsies and more elaborate stool purification techniques are rarely required. Patients with a clinical illness consistent with giardiasis but with multiple negative stool examinations for *Giardia* should undergo tests for *Cryptosporidium*.

Efficacious therapy against *Cryptosporidium* remains problematic. Nitazoxanide has a clinical efficacy of 72-88%, while the parasitological clearance rate is lower (60-75%). Its efficacy in immunocompromised hosts such as advanced HIV/AIDS patients remains unproven. In the United States, nitazoxanide is FDA approved for the treatment of cryptosporidiosis in immunocompetent persons ≥1 year of age. Paromomycin and high-dose azithromycin have modest efficacy in treating chronic cryptosporidiosis in immunocompromised patients. Subcutaneous octreotide helps control diarrhea in HIV/AIDS patients. Complete recovery is dependent on resolution of the immune deficit, as can occur with anti-HIV therapies. Immunosuppressive chemotherapy should either be delayed or transiently lowered if possible in a patient with cryptosporidiosis.

Prevention of fecal-oral transmission of *Cryptosporidium* oocysts can be achieved by strict personal hygiene, eating cooked food, and avoiding water theme parks, uncooked fruits and vegetables, oro-anal sexual exposure, and direct contact with animals, particularly calves and lambs. It is important to note that chlorination does not adequately kill the *Cryptosporidium* oocysts. Because of the lower parasite clearance rates, it is important to advise the patient to avoid public pools until symptom resolution and for at least 2 weeks after treatment. Retesting is unnecessary unless the patient is symptomatic. Boiling water for 1 minute is the best method of decontaminating water. In addition, using filters with 1 µm or smaller pore size are effective in removing the oocysts.

Balantidiasis

Balantidium coli is the only ciliated protozoan pathogen in humans. This parasite is very large (100 µm) and is easily identified in stool specimens. It is acquired by close contact with swine or, more rarely, transmitted within chronic care facilities for the developmentally disabled. It produces invasive disease of the colon with symptoms of colitis and dysentery. Tetracycline, iodoquinol, and high-dose metronidazole are all effective in treating balantidiasis.

OTHER PROTOZOAN PATHOGENS

Cystoisospora (Formerly Isospora) belli

Cystoisospora belli has been reported as a rare cause of enteritis. It is distributed worldwide but is more prevalent in South America and Africa. The clinical syndrome resembles giardiasis and is acquired by contact with contaminated water or food. Persistent diarrhea associated with *Cystoisospora* can occur in immunocompromised patients. Identifying the characteristic oocysts on modified acid-fast stool smears is diagnostic. Trimethoprim-sulfamethoxazole is the agent of choice; pyrimethamine may be useful in people allergic to sulfa. There are two reported cases of parasite clearance with nitazoxanide (not FDA approved for this indication).

Cyclospora cayetanensis

Cyclospora cayetanensis is an intestinal protozoan pathogen that causes diarrhea and is found in both developed and developing countries. It is presumably acquired through ingestion of contaminated water or food and not likely to be transmitted person-to-person. It has marked seasonal variation, tending to occur more in the late spring and summer months. The oocysts are detected by modified acid-fast (Ziehl–Neelsen) staining or by ultraviolet autofluorescence microscopy. The spherical cyst-like organisms measure 8-10 μm in diameter and are larger than *Cryptosporidium* oocysts.

Cyclospora infection in immunocompetent patients results in a prolonged self-limited watery diarrhea lasting up to 10 weeks. During the acute phase, upper abdominal symptoms, nausea, and fever accompany diarrhea. This may be followed by anorexia, weight loss, and fatigue. Symptoms may wax and wane for up to 4-8 weeks. Cases of cyclosporiasis in immunocompromised patients have been incompletely characterized, but the clinical presentation is similar to cryptosporidiosis. Cyclospora may be able to cause biliary tract disease among people with HIV/AIDS. The diagnostic differentiation between the two protozoan pathogens is significant, because cyclosporiasis responds to trimethoprim-sulfamethoxazole (adults, 160 mg trimethoprim and 800 mg sulfamethoxazole twice a day; children, 4 mg/kg trimethoprim and 20 mg/kg sulfamethoxazole twice a day) given for ≥3 days, whereas *Cryptosporidium* infections do not. Albendazole, trimethoprim, azithromycin, nalidixic acid, norfloxacin, tinidazole, metronidazole, quinacrine, tetracycline, and diloxanide furoate have no or limited activity on *Cyclospora*. Alternatives for patients allergic to sulfonamide include either desensitization to sulfonamide or treatment trial with ciprofloxacin based on a randomized controlled trial in HIV-infected patients with *Cyclospora* or *Cystoisospora*. Nitazoxanide has also shown broad in vitro activity against *Cyclospora* but needs clinical validation.

Similar to *Cryptosporidium*, *Cyclospora* is resistant to chlorination. Therefore, it is important to advise travelers regarding water precautions. Cyclosporiasis can be prevented by drinking boiled or bottled water, avoiding raw vegetables and fruits, and adhering to strict hand washing.

Dientamoeba fragilis

Dientamoeba fragilis is a flagellate protozoan that has been associated with a mild, nonspecific enteritis syndrome. Iodoquinol is the treatment of choice; tetracycline and paromomycin are alternatives.

POSSIBLE PATHOGENS

Blastocystis hominis

Blastocystis hominis is a common stool commensal (up to 19% of normal controls in the United States are colonized). There is evidence that heavy infestations may be associated with cramps, vomiting, dehydration, abdominal pain, sleeplessness, nausea, weight loss, lassitude, dizziness, flatus, anorexia, pruritus, and tenesmus.

B. hominis infections in primates have been cured with trimethoprim-sulfamethoxazole. In vitro susceptibility tests show that the following drugs may be effective, in descending order: emetine, metronidazole, nitazoxanide, furazolidone, trimethoprim-sulfamethoxazole, iodochlorhydroxyquin (Entero-Vioform), and pentamidine. Chloroquine and iodoquinol have also been reported as effective treatments.

The role of *B. hominis* as a human pathogen is still controversial. Some published reports, based on clinical and laboratory studies, have suggested that when *B. hominis*-associated diarrhea appears to respond to therapy, improvement may, in fact, be due to some other undetected organism that is actually causing the problem.

NONPATHOGENIC PROTOZOA

Numerous other species of protozoa can be detected in human feces, including nonpathogenic protozoa such as *Entamoeba coli*, *E. polecki*, *E. hartmanni*, *Iodamoeba bütschlii*, and *Endolimax nana*. At the present time identification of one of these organisms in the stool is a useful marker of exposure to fecal-contaminated food or water. Their presence should prompt a more exhaustive search for other intestinal pathogens.

FURTHER READING

Ali, S.A., Hill, D.R., 2003. Giardia intestinalis. Curr. Opin. Infect. Dis. 16, 453–460.

Anonymous, 2004. Tinidazole (Tindamax): a new anti-protozoal drug. Med. Lett. Drugs Ther. 46, 70–72.

Calderaro, A., Gorrini, C., Bommezzadri, S., et al., 2006. *Entamoeba histolytica* and *Entamoeba dispar*: comparison of two PCR assays for diagnosis in a non-endemic setting. Trans. Roy. Soc. Trop. Med. Hyg. 100, 450–457.

Centers for Disease Control and Prevention, 2004. Outbreak of cyclosporiasis associated with snow peas—Pennsylvania, 2004. MMWR 53, 876–878.

Ekdahl, K., Andersson, Y., 2005. Imported giardiasis: impact of international travel, immigration, and adoption. Am. J. Trop. Med. Hyg. 72, 825–830.

Fox, L.M., Saravolatz, L.D., 2005. Nitazoxanide: a new thiazolide antiparasitic agent. Clin. Infect. Dis. 40, 1173–1180.

Fotedar, R., Stark, D., Beebe, N., et al., 2007. Laboratory diagnostic techniques for *Entamoeba* species. Clin. Microbiol. Rev. 20, 532–534.

Gonzales, M.L.M., Dans, L.F., Martinez, E.G., 2009. Antiamoebic drugs for treating amoebic colitis. Cochrane Database Syst. Rev. (2), CD006085.

Haque, R., Mollah, N.U., Ali, I.K., et al., 2000. Diagnosis of amebic liver abscess and intestinal infection with the TechLab *Entamoeba histolytica* II antigen detection and antibody tests. J. Clin. Microbiol. 38, 3235–3239.

Haque, R., Mondal, D., Duggal, P., et al., 2006. *Entamoeba histolytica* infection in children and protection from subsequent amebiasis. Infect. Immun. 74, 904–909.

Herwaldt, B.L., 2000. *Cyclospora cayetanensis*: a review, focusing on the outbreaks of cyclosporiasis in the 1990's. Clin. Infect. Dis. 31, 1040.

Mejia, R., Vicuña, Y., Broncano, N., et al., 2013. A novel, multi-parallel, real-time polymerase chain reaction approach for eight gastrointestinal parasites provides improved diagnostic capabilities to resource-limited at-risk populations. Am. J. Trop. Med. Hyg. 88 (6), 1041–1047.

Nash, T.E., 2013. Unraveling how *Giardia* infections cause disease. J. Clin. Invest. 123 (6), 2346–2347.

Nash, T.E., Ohl, C.A., Thomas, E., et al., 2001. Treatment of patients with refractory giardiasis. Clin. Infect. Dis. 33 (1), 22–28.

Petri, W.A. Jr., Singh, U., 1999. Diagnosis and management of amebiasis. Clin. Infect. Dis. 29, 1117–1125.

Ribes, J.A., Seabolt, J.P., Overman, S.B., et al., 2004. Point prevalence of *Cryptosporidium*, *Cyclospora*, and *Isospora* infections in patients being evaluated for diarrhea. Am. J. Clin. Pathol. 122, 28–32.

Ross, A.G., Olds, G.R., Cripps, A.W., et al., 2013. Enteropathogens and chronic illness in returning travelers. N. Engl. J. Med. 368 (19), 1817–1825.

Rossignol, J.F., Ayoub, A., et al., 2001. Treatment of diarrhea caused by *Cryptosporidium parvum*: a prospective randomized, double-blind, placebo-controlled study of nitazoxanide. J. Infect. Dis. 184, 103–106.

Rossignol, J.F., Kabil, S.M., el-Gohary, Y., et al., 2006. Effect of nitazoxanide in diarrhea and enteritis caused by *Cryptosporidium* species. Clin. Gastroenterol. Hepatol. 4, 320–324.

Sohail, M.R., Fischer, P.R., 2005. Blastocystis hominis. Trav. Med. Infect. Dis. 3, 33–38.

Solaymani-Mohammadi, S.I., Singer, S.M., 2010. *Giardia duodenalis*: the double-edged sword of immune responses in giardiasis. Exp. Parasitol. 126 (3), 292–297.

Zaat, J.O.M., Mank, T.G., Assendelft, W.J.J., 2005. Drugs for treating giardiasis. Cochrane Libr. CD000217.

CHAPTER 33

Food Poisoning: Toxic Syndromes

Elaine C. Jong

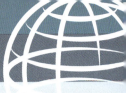

Once away from home, travelers are especially vulnerable to food-borne illness since with regard to food, they rely on the sourcing, processing, and culinary skills of others. Toxic syndromes due to food poisoning may occur after ingestion of foods that have been inadequately cooked, stored, or preserved. Knowledge of common food associations and clinical syndromes can help travelers to select safe foods or prompt them to seek help if they are stricken. Humans become intoxicated in two ways: after ingesting pre-formed toxins produced by bacteria present in the foods or by ingesting bacterial forms that proliferate in the gut and produce enterotoxins that are absorbed within the small intestine (the latter mechanism is also called a "toxical infection"). The bacteria commonly recognized as causes of food poisoning are ubiquitous in the environment and include *Clostridium perfringens*, *Staphylococcus aureus*, *Bacillus cereus*, and *Clostridium botulinum* (types A, B, and E).

Disease caused by pre-formed enterotoxins of *S. aureus* and *B. cereus* typically present as acute gastrointestinal illness. *C. perfringens* type A food poisoning also presents as acute gastrointestinal illness, but enterotoxin production occurs in the host following ingestion of the bacteria. Pigbel or necrotizing enteritis is a serious illness caused by *C. perfringens* type C. Botulism occurs when foods contain pre-formed toxins produced by *C. botulinum*; however, the clinical presentation usually involves neurological rather than gastrointestinal symptoms. Infant botulism is similar to *C. perfringens* in that toxin is produced after ingestion of contaminated food when *C. botulinum* spores germinate to produce bacteria that release intraluminal toxin during vegetative multiplication in the gut.

Table 33.1 summarizes the agents of food poisoning, including the incubation periods, clinical syndromes, and characteristic food associations. Websites providing reports of major outbreaks and information on food safety are given in **Table 33.2**.

FOOD POISONING PRESENTING AS GASTROINTESTINAL ILLNESS

The onset of symptoms is usually within hours after ingestion of contaminated food. In mild cases of food poisoning, vomiting, diarrhea, and abdominal cramping may be of short duration and resolve before the afflicted person seeks medical attention.

Etiology

C. perfringens type A infection has been identified as a common cause of food-borne disease in industrialized countries and is a leading cause of food poisoning cases in the United States, responsible for approximately 10% of food-borne illness associated with a known pathogen. *C. perfringens* spores germinate during cooking in stews, soups, gravies, and other meat or poultry dishes, and then if the food is allowed to cool at room temperature for a prolonged period (e.g., 12-14 hours) the *C. perfringens* bacteria proliferate. After ingestion, the actively growing (vegetative stage) bacteria multiply and then sporulate in the small intestine.

TABLE 33.1   Common Pathogens Causing Food Poisoning

Pathogen	Incubation	Characteristic Foods	Major Symptoms	Pathophysiology
Clostridium perfringens	6-24 h	Meat, poultry	Cramping abdominal pain,[a] diarrhea; vomiting and fever uncommon	Enterotoxin formed in vivo
Staphylococcus aureus	30 min to 8 h; usually 2-4 h	Creamy desserts, custards, salads, chopped hams, meats, baked goods	Vomiting,[a] cramping abdominal pain, diarrhea	Preformed enterotoxin
Bacillus cereus (emetic syndrome)	1-6 h	Rice, vegetables, meat ("fried rice syndrome")	Vomiting,[a] diarrhea; fever uncommon	? Preformed enterotoxin
Bacillus cereus (diarrheal syndrome)	6-24 h	Custards, cereals, puddings, sauces, meat loaf	Diarrhea[a], abdominal cramps, and vomiting; fever uncommon	? Preformed enterotoxin similar to ETEC LT toxin
Clostridium botulinum	2 h to 8 days; usually 12-48 h	Types A and B: improperly canned or preserved (pickled, cured, smoked) meats and vegetables; type E: smoked or preserved fish	Diplopia,[a] blurred vision,[a] photophobia[a]; dysphonia, dysarthria, weakness of tongue; nausea and vomiting; symmetric descending paralysis of motor and respiratory muscles that may progress rapidly	Preformed toxin

[a]Major distinguishing symptoms.
Adapted from: CDC-EIS, 2003. Compendium of Acute Foodborne and Waterborne Diseases. http://www.cdc.gov (accessed July 9, 2009).
ETEC, Enterotoxigenic Escherichia coli; LT, heat-labile.

TABLE 33.2   Web Sites for Food Safety and Outbreak Information

Centers for Disease Control and Prevention	http://www.cdc.gov/foodsafety
	http://www.cdc.gov/botulism
US Dept. of Agriculture Food Safety and Inspection Service	http://www.fsis.usda.gov
US Food and Drug Administration	http://www.cfsan.fda.gov
World Health Organization, Regional Food Safety Newsletter	http://www.who.int

C. perfringens bacteria entering the sporulation stage produce enterotoxin, which is then absorbed by the host.

Rare cases of fatal adult necrotizing enterocolitis have been reported in association with food-borne *C. perfringens* type A infections. Cases reported included previously healthy adults, although some reported cases had drug-induced constipation and fecal impaction that may have led to prolonged exposure of the colonic mucosal tissue to *C. perfringens* type A toxins and contributed to the development of illness.

S. aureus strains producing enterotoxin are usually inoculated from hands of infected human carriers into proteinaceous food products (e.g., creamy desserts and pastries, salads, meats) served or stored at room or refrigerator temperatures, conditions allowing staphylococcal proliferation and toxin production. Staphylococcal enterotoxins (A, B, C, D, and E) are relatively heat stable, so subsequent cooking of contaminated foods will not necessarily destroy them.

B. cereus is a ubiquitous soil bacterium present on rice, vegetables, and some meats. The illness ensuing from ingestion of *B. cereus*-contaminated food has been given the nickname "fried rice syndrome", as ingestion of fried rice was associated with the first recognized outbreaks. The ingredients and the cooking technique for this dish are especially conducive to illness-producing situations when fried rice is stored for prolonged periods at room temperature after cooking. The heat of cooking stimulates the *B. cereus* spores to germinate, and bacterial proliferation takes place in the food at room temperature, liberating enterotoxins. Flash cooking or brief reheating of the contaminated food before serving is not sufficient to inactivate the toxin nor kill the bacteria.

A short-incubation syndrome, with onset 2-9 hours after ingestion, is associated with the pre-formed toxin in the food. There is a long-incubation syndrome, with onset 6-14 hours after ingestion of contaminated food, associated with toxin elaborated by *B. cereus* bacteria proliferating within the gastrointestinal tract.

Diagnosis

A gastrointestinal illness characterized by a relatively rapid onset of symptoms after eating, and limited to 1 or 2 days, is likely to be food poisoning. Cramping abdominal pain is the hallmark of food poisoning caused by *C. perfringens*, and severe vomiting is the hallmark of food poisoning caused by *S. aureus*. *B. cereus* has two toxins, one causing a gastrointestinal illness with prominent vomiting (like *S. aureus* toxin) and one causing watery diarrhea (like the heat-labile toxin of enterotoxigenic *E. coli*). The diagnosis can be best confirmed if some of the original questionable food is available for laboratory testing. Laboratory testing of patient stool specimens, vomitus, and serum is laborious and is customarily performed by state public health department laboratories during large outbreaks. Commercially available enterotoxin kits available for *B. perfringens*, *S. aureus*, and *B. cereus* allow for rapid diagnosis, often before culture results are available.

Treatment

Antibiotics are of no known value in food poisoning, since onset of symptoms is related to a certain level of the given enterotoxin being present in the gut; once formed, the toxin can exert its biologic effect independently of the continued viability of the bacterial source.

Treatment is directed toward symptomatic relief of the nausea and vomiting and replacement of fluids and electrolytes lost in watery stools and emesis. Oral rehydration is described in Chapter 8. Rarely, nausea, vomiting, and diarrhea will be so severe that parenteral rehydration is necessary. Infants, the elderly, and the debilitated are most susceptible to complications from common food poisoning.

PIGBEL

Pigbel is a form of necrotizing enterocolitis (enteritis necroticans) caused by *C. perfringens* type C endemic in the Papua New Guinea highlands. The *C. perfringens* bacteria are ingested in contaminated pork and other foods and appear to colonize the intestinal tract of up to 70% of normal villagers.

Rapid intestinal proliferation of *C. perfringens* with production of β toxin follows ingestion of meat and/or other high-protein foods. If a person has inadequate levels of proteases, the β toxin cannot be destroyed and causes necrotizing enterocolitis. Children appear to be especially susceptible to pigbel owing to low levels of intestinal proteases associated with a chronic protein-deficient diet and a low level of immunity to β toxin. A staple of the village diet is sweet potato, which contains trypsin inhibitors and contributes to the problem.

In most cases, cytopathic intestinal damage from β toxin occurs early during *C. perfringens* proliferation. Symptoms of necrotizing enterocolitis (fever, abdominal pain, intestinal obstruction) may not be manifested until several days later, too late for neutralization of β toxin by administration of exogenous antitoxin to ameliorate the clinical course. A pigbel vaccine (Wellcome Labs) employing *C. perfringens* type C β toxoid appeared to offer protection among recipients in trials in the Papua New Guinea highlands, and the incidence of the disease dramatically decreased after vaccine programs during the 1980s. Sporadic cases still occur in Papua New Guinea, and cases of enteritis necroticans have been reported from poor communities in diverse geographic locations in Africa, Central and South America, the western Pacific, and Asia where poor food hygiene coupled with conditions of protein deprivation, staple diets containing trypsin inhibitors, and intermittent meat feasting set the stage for development of disease.

BOTULISM

C. botulinum bacteria produce extremely potent nerve toxins that humans are exposed to through ingestion of improperly preserved food or by absorption of the toxins from *C. botulinum*–contaminated wounds. Patients with botulism develop severe muscle weakness that starts in the head and progresses to the rest of the body, eventually resulting in complete loss of muscle function and the inability to breathe. Cases of food-borne botulism have been associated with a variety of foods, including home-canned foods (especially low-acid foods such as vegetables) and lightly preserved foods such as fermented, salted, or smoked fish and meat products. The foods implicated differ among countries and reflect regional and cultural differences in eating habits and food preservation techniques. Occasionally, commercially canned foods are implicated in botulism outbreaks. Examples of foods associated with botulism outbreaks are low-acid preserved vegetables such as green beans, spinach, mushrooms, beets, potatoes, and bamboo shoots; fish, including canned tuna; and meat products, such as ham, chicken, and sausage.

Etiology

The spore form of *C. botulinum* is commonly found in soils, aquatic sediments, and fish. The spores are heat resistant, but after a heat shock or other stimulus, the spores can germinate and the vegetative-state bacteria will proliferate under anaerobic conditions at a relatively high pH (>4.6), producing toxin. Of the eight immunologically distinct types of *C. botulinum* toxin, types A and B are responsible for most reported cases of food-borne disease, and type E has been associated with smoked fish. Types Cα, Cβ, and D have been isolated from animals, and types F and G are rarely isolated from human cases.

Clinical Presentation

Blurred vision, dysphagia, and dysarthria are common presenting complaints, rather than gastrointestinal symptoms. Symmetric cranial nerve palsies and descending flaccid paralysis of motor and autonomic nerves are the hallmarks of botulism. As the disease progresses, consciousness is maintained and there is no fever. Other causes of neurologic dysfunction that mimic botulism, such as stroke, the Guillain-Barré syndrome, and myasthenia gravis, must be considered and ruled out.

Diagnosis

The diagnosis of botulism is extremely tricky owing to the great variation in time between ingestion of the contaminated food and the onset of diagnostic symptoms. The usual incubation period is 12-48 hours, but symptoms may develop within 2 hours after the ingestion or appear more than a week afterward. A careful food history should be obtained for up to the 2 weeks prior to the development of illness. The presumptive diagnosis is made based on the development of compatible clinical findings, history of exposure to one of the suspect foods, and the elimination of other possible causes of the illness.

Diagnosis of botulism can be confirmed if the suspected food is still available. Toxin in the serum or feces of stricken patients can be detected by bioassay in laboratory animals. The most sensitive and widely accepted assay method for detection of botulinum neurotoxin is the mouse bioassay, which takes 4 days to complete. Rapid and sensitive in vitro detection methods are under development but are not yet available.

Treatment

In illness caused by *C. botulinum* toxin, prompt administration of polyvalent equine antitoxin is indicated as soon as possible after the clinical diagnosis has been made, although respiratory support for severe respiratory muscle weakness may be the most important critical intervention. In 2013, the Food and Drug Administration licensed Botulism Antitoxin Heptavalent (A, B, C, D, E, F, G)-(Equine)(Calgene), which can neutralize all seven of the botulinum nerve toxin serotypes known to cause botulism. Botulism antitoxin (BAT) is distributed in the United States through the Centers for Disease Control and Prevention (CDC) Drug Service. BAT is administered through slow intravenous infusion, which may take several hours; common side effects may include headache, fever, chills, rash, itching, and nausea. The horse serum components of BAT can rarely induce an anaphylactic reaction in the recipient or a delayed hypersensitivity reaction (serum sickness). When providing care to a patient with the presumed diagnosis of botulism, clinicians should contact the CDC to obtain BAT, for guidance on management and treatment, and for assistance with outbreak management, depending on the circumstances of the reported exposure.

Outbreak Management

In identified source outbreaks, contact tracing and publicity through the public health departments may help to prevent additional cases of illness and death. One reported outbreak of botulism in travelers was associated with food served at a restaurant and proved difficult to trace because of the widespread dispersion of the cases in two countries after the common food source was ingested.

An outbreak of botulism associated with home-canned bamboo shoots in northern Thailand in March 2006 illustrated some of the challenges of providing a medical response to a large outbreak. Botulism caused illness in 209 persons, required hospitalization of 134, and required mechanical ventilation in 42. Supplies of *Botulinum* antitoxin sufficient to treat 90 patients (103 vials) eventually were obtained from multiple international donors and commercial sources, but a lack of a pre-arranged emergency plan for global mobilization of the antitoxin resulted in delays of 5-9 days to acquire and deliver the product. There were no deaths in this outbreak, and the ability of Thai authorities to mobilize 42 ventilators and staff to manage the most severely affected patients probably prevented significant mortality in this outbreak, given the unavoidable delay in acquiring the antitoxin.

National and international agencies (CDC in Atlanta, National Laboratory in London, National Institute of Infectious Diseases in Tokyo, World Health Organization in Geneva, etc.) are the best sources for information about available supplies of *Botulinum* antitoxin, but there is no formal predefined protocol for global mobilization of the antitoxin at the time of writing.

Prevention of Botulism

Cooking foods at high temperatures will inactivate the toxin: boiling at 212° F (100° C) for 10 minutes or heating at 176° F (80° C) for 30 minutes. However, the *C. botulinum* spores can survive heating at 212° F (100° C) for several hours. Occasionally, ingested spores will proliferate in the human gastrointestinal tract and liberate enterotoxin that is absorbed by the host, causing symptoms. This latter mechanism is thought to account for long-incubation botulism and for infant botulism.

INFANT BOTULISM

This condition usually occurs in infants <6 months of age and results from inadvertent ingestion of C. botulinum spores, which germinate in the gut, proliferate, and release toxin. Infants with this condition may present with clinical symptoms of constipation, loss of appetite, weakness, altered cry, and loss of head control. Prevention consists of appropriate sterilization of homemade infant formulas. Raw honey contains spores of C. botulinum, and mothers are cautioned to not feed raw honey to their infants.

ADVICE TO TRAVELERS

Travelers are at special risk of food-borne illnesses including food poisoning because of increased exposure to foods prepared outside the home under unknown conditions of preparation and storage. Common advice for prevention of all food-borne illnesses includes selecting food that is freshly prepared, thoroughly cooked, and served piping hot or within 1 hour of preparation. For safety, chicken should be cooked to a temperature above 165°F (74°C), pork above 155°F (68°C), and ground beef above 155°F (68°C): rare or pink meat or poultry should not be consumed. The new instant-read digital food thermometers may be useful for checking the internal temperature of cooked meats and casseroles. Pre-cooked foods served warm or served from chafing dishes should be reheated to over 150°F (66°C) and held at that temperature. Pre-cooked foods served at room temperature, cold foods served in all-day buffets, and baked goods with creamy fillings should be avoided when possible during travel in less-developed areas. Cold foods and leftovers should be refrigerated below 45°F (7°C) until serving. Fermented, salted, or smoked fish and meat products should be avoided in general during travel, unless known to be obtained from reliable sources. Careful selection of food is the only way to avoid food poisoning, as the contaminated food may appear, taste, and smell like safe edible food.

FURTHER RESOURCES

Centers for Disease Control and Prevention, 2009. Clostridium perfringens infection among inmates at a county jail—Wisconsin, August 2008. MMWR 58, 138–141.
A macaroni and beef casserole from a commercial food supplier served for dinner to inmates at a county jail was identified as the most probable cause of nausea, vomiting, and diarrhea among more than 100 inmates. C. perfringens enterotoxin was present in submitted stool specimens and C. perfringens was isolated from a sample of the casserole. Improper food handling, cooking, storage, and reheating of the pre-cooked food were the most probable causes of the food contamination.

Centers for Disease Control and Prevention, 2013. Outbreak of staphylococcal food poisoning from a military unit lunch party—United States, July 2012. MMWR 62, 1026–1028.
A detailed report of the epidemiologic investigation of 22 cases of staphylococcal intoxication associated with improperly prepared and stored food at a lunch party at a military base. Isolation of S. aureus and staphylococcal enterotoxin A in the chicken, sausage, and rice casserole confirmed the diagnosis. Commercially available toxin detection kits for S. aureus and B. cereus are approved to directly test food samples; the test kit for C. perfringens enterotoxin is approved only for testing stool specimens.

Centers for Disease Control and Prevention (CDC), 2015. Surveillance for Foodborne Disease Outbreaks, United States, 2013, Annual Report. US Department of Health and Human Services, CDC, Atlanta, Georgia.
Of approximately 48 million cases of food-borne illnesses per year in the United States, 9.4 million are caused by known pathogens. Food-borne disease outbreaks for the year 2013 are reported by pathogen, food item, where consumed (home, restaurant, institution), and state, and whether hospitalization was required.

Scallon, E., Hoekstra, R.M., Angulo, F.J., et al., 2011. Foodborne illness acquired in the United States—major pathogens. Emerg. Infect. Dis. 17, 7–15.
Analysis and summary of US data from 2005 to 2008. An average of around 1 million cases per year of domestically acquired food-borne illness were caused by C. perfringens, approximately 250,000 cases by S. aureus, and 63,000 cases by B. cereus. There were 55 cases of C. botulinum. For comparison, nontyphoidal

Salmonella *spp. accounted for just over 1 million cases per year. The complexities and challenges of food-borne illness surveillance in the United States are discussed. Data from resource-limited countries are likely to be less complete.*

Sobel, J., Mixter, C.G., Kohe, P., et al., 2005. Necrotizing enterocolitis associated with *Clostridium perfringens* type A in previously health North American adults. J. Am. Coll. Surg. 201, 48–56.
C. perfringens *type A infections may be an unsuspected etiology in adult necrotizing enterocolitis.*

Ungchusak, K., Chunsuttiwat, S., Braden, C.R., et al., 2007. The need for global planned mobilization of essential medicine: lessons from a massive Thai botulism outbreak. Available at <http://www.who.int/bulletin/volumes/85/3/06-39545> (accessed July 26, 2015).
Rapid mobilization of botulism antitoxin for use in a massive international botulism outbreak presented many challenges.

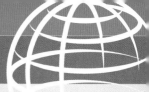

CHAPTER 34

Fish and Shellfish Poisoning: Toxic Syndromes

Elaine C. Jong

Toxic seafoods are causative agents in a number of gastrointestinal and neurologic illnesses. Historically, these illnesses were seen mainly in specific geographic locations, associated with local seafood products and affecting local resident populations. However, that situation has now changed remarkably: ever-increasing growth in international tourism and the global fish market that emerged over the past two decades have contributed to increased cases of seafood intoxication presenting as unfamiliar toxic syndromes among seafood consumers in non-endemic areas far distant from the seafood's place of origin and in returned international travelers. Thus it is important for all healthcare providers, especially emergency medicine personnel and primary care providers worldwide, to become familiar with the clinical presentations, mechanisms of toxicity, and currently accepted treatments for some of the more common seafood intoxications.

The focus of this chapter is on toxic syndromes in humans resulting from the inadvertent ingestion of toxin-contaminated fish or shellfish. Illnesses that may result from bacterial, viral, or parasitic contamination of food and water are discussed in Chapters 8, 22, 23, and 31-33.

Marine biotoxins are acquired by small herbivorous fish that eat algae; they are concentrated in the skin, musculature, and viscera (i.e., ichthyosarcotoxic), in the reproductive organs (i.e., ichthyotoxic), or in the blood (ichthyohemotoxic). Big carnivorous fish eat the little fish, and the toxin is conserved in increasing concentrations moving up the food chain. Of the nine kinds of ichthyosarcotoxism (based on types of fish), the most important are scombroid, ciguatera, and puffer fish (tetrodotoxin) poisoning. Botulism toxin E intoxication is briefly covered as part of the differential diagnosis of fish poisoning syndromes and is considered in Chapter 33.

Shellfish acquire marine biotoxins from filter feeding on algae. Four major toxic syndromes associated with bivalve mollusk consumption are major health and economic concerns: paralytic shellfish poisoning, neurotoxic shellfish poisoning, diarrhetic shellfish poisoning, and amnesic shellfish poisoning.

A patient's history of a specific seafood ingestion is crucial to establishing the diagnosis of fish or shellfish poisoning. Often patients will not easily recall the inciting meal, as in most cases there is no uniformly reliable appearance, smell, or taste that distinguishes contaminated seafood prior to ingestion and development of symptoms.

SCOMBROID FISH POISONING

Scombroid poisoning is the name given to the histamine-like reaction that occasionally results from the ingestion of improperly cooled and stored tuna and related species in the family Scombridae. These dark-meat fish include the skipjack tuna (*Euthynnus pelamis*), the bonito (*Sarda sarda*), the mackerel (*Scomber scombrus*), and the albacore (*Thunnus alalunga*). A nonscombroid fish, mahi-mahi (*Coryphaena hippurus*), can also become toxic and is actually

451

a commonly implicated fish in scombroid outbreaks in the United States. The Centers for Disease Control and Prevention reported two outbreaks of scombroid fish poisoning in late 2006, one in Louisiana and one in Tennessee. Both outbreaks were associated with tuna steaks imported from Indonesia and Vietnam, but consumed in Louisiana and Tennessee, respectively.

Fish become toxic after being caught, when inadequate cooling during transport and storage allows for bacterial proliferation. These bacteria (primarily *Morganella morganii* but also other bacteria such as *Escherichia*, *Proteus*, *Salmonella*, and *Shigella* species) degrade histidine present in the musculature of the fish to heat-stable histamine and a histamine-like substance termed saurine. Studies suggest that most symptoms are due to saurine, as histamine when given orally is poorly absorbed and chemically inactivated in the gastrointestinal tract. An exception may occur in patients treated with isoniazid for tuberculosis, as this medication inhibits histaminase in the gut and may make patients more susceptible to the histamine contained in scombrotoxic fish, thus accentuating the symptoms and signs of scombroid poisoning.

Scombrotoxic fish usually appear normal, but toxicity should be suspected if the fish tastes "peppery or sharp." *Within 30 minutes of ingestion of a toxic fish, a systemic histamine-like reaction occurs.* Symptoms and signs include headache, flushing, a burning or peppery taste in the mouth, abdominal cramps with nausea, vomiting, diarrhea, tachycardia, dry mouth, and occasionally urticaria, angioedema, and bronchospasm. Symptoms are transient, rarely lasting over 8-12 hours, and deaths are unusual. Diagnosis is clinical but can be confirmed by measuring the histamine content of the suspected fish, which is generally 20 mg/100 g of fish muscle, or higher (normal histamine content is <1 mg/100 g of fish muscle). Treatment consists of forced emesis and antihistamines. In addition to diphenhydramine (Benadryl), treatment with histamine-2 antagonists such as cimetidine (300 mg intravenous [IV]) or ranitidine (50 mg IV) may provide symptomatic relief. If symptoms are severe, the patient may require IV fluids, antiinflammatory steroids, aminophylline, and epinephrine as used for anaphylaxis-like reactions.

Prevention consists of storing the fish at less than 40° F (4.4° C) at all times between catching and consumption, according to food-safety recommendations.

CIGUATERA FISH POISONING

Ciguatera poisoning presents with acute gastrointestinal and neurologic symptoms following the ingestion of normally edible reef fish that contain ciguatoxins produced by the unicellular marine dinoflagellate *Gambierdiscus toxicus*. Most outbreaks occur in the Caribbean, the Indo-Pacific islands, and the Indian Ocean between 35° North and 35° South latitude. Although more than 425 species of fish are known to be occasionally toxic, the more commonly implicated fish include the barracuda (Sphyraenidae), red snapper (*Lutjanus bohar*), grouper, amberjack (*Seriola dumerili*), sea bass (Serranidae), surgeonfish (Acanthuridae), and moray eel (Muraenidae). Previously, ciguatera poisoning was rarely reported outside local communities within the endemic tropical latitudes; however, increasing numbers of cases are being seen in nontropical countries as the number of international tourists grows each year, and unwary travelers who ingested contaminated fish in endemic areas return home with persistent symptoms. Ciguatera poisoning has become a world health issue as reef fish caught in ciguatera-endemic areas are exported to distant non-endemic areas.

Ciguatoxin (gambiertoxin) is a nonprotein polyether toxin with water-soluble and lipid-soluble fractions. The toxins and their metabolites are accumulated in the musculature, liver, and viscera of herbivorous fish and are concentrated in the food chain when carnivorous fish feed on the smaller herbivorous fish. The toxins become more polar as they undergo oxidative metabolism and pass up the food chain. Increasing polarity of the toxin is associated with increased toxicity, and humans are exposed at the end of the food chain.

The main Pacific ciguatoxin (P-CTX-1) causes ciguatera poisoning at levels of 0.1 mcg/kg or higher in the flesh of carnivorous fish, whereas the main Caribbean ciguatoxin (C-CTX-1) is less polar and 10-fold less toxic than P-CTX-1. Ciguatoxin induces partial membrane depolarization by enhancing sodium ion permeability in voltage-dependent sodium channels in nerve cell membranes. A recent report suggests that the ciguatoxins and brevetoxin (involved in neurotoxic shellfish poisoning) may have a potent effect on TRPV1 channels, modulating thermal and pain sensation.

Ciguatoxins are not affected by heating, freezing, or drying, and toxic fish have normal taste, texture, and odor. *Symptoms develop 2-6 hours following ingestion of the fish* and last about 1 week but occasionally can extend for months or even years. Typically, patients develop gastrointestinal symptoms such as nausea, watery diarrhea, abdominal cramps, or vomiting. Persistent bradycardia lasting several days has also been reported. Distal paresthesias are common, and the teeth may feel numb or loose. A majority of victims note an unusual hot-cold sensory reversal, in which cold objects "burn" when handled. Asthenia and arthralgias are frequent, and 10-45% of patients develop pruritus, usually 1-3 days after fish ingestion. Erythematous skin rashes that may blister or desquamate can occur in up to 20% of patients. In severe instances, ataxia, paresis, paralysis, or transient blindness occurs, often in association with sinus bradycardia and hypotension. Deaths are generally the result of respiratory depression, coma, and convulsions.

Diagnosis is made clinically but can be verified by assaying for the toxin in the implicated fish, using a bioassay (mouse, cat, mongoose, or brine shrimp), an enzyme-linked immunosorbent assay, or a radioimmunoassay.

Treatment is supportive and consists of forced emesis, IV fluids if volume is depleted, and respiratory support if indicated. IV mannitol (1 gm/kg) was reported to ameliorate neurologic symptoms when given acutely, but subsequent studies did not confirm its efficacy. Other drugs that have been anecdotally reported to give symptomatic relief are amitriptyline (50 mg/day), tocainide (400 mg three times a day), and nifedipine (10 mg three times a day). Another published report described successful treatment of ciguatera poisoning symptoms with gabapentin, a drug structurally related to gamma-aminobutyric acid and usually employed as an antiepileptic or for treatment of chronic pain. Treatment with gabapentin, 400 mg orally three times daily for up to 5 weeks, was reported to relieve neurologic symptoms, pruritus, and sharp, shooting pains in the legs associated with ciguatera poisoning, even though treatment was initiated 1 month after the onset of symptoms.

PUFFER FISH POISONING (TETRODOTOXIN POISONING)

Puffer fish, porcupine fish, ocean sunfishes, and related species in the order Tetraodontiformes are frequently poisonous and may produce a severe neurologic illness following ingestion. This is a particular problem in Japan, Taiwan, and Southeast Asia where puffer fish (*fugu*) is a culinary delicacy. The intoxication has been rarely reported in the United States.

The toxicity is due to the accumulation of tetrodotoxin in the ovaries, liver, intestines, and, to a lesser extent, the musculature of the fish. The toxin is believed to originate from something the puffer fish ingests, but attempts to implicate specific species of algae, jellyfish, sponges, and so forth have not been definitive. A clear correlation does exist, however, between the reproductive season of the puffer fish and its likelihood of being poisonous.

Tetrodotoxin is a nonprotein aminohydroquinazoline compound with a heterocyclic structure. It is water-soluble and heat-resistant and does not alter the taste or appearance of the fish. It appears to be similar, if not identical, to tarichatoxin, present in the California newt, and also to a toxin present in the skin of *Atelopus* frogs in Costa Rica. Physiologically, tetrodotoxin is similar to saxitoxin and (see below) prevents the generation of action potentials by blocking the voltage-sensitive sodium channels in the membranes of nerves and muscle, but it has no effect on potassium conductance.

Most patients experience *signs and symptoms of tetrodotoxin poisoning within 6 hours of ingestion, but a few have experienced a delayed onset of up to 20 hours.* Signs and symptoms include profuse sweating and salivation, hypothermia, headache, tachycardia, and hypotension. Gastrointestinal symptoms of nausea, vomiting, diarrhea, or abdominal pain may or may not be present. The hallmark of puffer fish poisoning is neurologic: paresthesias that frequently progress to numbness, ataxia, tremor, and paralysis involving both cranial and peripheral nerves. Respiratory compromise and cardiac arrhythmias may result. Occasional patients have complete flaccid paralysis with absent corneal reflexes and dilated pupils but maintain consciousness; these patients require ventilatory support including intubation and mechanical ventilation. Mortality may reach 60%, but the prognosis is good with eventual full recovery if the patient survives the first 24 hours.

Diagnosis is made on clinical grounds. There is no effective antidote. If the patient is seen within 3 hours of ingestion, gastric lavage with 2 L of 2% sodium bicarbonate, followed by instillation of activated charcoal in 70% sorbitol solution, may help to remove toxin from the gastrointestinal tract. Patients require supportive care with special attention to the pulmonary status. Serial vital capacity tests should be done, and early intubation is recommended if there is evidence of inadequate ventilation. There are anecdotal reports of improvement with edrophonium, pralidoxime, and atropine.

Attempts in Japan to prevent the disease have included the requirement of a special license for both restaurants and cooks wishing to serve puffer fish. Only the musculature of the puffer fish can be served and that only during the nonreproductive season (winter months), when the fish are least likely to be toxic. Recreational fishermen in Asian and Southeast Asian waters should be educated as to the identification and potential toxicity of puffer fish and related species.

BOTULISM TOXIN E

Clostridium botulinum bacteria secreting botulism toxin type E have been reported as contaminants of improperly processed or smoked fish and fish eggs. Approximately 24-36 hours after ingestion of contaminated seafood, gastrointestinal symptoms may develop, followed in 3-7 days by cranial nerve dysfunction and symmetric descending weakness. The botulism toxin E blocks acetylcholine release at the neuromuscular junction. The diagnosis is made by clinical presentation and a history of eating preserved fish or fish eggs. Treatment consists of supportive care; heptavalent botulism antitoxin obtained from the CDC should be administered as soon as possible (Chapter 33).

PARALYTIC SHELLFISH POISONING

An unusual neurologic disorder that may follow shellfish ingestion is termed paralytic shellfish poisoning. The disease is primarily associated with the consumption of bivalve mollusks, such as clams, mussels, and oysters, but has also been reported following ingestion of gastropods, chitons, starfish, and crustaceans. Crab, abalone, and fin fish do not appear to be affected. The disease is mainly restricted to temperate climates, with most reported outbreaks in North America, Europe, and Japan, although cases have also occurred in South Africa, Papua New Guinea, and New Zealand.

The toxicity of paralytic shellfish poisoning is due to the accumulation of saxitoxin, a tetrahydropurine base, and related compounds in the shellfish. It does not affect the appearance or taste of the marine mollusks, nor is it effectively inactivated by cooking. Like tetrodotoxin, it blocks action potential generation by preventing sodium ion flow in nerve and muscle cell membranes.

Saxitoxin originates in a unicellular dinoflagellate known as *Gonyaulax*. Since bivalve mollusks are filter feeders, they concentrate the toxins from *Gonyaulax* in their digestive glands (the hepatopancreas). In the Alaska butter clam (*Saxidomus*), the saxitoxin is concentrated in the siphon as well. Toxicity of shellfish correlates with the bloom of this dinoflagellate, known colloquially as "red tide" due to discoloration of coastal waters. Along the Pacific Coast these usually occur between May and October. Toxicity lessens as the dinoflagellate population decreases, but complete detoxification of shellfish may take up to a year.

Symptoms usually occur within 30 minutes after ingestion of contaminated shellfish and include distal and oral paresthesias that may progress to numbness. A sensation of "floating," gross incoordination, and paralysis with respiratory compromise may develop. The case fatality rate is 8.5%.

Diagnosis is clinical, and treatment is supportive, as with other fish poisonings. Suspect shellfish can be analyzed in a mouse bioassay. Toxic shellfish have more than 4 MU (mouse unit)/g wet flesh (1 MU of saxitoxin is the amount that kills a 20-g mouse 15 minutes following intraperitoneal injection of a heated acid extract of the shellfish). Increasing application of liquid chromatography-mass spectrometry methods for the detection of marine biotoxins in seafood safety and surveillance programs will allow for faster analysis of toxic samples.

Prevention of paralytic shellfish poisoning requires public health measures, with routine surveillance and prompt closure of any beach to shellfish collecting when toxic levels of saxitoxin are detected. A Shellfish Safety Hotline (1-800-562-5632) gives information 24 hours a day on harmful algal blooms on Pacific Ocean beaches in Washington state; Oregon maintains its own hotline (1-800-449-2474).

NEUROTOXIC SHELLFISH POISONING (NONPARALYTIC)

Neurotoxic shellfish poisoning affects people who eat mollusks from red tides off the Florida coast. The contaminated shellfish contain brevetoxin from the dinoflagellate *Ptychodiscus brevis* in the red tides. About 1-6 hours after ingestion of contaminated shellfish, the affected person will experience paresthesias, reversal of hot and cold temperature sensation, ataxia, nausea, vomiting, and diarrhea. As mentioned above, both ciguatoxins and brevetoxin may act on TRPV1 channels in nerve cell membranes, affecting thermal and pain sensation. Treatment is symptomatic and supportive. When the toxin is aerosolized in rough surf, exposed people can develop a syndrome consisting of conjunctivitis, rhinorrhea, and a nonproductive cough.

DIARRHETIC SHELLFISH POISONING

Diarrhetic shellfish poisoning can occur in people *hours to days after ingesting contaminated mussels*. A published report of a large outbreak of diarrhetic shellfish poisoning in 2000 involving 120 people in northern Greece who ate mussels harvested from the Adriatic Sea following algal blooms illustrates the international scope of shellfish poisoning outbreaks. Mussels, like other bivalves, are filter feeders and can acquire okadaic acid, a dinophysistoxin-1 from toxic dinoflagellate algae, *Dinophysis acuminata*. The syndrome is characterized by nausea, vomiting, diarrhea, and cramps. Treatment is symptomatic and supportive.

AMNESIC SHELLFISH POISONING

Amnesic shellfish poisoning (domoic acid poisoning, mussel poisoning) is a toxic encephalopathy first described among people who ate contaminated mussels from cultivated beds in Prince Edward Island, Canada in 1989. The mussels contained domoic acid, a marine toxin produced by a marine diatom *Nitzschia pungens*. Environmental factors that favor the proliferation of the algae around certain marine areas allow the toxin to be accumulated by shellfish. Since the original syndrome was described, domoic acid has been detected periodically in razor clams and Dungeness crabs from the Olympic Peninsula in Washington state.

Domoic acid is related structurally to the excitatory amino acid neurotransmitter glutamate. Gastrointestinal symptoms (nausea, vomiting, abdominal cramps, and diarrhea) occur within 24 hours after the toxic ingestion, and neurologic symptoms (headache, seizures, hemiparesis, ophthalmoplegia, abnormal state of arousal ranging from agitation to coma, and antegrade memory loss) become manifest within 48 hours after the ingestion. In the Canadian outbreak, the gastrointestinal symptoms resolved after a day or two. However, after initial widespread neurologic dysfunction, the survivors had persistence of memory deficits and motor neuropathy. Treatment is symptomatic and supportive.

FURTHER READING

Bagnis, R., Kuberski, T., Langier, S., 1979. Clinical observations on 3009 cases of ciguatera fish poisoning in the South Pacific. Am. J. Trop. Med. Hyg. 28, 1067–1073.
A foundation paper, presenting a comprehensive analysis of ciguatera fish poisoning in the South Pacific.

Centers for Disease Control and Prevention, 2007. Scombroid fish poisoning associated with tuna steaks—Louisiana and Tennessee, 2006. MMWR 56, 817–819.
The tuna steaks originated in Asia but were ingested in Louisiana and Tennessee.

Centers for Disease Control and Prevention, 2013. Ciguatera fish poisoning-New York City, 2010–2011. MMWR 62, 61–65.
A report on six outbreaks and a single case of ciguatera fish poisoning involving a total of 28 people in the New York City area. Persons who became ill had eaten tropical reef fish in metropolitan NYC restaurants or had purchased the fish in area fish markets and supermarkets. Mislabeling, incorrect labeling, or misidentification of the fish and lack of recognition of the ciguatera fish poisoning syndrome by clinicians who were consulted contributed to a delay in diagnosis and in timely outbreak detection and notification.

Cuypers, E., Yanagihara, A., Rainier, J.D., et al., 2007. TRPV as a key determinant in ciguatera and neurotoxic shellfish poisoning. Biochem. Biophys. Res. Commun. 361, 214–217.
Research directed toward understanding the physiology of ciguatera (ciguatoxin) and neurotoxic shellfish poisoning (brevetoxin); transient receptor potential channels are a large group of ion channels located on plasma membranes and are calcium ion selective.

Economou, V., Papadopoulou, C., Brett, M., et al., 2007. Diarrheic shellfish poisoning due to toxic mussel consumption: the first recorded outbreak in Greece. Food Addit. Contam. 24, 297–305.
The mussels were harvested following an algal bloom in the Adriatic Sea.

How, C.K., Chern, C.H., Huang, Y.C., et al., 2003. Tetrodotoxin poisoning. Am. J. Emerg. Med. 21, 51–54.
Approach to treating puffer fish poisoning in the emergency department.

Hung, Y.M., Hung, S.Y., Chou, K.J., et al., 2005. Short report: persistent bradycardia caused by ciguatoxin poisoning after barracuda fish eggs ingestion in southern Taiwan. Am. J. Trop. Med. Hyg. 73, 1026–1027.

Johnson, R., Jong, E.C., 1983. Ciguatera: Caribbean and Indo-Pacific fish poisoning. West. J. Med. 138, 872–874.
A case of ciguatera in a returned Northwest traveler that was acquired in the Caribbean and caused persistent hot-cold reversal.

Perl, T.M., Bedard, L., Kosatsky, T., et al., 1990. An outbreak of toxic encephalopathy caused by eating mussels contaminated with domoic acid. N. Engl. J. Med. 322, 1775–1780.
Original medical report on the outbreak of mussel poisoning in Halifax, Nova Scotia that led to the discovery of amnesic shellfish poisoning.

Teitelbaum, J.S., Zatone, R.J., Carpenter, S., et al., 1990. Neurologic sequelae of domoic acid intoxication due to ingestion of contaminated mussels. N. Engl. J. Med. 322, 1781–1787.
Survivors of the original outbreak of amnesic shellfish poisoning were left with permanent neurologic sequelae.

CHAPTER 35

Approach to Tropical Dermatology

Andrea Kalus

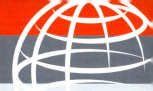

Travelers to tropical locations often encounter skin problems. They are among the top three reasons returning travelers seek medical care. Many of the skin diseases common in the tropics are also common in temperate climates, although they may be modified by factors related to climate, geography, and socioeconomic conditions.

In studies of returning travelers with cutaneous diseases, the most common conditions, in decreasing order of frequency, are cutaneous larva migrans (Chapter 37), pyodermas (Chapter 36), arthropod-induced dermatitis (such as scabies), myiasis, tungiasis (Chapter 37), and cutaneous leishmaniasis (Chapter 39). In addition to infectious skin problems the harsh environment of the tropics can also affect the skin through environmental factors, including increased heat and humidity as in miliaria, increased exposure to solar radiation (Chapter 36), biting arthropods, and exposure to new contact allergens and/or irritants (Chapter 36).

Some of the cutaneous diseases common among travelers to tropical areas, and endemic in local populations, are considered "neglected diseases." Scant comprehensive data exist about their prevalence, and there is little research comparing the relative efficacy of treatment options. Diagnosis in travelers' home countries can also be difficult because of the relative rarity of these diseases outside the tropical environment.

The evaluation of cutaneous lesions acquired in the tropics should follow general dermatologic principles, but with appropriate consideration of unique tropical disease etiologies. This chapter focuses on the basic approach to the patient with skin disease in or having returned from the tropics. A primer on topical therapy is also included.

CLINICAL APPROACH

The evaluation of the patient with a chief complaint of skin lesions or rash should include a systematic approach with physical examination, history, and appropriate diagnostic tests. In contrast to most general medical providers, dermatologists rely mostly on visual inspection of the skin, noting primary lesion morphology and distribution. History and laboratory tests are often used to confirm a specific diagnosis or narrow a differential diagnosis made from physical examination.

The examination of the skin should be performed in good light. Whenever possible, the entire skin surface should be examined, including the hair, scalp, nails, and mucous membranes. In certain instances, it may also be important to examine the patient for lymphadenopathy and organomegaly.

A precise description of findings allows the rash to be categorized into general groups, limiting diagnostic possibilities. *Primary* changes— those directly due to the disease process— should be distinguished from *secondary* changes, which are modifications occurring over time as the result of external factors, such as rubbing, scratching, or superimposed bacterial infection. Secondary changes include scale, crusts, excoriations, and lichenification. The common types of primary lesions are defined as in **Box 35.1**.

457

Box 35.1   Common types of primary lesions

- *Macules* are focal alterations in skin color <10 mm in diameter without any change in texture or thickness
- *Patches* are similar nonpalpable color changes >10 mm in diameter
- *Papules* are solid elevated lesions <10 mm in diameter
- *Plaques* are solid elevations >10 mm in diameter
- *Nodules* are solid masses located more deeply within the skin and can be of any size
- *Vesicles* are clear, fluid-filled blisters <5 mm in diameter
- *Bullae* are clear, fluid-filled blisters >5 mm in diameter
- *Pustules* are filled with opaque purulent material
- *Erosions* are shallow depressions with loss of partial or full thickness epidermis; may be a ruptured vesicle
- *Ulcers* are deeper areas of epithelial loss, into the dermis or even the fat
- *Scale* is visible accumulation of stratum corneum and may be a primary or secondary change.

Important points of the history include a list of countries visited, duration of time in each location, whether urban or rural areas were visited, and information about specific activities (e.g., fishing, camping). Specific details about the skin problem should include a description of the onset and evolution of the lesions, associated symptoms, and all forms of treatment used, including nonprescription treatment. A history of antecedent trauma, insect bite, suspected precipitating factors, exposure to animals, similar rash in companions, and personal or family history of similar or other skin disease should be explored.

Diagnostic tests are often needed to supplement physical diagnosis. These include Gram stain, mineral oil test for scabies, potassium hydroxide (KOH) examination, and skin biopsy. The KOH examination is a quick, easy, and inexpensive test in the diagnosis of fungal infections. The technique is discussed with dermatophyte infections (Chapter 38). Gram stain is invaluable for diagnosis of bacterial and some fungal (e.g., *Pityrosporum*) skin infections.

Skin biopsy may be necessary in certain cases to establish the diagnosis. An established lesion without manipulation should be selected to minimize secondary changes. The skin should be prepared with antiseptic and anesthetized with lidocaine. Most dermatologists use 3- or 4-mm biopsy punches, but an incisional biopsy is also appropriate, particularly for deep lesions. Many dermatologists elect to close the biopsy wound with non-absorbable suture, although that is not absolutely necessary. If an unusual infectious agent is suspected, it is important to notify the pathologist so that special stains can be done on the skin biopsy specimen. A separate biopsy can be sent to the microbiology laboratory in a sterile container or microbiology collection tube for bacterial and fungal culture. Increasingly, molecular biology tools such as polymerase chain reaction are used to identify infectious etiologies, and these tests can be performed on biopsy specimens.

GENERAL DERMATOLOGIC TREATMENTS

Specific therapy for dermatologic diseases requires a specific diagnosis and is discussed with each disease entity in other chapters. Two aspects of dermatologic therapy, compresses and topical steroids, are discussed here.

Compresses are used to provide nonspecific relief in inflammatory dermatoses and to gently lift crust from weeping lesions. Compresses are made of several layers of cotton cloth such as tea towels that are soaked in a solution and partially wrung out. The active ingredient in most solutions used for compresses is water, although bacteriostatic or drying agents,

TABLE 35.1	Topical Steroid Strength Groups
Low potency	Hydrocortisone 1% cream or ointment
	Desonide 0.05% cream or ointment
Medium potency	Triamcinolone acetonide 0.1% cream or ointment
	Fluocinolone 0.01% cream or solution, 0.025% ointment
	Mometasone 0.1% cream or ointment
High potency	Fluocinonide 0.05% cream or ointment
	Clobetasol 0.05% cream or ointment
	Desoximetasone 0.25% cream or ointment

such as aluminum acetate (Burow solution), are frequently added. The compress is placed on the lesion and left in place for 10-15 minutes, then removed, soaked, wrung out, and replaced. The brief time on the lesion allows evaporative cooling and removes some exudate. The compress should be applied repeatedly for 15-20 minutes several times a day, more often for exudative lesions. Wet dressings should not be left on the skin for long periods, since they may macerate surrounding healthy tissue.

Topical steroids are highly effective agents for reducing the cutaneous immune response and are widely used in treating inflammatory conditions. A large number of products are available, varying greatly in potency and potential to produce side effects. In addition, different vehicles are available, including creams, ointments, lotions, solutions, gels, and sprays. It is convenient to know products of low, medium, and high potency in either cream or ointment form. Low-potency steroids are used in those areas most susceptible to topical steroid side effects: the face, axillae, groin, and genitals. Side effects of topical steroids include atrophy, telangiectasia, striae, and steroid-induced rosacea. Medium-potency steroids are used for most other body locations, except for severe or refractory conditions, which are treated with high-potency steroids.

In general, the drier the skin condition, the more hydrophobic the topical steroid vehicle should be. In descending order of greasiness are ointments, creams, lotions, and solutions. Gels, sprays, and solutions are essentially equivalent in their low or no oil content. Solutions are useful for scalp involvement. **Table 35.1** provides a simplified list of steroid preparations in each potency class.

Knowing the quantity of topical steroid to prescribe is also useful. Topical steroids should be applied sparingly in a thin layer and are usually dosed twice daily. A dose of 30 g of an agent is usually enough to cover an average adult's total body surface area once. Based on this amount, one can roughly estimate a desired quantity to prescribe. Container sizes typically are 15, 30, 60, 120, and 240 g; 1-lb and 1-kg sizes are available in some formulations. Prescribing large quantities with refills of high-potency topical steroids is not recommended.

FURTHER READING

Freedberg, I.M., Eisen, A.Z., Wolff, K., et al., 2003. Fitzpatrick's Dermatology in General Medicine, fifth ed. McGraw-Hill, New York.

Tyring, S.K., Lupi, O., Hengge, U.R., 2005. Tropical Dermatology. Elsevier, New York.

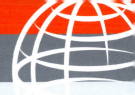

CHAPTER 36

Acute Skin Reactions and Bacterial Infections

Ellen Thompson and Andrea Kalus

Acute skin reactions are often symptomatic and account for many of the skin-related complaints of travelers. Sunburn and other ultraviolet (UV) light reactions, bacterial infections, medication-related rashes, dermatitis, and insect bites and stings are all common. These occur with brief exposure to environmental hazards or drugs. In many cases, they can be prevented.

SUNBURN AND OTHER ULTRAVIOLET LIGHT REACTIONS

The intensity of UV radiation from the sun is related to season, latitude, and time of day. The amount of UV light reaching the earth's surface is greater in the tropics. This can lead to *sunburn* or *photosensitive drug eruptions* or unmask or aggravate *photosensitive diseases*, such as solar urticaria, polymorphous light eruption, porphyria, discoid and systemic lupus erythematosus, and dermatomyositis. A number of medications when combined with UV light in vivo can cause photosensitive drug eruptions (see **Table 36.1**). UV light can also trigger recurrent *herpes simplex*. Over the long term, UV exposure promotes premature skin aging and skin cancer.

Etiology

Sunburn is chiefly caused by UVB radiation (290-320 nm), while photoaging and sun-related skin cancers is attributed to UVA radiation (320-400 nm). UVA also penetrates most glass, such as untreated windows of vehicles. Individual tolerance to sun exposure is a function of skin pigmentation, genetic ability to synthesize melanin in response to UV light, and metabolic and pharmacologic factors.

Prevention

Avoidance of the sun is the ultimate protection against UV-induced conditions. The highest intensity of light occurs between 10 a.m. and 4 p.m., so limiting UV exposure during this period is helpful. Brimmed hats, long-sleeved shirts, and long pants can cover the largest areas of exposed skin. Lightweight, UV-protectant clothing designed for hot weather is available at most sporting goods stores. Sunglasses with UV-protectant lenses will limit sun-related effects on the eyes, which can sometimes go unnoticed. Sunglasses without UV protection, meanwhile, can contribute to increased sun damage to the eyes.

When shading exposed areas is not possible, sunscreen can be used to protect the skin. Choose a product with a sun protection factor (SPF) of 30 and look for sunscreens labeled as "broad spectrum." This indicates they provide protection against both UVA and UVB wavelengths. Products may be labeled "water resistant" for either 40 or 80 minutes but then lose effectiveness. Optimal protection requires application 15-20 minutes before sun exposure. The product should be applied liberally; 1 ounce is recommended for a full-body application. The average person uses less than half of the recommended amount to achieve the advertised protection. Reapplication during the day is necessary to maintain protection, particularly after swimming or perspiring heavily. Lip protection against UV light can be provided with specially formulated lip sunscreens.

TABLE 36.1   Drug Eruption Patterns

Reaction Type	Onset	Features	Common Causes
Exanthematous (maculopapular)	About a week after introduction of a new drug	Most common, starts on the trunk with centrifugal spread. Often accompanied by low fever, pruritus. Resolves in 1-2 weeks.	Antibiotics: penicillins, cephalosporins, sulfamethoxazole NSAIDs, some anti-epileptics, among many others
Photosensitive	3-6 h after sun exposure; phototoxic within 1 day of exposure; photoallergic	Sun-exposed distribution with sharp outlines. Naturally shaded areas spared (upper eyelids and below chin and nose). May appear as exaggerated sunburn or vesicular rash.	*Antibiotics*: quinolones, sulfonamides, tetracyclines (esp. doxycycline), trimethoprim Antimalarials: chloroquine, quinine, quinidine. Antifungals: griseofulvin Antiemetics: prochlorperazine Diuretics: furosemide, thiazide NSAIDs Amiodarone Sunscreens: PABA, oxybenzone
Urticaria (hives), angioedema, anaphylaxis	Initial reaction appears in days, but repeated exposure shortens the onset to minutes to hours	Ranges in severity from urticarial to life-threatening angioedema (compromising airway) or anaphylaxis	Antibiotics (especially penicillins), NSAIDs, blood products, opioids/anesthetics, antifungals (fluconazole and ketoconazole); radiocontrast; vaccines containing egg protein; pollen vaccines; ACE inhibitors

ACE, Angiotensin converting enzyme; *NSAIDs*, nonsteroidal anti-inflammatory drugs; *PABA*, para-aminobenzoic acid.

Broad-spectrum coverage can be achieved by including complementary chemicals that absorb UVA and UVB light and/or by physical agents such as zinc oxide or titanium dioxide, which scatter UVA and UVB light. UVA protection is provided by avobenzone and oxybenzone, among other chemicals. UVB protection is provided by aminobenzoic acid, homosalate, octisalate, and octinoxate. Sun blocks often combine these chemicals and/or include titanium dioxide and zinc oxide to provide broad-spectrum coverage. Newer broad-spectrum agents are now available, such as Mexoryl. Some caution should be used with spray sunscreen. Dispersion by wind and failure to rub in sprayed product may lead to less photoprotection than is provided by traditional lotions (**Fig. 36.1**). Accidental inhalation of sprayed products presents another risk.

Self-tanning products (spray or creams) do not impact melanin synthesis and provide no sun protection. Pre-travel tanning is not recommended. It provides only minimal protection and can actually increase overall UV exposure.

Treatment

Sunburn treatment options are directed at symptom control and are minimally effective. The most important first step after a burn is to limit further UV exposure through implementing above-mentioned prevention methods of sun avoidance and sun protection.

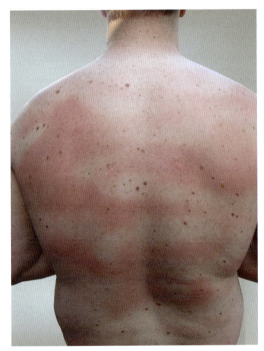

Fig. 36.1 Geographic sunburn after inadequate application of a spray sunscreen. (Courtesy of Corrine Hecht, MD.)

Mild sunburn is treated with nonsteroidal anti-inflammatory drugs and cool compresses, topical calamine, or aloe-based gels. Topical steroids have not demonstrated effectiveness in trials even though they are sometimes recommended.

Severe sunburn often does not respond to the aforementioned measures. Though not commercially available in the United States, topical indomethacin or diclofenac has been reported to be effective in reducing erythema and tenderness when applied soon after exposure. While prednisone seems to be ineffective at lessening the cutaneous sequelae of sunburn, it may improve the systemic symptoms of fever and headache that can occur with severe sunburn. Brief treatment with 40-60 mg/day for 3-4 days may be used.

DERMATITIS IN TRAVELERS

Dermatitis is a general term for superficial inflammation of the skin and can be further classified according to etiology and clinical features. Common types include atopic dermatitis, contact dermatitis, nummular dermatitis, seborrheic dermatitis, and hand or dyshidrotic dermatitis.

Contact dermatitis is responsible for the majority of new onset dermatitis in travelers. Contact dermatitis is further divided into irritant and allergic etiologies. *Irritant contact dermatitis* occurs on contact with an agent capable of causing injury and inflammation in most, if not all, people. *Allergic contact dermatitis* occurs in sensitized individuals (e.g., poison ivy or oak).

Etiology

Irritant contact dermatitis is caused by soaps, solvents, detergents, cleansers, cutting oils, and acid or alkaline solutions. Excessive hand washing is an example of chronic irritant contact dermatitis caused by soaps and frequent wetting of the skin. Individual susceptibility to any irritant varies greatly.

Allergic contact dermatitis can result from exposure to an enormous array of chemical compounds but requires specific sensitization. The most common sensitizers include nickel, fragrances, rubber, formaldehyde, paraphenylenediamine, ethylenediamine, and neomycin. It is important to remember that many products sold for use on the skin contain sensitizers such as neomycin, benzocaine, ethylenediamine, fragrances, and lanolin.

Some topical agents can act in concert with UV light to produce *photocontact dermatitis*. This includes fragrances and, ironically, sunscreen agents, such as PABA and oxybenzone, which can cause photosensitive reactions.

Plant dermatitis (*phytodermatitis*) is a subset of contact dermatitis of particular importance to those traveling to rural areas. Many plants in a number of different families produce sensitizing chemicals. Poison ivy, poison oak, and poison sumac are members of the family Anacardiaceae and produce a resin capable of sensitizing 70% of the population. Related plants containing cross-reacting chemicals include the Japanese lacquer tree (*Rhus verniciflua*), the India marking nut tree, raw cashew shells (*Anacardium occidentale*), mango rind (*Mangifera indica*), and the fruit of the ginkgo (*Ginkgo biloba*). Causes of plant dermatitis depend on the local flora. Mango dermatitis is the most common plant dermatitis in Hawaii. Philodendron is the most common cause in India. Primrose is a frequent sensitizer in Europe.

Phytophotodermatitis is a sun-induced plant dermatitis. Celery, limes, lemons, parsley, figs, and others contain natural psoralens that can incite a phototoxic reaction when contact with these plants is followed by sun exposure. Cases of systemic phototoxicity after ingestion of these plants followed by UV exposure have been reported.

Clinical Features

The primary lesions of dermatitis are erythematous papules and vesicles. In severe cases, bullae form and papules coalesce into plaques. Chronic lesions show scale, secondary changes of lichenification, and, sometimes, bacterial superinfection. Pruritus is a constant feature of dermatitis. Contact dermatitis is distributed in sites of contact. The thicker skin of the palm and soles is more resistant. Allergic reactions may be spread with the hands to other sites of the body, such as the face, eyelids, and genitals. Plant dermatitis classically shows linear blisters where the skin brushed against the causative plant.

Diagnosis

Dermatitis is usually diagnosed clinically. Establishing the cause of contact dermatitis requires a careful history on exposure to plants, soaps, chemicals, topical medications, and the activities associated with the dermatitis. Patch testing is invaluable in establishing the etiology of allergic contact dermatitis.

Differential diagnosis of dermatitis includes scabies, insect bites, drug eruptions, swimmer's itch (cercarial dermatitis), atopic dermatitis, and psoriasis.

Treatment

Dermatitis of any etiology is treated in a similar manner. Known offending agents are avoided and protective clothing or gloves may be helpful when the person must continue activities associated with the dermatitis. Mild cases of dermatitis are treated with mid-potency topical steroids. Weeping or exudative lesions should be compressed with tap water or Burow's solution (see Chapter 35) for 15-30 minutes, four times a day, followed by topical steroids. Severe contact dermatitis is treated with prednisone 40-60 mg/day (adult dose), tapering the dose over 2-3 weeks. In allergic contact dermatitis, stopping prednisone too soon often results in recurrence. If a sensitized person contacts a known allergen, the skin should be promptly washed with soap and water. If secondary bacterial infection is present, it should be treated with antibiotics effective for *Staphylococcus* and *Streptococcus* spp.

DRUG ERUPTIONS

Cutaneous reactions to drugs are common and can be serious. Travelers frequently take new medications, either as prophylaxis or as therapy for acquired symptoms. Consider an at-home trial of drugs prior to travel. New reactions from long-standing medications may also occur due to intense tropical sunlight. Patients who are told that their medications place them at higher-than-usual risk of photoreactions may be motivated to take extra UV precautions, so providers should review medication lists with this issue in mind before their patients depart.

Clinical Features

Common presentations and etiologies of drug eruptions are listed in **Table 36.1**.

Diagnosis

Take a careful history, inquiring about over-the-counter and herbal/complementary medicines, including the date started. Exanthematous eruptions may be initially confused with viral exanthems. Urticaria may be caused by foods, parasitic and viral infections, or physical agents and often occurs idiopathically. The differential diagnosis of drug-induced photoeruptions includes other photosensitive rashes, such as polymorphous light eruption, lupus erythematosus, and some porphyrias.

Treatment

- Discontinue non-essential drugs.
- Antihistamines
  - Hydroxyzine: 25 mg by mouth every 4-6 hours
  - Diphenhydramine: 25-50 mg by mouth every 4-6 hours
  - Cetirizine: 10 mg/day (a less sedating option).
- Topical steroids for symptomatic relief
- Refer urgently to dermatology if mucous membranes are involved (mouth, vagina, conjunctiva) or if skin blisters.

ARTHROPOD BITES AND STINGS

Arthropod bites and stings are common dermatologic complaints of tropical travelers. Clinical symptoms result from hypersensitivity to arthropod antigens, toxic effects of venoms, or both. Important venom-producing arthropods include some species of spiders, Hymenoptera (bees and wasps), ants, centipedes, and scorpions. Nonvenom-producing, biting arthropods include species of flies, mosquitoes, bedbugs, fleas, mites, lice, and ticks (see also Chapter 20 and Chapter 24 for discussion of tick-borne tropical infections).

Etiology and Clinical Features

There are many biting *spiders*, but several are worth special mention. The black widow spider, *Latrodectus mactans*, and other *Latrodectus* spp. are found worldwide. *L. mactans* is best identified by the red hourglass shape on the ventral abdomen. The bite is often painless, but a neurotoxin, α-lactotoxin, can cause systemic symptoms including muscle spasms, headache, abdominal pain, nausea, and hypotension, which can progress to shock and death.

Loxosceles spp., including the brown recluse spider, are found in North and South America, have a violin shape on the cephalothorax and produce venom containing sphingomyelinase D, causing extensive local skin and soft tissue necrosis. *Brown recluse spider* bites cause a mild urticarial reaction in the majority of cases. Some bites cause severe local reactions characterized by an expanding bulla with surrounding pallor followed by cyanosis and necrosis within 48-72 hours. Systemic involvement is rare but may be fatal and includes disseminated intravascular coagulation, hemolysis, and renal failure.

The wandering spider, *Phoneutria nigriventer*, is a large South American spider measuring 3 cm in body length and produces a potent neurotoxin.

Hymenoptera include bees, wasps, hornets, yellow jackets, and ants and cause painful reactions from venom injected from a posterior stinger. Half of the fatal envenomations in the United States are due to Hymenoptera. Honeybees produce venom containing histamine, phospholipase A, hyaluronidase, and other constituents. Stings produce a painful wheal that subsides over a few hours. In sensitized individuals, urticaria, laryngeal edema, bronchospasm, and anaphylaxis begin immediately. Less common systemic manifestations include toxic reactions from large numbers of simultaneous stings or a serum sickness-like syndrome that follows the sting by days to weeks.

Solenopsis invicta, the imported fire ant, is common in the southern United States, Argentina, Uruguay, and Brazil. *Fire ant* stings may cause anaphylaxis but usually produce local reactions. Stings cause an immediate wheal, which becomes a vesicle and then a sterile pustule over 12-24 hours.

Many species of *scorpions* are found in arid regions of the tropics and subtropics. Fatal stings are usually seen in children in areas where species produce neurotoxic venom. Scorpion stings cause a painful local reaction, occasionally with some necrosis. Some species produce venom that can induce sympathomimetic, parasympathomimetic, and neurologic symptoms. Infants and children are at highest risk for fatal reactions. Antivenoms are available for some scorpion toxins; however, there are often little data on their benefits, and risks include anaphylactic reaction.

Other arthropods that normally cause more localized responses include the *Scolopendra* centipedes of Hawaii and western United States, biting flies of many varieties found worldwide, fleas (including *Tunga penetrans*; see Chapter 37), bedbugs, and human ectoparasites (Chapter 37). *Bedbug bites* usually occur on the face, arms, ankles, or buttocks and are often arranged in a cluster or line of two or three bites. The appearance of individual bites ranges from small hemorrhagic puncta to papular urticaria that last for several days. The bites themselves occur at night and are typically painless. Bedbugs move from crevices in furniture to the human host for only a few minutes to feed and then retreat.

In addition to bites and stings, simple contact with Lepidoptera (butterflies, moths, and their caterpillars) can cause a pruritic erythematous papular rash within hours of contact. Caterpillar and moth species worldwide have been linked to reactions including conjunctivitis, keratitis, iritis, and pharyngitis.

One particularly dangerous species, the *Lonomia obliqua*, or giant silkworm moth of South America, can cause a fibrinolytic reaction similar to disseminated intravascular coagulation, which can be fatal. Another dangerous species, the *Premolis* caterpillar, lives on rubber trees in the Amazon. Repeated contact with its bristles can cause a periarticular fibrosis with permanent disfiguration.

Diagnosis

Stings usually present no problem with diagnosis because of the immediate pain. Bites may be more difficult to diagnose if the injury is painless or occurs during sleep. The pruritic papules of typical bites may resemble other hypersensitivity reactions, such as urticaria or dermatitis. Patients presenting with an unwitnessed "spider bite" often have community-acquired methicillin-resistant Staphylococcus aureus (MRSA) skin infection. Bullous or necrotic reactions may mimic other rashes. Definitive diagnosis is possible only if the bite is observed. In unresolved situations a biopsy may be helpful.

Treatment

Most papular and mild bullous reactions are self-limited and can be treated with compresses and topical steroids or oral antihistamines for pruritus. As with all penetrating skin injuries, tetanus prophylaxis should be given if the patient's status is not up-to-date.

Angioedema can be treated with prednisone 30-40 mg/day for several days. More severe generalized urticarial reactions or anaphylaxis are treated promptly with epinephrine 0.3-0.5 mg subcutaneously, repeated every 15-20 minutes. Most patients respond within one or two doses. Intravenous epinephrine may be necessary if hypotension persists despite these measures.

Black widow spider reactions may require hospitalization and treatment with analgesics, muscle relaxants, intravenous calcium, and supportive care. An equine antivenom is available in several countries.

Brown recluse spider bites are usually benign and can be treated symptomatically. Ice and elevation are used for symptomatic relief. Dapsone may prove useful to treat related tissue necrosis. To prevent treatment toxicity, glucose 6-phosphate dehydrogenase status should be evaluated prior to treatment with dapsone. A surgical approach is potentially harmful and should be avoided. Systemic reactions may be life threatening and require hospitalization for supportive care. Antivenom is not available in the United States but is available for South American recluse bites where the reaction is often more severe.

Scorpion stings are treated by local wound care, ice packs, and antihistamines. The Food and Drug Administration recently approved the scorpion antivenom Anascorp, or Centruroides immune F(ab)2, for envenomations resulting in serious clinical symptoms. Antihypertensives or anticonvulsants may be needed for supportive care.

Hymenoptera stingers (from bees, yellow jackets, wasps, or fire ants) should be removed as quickly as possible. While forceps are suggested, they should be applied to the shaft of the stinger immediately proximal to the skin, to avoid squeezing more venom into the patient from the venom sack attached to the stinger. When no instruments are available, an alternative is to scrape off the stinger.

Butterfly and moth (Lepidoptera) bristles, often invisible, can be removed with cellophane tape. Clothing that has been in contact with the moth or caterpillar should be removed and washed, and exposed skin should be washed.

Prevention

People with a history of severe sting reactions at risk of further exposure can undergo venom desensitization. All people with a history of severe reactions, whether or not they have undergone desensitization, should carry kits including antihistamines and a syringe of epinephrine. Epinephrine auto-injectors are commercially available and should be prescribed pre-departure. These devices are sensitive to high temperatures and should be kept within the temperature range on the package insert (e.g., never in a car parked in the sun).

Protective clothing, insect repellant, and even repellant-treated clothing can all help prevent some stings and bites (see Chapter 6). However, insect repellents have no effect on spiders or bees.

Control of bedbugs involves treating crevices in walls and furniture with an insecticide, such as 0.5% lindane or 2% malathion, or spraying bed nets with a permethrin-containing insecticide.

Bacterial Skin Infections

Bacterial infections of the skin are a major problem in the tropics and a common problem among travelers. One study of travelers returning to France found that bacterial infections were the second most common presenting skin condition after cutaneous larva migrans (Chapter 37).

The high prevalence of bacterial infections in tropical climates is attributed to the warm, humid environment and can be worsened by close contact and poor hygiene. Other predisposing factors include insect bites, traumatic lesions, and other dermatoses such as contact dermatitis and scabies. Infections caused by staphylococci and streptococci are far more common in the tropics than are the exotic "tropical diseases."

PYODERMA

Pyoderma refers to superficial bacterial infectious syndromes involving the skin and follicular structures such as impetigo (including bullous or ulcerative forms), folliculitis, furunculosis, paronychia, erysipelas, and cellulitis.

Etiology

Staphylococcus aureus (both MRSA and methicillin-susceptible [MSSA]) and group A streptococci (GAS) are common causes of pyoderma.

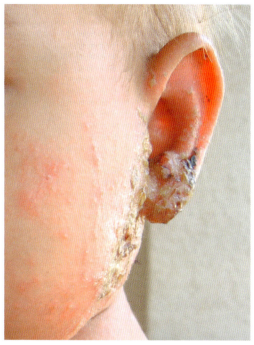

Fig. 36.2　**Pustules and honey-colored crusting on the ear of a child with impetigo.** (Courtesy of Michi Shinohara, MD.)

Clinical Features

Impetigo is an exceedingly common condition seen primarily in children. Invasion of the skin by pathogenic *S. aureus* or GAS often follows minor trauma. An isolated, erythematous papule or pustule accounts for the initial lesion. The primary lesion rapidly gives rise to a distinctive amber- or "honey"-crusted erosion with or without an erythematous border (**Fig. 36.2**). Pruritus may accompany the lesions, and regional lymphadenopathy may be present. The condition usually affects the central face around the nares and lips but can occur anywhere.

Bullous impetigo is a superficial blistering condition caused by the elaboration of a toxin *S. aureus*. Children are most frequently affected. Bullous impetigo presents as flaccid, well-demarcated bullae without surrounding erythema that arise rapidly from vesicles, often in intertriginous areas. The bullae rupture spontaneously in 1 or 2 days, leaving shallow erosions covered by a light brown, varnish-like crust.

Impetiginization describes when *S. aureus* or GAS secondarily infects skin that has been compromised by a pre-existing dermatosis. Atopic dermatitis, contact dermatitis, insect bites, dermatophyte infection, and infestations with mites or lice are frequent precursors. Lesions present as focal or widespread papules or plaques with honey-colored crusts. Close observation at the periphery may reveal the primary lesions of the underlying dermatosis.

Folliculitis is an infection of the hair follicle most often caused by *S. aureus*. Superficial folliculitis presents as follicle-based 1- to 2-mm pustules on an erythematous base, often with a central protruding hair shaft. The most frequent areas involved are the scalp, thighs, buttocks, axillae, and, in men, the beard, where it is called folliculitis barbae or sycosis barbae.

Furunculosis refers to isolated or multiple cutaneous infections centered on hair follicles with pus extending through the dermis, forming an abscess in the subcutaneous tissue. They occur most often in areas of friction and/or perspiration such as the axillae and buttocks. They present as painful, erythematous papules or nodules, with or without an obvious central follicular ostium. After several days, the lesion may come to a point and drain purulent material. A carbuncle refers to several communicating furuncles. Both furuncles and carbuncles are commonly referred to as "boils."

Ecthyma is often a deeper extension of untreated impetigo or folliculitis that presents as 5- to 15-mm punched-out erosions with elevated, erythematous borders. A densely adherent, thick serum crust overlies each lesion, giving a characteristic appearance. Regional lymphadenopathy is common. Lesions are most common on the buttocks and legs but can occur anywhere.

Acute paronychia is a suppurative infection of the proximal and lateral nail folds. It often follows a break in the skin resulting from minor trauma. *S. aureus* or *S. pyogenes* are the most common pathogens in acute paronychia. The presentation is that of an exquisitely tender, hot, erythematous nail fold, with or without frank abscess formation.

Erysipelas is an infection of the skin and superficial lymphatic channels usually due to GAS. It classically presents as a well-demarcated, brightly erythematous, hot, tender indurated plaque on the face or lower extremities. The pathogenic organisms gain entry into the skin via minor trauma, including pre-existing dermatitis.

Cellulitis may result from untreated erysipelas, but usually arises de novo, and is an infection of the deeper cutaneous and subcutaneous tissues. Cellulitis differs from erysipelas clinically by having indistinct borders and less pronounced brawny edema. Either GAS or *S. aureus* can cause cellulitis, although in the absence of a drainable focus of pus, GAS is the leading cause.

Diagnosis

Diagnosis of the various pyodermas is usually made primarily on clinical findings, and cultures are often unnecessary. Impetigo contagiosa may be difficult to differentiate from an exudative dermatitis, which may also have a crust. Bullous impetigo should be distinguished from other blistering disorders, such as bullous arthropod bites, pemphigus vulgaris, bullous pemphigoid, acute vesicular dermatitis, erythema multiforme, and bullous drug reactions.

Folliculitis, although most often caused by Gram-positive cocci, has many causes including chemical irritants, yeasts (*Candida* and *Malassezia*), Gram-negative bacteria (*Pseudomonas* spp., so-called hot tub folliculitis), dermatophytes, herpes simplex virus, pseudofolliculitis barbae, and various drug eruptions.

Hidradenitis suppurativa should be considered if furuncular lesions are localized to the axillae, groin, or intergluteal cleft. Furuncular myiasis (see Chapter 37) must be considered in anyone presenting with furunculosis after travel to an endemic area.

Treatment

See **Figure 36.3.**

- Superficial infections: topical antimicrobials such as mupirocin applied several times a day is recommended, as well as warm compresses that promote drainage. This treats both GAS and *S. aureus* infections.
- Nonpurulent skin infections (e.g., cellulitis): GAS should be covered. A first-generation cephalosporin or a penicillinase-resistant penicillin is first-line therapy. Clindamycin may be substituted for patients with a true beta-lactam allergy (although these are actually rare).
- Purulent skin infections: *S. aureus* (both MRSA and MSSA) is most likely. Incision and drainage may be necessary—and sufficient—for infections involving furuncles or abscess. Incision and drainage alone is almost always appropriate for staphylococcal abscesses or boils, and patients with these very rarely require antibiotics at all. However, patients

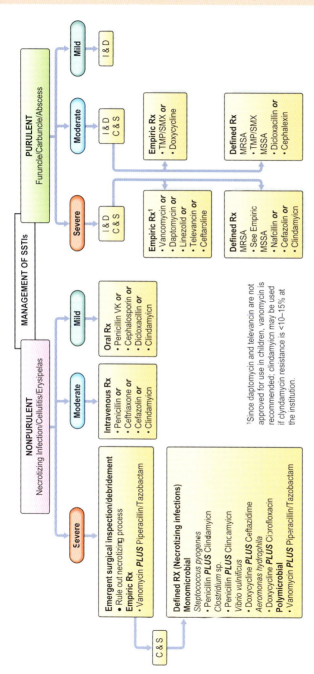

Fig. 36.3 Infectious Diseases Society of America algorithm guidelines. *C & S,* Culture and sensitivity; *I & D,* incision and drainage; *MRSA,* methicillin-resistant *Staphylococcus aureus; MSSA,* methicillin-susceptible *S. aureus; SSTIs,* skin and soft tissue infections; *TMP/SMX,* trimethoprim-sulfamethoxazole. (From: Stevens, D.L., Bisno, A.L., Chambers, H.F., et al., 2014. Practice guidelines for the diagnosis and management of skin and soft tissue infections: 2014 update by the Infectious Diseases Society of America. Clin. Infect. Dis. 59 (2), 147–159.)

presenting with multiple lesions, large areas of cellulitis, immune suppression, and any systemic symptoms of disease should be treated with systemic antibiotic therapy, such as empiric trimethoprim-sulfamethoxazole, or a tetracycline, plus a first-generation cephalosporin. Clindamycin alone provides less reliable MRSA coverage. Pus should be sent for culture and sensitivity, and antibiotics focused based on results. Parenteral antibiotics may be necessary in people showing systemic disease (fever and chills).

PYOMYOSITIS

Etiology

Pyomyositis, or purulent infection of skeletal muscle, is caused predominately by *S. aureus* but may also be due to streptococci along with other more rare causes.

Epidemiology

Pyomyositis occurs in tropical areas and is a rare but increasing problem in temperate climates. Most cases occur in children or young adults; males are affected more often than females. Up to 50% of cases are associated with a history of trauma to the affected muscles. Other predisposing factors include toxocariasis, immunodeficiency (specifically human immunodeficiency virus), malnutrition, and injection drug use.

Clinical Features

The characteristic features of pyomyositis are pain and tenderness of the involved muscle, fever, and leukocytosis. The most frequently affected muscles include those of the thigh, calf, deltoid, buttocks, iliopsoas, pectoral, and latissimus dorsi. The first week or two of infection is characterized by localized pain, with "woody" muscle texture on palpation. Two to three weeks after initial symptoms present, fever and extreme muscle tenderness is common. Many patients seek care at this point. A deep abscess can often be detected, and pus can be drained from it. Without treatment patients can worsen to a toxic stage with many life-threatening complications including septic shock, septic emboli, endocarditis, pneumonia, and renal failure.

Diagnosis

Differential diagnosis includes muscle hematoma, deep venous thrombosis, thrombophlebitis, neoplasm, and sickle cell crisis. Iliopsoas pyomyositis may mimic appendicitis. Diagnosis is made by recovery of pus from the affected muscle by needle aspiration or surgical exploration. Magnetic resonance imaging, computed tomography, and ultrasound, especially during the purulent stage, aid in diagnosis.

Treatment

In the earliest stage of disease systemic antibiotics can be curative, but most patients present in later stages when treatment requires surgical drainage and parenteral antibiotics. Antibiotic therapy should be guided by cultures. Pending results, empirical therapy should be directed to cover *S. aureus*, including MRSA. In immunocompromised patients, broader coverage for Gram-negative and anaerobic organisms should be provided.

Skin Ulcers

Skin ulcers in the tropics may be the result of bacterial infections not often encountered in temperate climates. Six bacterial causes are discussed in the following section.

Buruli Ulcer

Buruli ulcer (also known as Bairnsdale ulcer) is a painless skin ulcer caused by a slow growing acid-fast bacillus, *Mycobacterium ulcerans*. It is the third most common mycobacterial disease and may soon overtake leprosy for overall worldwide disease burden.

Epidemiology

Buruli ulcer occurs in tropical, humid environments in areas with stagnant swampy water and often in rural and remote areas. It is most common in West Africa but also found in

Mexico, South America, Australia, Papua New Guinea, and Japan. Cases acquired by travelers have been reported. Disease rates in some endemic populations range as high as 16-22%. While the mode of transmission has not been established, it is thought to involve direct contact with contaminated soil or water. Young people are most often affected, with the usual age of infected persons ranging from 4 to 22 years.

Clinical Features

Lesions of Buruli ulcer present as firm, nontender, mobile subcutaneous nodules, usually on an extremity after local trauma. Pruritus often accompanies this early lesion. In 1 or 2 months, toxin production causes necrosis of the nodules and underlying tissue and an indolent, generally painless ulcer with indurated, undermined borders and substantial fat necrosis without involving deeper tissue. Ulcers heal spontaneously after months or years with significant scarring, contractures, and limb deformities. Infection is not accompanied by systemic illness or regional lymphadenopathy, and fatalities are rare.

Diagnosis

The diagnosis is often made clinically. The acid-fast bacilli may be demonstrated by Ziehl–Nielsen staining of swabs or biopsies from the undermined ulcer border. Cultures may take as long as 8 weeks to turn positive.

Differential diagnosis includes other infections such as tropical ulcer (see below), cutaneous tuberculosis, leprosy (Chapter 40), leishmaniasis (Chapter 39), and fungal infections (Chapter 38). Other non-infectious ulcerating conditions, such as pyoderma gangrenosum and venous stasis, should be considered.

Treatment

Size at presentation will determine treatment. Prolonged courses of antibiotics can be helpful and may be combined with surgery. Combination therapy with streptomycin, clarithromycin, fluoroquinolones, and rifampin has been effective. Early lesions may be treated by excision and closed primarily or with grafting.

Tropical Ulcer

Tropical ulcer (also called tropical phagedenic ulcer or Malabar ulcer) is a condition in which a large, painful, ulcer forms rapidly on areas of skin prone to trauma. The majority of tropical ulcers appear on the leg. The etiology of this condition is believed to be polymicrobial infection with anaerobes (especially *Fusobacterium* spp.) in early disease and spirochetes in later infection. Ulcer formation is associated with malnourishment and underlying chronic disease.

Epidemiology

Tropical ulcer occurs in most hot, humid tropical regions of the world, including Africa, India, and the Western Pacific region.

Clinical Features

Lesions are most common on the lower extremities, and usually solitary. Ulcers begin as an erythematous papule or hemorrhagic bulla that breaks down within 7-10 days to form a large, well-demarcated, cup-shaped ulcer with an indurated, undermined border. The ulcer is painful and foul-smelling, and its granulating base is often covered by a yellowish membrane. Left untreated, ulcers may be deep enough to involve periosteum of underlying bone. Patients may be febrile and systemically ill, but regional lymphadenopathy is rare. With time, the ulcer may heal with significant scarring and functional disability. In some cases, ulcers have been known to persist for 10 years or more.

Diagnosis

This is a diagnosis of exclusion of other skin infections such as those included in this section (especially Buruli ulcer) and conditions such as cutaneous tuberculous, leishmaniasis, venous stasis, and pyoderma gangrenosum.

Treatment

Underlying nutritional deficiencies or chronic disease should be addressed. Local care for the ulcer includes rest, elevation, and local wound care with appropriate bandages or compresses. Antibiotics, most frequently penicillin, metronidazole, or a tetracycline, are administered until healing occurs. Reconstructive surgery and grafting may be required.

CUTANEOUS DIPHTHERIA

Diphtheria (veldt sore), while not commonly seen in temperate regions, is still endemic in many tropical countries.

Epidemiology

Cutaneous diphtheria often occurs in unvaccinated children and has been associated with skin trauma, often associated with infected insect bites. In some instances, the lesions act as reservoirs of the infectious agent and may cause respiratory and cutaneous infections in contacts. The bacteria may also be found in dust and fomites.

Clinical Features

Cutaneous diphtheria usually begins as a small papule or vesicle, often at the site of a minor skin wound. In 2-5 days the vesicle breaks down to form a well-demarcated shallow, painful, punched-out ulcer with elevated borders and surrounded by a rim of erythema. The base of the ulcer is covered by an adherent gray membrane. The ulcer may enlarge gradually and become anesthetic. The ulcer rarely exceeds 3 cm.

Diagnosis

Diagnosis can be confirmed by culture of swabs taken from the ulcer base. In chronic cases, a mixed infection is often present, and *Staphylococci* are frequently cultured from the same lesions.

Treatment

Treatment of cutaneous diphtheria consists of diphtheria antitoxin (if toxigenic) and a 2-week course of systemic antibiotics (erythromycin or penicillin). This is a reportable condition, and close contacts should be screened and offered prophylaxis with antibiotics and a diphtheria immunization booster if the index strain is found to be toxigenic.

CUTANEOUS TULAREMIA

Cutaneous tularemia (ulceroglandular fever) is the most common presentation of *Francisella tularensis*, a highly virulent, pleomorphic, Gram-negative coccobacillus. In the cutaneous form, the bacteria are transferred from infected animal reservoirs (often rabbits or hares), by the bite of an arthropod, or by direct contact with the blood or tissue of an infected animal.

Epidemiology

Tularemia is endemic in many areas of the northern hemisphere, including the United States, Canada, the Nordic countries, and Japan; it is also seen in Mexico and Central America. Many cases are reported in hunters, who become infected while skinning infected animals. The eyes may become involved if bacteria inoculate that area. Pneumonic tularemia is a serious but separate clinical entity, arising when bacteria are directly inhaled (e.g., infected ground rodent is aerosolized by a lawn mower).

Clinical Features

The incubation period of cutaneous tularemia is 3-5 days. The initial lesion, a red, painful nodule, usually appears 1 or 2 days after the onset of a high fever, headache, chills, myalgia, and prostration. Within a few days, the nodule rapidly becomes pustular and then breaks down to form a well-demarcated ulcer. The ulcer often heals spontaneously, leaving a small scar. Within a few days of the onset of the disease regional lymph node enlargement and tenderness develops (ulceroglandular tularemia), often prompting the patient to seek medical attention.

Diagnosis

The diagnosis of tularemia is suggested by the history of exposure to wild rabbits, rodents, or ticks and the associated finding of a small skin ulcer with central eschar and significant, tender lymphadenopathy.

Diagnosis can be confirmed by a serum microagglutination test or through identification (using fluorescent antibodies) of *F. tularensis* in smears from the base of the ulcer. Bacteria are highly virulent. Laboratory workers should be notified if cultures are to be attempted.

Treatment

- Mild disease: doxycycline 100 mg, twice daily for 14 days
- Moderate or severe disease: streptomycin 10 mg/kg intramuscularly every 12 hours for 7-10 days (not to exceed 2 mg/daily), or gentamicin 5 mg/kg daily in three divided doses intramuscularly or parenterally for 7-10 days.

CUTANEOUS ANTHRAX

Anthrax is a zoonotic illness caused by *Bacillus anthracis*, an aerobic spore-forming Gram-positive bacillus. There are three major clinical forms of the disease (cutaneous, pulmonary, and gastrointestinal), with the cutaneous form being the most common. Cutaneous anthrax is usually acquired from inoculation through a minor skin wound or abrasion, often during skinning sheep or other livestock. Although systemic forms of anthrax are often fatal, when treated appropriately the cutaneous type of the disease causes death in <1% of cases.

Epidemiology

Cutaneous anthrax has been found in tropical and subtropical regions of Africa, South and Central America, the Caribbean Islands, and the Philippines. Most cases are found in people with direct contact with animal hides.

Clinical Features

Cutaneous anthrax begins as a small painless skin nodule within 1 week after bacterial or spore invasion, usually through a minor wound. Lesions are found most commonly on the head or neck and the upper extremities. Within 2-3 days, the nodule becomes a blister, and then breaks down to form a shallow, painless ulcer with an edematous border. The ulcer base becomes covered by a characteristic black eschar. Systemic symptoms are not common, although regional lymph node enlargement is noted. In untreated cases, the eschar loosens and falls off after 2-3 weeks, and the ulcer then heals, usually without scar formation.

Diagnosis

The diagnosis is suggested by the clinical appearance of the lesion, especially the presence of a typical black eschar covering the ulcer. It can be confirmed by the demonstration of the Gram-positive bacilli in a smear taken from the ulcer under the eschar or in tissue removed by biopsy. *B. anthracis* may also be cultured; immunohistochemical stains are available for its identification in tissue specimens.

Treatment

Skin infection caused by *B. anthracis* is susceptible to most antibiotics. A 7- to 10-day course of ciprofloxacin (500 mg twice daily) or doxycycline (100 mg twice daily) is recommended. Infection cannot spread from person to person, thus no special precautions are indicated when caring for patients with any form of anthrax. However, laboratory personnel should be notified when this condition is suspected, because it can be spread when grown in culture.

CUTANEOUS MELIOIDOSIS

Skin lesions may be a prominent feature of melioidosis (also known as Whitmore disease), an infection caused by the pleomorphic Gram-negative bacillus *Burkholderia pseudomallei*. The disease may be divided into three clinically distinct patterns: localized, septicemic, and pulmonary. Skin lesions are a feature of both the septicemic and acute localized forms.

B. pseudomallei have been isolated from soil, mud, and surface water and abound in rice paddies and marshes. Infection in humans is thought to arise mainly from bacteria in the environment that enter the skin through small wounds and abrasions.

Epidemiology

Melioidosis is endemic in several countries in Southeast Asia and is distributed widely elsewhere in the tropics, including Central and South America and the Caribbean Islands, Australia, Africa, and the Middle East. The disease has been increasingly recognized as a hazard to those who travel "off road" as backpackers or eco-tourists. Diabetes mellitus is a risk factor for the disease.

Clinical Features

The skin signs of melioidosis range from localized cutaneous ulcers thought to occur at the site of percutaneous inoculation to multiple pustules or caseous nodules that appear widely over the skin surface as an expression of the septicemic form of infection. The incubation period appears to be influenced by the amount of inoculum and may vary widely, although it generally falls within 2-21 days from the date of the initial inoculation.

The skin lesions in localized melioidosis usually take the form of an ulcerated indurated plaque on an exposed area of the body. These lesions tend to be chronic and often drain a serosanguineous fluid. Cutaneous melioidosis may also appear as widespread miliary pustules in the septicemic form of the disease. Rarely, skin lesions of melioidosis may present as deep subcutaneous abscesses.

Disease severity can range from subclinical and localized skin infection described above to systemic disease including high fever, rigors, and sometimes confusion, stupor, jaundice, and diarrhea. It can also reactivate body-wide at times of stress, as has occurred in American veterans of the Vietnam War years after their initial infection.

Diagnosis

The skin signs of cutaneous melioidosis are not specific, and several other infectious processes should be considered, including tularemia, nocardiosis, and anthrax. The diagnosis may be suspected, however, in patients who show chronic indurated draining skin ulcers, with relevant travel history.

Smears from ulcers or abscesses yield Gram-negative bacilli, which show a characteristic bipolar "safety pin" pattern with Wright's stain. *B. pseudomallei* also can be grown in culture, and an indirect hemagglutination assay may be available in the countries where the disease is endemic. Because it can be spread to laboratory personnel, they should always be notified when this diagnosis is considered.

Treatment

Although *B. pseudomallei* is usually susceptible to most antibiotics, it is recommended that specific susceptibility tests be done on each isolate. A treatment regimen of ceftazidime or imipenem (during an initial hospital stay) followed by an outpatient course of chloramphenicol, trimethoprim-sulfamethoxazole, and doxycycline, for up to 20 weeks, has been shown to reduce mortality by 50%. Healthcare workers should use standard precautions when caring for these patients.

FURTHER READING

Chauhan, S., Jain, S., Varma, S., et al., 2004. Tropical pyomyositis (myositis tropicans): current perspective. Postgrad. Med. 80, 267–270.

De Benoist, A.C., White, J.M., Efstratiou, A., et al., 2004. Imported cutaneous diphtheria, United Kingdom. Emerg. Infect. Dis. 10, 511–513.

Dobos, K.M., Quinn, F.D., Ashford, D.A., et al., 1999. Emergence of a unique group of necrotizing mycobacterial diseases. Emerg. Infect. Dis. 5, 367–378.

Elston, D.M., 2004. Prevention of arthropod-related disease. J. Am. Acad. Dermatol. 51, 947–954.

Godyn, J.J., Siderits, R., Dzaman, J., 2004. Cutaneous anthrax. Arch. Pathol. Lab. Med. 128, 709–710.

Gould, J.W., Mercurio, M.G., Elmets, C.A., 1995. Cutaneous photosensitivity diseases induced by exogenous agents. J. Am. Acad. Dermatol. 33, 551–573.

Haddad, V. Jr., Cardoso, J.L., Lupi, O., et al., 2012. Tropical dermatology: venomous arthropods and human skin: part I: Insecta. J. Am. Acad. Dermatol. 67 (3), 331.e1–331.e14.

Hay, R.J., Adriaans, B.M., 1998. Bacterial infections. In: Champion, R.H., Burton, J.L., Burns, D.A. (Eds.), Textbook of Dermatology, vol. 2, sixth ed. Blackwell, London.

Kemp, E.D., 1998. Bites and stings of the arthropod kind. Treating reactions that can range from annoying to menacing. Postgrad. Med. 103, 88.

Larson, J.L., Clark, R.F., 1999. Plant toxins in the tropics. In: Guerrant, R.L., Walker, D.H., Weller, P.F. (Eds.), Tropical Infectious Diseases: Principles, Pathogens, and Practice. Churchill Livingstone, Philadelphia, p. 155.

Lee, P.K., Zipoli, M.T., Weinberg, A.N., et al., 2003. Pyodermas: *Staphylococcus aureus*, *Streptococcus*, and other gram-positive bacteria. In: Freedberg, I.M., Eisen, A.Z., Wolff, K. (Eds.), Fitzpatrick's Dermatology in General Medicine, sixth ed. McGraw-Hill, New York.

Lupi, O., Madkan, V., Tyring, S.K., 2006. Tropical dermatology: bacterial tropical diseases. J. Am. Acad. Dermatol. 54 (4), 559–578.

Naafs, B., 2006. Allergic skin reactions in the tropics. Clin. Derm. 24, 158–167.

Prussick, R., Knowles, S., Shear, N.H., 1994. Cutaneous drug reactions. Curr. Probl. Dermatol. 6, 81.

Rietschel, R.L., Fowler, J.F., 1997. Fisher's Contact Dermatitis, fourth ed. Williams & Wilkins, Baltimore.

Robinson, D.C., Adriaans, B., Hay, R.J., et al., 1988. The clinical and epidemiologic features of tropical ulcer (tropical phagedenic ulcer). Int. J. Dermatol. 27, 49.

Senol, M., Ozcan, A., Karincaoqlu, Y., et al., 1999. Tularemia: a case transmitted from a sheep. Cutis 63, 49–51.

Sissolak, D., Weir, W.R., 1994. Tropical pyomyositis. J. Infect. Dis. 29, 121.

Sizaire, V., Nackers, F., Comte, E., et al., 2006. *Mycobacterium ulcerans* infection: control, diagnosis and treatment. Lancet Infect. Dis. 6, 288–296.

Skin Cancer Foundation. www.skincancer.org.

Stevens, D.L., Bisno, A.L., Chambers, H.F., et al., 2014. Practice guidelines for the diagnosis and management of skin and soft tissue infections: 2014 update by the Infectious Diseases Society of America. Clin. Infect. Dis. 59 (2), 147–159.

Thng, T.G., Seow, C.S., Tan, H.H., et al., 2003. A case of nonfatal melioidosis. Cutis 72, 310–312.

Wilson, D.C., King, L.E., 1999. Arthropod bites and stings. In: Freedberg, I.M., Eisen, A.Z., Wolff, K. (Eds.), Fitzpatrick's Dermatology in General Medicine, fifth ed. McGraw-Hill, New York.

Wright, S.W., Wrenn, K.D., Murray, L., et al., 1997. Clinical presentation and outcome of brown recluse spider bite. Ann. Emerg. Med. 30, 28–32.

Zhu, Y.I., Stiller, M.J., 2002. Arthropods and skin diseases. Int. J. Derm. 41, 523–549.

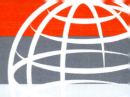

CHAPTER 37

Ectoparasites, Cutaneous Parasites, and Cnidarian Envenomation

Ellen Thompson and Andrea Kalus

This chapter describes common infestations by ectoparasites, including mites, lice, ticks, creeping eruption (cutaneous larva migrans), maggots (myiasis), and jiggers (tungiasis). Waterborne swimmer's itch (cercarial dermatitis) and jellyfish, or cnidarian ("nye-*dare*-ee-uhn"), envenomation are also discussed.

Living in close quarters, hiking, camping, visiting beaches, and swimming can increase exposure to many of these organisms. Avoiding contact with sand and soil, using chemical insect repellents, wearing long sleeves, pants, and shoes, as well as using bed nets, can aid in preventing many of these diseases.

ECTOPARASITES

Scabies

Etiology

Scabies is caused by the nearly microscopic human "itch mite" *Sarcoptes scabiei* var. *hominis*. Scabies causes intense pruritus, generally developing several weeks after infestation, with itching that worsens at night. Scabies is spread by skin-to-skin contact and rarely via contaminated clothing, bedding, or other fomites. The scabies mite lives for about a day away from a human host.

Mites burrow into the skin's outer layer and lay 2-4 eggs along the burrow path each day. A single female can lay up to 40 eggs. The time from ovum to mature mite is about 10-14 days. This cycle can repeat indefinitely, though some people can clear the infestation through their own immune response.

Epidemiology

Scabies occurs worldwide and is epidemic in much of the tropics. People of all ages are affected. Prevalence in the developing world is estimated at 10% in the general population and up to 50% among children. Crowding is a likely important factor, because scabies is highly contagious through skin-to-skin contact.

Clinical Features

In most people, lesions and pruritus develop several weeks after infestation due to a delayed-type hypersensitivity immune response to the mites, ova, saliva, and/or feces. Secondary papules, pustules, and/or vesicles are often present. The distribution of lesions includes finger webs, flexor surfaces of the wrists, axillae, breasts, umbilicus, genitals, buttocks, and feet. Burrows are 3-5 mm, threadlike, linear lesions seen typically in the finger webs, on the wrists, and on the glans penis. Secondary bacterial infection is common, and impetigo occurring in the aforementioned distribution suggests scabies.

In temperate climates, the face and scalp are spared except in infants and the elderly. In the tropics, the scalp and face may be involved; secondary infection is more frequent; and burrows are often absent. Crusted scabies (formerly called "Norwegian scabies"), in which thousands to millions of mites are present on an immune-compromised host, may occur anywhere on the body, although an acral distribution is common. Hyperkeratotic plaques and crusts predominate, resembling psoriasis. Burrows are obscured by overlying crusts, and, surprisingly, pruritus is often mild or absent.

Diagnosis

Identification of burrows in a typical distribution can make a clinical diagnosis. But burrows are not always present and are less common in tropical climates. Exposure history and typical distribution of lesions can also be used to make a clinical diagnosis.

A definitive diagnosis of scabies is made by identification of the mite, eggs, or feces in skin scrapings. Take scrapings from burrows whenever possible: with a scalpel blade coated with mineral or immersion oil, scrape the lesions firmly enough to cause pinpoint bleeding. Place the scrapings on a slide with a coverslip and then examine under a low-power objective lens. Sensitivity is dependent on experience; failure to find evidence of mites cannot rule out scabies.

Treatment

All household members and intimate contacts should be treated simultaneously, even if asymptomatic, to avoid reinfestation.

- Permethrin 5% cream offers a high cure rate and minimal toxicity. It is safe for infants >2 months old. Apply 30-50 mL from the neck down, leave 8-12 hours, then wash. One treatment is generally effective, but it can be reapplied after 5-7 days.
- Lindane 1% is a second-line topical treatment but is banned in some countries due to neurotoxicity presenting as seizures and neuromuscular rigidity, usually affecting children or elderly patients. It is applied like permethrin. Avoid using in infants and young children; it is not recommended for women who are pregnant or nursing.
- Ivermectin is an oral alternative with increasing popular use and is well tolerated. A single dose of 200 µg/kg body weight is as effective as lindane, and two doses, 2 weeks apart, is as effective as permethrin.
- An alternative treatment for infants <3 months includes 10% crotamiton cream, applied on two consecutive nights and washed off 48 hours after the second treatment. A second treatment in 2 weeks may be given.
- 5-10% sulfur ointment is commonly used in Africa and South America; it is safe for infants and is the treatment of choice for pregnant women.

Clothing and linens should be washed in hot water at the time of treatment. Nonwashable clothing should not be worn for 3-5 days. Household fumigation is not necessary.

Lice

Etiology

Head lice (pediculosis capitis) and body lice (pediculosis corporis) are caused by the human louse *Pediculus humanus*, a light-gray insect, 3-4 mm long, that feeds on blood. The head and body subspecies are practically identical, with distinct patterns of infestation. All forms of lice require a human host to survive and would die after 2-3 days without feeding.

Female head lice live on the scalp for 3-4 weeks and lay about 10 eggs, or nits, a day. Nits are deposited on the base of the hair shaft and incubate for 7-12 days; female nymphs mature in roughly another 10 days. The total number of adult lice is usually less than 10 at any time, and the infestation is primarily at the back of the head. Body lice live in the seams of clothing and move to the body transiently to feed.

Phthirus pubis lice, or pubic lice, are 1-2 mm and brown in color. Pubic lice live on pubic hair but may be found on any body hair and on eyelashes and eyebrows. Nits take about a week to hatch and another 2-3 weeks to mature.

Epidemiology

Head lice are found worldwide, are common among children across socioeconomic classes, but are associated with poor hygiene and crowding when present on adults.

Body lice occur worldwide in conditions of poor hygiene, especially where clothing is not changed and washed regularly. Transmission occurs through close body contact or sharing infested clothing. Lice may live for several days on clothing or bedding, but routine laundering will kill them. Body lice are vectors for typhus (*Rickettsia prowazekii*), trench fever (*Bartonella quintana*), and relapsing fever (*Borrelia recurrentis*).

Sometimes called crabs, pubic lice are primarily transmitted sexually and also endemic worldwide. In regions where pubic hair shaving is common, this condition has become very unusual.

Clinical Features

Head lice cause pruritus of the scalp, and scratching leads to excoriations. Further complications include furunculosis or impetigo. Scalp pyoderma should prompt an inspection for head lice.

The hair is often matted or lusterless, and regional lymph nodes may be enlarged. Light-gray adults and nymphs can be seen crawling among the hair and nits are usually apparent on examination. Nits are 0.5-mm ovals cemented to individual hairs where the shaft emerges from the scalp and grow out with the hair. Nits are initially translucent near the base of the hair shaft, where they are first laid, but after they hatch, when they have grown about 1 cm from the scalp, they appear white.

Body lice produce generalized pruritus, with excoriations usually worse over the back, shoulders, and arms. In contrast to scabies and head lice, the head, hands, and feet are spared. Typical lesions are excoriated papules with or without secondary bacterial infection. Lice and nits are not found on the body but may be seen in clothing.

Pubic lice cause pruritus from the umbilicus to the mid-thighs, most severely in the pubic area. Finding the tiny lice or nits may require a careful search. Often, no skin lesions are present, but excoriations or small bluish macules, called maculae caeruleae, are seen occasionally. These are thought to be hemosiderin deposition from bite trauma.

Diagnosis

For travelers in tropical areas, it is important to distinguish nits from white and black piedra, a fungal infection that can appear similar to nits (Chapter 38). White piedra loosely adheres to hair shafts, as opposed to nits, which are strongly attached. White piedra tends to affect the axillae, groin, and face more often than the scalp. Black piedra commonly occurs in the scalp and facial hair, can be similarly sized to nits, and is strongly attached to the hair. Visualization with a KOH preparation and microscopic inspection will reveal characteristic septate hyphae, distinguishing black piedra from lice.

Lice are diagnosed by finding the louse or nits. The use of a hand lens may aid diagnosis.

Treatment

Head lice

All topical treatments should be reapplied at about 7 days to prevent reinfestation.

- 10-minute application of 1% permethrin shampoo, which is repeated at 7 days.
- 0.5% malathion lotion left on for 8-12 hours, used in cases of permethrin resistance (not for use in children under the age of 2)
- For those who fail to respond to topical treatment, drug resistance may be the cause; in this case, use ivermectin (single dose of 200 μg/kg body weight) and ensure that all close contacts have been treated as well.
- Bed linens and hats should be laundered or dry-cleaned.

Body lice
- Bathe the body and wash all clothing or apply insecticide powder to the inner surface of clothing. DDT powder or 1% malathion powder is effective.

Pubic lice
- 10-minute application of 1% permethrin shampoo from the axillae to the thighs
- 10-minute application of 1% pyrethrin with piperonyl butoxide, as above
- 0.5% malathion lotion left on for 8-12 hours
- Sexual partners should be treated simultaneously to prevent reinfestation. Sexual partners from the previous month should be contacted. Evaluate patients for other possible sexually transmitted infections.
- Eyelashes cannot be treated with the above chemical remedies. In this location treatment is with thick application of petrolatum or other occlusive ointment twice a day for 10 days, accompanied by mechanical removal of lice and nits.

Topical 0.1% triamcinolone or other low-potency topical steroid may be used for symptomatic itch relief. In all cases bacterial superinfection should be considered and treated where appropriate.

CUTANEOUS LARVA MIGRANS

Cutaneous larva migrans is caused by invasion into the skin by the larvae of animal hookworms.

Etiology

The most common cause is the larva of the dog and cat hookworm, *Ancylostoma braziliense*. Eggs, passed in the stool of the animal, mature into infective larvae in the soil. These larvae penetrate the skin of humans and produce serpiginous lesions by burrowing aimlessly through the skin. They are not able to penetrate deeper and continue their life cycle in humans, so we are dead-end hosts. If untreated, the larvae usually die within 2-8 weeks.

Epidemiology

The disease occurs in warm and humid conditions throughout the world. Infections peak during rainy seasons. The most important risk factor is skin exposure to soil contaminated with dog or cat feces. In travelers, this typically occurs when walking barefoot, such as on beaches. Feet are most often affected, but any skin exposure to contaminated soil can result in infection.

Clinical Features

After larval penetration, mild itching and nonspecific papules may occur and subside. After 1-3 days the larva begins to migrate, leaving a tortuous, raised, linear track marked by pruritus and erythema (**Fig. 37.1**). The lesion advances a few millimeters to several centimeters each day, and there may be resolution of the older parts of the track. Multiple lesions are common. Excoriation and secondary infection are seen.

Diagnosis

The diagnosis is usually made clinically when a characteristic lesion appears in a person with a history of possible exposure. Biopsy often fails to demonstrate the organism, which usually lies 1-2 cm beyond the leading edge of the track.

Treatment

- Ivermectin: one oral dose (200 μg/kg body weight)
- Albendazole: 400 mg orally for 3-7 days
- Thiabendazole: 10-15% topically three times daily for 5-7 days.

Topical 0.1% triamcinolone or other low-potency topical steroid may be used for symptomatic itch relief. Bacterial superinfection should be considered and treated where appropriate.

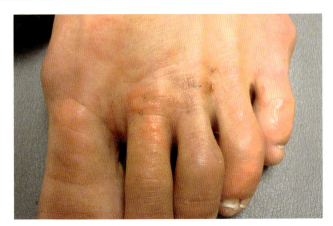

Fig. 37.1   Cutaneous larva migrans. Note the serpiginous track on the little toe.

MYIASIS

Myiasis refers to infestation by the larvae of flies. Animals, including livestock, are more typical hosts, but humans can also function as hosts. The larvae mature over several weeks to 2 months. Infestation sites are characterized by intermittent pain and irritation, often accompanied by exudate, and may not present until travelers have returned home. Patients may report a sensation of movement under the skin.

The three cutaneous forms are furuncular myiasis, dermal myiasis, and wound myiasis, with some overlap among these and with cutaneous larva migrans. Furuncular myiasis occurs primarily in Mexico, Central and South America, and Africa and may be found among travelers returning from these areas. Dermal myiasis occurs in Central and South America and is a variant of cutaneous larva migrans. Wound myiasis is a ubiquitous condition that occurs whenever flies deposit eggs into an open wound or ulcer, which then develop into larvae. Most infestations are superficial. However, infestation by several species of screw-worm flies results in dangerous sequelae due to the tendency of the larvae to penetrate deep tissue.

Etiology, Epidemiology, and Clinical Features

Furuncular Myiasis

Furuncular myiasis in Mexico and Central and South America is caused by the human botfly, *Dermatobia hominis*. This 1.5-cm-long yellow-brown fly catches other biting insects such as mosquitoes in midair and attaches its eggs to their bodies. When the biting insect feeds, the eggs hatch and the larvae enter, often through the puncture wound. The larvae develop in the dermis, breathing through an opening (pore) in the skin. Botfly myiasis may occur on any exposed surface but commonly is found on the scalp as single or multiple 2- to 3-cm domed erythematous papule(s) with a central pore. Careful inspection may reveal movement beneath. Lesions can produce paroxysmal pain and pruritus and can lead to secondary infection. Larvae leave the host after 5–10 weeks.

African furuncular myiasis is due to the tumbu fly, *Cordylobia anthropophaga*. Tumbu fly larvae infestations are more common during rainy seasons, when fly populations rise. They develop from eggs that have been laid on shady ground or on objects such as clothes or diapers hung out to dry. Larvae hatch and can live up to 9 days before finding a host. They are sensitive to warmth and vibration, allowing them to find a host. They penetrate human skin quickly, typically at the head, neck, breast, or back, or any areas in contact with contaminated clothing. Larvae mature and vacate the host after 8-12 days; in the meantime, they produce a boil-like lesion, often accompanied by exudate and pruritus. Heavy infestation can also cause fever and malaise.

Rare cases of North American furuncular myiasis have been associated with endemic botflies (*Cuterebra* species).

Dermal myiasis

Gasterophilus species of horse fly cause creeping eruptions worldwide. *Hypoderma ovis* and *Hypoderma lineatum* are cattle bot flies found in the Northern Hemisphere causing presentation similar to cutaneous larva migrans.

Wound myiasis

Most wound myiasis consists of superficial infestation of existing wounds or ulcers. However, two varieties of screwworm can cause deeper and more serious infestation. The *Cochliomyia hominivorax*, or New World screwworm (blowfly larvae) is found in parts of South and Central America and some Caribbean islands. Human infestation is rare but can be fatal because larvae penetrate deep tissue. Also, larvae are laid in multiple batches, with mature flies attracted back by a scent given off by maturing larvae. This can result in as many as 3000 larvae at a given site. The blowfly responsible for the New World screwworm has a blue-green body and is slightly larger than a housefly. It produces pink larvae that can reach 2 cm in length. The *Chrysomya bezziana*, or Old World screwworm, is found in tropical Africa and parts of Asia, including Indonesia and the Philippines, as well as New Guinea. The mature screwworm fly is 8-12 mm, with a blue-green body and two stripes across the thorax.

Diagnosis

Diagnosis requires identification of larvae. Consider myiasis in patients returning from affected countries presenting with lesions resembling boils. Typically a pore is maintained to allow larvae to breathe, and sometimes feces or bubbles can be seen in the exudate. Myiasis lesions in which infected patients feel sense of movement are more easily diagnosed.

Treatment

- First, try to prevent exposure with physical and chemical protection from biting insects, and iron all air-dried clothes in areas of tumbu fly myiasis to kill larvae before wearing the clothes.
- There is no medical treatment for myiasis; the larvae may be left to mature and fledge on their own, usually without harm to the host, or they can be extracted. Patients usually opt for extraction.
- If office visit time allows, apply an occlusive substance such as petroleum jelly over the air holes to block the air supply to larvae. Within an hour this should agitate them and drive them to the surface, where they may be more easily grasped with forceps and removed. If time is limited, apply a small occlusive adhesive bandage over each lesion. The bandage is peeled off after 3-4 days, and the dead (asphyxiated) larva can be extracted from the burrow. This technique may be expeditious for patients with multiple lesions.
- Surgical extraction may be necessary, particularly in the case of deeper burrowing screwworms. Extraction of the Old World screwworms can be complicated by the presence of spiny processes.

TUNGIASIS

Etiology

Tungiasis is caused by *Tunga penetrans*, a tiny sand flea, known as the nigua, chigoe, or jigger flea. Dogs, cats, pigs, cows, and rats are known reservoirs. The fertilized female flea burrows into the bare skin of the host, where it resides beneath the stratum corneum of the epidermis and feeds on blood. It maintains a connection to the outside and discharges feces and lays eggs through this connection. Over the course of a few weeks, the female discharges 100 eggs or more. The flea dies within the epidermis and is sloughed off over time.

Epidemiology

Tungiasis is indigenous in Central and South America, the Caribbean islands, sub-Saharan Africa, India, Pakistan, and in the Indian Ocean islands of Madagascar and the Seychelles.

Clinical Features

Penetration by the flea occurs typically around the toenail or in interdigital spaces, as well as other areas of the foot, in patients who wear open shoes. It may cause pruritus, typically without visible manifestations. Five days later, small white papules or nodules appear, with a black point that corresponds to the fleas' connection to the outside. As the flea engorges, pain increases. The nodule can reach a diameter of up to 1.2 cm. This also corresponds to the time when the flea releases ova. She then dies, resulting in a black scab that heals spontaneously. Lesions can also ulcerate and are prone to superinfection. Multiple or numerous infestations can cause significant deformity.

Diagnosis

Diagnosis can be difficult outside the endemic area, where it may be misidentified as a wart, insect bite, or inflammation due to a splinter or foreign body. Diagnosis should be made by removing and identifying the flea.

Treatment

- Removal of the flea is easier in the earlier stages of infection. Use a sterile needle or curette, accompanied by careful cleaning of the area. Later stages may necessitate an incision to remove the flea. Rupture of the egg sac is not harmful to the patient and can be handled with copious lavage; however, it is important to remove the entire flea, whether intact or not.
- Topical and systemic treatments have been ineffective. Recently, application of low-viscosity silicone oils such as NYDA dimeticone has been promising. This is believed to smother the flea.
- Secondary bacterial infection should be treated with appropriate antibiotics.
- To prevent infection in endemic areas, wear shoes and inspect feet routinely.

TICK BITES

Ticks are blood-sucking insects that can cause significant local and systemic reactions and are vectors for a variety of viral and bacterial diseases.

Etiology

Ticks are ectoparasites found worldwide, encompassing more than 800 recognized species. Ticks feed by anchoring mouth parts in the skin and inserting a hollow proboscis to suck blood. They are members of the class Arachnida and are divided into two families: Ixodidae, or hard-bodied ticks, and Argasidae, or soft-bodied ticks.

Ixodidae live in forest and grassland areas, attach to warm-blooded hosts, and remain on the skin for days to weeks before dropping off. Ixodid ticks are vectors for Lyme disease (Chapter 24), ehrlichiosis, Rocky Mountain spotted fever, babesiosis, Colorado tick fever, tick-borne encephalitis, and other infectious diseases. The Argasidae are mainly parasites of birds and live in nesting areas. They feed rapidly at night, often on several hosts in succession. Argasid ticks are vectors for relapsing fever and other illnesses.

Clinical Features

Tick bites are usually painless and unnoticed. Argasid ticks feed only transiently at night, and thus are virtually never discovered by patient or physician. The ixodid tick body may be noticed incidentally on the skin as a pea-sized tumor. Urticarial papules and pruritus may occur, calling attention to the tick. These papules subside within a few days after removal.

Argasid ticks cause more frequent inflammatory or papular reactions, which subside over several weeks. One Argasid species, *Ornithodoros tholozani*, produces deep red macules or papules with a central punctum at the bite site.

Tick bite granuloma is a persistent pruritic reaction occurring at the site of attachment of the tick. In some cases, tick bite granuloma is associated with retention of mouth parts in the skin. These granulomas are firm, slightly erythematous nodules that persist for months or years.

Tick fever is a systemic reaction with fever, headache, vomiting, and abdominal pain. This occurs after several days of attachment by the tick and subsides within 12-36 hours after its removal.

Tick paralysis is a rare, potentially fatal systemic reaction caused by the bite of several species of ticks endemic to western North America and Australia. Paralysis is attributed to a toxin elaborated by the tick. The reaction begins after 5-6 days of attachment, accompanied by irritability and sometimes low-grade fever. An ascending lower motor neuron paralysis develops rapidly and may lead to death from bulbar paralysis or aspiration. Symptoms abate rapidly after removal of the tick.

Diagnosis

Diagnosis is easiest if the tick is found attached to the skin. Otherwise tick bite reactions can be difficult to distinguish from reactions to other biting insects. Tick bite granuloma is distinguished from many other granulomatous processes by the intense pruritus that is present, but biopsy may be necessary.

Treatment

When traveling in tick-infested areas, wear light-colored clothing, because ticks are typically dark in color, which aids in spotting them before attaching to skin. Tuck pant cuffs into socks. Insect repellents containing DEET or picaridin and permethrin spray applied to clothing also offer some protection.

Treatment

- Grasp the tick as close to the skin as possible with tweezers, small forceps, or protected fingers. Apply steady traction perpendicular to the skin surface. Avoid pressure on the tick body. Tick fever and tick paralysis are treated by removal of the tick and supportive measures.
- Tick bite granuloma responds to intralesional steroids.
- Antibiotic prophylaxis after tick bites is controversial and should be considered only in select circumstances (see Chapter 24).

CERCARIAL DERMATITIS

Cercarial dermatitis, also known as swimmer's itch, is a self-limited, common parasitic infection in which humans are dead-end hosts. The number of outbreaks reported is increasing worldwide.

Etiology

Cercarial dermatitis is caused by penetration of the skin by avian schistosomal larval forms called cercariae. Snails infected with schistosome (blood fluke) species shed the infective cercariae into the water. The cercariae penetrate the wet skin of warm-blooded animals, including people. The cercariae can penetrate the upper layers of human skin but are unable to enter the vascular system, and soon die. In contrast, pathogenic species of schistosomes can enter the vascular system, where maturing flukes cause systemic disease (see Chapter 48).

Epidemiology

Cercarial dermatitis occurs worldwide where either fresh or saltwater is heavily contaminated with infected avian feces. People are exposed by swimming or wading in contaminated water.

Clinical Features

There are two phases to cercarial dermatitis: transient symptoms soon after exposure and delayed symptoms. Penetration of cercariae is accompanied by a prickling sensation and urticarial wheals, which resolve. Hours later, pruritic macules, papules, or vesicles may develop in the same sites. Recurrent infections result in increased inflammatory response. These lesions reach maximal intensity 2-3 days after infection and then subside within 1-2 weeks. Secondary bacterial infection can occur in excoriated lesions. Subsequent attacks tend to become more severe. Cercarial dermatitis usually spares areas covered by clothing, in contrast to seabather's eruption (discussed later in this chapter).

Diagnosis

Diagnosis rests on the history of exposure to contaminated water and typical clinical findings. Differential diagnosis includes insect bites, contact dermatitis, and scabies.

Treatment

- Immediate rubbing of the skin with a towel after leaving the water may remove adherent cercariae before they can penetrate the epidermis.
- Mild cases can be treated with compresses and topical steroids. Severe cases may require a brief course of systemic steroids.
- Secondary infection should be treated with appropriate antibiotics.
- Antiparasitic medications are not necessary.

CNIDARIAN ENVENOMATION

People swimming or wading in seawater are at risk for envenomation by cnidarians ("seabather's eruption"). Reactions to envenomation can range from very mild to fatal.

Etiology

The phylum Cnidaria includes more than 9000 invertebrate species that are most abundant in tropical waters, including sea anemones, coral, and jellyfish. By definition, all are capable of stinging their prey, but consequences in humans are usually subclinical or minor irritation; a few species, however, may cause dangerous envenomation. The injuries caused by Cnidaria are due to venom-laden organelles called nematocysts, containing a coiled filament with a barbed end. With the proper stimulus, these embed in the skin, discharging venom. Tentacles stuck to the skin often contain undischarged nematocysts that can be triggered by pressure or fresh water. Other stinging sea animals include sea urchins, sea anemones, sponges, stingrays, sea cucumbers, catfish, lionfish, and cone snails. True coral may cause stinging and can also cause foreign body granulomas.

Epidemiology

People in contact with seawater, or those walking on the beach in contact with washed-up jellyfish, are at risk for cnidarian stings. All ages are affected, but most severe or fatal reactions occur in children.

Clinical Features

Cnidarian stings present with a wide range of cutaneous and systemic features (**Table 37.1**). The severity depends on the number of nematocysts discharged into the skin, the nature of the venom, and the sensitivity of the victim. The best known is the Portuguese man-of-war, while the most deadly is the box jellyfish. The majority, however, cause only mild to moderate irritation.

Symptoms begin immediately or soon after contact and include stinging or burning pain, which may be severe. Pruritic or painful urticarial papules may become vesicular or bleed. Any part of the body can be affected, but because tentacles can become trapped in the fabric of water-permeable swimwear, lesions tend to cluster in areas that were covered during the swim. Lesions are typically distributed along a linear pattern (**Fig. 37.2**). Systemic reactions are variable among species and can include generalized urticaria, muscle spasms, anaphylaxis, and cardiovascular collapse.

TABLE 37.1 Common or Clinically Important Cnidarian Stings

Species	Distinguishing Features	Location	Clinical Effects and Considerations
Portuguese man-of-war, *Physalia physalis*	30-cm "sail" and 10-m long tentacles	Tropical Atlantic and Indo-Pacific	Cutaneous: "whip" lesions, wheals >7 cm Necrosis after 24 h Systemic: arrhythmia, headaches, fatalities associated
Bluebottle (or Indo-Pacific Portuguese man-of-war), *Physalia utriculus*	4-5 m long	Tropical Indo-Pacific, Australian, South Atlantic	Cutaneous: local pain, wheals, vesicles Systemic: none confirmed
Box jellyfish, *Chironex fleckeri*		Mainly Indo-Pacific and Australian tropical and subtropical waters, concentrated around northern Australia, with reports in east Pacific and Atlantic (Related *C. quadrigatus* found in Indo-Pacific including northern Australia, the Philippines, Malaysia, and Japan. The related Chiropsalmus *quadrumanus* is found in the Gulf of Mexico and in Brazilian coastal water.)	Special toxins: cardiotoxin and necrotoxin Cutaneous: massive wheals, vesicles persisting for 10 days resulting in scarring Systemic: 20% of stings are fatal. Arrythmia, cardiac arrest, hypotension, pulmonary hypertension Envenomations involving 6 m of total tentacle length may result in immediate loss of consciousness and 15 m of tentacle length of envenomation may be fatal. **Important: A single antivenom is made by Commonwealth Serum Laboratory based in Australia and is sold directly to consumers in some countries.**
Irukandji jellyfish, *Carukia barnesi* (and some related species)	Tiny jellyfish, up to 3 cm	Found in northern Australia October–May. Rare cases in southern Australia, Hawaii, Florida, Papua New Guinea, and Thailand.	Special toxins: mechanism unknown, possibly related to catecholamine release Cutaneous: oval erythematous area of 5-7 cm surrounded by papules Systemic: Several deaths reported. **Irukandji syndrome:** backache, hypertension, headache, muscle cramps, nausea, and vomiting **Important: Acetic acid/vinegar may amplify the effect.**
Fire coral, *Millepora*		Shallow reefs of tropical Atlantic and Caribbean	
Sea nettles *Chrysaora* and *Cyanea*		Worldwide	Cutaneous: frequent cause of less severe stings
Thimble jellyfish, *Linuche unguiculata*, or sea anemone, *Edwardsiella lineata*		Bahamas, Bermuda, Philippines, Florida (USA), Thailand, Brazil, New Zealand	Cutaneous: causes "seabather's eruption," severely pruritic erythematous lesions. Thought to be caused by larvae trapped against the skin in clothing or hair, releasing nematocysts when they desiccate and die.

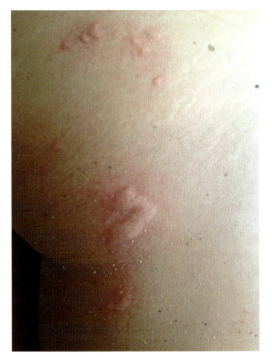

Fig. 37.2 **Linear urticarial papules and plaques following acute cnidarian sting.** (Courtesy of Jennifer Gardner, MD.)

Diagnosis

Cnidarian envenomation should be suspected whenever pain or itching begins during or after contact with seawater. A specific history of activities may help to distinguish between envenomation by free-floating or sessile forms. The pattern of skin lesions may also be helpful in identifying the causative organism, if it was not seen. The tentacles of the Portuguese man-of-war produce a characteristic whiplash appearance. Fragments of tentacles may adhere to the skin. Different species can be identified by microscopic examination of the nematocysts after removal by pressing cellophane tape against the skin.

Treatment

- The first step is to prevent further envenomation. Rinse the area with seawater to remove nematocysts. Fresh water may trigger further injection of venom.
- Hot water immersion (40-41° C) has been effective in relieving pain.
- Nematocysts may be inactivated with 5% acetic acid (household vinegar), although unexpected discharge of venom may occur.
- Tentacles and unseen nematocysts can be removed by unidirectional scraping with a thin firm object, such as a credit card, through a shaving motion along the affected area.
- Local reactions are treated with compresses, analgesics, and antihistamines if pruritus is prominent.
- A specific antivenom is available for stings by the box jellyfish *Chironex fleckeri* (Commonwealth Serum Laboratory, Melbourne, Australia).

- Severe cases of cutaneous pain and swelling may require a short course of systemic corticosteroid therapy.
- Ulcerated lesions may become secondarily infected and require antibiotics.
- Anaphylaxis is treated with standard supportive measures. Calcium gluconate or diazepam is sometimes used to control muscle spasms.

People planning activities involving significant water exposure in unknown waters, such as scuba diving, should inquire about local hazardous species. Cnidarians found washed ashore should not be handled. Swimmers, divers, and others participating in water activities where risks of cnidarian envenomation exist should wear protective gloves, footwear, and other garments such as wetsuits that are too thick to allow nematocyst penetration.

FURTHER READING

Blackwell, V., Vega-Lopez, F., 2001. Cutaneous larva migrans: clinical features and management of 44 cases presenting in the returned traveler. Br. J. Derm. 145, 434–437.

Burke, W.A., 2002. Cnidarians and human skin. Dermatol. Therapy 15, 18–25.

Cegolon, L., Heymann, W.C., Lange, J.H., et al., 2013. Jellyfish stings and their management: a review. Mar. Drugs 11, 523–550.

Dehecq, E., Nzungu, P.N., Cailliez, J.C., et al., 2005. *Cordylobia anthropophaga* outside of Africa: a case of furuncular myiasis in a child returning from Congo. J. Med. Entomol. 42, 187–192.

Feldmeier, H., Heukelbach, J., 2009. Epidermal parasitic skin diseases: a neglected category of poverty-associated plagues. Bull. World Health Organ. 87 (2), 152–159.

Fisher, A.A., 1987. Toxic and allergic reactions to jellyfish with special reference to delayed reactions. Cutis 40, 303–305.

Francescone, F., Lupi, O., 2006. Myiasis. In: Tyring, S.K. (Ed.), Tropical Dermatology. Elsevier, New York.

Heukelbach, J., Feldmeier, H., 2008. Epidemiological and clinical characteristics of hookworm-related cutaneous larva migrans. Lancet Infect. Dis. 8 (5), 302–309.

Heukelbach, J., Feldmeier, H., 2006. Scabies. Lancet 367 (9524), 1767–1774.

Horak, P., Kolarova, L., 2001. Bird schistosomes: do they die in mammalian skin? Trends Parasitol. 17, 66–69.

Macias, P.C., Sashida, P.M., 2000. Cutaneous infestation by *Tunga penetrans*. Int. J. Dermatol. 39, 296–298.

Mashek, H., Licznerski, B., Pincus, S., 1997. Tungiasis in New York. Int. J. Dermatol. 36, 276–278.

Mulvihill, C.A., Burnett, J.W., 1990. Swimmer's itch: a cercarial dermatitis. Cutis 46, 211–213.

Ottuso, P., 2013. Aquatic dermatology: encounters with the denizens of the deep (and not so deep): a review. Part I: the invertebrates. Int. J. Dermatol. 52, 136–152.

Tamir, J., Haik, J., Orenstein, A., et al., 2003. *Dermatobia hominis* myiasis among travelers returning from South America. J. Am. Acad. Dermatol. 48, 630–632.

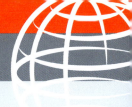

CHAPTER 38

Fungal Skin Infections

Andrea Kalus

Residents and travelers experience a variety of fungal infections of the skin. Many are not unique to the travel location, but the heat and humidity of the tropical environment increases susceptibility to these infections. In addition, inoculation with endemic fungal pathogens can result in deep fungal infections of the skin and subcutaneous tissues. In some cases presentation is delayed until travelers have returned to their home country.

Fungal infections of the skin (mycoses) are broadly divided into superficial and subcutaneous, based on the depth of involvement in the skin. Etiologies vary by presentation.

SUPERFICIAL CUTANEOUS MYCOSES

Superficial cutaneous mycoses invade the outer layer of skin (stratum corneum), hair, or nails. Dermatophytes and *Candida* species are the primary organisms responsible for the superficial mycoses, and immune response of the host may be minimal.

Dermatophyte Infections (Dermatophytoses)

Dermatophyte infections are due to fungal species in three genera: *Trichophyton*, *Microsporum*, and *Epidermophyton*. Worldwide, *Trichophyton rubrum* is the most common cause of dermatophyte infection, but in many instances the same clinical presentation can be caused by dermatophytes from different genera.

Epidemiology

The epidemiology of dermatophyte infection is different for each clinical presentation and geographic area. For example, tinea pedis and nail infections are uncommon before puberty, whereas tinea capitis is primarily a disease of childhood. Dermatophyte infections are enhanced by heat and humidity, and travelers to the tropics may note an exacerbation of a pre-existing infection. Sources of dermatophyte infection include soil, animal reservoirs, and human-to-human transmission.

Clinical Features

Tinea capitis, or "ringworm" of the scalp, is mainly a disease of children caused by *Microsporum* or *Trichophyton* species. *Trichophyton tonsurans*, *Microsporum canis*, and *Microsporum audouinii* are most common.

The condition presents with hair loss (alopecia), usually with scale. Patchy areas of broken hairs covered by white scales can resemble seborrheic dermatitis. When tinea capitis invades the hair shaft the scalp shows a characteristic "black-dot" pattern, in which hairs broken off at scalp level resemble comedones within patches of alopecia. Lymphadenopathy is frequently present and can help differentiate from non-infectious causes of hair loss.

Inflammatory tinea capitis occurs in the setting of tinea infection coupled with a brisk host inflammatory response. A boggy inflamed plaque (kerion) may form, which is associated with systemic symptoms, including fever, pain, and regional lymphadenopathy. Permanent hair loss may occur.

Tinea favosa (favus) is a special type of chronic and progressive inflammatory infection on the scalp most frequently caused by *Trichophyton schoenleinii*. This variant is seen in Asia, Africa, the Middle East, and South America. It is characterized by permanent hair loss and inflammation of the scalp, which becomes covered by matted hair with dense, yellow, follicular, cup-shaped crusts (scutula) that have an unpleasant odor.

Tinea corporis, or "ringworm," affects all ages and is recognized by annular, thin plaques, with erythema and scale most prominent at the advancing border (**Fig. 38.1**). Lesions spread outward with central clearing. There may be multiple areas involved, but widespread involvement is unusual. The plaques vary in size from a few millimeters to many centimeters in diameter. Pruritus is variable. In some cases there is follicular involvement presenting with papules and pustules, especially at the advancing border. Differential diagnosis of tinea corporis includes psoriasis, nummular eczema, pityriasis rosea, subacute cutaneous lupus, and secondary syphilis.

Tinea imbricata is an unusual variant of tinea corporis caused by *Trichophyton concentricum* that is endemic in the South Pacific, Southeast Asia, and Central and South America. This presentation is chronic and results in the development of multiple large, loosely adherent scales covering large areas of the body that coalesce to form lacy concentric patterns similar to wood grain.

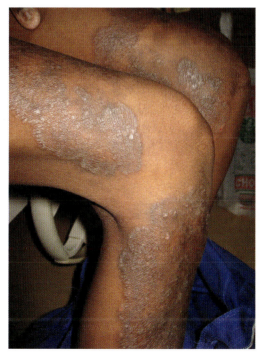

Fig. 38.1   Sharply demarcated plaques with central clearing and accentuation of the advancing border in tinea corporis. (Courtesy of Nicholas Compton MD.)

Tinea cruris, or "jock itch," usually occurs in adult males and may be accompanied by tinea pedis. It is caused by *Epidermophyton floccosum*, *Trichophyton rubrum*, or *Trichophyton mentagrophytes*. The infection begins as an erythematous scaling patch involving intertriginous areas of the groin folds and inner thighs. Although it may extend on the lower abdomen and gluteal region, the scrotum is usually spared. There is mild erythema, with a well-demarcated scaly border. Differential diagnosis includes seborrheic dermatitis, erythrasma, intertrigo, candidiasis, and psoriasis.

Tinea pedis, or "athlete's foot," is the most common location for dermatophyte infections. Clinical variants of tinea pedis include maceration and scale of the interdigital spaces and mild diffuse erythema and scale of the foot in a moccasin distribution. A vesicular presentation with 1-2 mm dried vesicles of the plantar surface, commonly on the mid foot, may occur. Differential diagnosis includes contact dermatitis and psoriasis.

Onychomycosis, or dermatophyte infection of the nail, results in nail plate thickening, dystrophy, and subungual debris of one or several nails. Toenails are affected more often than fingernails. Many organisms may cause onychomycosis, including nondermatophytes. When dermatophytes are the culprit, then concurrent tinea pedis is usually the source of the nail infection. Differential diagnosis includes psoriasis, lichen planus, candidiasis, and hereditary nail dystrophies. In diabetic individuals dermatophyte infections of the nails and feet create a portal of entry for bacterial infections, putting them at risk for cellulitis, especially due to streptococci.

Diagnosis

In all forms of dermatophyte infection, diagnosis rests on demonstrating the fungus, either by KOH examination of scrapings or by culture. The KOH examination is a simple, rapid diagnostic tool. A sample is taken of scale at the active border of skin lesions, of subungual debris in onychomycosis, or of hairs in tinea capitis. The sample is placed on a microscope slide, covered with a few drops of 10-20% KOH and a coverslip, then heated briefly to lyse keratinocytes and reveal the KOH-resistant fungal structures. The specimen is examined for hyphae using the ×10 objective with the condenser lowered. Culture for dermatophytes often requires 2-6 weeks' growth to identify the fungal species.

Treatment

Topical therapy

Topical therapy is usually adequate for tinea pedis, tinea cruris, and limited forms of tinea corporis. Topical agents include imidazoles (clotrimazole, miconazole, ketoconazole, and econazole), the allylamine terbinafine, and other agents (ciclopirox, naftifine, and tolnaftate). These agents are usually applied as creams twice daily until clearing occurs. Avoid topical steroid use in these conditions, as it can worsen infection.

Systemic therapy

For tinea capitis, oral treatment is required; griseofulvin is effective therapy. The newer antifungals terbinafine, itraconazole, and fluconazole have been shown to be efficacious and safe alternatives to griseofulvin.

- Griseofulvin single or divided daily dose, 20 mg/kg/day for 6-12 weeks
- Terbinafine: patient weight >35 kg, 250 mg/day for 2-4 weeks; patient weight <25 kg, 125 mg/day for 6 weeks
- Itraconazole: 5 mg/kg per day for 4-6 weeks or pulse dosing of 5 mg/kg per day for 1 week each month for 2-3 months.

Duration of therapy with these agents is adjusted based on clinical response. Adjunctive use of antifungal shampoos (selenium sulfide or ketoconazole) often hastens the clinical response and may help prevent spread of infection to others.

Systemic therapy is indicated for recalcitrant or widespread tinea corporis, cruris, and pedis. The following regimens (adult doses) have been used:

- Terbinafine: 250 mg daily for 2 weeks
- Fluconazole: 50-100 mg daily or 150 mg once a week for 2-3 weeks

- Itraconazole: 100 mg daily for 2 weeks or 200 mg daily for 7 days.
  Onychomycosis is treated systemically. The following regimens have been used:
- Terbinafine: 250 mg/day for 6 weeks in fingernails and 12 weeks in toenails
- Itraconazole: 200 mg orally twice a day for 7 days/month for 3 months for toenails (two pulses for fingernails) or 200 mg orally daily for 12 weeks
- Fluconazole: 150-200 mg orally weekly for 9 months for toenails (6 months for fingernails).

The imidazole antifungals (ketoconazole, itraconazole, and fluconazole) have significant drug interactions; review the patient's medications for conflicts before prescribing.

Tinea Nigra

Tinea nigra is an uncommon superficial mycosis, often grouped with the dermatophytes, but caused by the melanin-producing dimorphic yeast *Hortaea werneckii*. The organism lives in soil, sewage, decaying vegetation, and also has been found on shower stalls in humid environments.

Epidemiology

Tinea nigra is a rare condition found in warm and humid climates, thought to be contracted from soil or decaying vegetation. The disease has been reported mainly in Central and South America, although cases have been identified in the southern United States, Africa, and Southeast Asia. Inoculating the organism into the skin with minor trauma has produced experimental infections, and this is believed to be the probable mechanism for natural infection. Lesions slowly develop over years and have been observed in travelers to endemic areas.

Clinical Features

The typical lesion is a well-demarcated, asymptomatic, brown to black patch of the palmar or plantar skin, resembling a stain. The lesions may resemble junctional nevi or acral lentiginous melanoma; however, the pigment may be partly removed by shaving off the most superficial stratum corneum layer of the skin. It occurs most commonly on the palms, but feet and other areas can be involved.

Diagnosis

KOH preparation of skin scrapings reveals hyphae. If a skin biopsy is done, the pigmented organisms can be seen in the stratum corneum.

Treatment

Tinea nigra is effectively treated with twice daily applications of imidazole or ciclopirox. Topical tolnaftate and oral griseofulvin are reported to be ineffective.

Conditions Caused by *Malassezia*

Malassezia furfur and *Malassezia globosa* are lipophilic fungi and part of the normal human microbiome. It is believed they play a pathogenic role in several dermatologic conditions, including seborrheic dermatitis, tinea (pityriasis) versicolor, and *Malassezia* (*Pityrosporum*) folliculitis. The latter two conditions are discussed here.

Tinea Versicolor

Tinea versicolor (pityriasis versicolor) is a common, usually asymptomatic superficial fungal infection that thrives under conditions of warmth and increased moisture.

Epidemiology

It is primarily a condition of adolescents and young adults, although those of any age may be affected. In some tropical populations, prevalence may exceed 50% among young adults. Infection is believed to reflect changes in host flora, and therefore person-to-person transmission is thought not to occur. Travelers to the tropics may experience their first episode of tinea versicolor.

Clinical features

The lesions of tinea versicolor are round or oval macules that coalesce into larger patches. They have a fine scale that sometimes is evident only when the lesion is scraped during the physical examination. In untanned Caucasians lesions may be subtly fawn brown and go unnoticed. The yeast blocks melanin synthesis in the skin and also produces a skin bleaching agent. With ultraviolet exposure a hypopigmented spotted appearance is enhanced due to contrast with the darkened surrounding skin (**Fig. 38.2**). Lesions are typically distributed over the shoulders, chest, and back, and occasionally on the neck. Pruritus is usually absent.

Diagnosis

In tinea versicolor, the clinical presentation is often sufficient to make the diagnosis. A KOH examination of scale scraped from lesions invariably shows the organisms and confirms the clinical suspicion. They are seen as short, curved hyphae and spherical yeast, giving a characteristic "spaghetti and meatballs" appearance.

The ease of confirming the diagnosis makes differential diagnosis less important. However, the appearance of hypopigmented lesions in the tropics may raise concerns of Hansen's disease (Chapter 40), in which hypopigmented lesions are anesthetic, or vitiligo, in which the lighter areas are not covered by scale and are completely depigmented rather than merely lighter in color.

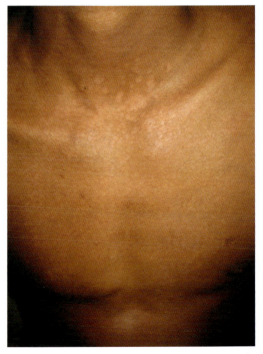

Fig. 38.2 **Hypopigmented and slightly pink macules on the chest in tinea versicolor.** (Courtesy of Nicholas Compton MD.)

Treatment

Topical

Many topical medications are effective in treating tinea versicolor, but recurrence is common. Even after successful treatment, pigment changes often take several months to return to normal. The following treatment regimens have been used successfully:

- 2.5% selenium sulfide shampoo: applied to affected areas for 10-15 min, then rinsed off. The application is repeated two times per week for 2-4 weeks.
- Various azole antifungal creams or lotions, including ketoconazole, miconazole, econazole, clotrimazole, and terbinafine: twice daily for 2 weeks.
- Oral treatment is sometimes required when topical therapy is impractical and success with multiple approaches is reported. One regimen is fluconazole 300 mg per week for 2 weeks.

Pityrosporum (Malassezia) *Folliculitis*

Pityrosporum folliculitis is a pruritic, follicular eruption caused by *Malassezia* spp. This disorder thrives in warm, humid climates especially on areas of the body covered by occlusive clothing. On biopsy prominent follicular dilation and inflammation is seen, owing to increased colonization with the fungi.

Epidemiology

Malassezia folliculitis usually affects young adults from the post-pubertal teens to the mid-30s, although it has been reported in children and the elderly. Predisposing factors include immunosuppression, corticosteroid therapy, and diabetes.

Clinical features

In temperate climates, *Malassezia* folliculitis characteristically presents as multiple monomorphic, pruritic, follicular papules and pustules distributed about the chest, upper back, and occasionally the proximal extremities.

Diagnosis

Diagnosis is best made by demonstrating the yeast in the follicular plug from one of the papules by direct microscopy using either 10-20% KOH or Gram stain. Serial sections of punch biopsies stained for fungi will also reveal numerous yeast forms in dilated follicles, but this is rarely necessary.

The differential diagnosis includes other types of folliculitis, including bacterial (staphylococcal) and candidal folliculitis, and acne vulgaris. Gram stain of an unroofed pustule helps to differentiate *Malassezia* folliculitis from other folliculitides. Acne vulgaris rarely has the prominent pruritus associated with the *Pityrosporum* folliculitis.

Treatment

Many topical regimens have been used effectively; there is no consensus on the best regimen. Adjunctive oral therapy is usually reserved for widespread cases or those unresponsive to topical therapy. The following regimens have been used successfully, although recurrences are common:

- 2.5% selenium sulfide shampoo: applied to affected areas for 10-15 minutes, then rinsed off. The application is repeated two times per week for 2-4 weeks.
- Various azole antifungal creams or lotions, including ketoconazole, miconazole, econazole, clotrimazole, and terbinafine: twice daily for 2 weeks.
- Itraconazole: 200 mg daily for 7 days.

Cutaneous Candidiasis

Candida albicans is part of the normal human mucosal flora. Under certain conditions and given various predisposing host factors, *C. albicans* and other less common species of *Candida* may become pathogenic, giving rise to several distinct clinical diseases. In addition to mucosal infections, candidiasis can occur as a cutaneous-only infection and as a systemic infection with cutaneous findings. Mucosal and cutaneous candidiasis are discussed here.

Epidemiology

The various clinical presentations of cutaneous candidiasis are quite common, with the greatest prevalence in newborns and elderly persons. In tropical climates, increased temperature and humidity, coupled with occlusive clothing, predispose travelers to cutaneous candidal infections. Other associated risk factors include diabetes, immunosuppression, corticosteroid therapy, and antibiotic use.

Clinical features

Oral candidiasis presents as "thrush" with white to gray, curd-like pseudomembranes overlying a shiny, brightly erythematous, painful mucosal surface on the buccal mucosa, palate, tongue, or gingivae. Differential diagnosis includes leukoplakia, in which the white mucosal plaques cannot be dislodged, and retained food particles that lack the underlying tenderness and erythema.

Less common oral presentations include the following:

- *Acute atrophic glossitis*: tender, shiny erythema of the dorsal surface of the tongue with loss of the normal papillae, seen most commonly in the setting of antibiotic or corticosteroid use.
- *Angular cheilitis* (*perlèche*): painful fissuring and erythema at the commissures of the lips.

Candidal vulvovaginitis occurs commonly in women and presents as a thick, white, vaginal discharge, often with associated pruritus, burning, and dysuria. The skin of the vulva often shows bright confluent erythema with scale and satellite papules and pustules. Speculum examination of the vaginal vault reveals brightly erythematous patches of vaginal mucosa with a "cottage cheese"-like vaginal discharge. Vulvovaginal involvement may extend to involve the perineum and crural folds, resulting in candidal intertrigo. *Candidal balanitis* usually occurs in uncircumcised men as confluent areas of moist, bright erythema with slight scale on the glans and prepuce. Candidal balanitis may spread to involve the scrotum and crural folds.

Candidal intertrigo is a common condition occurring in closely apposed skinfolds where there is a microenvironment of increased heat, humidity, and friction. Bright red, moist erythematous patches, usually with slight peripheral scale and satellite papules and pustules, occur symmetrically in the skin folds of the axillae, in the inframammary area, beneath the abdominal pannus, in the intergluteal fold, or in the crural folds. In infants, the skin folds of the anterior neck can be involved. Obesity, occlusion of the skin, and diabetes mellitus are common predisposing factors. Differential diagnosis includes psoriasis and seborrheic dermatitis, which should have findings consistent with these diagnoses in other areas. Tinea infection can involve the crural folds and would be distinguished by long, septated hyphal elements without yeast forms on KOH examination. Erythrasma, a bacterial infection caused by *Corynebacterium minutissimum*, has dull, red-brown, well-demarcated patches with fine scale; lacks satellite lesions and fungal elements on KOH scrapings; and shows a characteristic coral red fluorescence on Wood's lamp examination.

Diagnosis

Diagnosis can often be made clinically, but KOH examination of scrapings from mucosa or skin shows characteristic budding yeast cells and pseudohyphae. Culture is rarely necessary.

Treatment

All uncomplicated cutaneous candidiases respond well to most topical agents, including nystatin and azole antifungals. These agents come in various forms, including solutions, lotions, creams, powders, tablets, and troches. Creams and powders work well for intertrigo; measures to reduce occlusion and friction help prevent recurrence. Tablets and troches are best suited for oral candidiasis. Although topical agents work quite well for vulvovaginal candidiasis, fluconazole as a 150-mg, one-time oral dose is often used and preferred by patients.

It is important to search for and treat any underlying illness. The presence of oral thrush in an otherwise healthy individual should prompt an investigation of human immunodeficiency virus risk factors and appropriate testing when indicated.

Piedra

Piedra is a superficial fungal infection of the hair shaft seen most commonly in tropical climates. It presents in two distinct clinical varieties, black piedra and white piedra, caused by *Piedraia hortae* and *Trichosporon* species, respectively.

Epidemiology

Black piedra occurs in the tropical regions of the Americas and Southeast Asia. White piedra has a broader distribution, including Africa, Europe, and Japan. Both types show equal age and sex distribution.

Clinical features

Black piedra presents as asymptomatic, microscopic to 1 mm or larger, dark, firmly adherent, concretions on hair shafts of the scalp or, less commonly, the beard. White piedra also presents as asymptomatic concretions or nodules on the hair shafts, although these are lighter in color (white to light brown) and can be easily detached, unlike those of black piedra. White piedra involves facial and genital hair more often than scalp hair. In both forms, affected hair shafts may be weakened and fracture easily.

Diagnosis

Clinical inspection of the hair shafts and demonstration of fungal elements on KOH examination make the diagnosis in both forms of piedra. Culture of the organism can be problematic, so communication with the laboratory may aid in the accuracy of diagnostic testing.

Differential diagnosis includes lice (see Chapter 37), seborrheic dermatitis, trichomycosis axillaris, and inverse psoriasis. In trichomycosis axillaris, a benign infection of axillary or pubic hair by *Corynebacterium* species, yellow-tan deposits form on hair shafts. This disorder may be difficult to distinguish visually from white piedra, but KOH examination of the hair deposits will demonstrate the hyphae of *Trichosporon* in white piedra.

Treatment

Piedra is readily treated by cutting or shaving the affected hairs. Ketoconazole shampoo is an adjunctive treatment. In persistent cases oral itraconazole and terbinafine have been tried. *Trichomycosis axillaris* responds to topical clindamycin or benzoyl peroxide.

SUBCUTANEOUS MYCOSES

Subcutaneous mycoses are a group of uncommon localized fungal infections of the deep tissues caused by several species of fungi. These infections are seen mainly in the tropics and are thought to arise after endemic fungal organisms are directly implanted into the skin from a puncture wound or following an abrasion. Included in this group are chromoblastomycosis, mycetoma, sporotrichosis, and lobomycosis.

Chromoblastomycosis

Chromoblastomycosis (or "chromomycosis") is a chronic fungal infection of the skin and subcutaneous tissue caused by any of several pigmented fungi normally found in soil and wood, including species within the genera *Fonsecaea*, *Cladophialophora*, and *Phialophora*. These organisms are pigmented molds that produce identical clinical infections, and all appear in tissue sections as small (4-6 μm), brown-colored spherical forms, hence the name *chromo-*blastomycosis. They can be distinguished in culture.

Epidemiology

Chromoblastomycosis occurs worldwide but is most common in tropical areas of the Americas, Africa, and Asia. It is also regularly reported in Japan and Australia. The majority of cases occur in male farm workers in rural areas. Persons of all ages may be affected, but most cases occur in adults.

Clinical Features

Lesions typically begin as a unilateral, solitary, warty nodule, most often on the limbs (especially lower leg or foot), which evolves slowly to a large tumorous plaque that ulcerates. Satellite lesions occur around the primary lesion and may form along lymphatic channels. Lesions are frequently exophytic and friable, with lobulated, keratotic surfaces. The disease progresses slowly over many years and may involve an entire extremity. Local edema of the extremity often appears, with secondary bacterial infection and lymphadenitis. Pain is uncommon in the absence of bacterial infection. Untreated infections may persist more than 20 years. In rare cases, dissemination occurs with central nervous system (CNS) or visceral involvement.

Diagnosis

The diagnosis of chromoblastomycosis rests on demonstrating the causative organism on histologic sections with confirmation of the pathogenic species by culture. Biopsy for histology and culture should be taken from the active border of a lesion. Histology shows a nonspecific granulomatous and neutrophilic response and often the pigmented organisms ("copper pennies" known as "Medlar bodies"), which are diagnostic. Culture often takes 2-4 weeks. Serologic tests are not helpful.

Differential diagnosis includes other granulomatous processes, such as sporotrichosis, leishmaniasis, blastomycosis, and leprosy. Rarely, chronic lesions can undergo malignant transformation to squamous cell carcinoma.

Treatment

Chromoblastomycosis is not reliably responsive to medical therapy. With early treatment, cure can be achieved, but in advanced disease relapses are expected. Optimal treatment for the disease is still debated, but extended courses of itraconazole, terbinafine, and posaconazole have been used.

- Itraconazole: 200-400 mg/day
- Terbinafine: 250-1000 mg/day
- Posaconazole: 800 mg/day.

Amphotericin B and fluconazole are ineffective, and ketoconazole is not recommended due to toxicity with prolonged treatment. Treatment is lengthy with courses of 6-12 months, and drug resistance may develop during therapy. Combinations of multiple drugs, or drug therapy combined with physical approaches such as cryotherapy, application of heat, and ALA-PDT, are used with some effectiveness. Surgical approaches can be considered if the lesions are small.

Mycetoma

Mycetoma, also called "Madura foot," is a chronic and slowly enlarging infection that starts in the skin but ultimately is destructive to the subcutaneous tissue and muscle with eventual loss of function. Etiologies are certain fungi (eumycetoma) or filamentous bacteria (actinomycetoma). Occasionally the infection may extend to underlying bone. Mycetoma has three characteristic features: tumor formation, draining fistulas, and expelled granules ("grains").

The vast majority of cases of eumycetoma are caused by *Madurella mycetomatis*. Many other fungal species have been reported. Actinomycetoma may be caused by aerobic species of the actinomycetes, including *Nocardia*, *Streptomyces*, and *Actinomyces*.

Epidemiology

Mycetoma is caused by inoculation of the causative organism into the skin through trauma. The disease was initially described in India but is now found in Africa (especially Sudan, Senegal, and Somalia), Mexico, Central and South America, and Southeast Asia. Mycetoma mainly occurs in persons working barefoot in soil or vegetation and is usually contracted from fungal elements entering the skin through a puncture wound caused by a splinter or thorn. The vast majority of cases occur in young men.

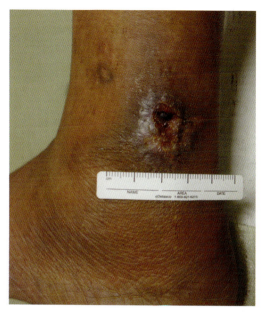

Fig. 38.3 Early actinomycetoma ulcer with nearby satellite lesion in a traveler.

Clinical Features

The usual site of inoculation is the foot, but the hands or other areas may be affected. After a latent period of one to several months, a painless subcutaneous nodule develops and slowly enlarges. The lesion progresses to form a large tumor with sinus tracts draining bloody or purulent material (**Fig. 38.3**). The lesion invades slowly by local extension to fascia and muscle and may eventually involve bone. Systemic symptoms are rare and pain is surprisingly infrequent, present in only about one-third of patients.

The sinus drainage typically contains granules, 0.1-5.0 mm in size, which may be white, pink, yellow, brown, or black, depending on the causative organism. Lesions tend to be progressive over many years, and late complications include functional loss, amyloidosis, and sepsis.

Diagnosis

The typical features of *swelling*, *fistula formation*, and *granules* may allow a clinical diagnosis. Specific diagnosis requires examination of the granules with culture. Granules may be obtained from drainage material or biopsy tissue. The most suitable granules for culture of fungi and actinomycetes are taken from the base of a biopsy specimen. Granules may also be crushed and examined in KOH microscopically. The hyphae of eumycetoma are distinguishable from the thin filaments of actinomycetoma.

Biopsy of the lesion will also show the organisms on histologic sections and is useful in ruling out neoplasms that may be in the clinical differential diagnosis. Radiographic imaging can help determine if osteomyelitis is present.

Treatment

Treatment varies based on the causal agent, the affected region, and the degree of invasion. Surgical excision is often recommended for early lesions, and in advanced cases amputation may be necessary. Surgery should be accompanied by medical treatment because of the risk of recurrence even with wide-margin amputations. Actinomycetoma responds more favorably with fewer recurrences than does eumycetoma. *Nocardia* spp. are treated for several months with trimethoprim-sulfamethoxazole, often combined with dapsone; in severe cases imipenem or amikacin is added. Standard therapy for eumycetoma is itraconazole and terbinafine, sometimes in combination. Avoiding walking barefoot in endemic areas and early wound disinfection is mandatory for prevention.

Sporotrichosis

Sporotrichosis, caused by the fungus *Sporothrix schenckii*, is a fungal infection of the skin, lymphatics, and subcutaneous tissue, which rarely becomes disseminated. *S. schenckii* is found in soil and plant debris in both temperate and tropical climates.

Epidemiology

Sporotrichosis occurs worldwide but is more common in warm, humid climates, with the highest rates of infection occurring in Mexico, Brazil, and South Africa. Infection occurs by inoculation into sites of trauma, and most cases arise in persons whose work predisposes to injury with infected material (e.g., gardeners, florists, and farm workers). An outbreak of 3000 cases was reported in South African mine workers who were exposed by rubbing against infected timber. In the United States, cases occur most often in rose gardeners and nursery workers who handle sphagnum moss.

Clinical Features

The primary lesion occurs at the site of inoculation as a painless dermal nodule that usually breaks down to form a ragged ulcer. The initial lesion may persist for weeks to months or may heal and disappear, only to be followed by further symptoms. In most cases, additional small, dusky red, painless nodules appear over weeks to months along the regional lymphatics. These may also ulcerate and form fistulae. Occasionally, the primary lesion is not followed by regional spread. These solitary lesions may become granulomatous plaques, which often develop smaller peripheral satellite lesions. Lesions may persist for years without therapy. Rarely, dissemination occurs to lungs, bone, CNS, and skin, usually in immunocompromised patients.

Diagnosis

The clinical picture of a painless, indurated ulcer on the hand, which is followed by subsequent lesions along regional lymphatics, should strongly suggest sporotrichosis. The diagnosis is established by isolating the organism, usually from a biopsy specimen. The histology of biopsied lesions shows a mixed granulomatous response but rarely reveals the organism. Fungal culture of biopsy material is the most reliable means of diagnosis, and cultures to rule out the other infections listed previously should always be performed concomitantly.

Lymphatic nodules can also be caused by atypical mycobacteria, particularly *Mycobacterium marinum*, nocardiasis, and tularemia. Solitary lesions must be distinguished from cutaneous tuberculosis, other deep fungi, anthrax, tularemia, and carcinoma.

Treatment

Medical treatment is usually effective. Itraconazole, 100-200 mg daily for 3-6 months, is recommended. Alternatives are terbinafine 500 mg twice per day or saturated solution of potassium iodide (SSKI). Standard therapy starts with 0.5-1 mg/day and is increased to an effective dose of 4-6 mg/day. Although SSKI is inexpensive and effective, patients often do not tolerate it due to associated side effects of hypersalivation and nausea. Finally, hyperthermia has been used to treat the localized form of the disease. Regardless of the therapy chosen, treatment should continue for at least 4 weeks after the resolution of clinical disease.

Lobomycosis

Lobomycosis (keloidal blastomycosis) is an uncommon localized infection of the skin caused by *Lacazia loboi*. In the skin, the fungus takes the form of a spherical intracellular yeast.

Epidemiology

Lobomycosis occurs most commonly in residents and travelers to the Amazon rainforest. It has also been seen in individuals from Central America and Mexico, with sporadic cases seen in France and the United States. The natural reservoir for the organism has not been identified, and the disease is usually seen in young men working in the rural forest. In addition to humans, bottlenose dolphins are infected in the wild.

Clinical Features

Lobomycosis usually begins as small papules or plaques grouped together on areas of exposed skin, most commonly ears, arms, or legs. The early lesions gradually evolve into shiny keloid-like nodules, which usually are either asymptomatic or cause mild itching. Proximal lymph nodes may also be involved. The disease tends to be chronic. Fully formed skin lesions may resemble the nodules of leprosy or sarcoid.

Diagnosis

The diagnosis is suggested by the clinical findings and confirmed by skin biopsy that shows distinctive fungal organisms embedded in histiocytic and giant cell granulomas. The fungi consist of round or lemon-shaped spheres, distributed singly or in short chains. So far culture attempts have been unsuccessful.

Treatment

Treatment generally consists of wide surgical excision of the lesions. Limited success has been reported with clofazimine, itraconazole, and posaconazole.

FURTHER READING

Abdel-Razek, M., Fadaly, G., Abdel-Raheim, M., et al., 1995. Pityrosporum (*Malassezia*) folliculitis in Saudi Arabia: diagnosis and therapeutic trials. Clin. Exp. Dermatol. 20, 406.

Ameen, M., 2009. Chromobastomycosis: clinical presentation and management. Clin. Exp. Dermatol. 34, 849–854.

Brun, A., 1999. Lobomycosis in three Venezuelan patients. Int. J. Dermatol. 38, 298–305.

Ely, J.W., Rosenfeld, S., Stone, M.S., 2014. Diagnosis and management of tinea infections. Am. Fam. Med. 90, 702–710.

Faergemann, J., 1998. Pityrosporum infections. In: Elewski, B.E. (Ed.), Cutaneous Fungal Infections, second ed. Blackwell, Malden, MA.

Gip, L., 1994. Black piedra: the first case treated with terbinafine. Br. J. Dermatol. 130, 26–28.

Gueho, E., Boekhout, T., Ashbee, H.R., et al., 1998. The role of *Malassezia* species in the ecology of human skin and as pathogens. Med. Mycol. 36, S220.

Gupta, G., Burden, A.D., Shankland, G.S., et al., 1997. Tinea nigra secondary to *Exophiala werneckii* responding to itraconazole. Br. J. Dermatol. 137, 483–484.

Gupta, A.K., Hofstader, S.L., Adam, P., et al., 1999. Tinea capitis: an overview with emphasis on management. Pediatr. Dermatol. 16, 171–189.

Hay, R.J., 1999. The management of superficial candidiasis. J. Am. Acad. Dermatol. 40, S35.

Hay, R.J., Moore, M., 1998. Mycology. In: Champion, R.H., Burton, J.L.Burns, D.A. (Eds.), Textbook of Dermatology, vol. 2, sixth ed. Blackwell Science, London.

Hsu, L.Y., Wijaya, L., Ng, E.S.T., et al., 2012. Tropical fungal infections. Inf. Dis. Clin. North Amer. 26, 497–512.

Jacinto-Jamora, S., Tamesis, J., Katigbak, M.L., 1991. Pityrosporum folliculitis in the Philippines: diagnosis, prevalence, and management. J. Am. Acad. Dermatol. 24, 693–696.

Martin, A.G., Kobayashi, G.S., 1999a. Superficial fungal infection: dermatophytosis, tinea nigra, piedra. In: Freedberg, I.M., Eisen, A.Z., Wolff, K. (Eds.), Fitzpatrick's Dermatology in General Medicine, fifth ed. McGraw-Hill, New York.

Martin, A.G., Kobayashi, G.S., 1999b. Yeast infections: candidiasis, pityriasis (tinea) versicolor. In: Freedberg, I.M., Eisen, A.Z., Wolff, K. (Eds.), Fitzpatrick's Dermatology in General Medicine, fifth ed. McGraw-Hill, New York.

Nenoff, P., Sande, W.W.J., Fahal, A.H., et al., 2015. Eumycetoma and actinolycetoma: an update on causative agents, epidemiology, pathogenesis, diagnostics and therapy. J. Eur. Acad. Dermatol. Venereol. 29 (10), 1873–1883. Epub.

Pappas, A.A., Ray, T.L., 1998. Cutaneous and disseminated skin manifestations of candidiasis. In: Elewski, B.E. (Ed.), Cutaneous Fungal Infections, second ed. Blackwell, Malden, MA.

Rivitti, E.A., Aoki, V., 1999. Deep fungal infections in tropical countries. Clin. Dermatol. 17, 171–190.

Rodriguez-Toro, G., 1993. Lobomycosis. Int. J. Dermatol. 32, 324–332.

Sivaraman, D., Thappa, D.M., Karthikeyan, H., et al., 1999. Subcutaneous phycomycosis mimicking synovial sarcoma. Int. J. Dermatol. 38, 916–925.

Sobera, J., Elewski, B.E., 2003. Fungal diseases. In: Bolognia, J.L., Jorizzo, J.L., Rapini, R.P. (Eds.), Dermatology. Mosby, London.

Talhari, S., Cunha, M.G., Schettini, A.P., et al., 1988. Deep mycoses in the Amazon region. Int. J. Dermatol. 27, 481–484.

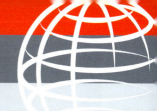

CHAPTER 39

Leishmaniasis

Frederick S. Buckner and Eli Schwartz

The leishmaniases are a group of chronic cutaneous, mucocutaneous, and visceral diseases caused by infection with one of several species of the protozoan parasite *Leishmania*. Members of the genus *Leishmania* are obligate intracellular parasitic protozoa in the family Trypanosomatidae. They exist as elongate, 10-15 μm, flagellated forms called promastigotes in their sand fly vectors. When an infected sand fly bites a mammalian host, it injects the promastigotes into the wound with its saliva. Tissue macrophages phagocytize the organisms, which then transform into round or oval, 2-3 μm nonflagellated forms called amastigotes. The amastigotes undergo successive asexual division until the macrophage ruptures, releasing the amastigotes, which enter other macrophages. When a sand fly bites an infected mammalian host, it ingests amastigote-laden macrophages along with its blood meal. The amastigotes transform into promastigotes and reproduce in the gut of the fly before migrating to the proboscis of the fly to complete the cycle with the next fly bite.

Hematophagous female sand flies in the genus *Phlebotomus* in the Old World and *Lutzomyia* and *Psychodopygus* in the New World transmit the *Leishmania* organisms (**Fig. 39.1**). Several nonhuman mammals serve as reservoirs for leishmaniasis, including domestic and wild canines and various rodents, depending on the geographic distribution and the species of *Leishmania* involved.

Currently, experts recognize over a dozen species, some of which they group into complexes of closely related species (i.e., the New World *L. mexicana* and the *L. viannia* complexes).

CLINICAL MANIFESTATIONS

There are three major clinical manifestations:

- Cutaneous leishmaniasis
- Mucocutaneous leishmaniasis
- Visceral leishmaniasis.

CUTANEOUS LEISHMANIASIS

Based on its geographic distribution, cutaneous leishmaniasis can be divided into Old World (including Southern Europe, the Middle East, parts of Southwest Asia, and Africa) and New World leishmaniasis (from the southern United States through Latin America to the highlands of Argentina). This distribution has clinical relevance, since Old World species cause mostly benign and often self-limiting cutaneous disease, while New World species cause a broad spectrum of manifestations, from benign to severe, including mucosal involvement.

Cutaneous leishmaniasis is a chronic ulcerative, frequently self-healing, skin infection. The worldwide distribution is shown in **Figure 39.2**. Local peoples apply many common names to this disease (see below). Depending on the species involved, the infecting organisms may spread by direct extension or metastasis to involve the mucosa of the upper

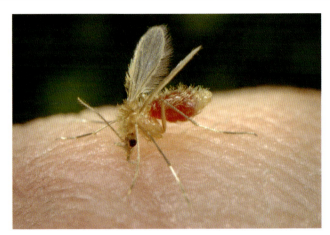

Fig. 39.1 The sand fly vectors of leishmaniasis are very small, only 2-3 mm (1/8 inch) in length. The photograph shows a *Phlebotomus papatasi* sand fly. (From http://phil.cdc.gov/phil/details.asp?pid=10275. Photo by J. Gathany, courtesy of CDC/Frank Collins.)

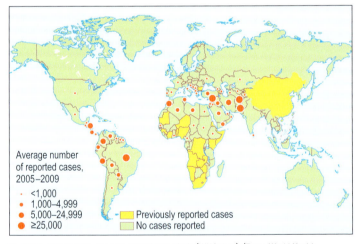

Fig. 39.2 **Distribution of cutaneous leishmaniasis (WHO data).** (From: World Health Organization, 2010. First WHO Report on Neglected Tropical Diseases: Working to Overcome the Global Impact of Neglected Tropical Diseases. Available at <http://whqlibdoc.who.int/publications/2010/9789241564090_eng.pdf>.)

respiratory tract (mucocutaneous leishmaniasis), resulting in painful disfigurement or even death.

Old World Cutaneous Leishmaniasis (OWCL)

Common names include Oriental sore, Rose of Jericho, Delhi boil, and Aleppo boil.

Etiology and Epidemiology

OWCL is caused by four species: *L. major*, *L. tropica*, *L. aethiopica*, and *L. infantum*.

L. major causes rural, wet, and zoonotic cutaneous leishmaniasis. The animal reservoirs are desert rodents. It is endemic in desert areas of northern Africa, Central Asia, the Sudan, and the Middle East. In certain communities, local prevalence may approach 100% and travelers may be affected.

L. tropica usually causes urban, dry, and more often anthroponotic cutaneous leishmaniasis. Experts now think that in some places (e.g., Afghanistan) humans are the primary host and may serve as a reservoir. In a recent outbreak in Israel, rock hyraxes were found to be the reservoir. Endemic areas include urban areas of the Mediterranean basin, Central Asia, and the Middle East.

L. aethiopica occurs mainly in Ethiopia and Kenya in rural mountain areas. Hyraxes, distant relatives of elephants, serve as the animal reservoir.

L. infantum occurs in the Mediterranean basin, China, Central Asia, and the Middle East. Adults infected with this species tend to develop a mild self-limited cutaneous disease, whereas infants tend to develop visceral disease. Infection can occur person-to-person among intravenous drug users sharing syringes. Animal reservoirs include domesticated and wild canines.

Clinical Features

Following inoculation by the sand fly, characteristic skin lesions generally appear within 6 weeks but may be delayed for prolonged periods depending on the size of the inoculum. The lesion begins as a small, pruritic, erythematous papule that slowly enlarges and breaks down to form a small ulcer or is sometimes a nodular lesion. Lesions may be single or multiple and occur on exposed skin surfaces. Ulcers persist for a variable time (measured in months) and heal slowly with scarring.

L. major often causes multiple lesions with an exudative base (**Fig. 39.3**). The infection runs a more rapid course, and the lesions may heal in 6 months. Spread to regional lymph nodes is rare.

L. tropica usually causes a single, more indolent ulcer that may require over 1 year for spontaneous healing. Internal organ involvement ("viscerotropic" infection) with *L. tropica* has been demonstrated in six US soldiers returning from prolonged deployment in the Middle East during the Gulf War.

L. aethiopica produces an even more indolent ulcer that may persist for several years. Diffuse cutaneous leishmaniasis, an anergic state with extensive skin infiltration by organisms resembling lepromatous leprosy, occurs in approximately 20% of endemic *L. aethiopica* infections.

New World Cutaneous Leishmaniasis (NWCL)

Common names include American cutaneous leishmaniasis, chiclero ulcer, espundia, bush yaws, uta, and picadura de pito.

Etiology and Epidemiology

NWCL is a disease of rural forest and jungle areas of most of Central and South America. Forest workers, agricultural workers, and others in rural, forested areas are primarily at risk. Several species belonging to the *L. viannia* and *L. mexicana* complexes cause NWCL (**Table 39.1**). Species from either complex may be principal causes of leishmaniasis in a given area. Both complexes are pathogenic throughout the range of disease in the New World, with the exceptions of southern Texas and the Dominican Republic, where *L. mexicana* is the

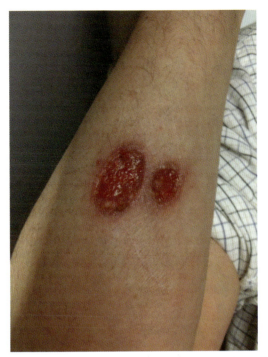

Fig. 39.3 Forearm lesions due to *L. major* in a defense contractor based in Iraq. (Photo by author, Fred Buckner.)

TABLE 39.1	New World Cutaneous Leishmaniasis
Subgenus	**Common Species**
Viannia	*L. (V.) brasiliensis*
	L. (V.) guyanensis
	L. (V.) panamensis
	L. (V.) peruviana
Mexicana	*L. mexicana*
	L. amazonensis
	L. venezuelensis

sole identified species. Animal reservoirs include foxes, sloths, and forest rodents, depending on the species.

Clinical Features

Cutaneous lesions may resemble those of OWCL with a few distinctive differences. Lesions tend to be larger, up to 7 cm in diameter, with an elevated, indurated border that is mostly ulcerative (**Fig. 39.4**). In addition, subcutaneous nodules with sporotrichoid distribution may be present, as well as regional lymphadenopathy. The cutaneous lesions heal very

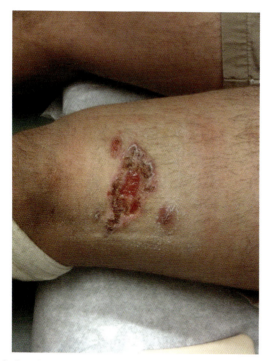

Fig. 39.4 Lesions above the knee in a traveler to Costa Rica with *L. panamensis* infection. Note the satellite lesions. (Photo by author, Fred Buckner.)

slowly, and they may spread to the oropharyngeal mucosa, causing mucocutaneous leishmaniasis.

Chiclero ulcer refers to cutaneous disease found in the Yucatan, Belize, and Guatemala caused primarily by *L. mexicana*. Lesions tend to be solitary and occur most frequently on the ear. Ear ulcers may persist for many years before healing and may result in destruction of the ear. Lesions in other skin areas often heal within 6 months. Mucosal spread is rare with *L. mexicana*.

Mucocutaneous leishmaniasis results primarily from infections caused by *L. (Viannia) brasiliensis*. The cutaneous lesions spread along lymphatics, resembling sporotrichosis, and mucosal disease occurs in 5–10% of cases. Mucosal involvement occurs by metastatic spread of infection from the skin and presents months to years after the initial cutaneous lesions. It typically begins as erythema, edema, and ulceration of the nasal septum, with gradual extension to the palate, pharynx, and larynx. Occasionally, the anus and other mucosal sites may be involved. This destructive, granulomatous process of the soft tissue can involve cartilage but not bone. Perforation of the nasal septum and collapse of the nasal bridge is typical, giving the so-called tapir nose. Mucosal disease is progressive and mutilating and may be fatal. The severe form of mucosal disease is called *espundia*.

Diffuse cutaneous leishmaniasis occasionally occurs and is similar to this form of OWCL.

Diagnosis of Cutaneous Leishmaniasis

Cutaneous leishmaniasis should be considered in patients with characteristic nonhealing skin lesion(s) with the appropriate exposure history. Frequently, patients have been treated with antibiotics without benefit. The differential diagnosis includes cutaneous fungal infection (sporotrichosis, histoplasmosis, coccidioidomycosis, etc.), mycobacterial infection (including nontuberculous mycobacterial infections such as *M. fortuitum*, *M. abscessus*, and *M. marinum*), leprosy, and skin cancer, particularly squamous cell carcinoma.

A definitive diagnosis requires tissue obtained by scrapings or punch biopsy. When the face or other sensitive sites are involved, needle aspirates can be obtained using small amounts of nonbacteriostatic normal saline. Tissue should be submitted for histology, culture, and, most importantly, molecular diagnostic analysis. Histology from touch preparations, aspirates, or tissue sections can reveal the amastigotes within macrophages. On Giemsa stain, these 2-3 μM oval structures contain a bar-shaped organelle, the kinetoplast, adjacent to the cell nucleus. Observing these structures establishes the diagnosis of leishmaniasis; however, species identification that is critical for clinical management decisions requires culture or molecular diagnostics.

A variety of specialized culture systems are available for biopsies, skin scraping, or needle aspirates. Promastigotes that grow can be subjected to species identification by biochemical or molecular techniques. The cultures are usually held for 4 weeks before they are considered negative. However, polymerase chain reaction (PCR) has become the test of choice for establishing the diagnosis of cutaneous leishmaniasis. DNA is extracted from punch biopsy specimens or needle aspirates and subjected to PCR and sequencing. Importantly, the results can be available in 2-3 days. Sensitivity ranges from 89 to 100%. It is uncommon for the direct PCR to be negative and cultures to be positive. DNA sequence methods have largely replaced biochemical methods (isoenzyme analysis) for species identification, since it is faster.

Drug susceptibility testing for *Leishmania* clinical isolates is not available.

The leishmanin skin test (Montenegro test) gives evidence of present or past infection and is usually positive 3 months after onset of lesions except in the diffuse form. It involves a subcutaneous injection of a given inoculum of killed promastigotes and is read at 48 hours after application. A response of ≥5 mm is positive.

Serologic tests are available in some centers, but their role in the diagnosis of cutaneous leishmaniasis is very limited.

Treatment

Few infectious diseases are as complex as cutaneous leishmaniasis when it comes to clinical management. Treatments can be lengthy, expensive, and toxic, so it is important to establish a parasitological diagnosis before initiating therapy. Furthermore, appropriate management depends on the species of *Leishmania* involved, therefore the diagnostic test should be one that provides species identification (discussed above). Even with species information available, there are inadequate clinical studies to always guide the best management. Individual circumstances will influence management decisions, such as the number, location, and age of the lesions. Three levels of management may be considered for cutaneous leishmaniasis.

1. For mild disease caused by less aggressive species, observation alone may be appropriate, particularly when considering the potential toxicity of drugs.
2. The next level involves local treatment such as topical ointments or intralesional injections with antileishmanial drugs. For practitioners in the United States, this approach is not commonly used due to the unavailability of approved drugs/formulations for this application. Other local treatment options include cryotherapy or thermotherapy, which have advocates under certain circumstances but require a certain level of skill and experience for optimal use.
3. Finally, systemic treatment (oral or intravenous [IV]) is recommended when local therapy is not an option or inappropriate. The indications for systemic treatment are summarized in **Table 39.2.**

Treatments for specific forms of cutaneous leishmaniasis are discussed below. Many of these treatments are dictated by local experiences, where options may be limited by

TABLE 39.2	Indications for Systemic Treatment for Cutaneous Leishmaniasis

- Lesion caused by *Viannia* subspecies (especially *L. (Viannia) brasiliensis*)
- Metastatic spread to lymph nodes
- Localization in the face
- Multiple lesions
- Chronic ear infection (chiclero, *L. mexicana*)

availability and cost of certain drugs. **Table 39.3** summarizes the doses and other details of the various treatment options.

Treatment of OWCL

For *L. major* local treatment is preferred. Where available, 15% paromomycin/12% methylbenzethonium chloride ointment is proven to be effective. Local infiltration with sodium stibogluconate is used in Europe and in Israel but has not been approved in the United States. Cryotherapy with liquid nitrogen can be used with relatively new and small lesions (<3 mm). Close observation is reasonable for mild cases of *L. major* infection, since it very rarely metastasizes and usually self-heals within a few months. When systemic therapy is indicated due to extensive disease or the location of lesions on face, hands, or feet, then IV antimony is most often used, although small studies suggest a role for liposomal amphotericin B. Fluconazole has been used successfully in Saudi Arabia but seems to be less effective in cases from North Africa or Iraq. There are not enough data available to support the use of miltefosine for *L. major*.

Whereas *L. major* infection can resolve without treatment in months, *L. tropica* infection tends to be slower healing and usually warrants antiparasitic treatment. *L. tropica* is thought to be less responsive to paromomycin ointment, therefore it is common practice to treat with intralesional sodium stibogluconate. Local thermotherapy (discussed further below) has been used with some success. When parenteral therapy is indicated, either sodium stibogluconate or liposomal amphotericin B are the best options. A role for miltefosine is uncertain.

Treatment of NWCL

Cutaneous leishmaniasis that is acquired in the Americas should be diagnosed as being caused by species in the *Viannia* complex (i.e., *L. braziliensis*, *L. guyanensis*, *L. panamensis*, or *L. peruviana*) versus the Mexicana complex (i.e., *L. mexicana*, *L. venezuelensis*, or *L. amazonensis*). The former tends to be more destructive and has higher potential for causing mucosal leishmaniasis, thus systemic therapy is usually indicated. Traditionally, parenteral antimony has been used for infections caused by *Viannia* species. However, recent studies show that oral miltefosine has high success rates (75-88%). An exception may be cases acquired in Guatemala where miltefosine success rates were only 45%. There is also growing experience with the successful use of liposomal amphotericin B for cutaneous leishmaniasis due to *Viannia* complex species. Better availability and shorter courses make liposomal amphotericin B preferable to sodium stibogluconate (at least in the United States), although high cost is a factor.

When a diagnosis of NWCL is made due to *L. mexicana*, either a "wait and see" approach or local therapy are considerations. Local therapy usually consists of injections of antimony combined with cryotherapy. Systemic antimony provides high cure rates when required. Infections due to *L. amazonensis* are usually treated either locally or systemically. There are limited data on the use of miltefosine, so parenteral antimony or liposomal amphotericin B is preferable.

Patients with cutaneous leishmaniasis should be reevaluated 6 weeks after the treatment course is completed, and if lesions are not improved by at least 75%, retreatment or

TABLE 39.3 Treatment Options for Leishmaniasis[a]

	Therapy	Route of Administration	Dose	Directions	Pros	Cons
Local therapy	Paromomycin ointment	Topical	15% paromomycin/12% methylbenzethonium chloride	Twice per day for 10-20 days	Topical	Not available in USA except through compounding
	Sodium stibogluconate	Intralesional injection	0.5-2.0 mL of 100 mg/mL pe-tavalent antimony	Intralesional every 3-7 days until healed	Local	Special skills required; drug not available in USA
	Cryotherapy (liquid nitrogen)	Cotton tipped applicator	Freeze-thaw-freeze	Repeat on 3-week cycles up to 3 times	Local	Special skills required; appropriate only with small lesions
	Thermotherapy	Thermal prongs	30-sec intervals in grid pattern over lesion	1-3 treatments	ThermoMed instrument is FDA approved	Special skills required; painful (local anesthesia required)
Oral therapy	Miltefosine	Oral	50 mg	BID (30-44 kg) or TID (>45 kg) × 28 days	FDA approved for cutaneous leishmaniasis; oral route	Gastrointestinal side effects; teratogenic
	Fluconazole	Oral	400-600 mg	Daily × 6 weeks	Oral; well-tolerated	Limited track record of success
	Ketoconazole	Oral	600 mg	Daily × 4 weeks	Oral	Limited track record of success
Parenteral therapy	Sodium stibogluconate	IV or IM	20 mg/kg/day	Daily × 10-20 days	Available through CDC; standard of care	High toxicity; provided via IND in USA
	Meglumine antimoniate	IV or IM	20 mg/kg/day	Daily × 10-20 days	Long track record	Not available in USA
	Amphotericin B deoxycholate	IV	0.5-1.0 mg/kg	Every other day × 20-30 days	Less expensive than AmBisome	Toxic; long duration of treatment
	Liposomal amphotericin B (AmBisome)	IV	3 mg/kg	5-7 daily doses	Shorter course, better tolerated than antimony	Expensive
	Pentamidine	IV	2-4 mg/kg	Every other day × 4-7 doses		Toxic; limited indications

[a]See text for indications.

CDC, Centers for Disease Control and Prevention; *IM*, intramuscular; *IND*, investigational new drug; *IV*, intravenous.

alternative treatment should be considered. After completion of treatment, lesions should be monitored for relapse for 1 year.

Mucosal leishmaniasis tends to be difficult to treat. Parenteral antimony (20 mg/kg per day of sodium stibogluconate for 28 days) gives cure rates approximating 60%. A study in travelers has shown that liposomal amphotericin B 3 mg/kg IV given daily for 5 days with another dose at day 10 is very effective. This treatment was given first only to cases of stibogluconate failure but was later used as primary treatment with high cure rates. However, because of the strong potential for relapse, it is recommended that mucosal lesions be followed for several years after completion of drug therapy.

VISCERAL LEISHMANIASIS

Visceral leishmaniasis, or kala-azar, results from infection with *L. donovani* in Africa and India, *L. infantum* in the Mediterranean basin, and *L. chagasi* in the New World. It, like the cutaneous leishmaniases, is transmitted by the bite of phlebotomine sand flies. Reservoir animals include various rodents and domesticated or wild canines, except in India where man is the only known reservoir.

Clinicians practicing in North America or Europe are less likely to see cases of visceral leishmaniasis than cutaneous leishmaniasis. Nonetheless, visceral leishmaniasis should be suspected in residents of or recent travelers to endemic areas (**Fig. 39.5**) who present with *intermittent fever, anemia,* and *marked hepatosplenomegaly*—a syndrome evocative of lymphoma. Occasionally, military groups have experienced epidemics; for example, kala-azar occurred in British soldiers in India. Visceral leishmaniasis has been reported in US veterans of the Gulf War, although most of the latter cases appear to have been due to *L. tropica*. Infection can result from brief exposure in an endemic area.

Clinical Features

Kala-azar arising in different regions may show many variations in its clinical and epidemiologic appearance. A cutaneous nodule often develops at the site of the parasite inoculation

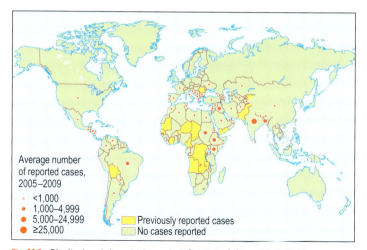

Fig. 39.5 Distribution of visceral leishmaniasis (WHO data). (From: World Health Organization, 2010. First WHO Report on Neglected Tropical Diseases: Working to Overcome the Global Impact of Neglected Tropical Diseases. Available at <http://whqlibdoc.who.int/publications/2010/9789241564090_eng.pdf>.)

in the African and Central Asian forms of the infection. Often this will have resolved before clinical illness develops. After an incubation period of 2-6 months, systemic manifestations develop insidiously, although the presentation may occasionally be abrupt. The earliest symptom is fever. On physical examination, the liver and spleen are large, firm, and non-tender. Lymphadenopathy is more frequently reported in the Mediterranean countries, East Africa, and China. Brazilian and Mediterranean kala-azar occur more frequently in children. Oral and nasopharyngeal lesions may occasionally be seen in the Sudan, East Africa, and India.

The clinical manifestations of kala-azar are due to the invasion of the reticuloendothelial cells of the spleen, liver, bone marrow, and skin and the subsequent multiplication of amastigotes within the cells. Untreated infections become chronic; in addition to the above physical findings, patients typically become markedly wasted. Patients with light-colored skin may develop a grayish cast—"kala-azar" is a Hindi name meaning "black fever."

Untreated visceral leishmaniasis may be complicated by intercurrent infections such as pneumonia, pulmonary tuberculosis, and dysentery; these often prove fatal. Some patients die from gastrointestinal hemorrhage.

The clinical presentation of visceral leishmaniasis in patients with acquired immunodeficiency syndrome (AIDS) is felt to be similar to the presentation in hosts without human immunodeficiency virus (HIV). Fever, splenomegaly, and pancytopenia are common. Involvement of the gastrointestinal tract is more common in AIDS patients. Abundant parasite-laden macrophages are found in the submucosa from the esophagus to the rectum. However, these patients typically respond poorly to treatment and have a high mortality rate.

Long after apparently successful treatment, some patients in India and East Africa develop post-kala-azar dermal leishmaniasis, a condition that resembles leprosy and features depigmented or nodular cutaneous lesions.

Diagnosis

The diagnosis of visceral leishmaniasis should be suspected in individuals presenting with characteristic signs and symptoms who have emigrated from or visited an area where leishmaniasis is endemic.

Laboratory studies reveal anemia, leukopenia, neutropenia, and occasionally thrombocytopenia. The eosinophil count is also low. A marked hyperglobulinemia due to increased IgG is usually present.

Microscopic examination and culture of bone marrow aspirates provide the best methods for reaching a definitive diagnosis of visceral leishmaniasis. Splenic aspiration is described in the literature but is discouraged due to risk of hemorrhage. In visceral leishmaniasis cases, serologic testing might be useful for diagnosis, followed by monitoring the response to treatment.

The introduction of PCR improves diagnostic sensitivity in bone-marrow aspirates. Recently it was also shown that the sensitivity of PCR of peripheral blood samples was similar to PCR of bone marrow aspirate (98%).

Treatment

In the absence of treatment, mortality from visceral leishmaniasis is >90%, thus systemic treatment is essential. The treatment options will depend on the availability and cost of drugs, likelihood of resistance, and host factors (particularly HIV status).

Liposomal amphotericin B (AmBisome), where it is affordable, has become the treatment of choice. Studies in India demonstrate cure rates of 96-100% with total doses of 14-20 mg/kg. The dose approved by the US Food and Drug Administration (FDA) is 3 mg/kg on days 1-5, 14, and 21, for a total of 21 mg/kg. In attempts to find the minimal dose, studies in India have shown a single dose of 7.5 mg/kg gave a 90% cure rate at 6 months. Higher cumulative doses (up to 60 mg/kg) are needed when treating HIV-infected patients. Liposomal amphotericin B is preferable to amphotericin B deoxycholate due to shorter course and less nephrotoxicity. Even so, liposomal amphotericin B is associated with infusion-related toxicity and nephrotoxicity and must be used with close supervision.

Parenteral antimony (sodium stibogluconate or meglumine antimoniate) has been a standard treatment for decades, but spreading resistance (mainly in India) is limiting its use. The side effects are significant, including myalgia, arthralgia, nausea, vomiting, rash, pancreatitis, and potentially fatal cardiotoxicity. Electrocardiograph monitoring is mandatory. Unless cost constraints are overriding, liposomal amphotericin B is preferred to antimony. Antimony is not FDA approved but can be appropriated through the Centers for Disease Control and Prevention (CDC) under an investigational new drug protocol. US providers will typically need to obtain institutional review board approval from their local institution. The current regimen recommended by the CDC is 20 mg/kg per day for 28 days; it is better tolerated intravenously, although it can be given intramuscularly. Patients typically feel better within 1 week of beginning treatment, but it may take weeks for laboratory values to normalize and months before splenomegaly resolves. Accurate assessment for complete cure mandates follow-up at frequent intervals over a 1-year period.

Miltefosine is an oral option for treating visceral leishmaniasis that has become available in the past decade. It was approved by the FDA in 2014. Cure rates in Indian studies are 94-97%. The standard regimen is 2.5 mg/kg/day for 28 days (available in 50-mg capsules). The oral route of administration is an obvious advantage, although 65% of patients experience vomiting. Importantly, miltefosine is teratogenic and needs to be used with extreme caution in woman of reproductive age. Resistance is an emerging problem in parts of India.

Parenterally administered paromomycin is a new and less expensive alternative for treating visceral leishmaniasis, although it is not approved in the United States. It is administered by the IV or IM route for 21 days. Indian studies show cure rates in the range of 88-95%. Adverse effects are relatively uncommon, although signs of hepatotoxicity, ototoxicity, and nephrotoxicity need to be monitored.

Due to increasing drug resistance, combination chemotherapy is emphasized, particularly in endemic regions. Reported combinations include liposomal amphotericin B plus miltefosine or paromomycin plus sodium stibogluconate.

Prevention of Leishmaniasis

Avoidance of sand flies (**Fig. 39.1**) is the essence of prevention. These insects are especially active at dusk and dawn. In areas of transmission, persons should wear protective clothing and apply insect repellent to exposed skin. Sleep in well-screened areas, although the sand flies can pass through screens or bed nets that are not closely woven. Apply pyrethroid-containing insecticide to clothing, bed nets, screens, and so on. No preventative vaccine or prophylactic drugs are available.

FURTHER READING

Blum, J., Lockwood, D.N., Visser, L., et al., 2012. Local or systemic treatment for New World cutaneous leishmaniasis? Re-evaluating the evidence for the risk of mucosal leishmaniasis. Int. Health 4 (3), 153–163.

Dorlo, T.P., Balasegaram, M., Beijnen, J.H., et al., 2012. Miltefosine: a review of its pharmacology and therapeutic efficacy in the treatment of leishmaniasis. J. Antimicrob. Chemother. 67 (11), 2576–2597.

Gonzalez, U., Pinart, M., Rengifo-Pardo, M., et al., 2009. Interventions for American cutaneous and mucocutaneous leishmaniasis. Cochrane Database Syst. Rev. (2), CD004834.

Gonzalez, U., Pinart, M., Reveiz, L., et al., 2008. Interventions for Old World cutaneous leishmaniasis. Cochrane Database Syst. Rev. (4), CD005067.

Herwaldt, B.L., 1999. Leishmaniasis. Lancet 354, 1191–1199

Hodiamont, C.J., Kager, P.A., Bart, A., et al., 2014. Species-directed therapy for leishmaniasis in returning travellers: a comprehensive guide. PLoS Negl. Trop. Dis. 8 (5), e2832.

Morizot, G., Kendjo, E., Mouri, O., et al., 2013. Travelers with cutaneous leishmaniasis cured without systemic therapy. Clin. Infect. Dis. 57 (3), 370–380.

Murray, H.W., 2012. Leishmaniasis in the United States: treatment in 2012. Am. J. Trop. Med. Hyg. 86 (3), 434–440.

Solomon, M., Baum, S., Barzilai, A., et al., 2007. Liposomal amphotericin B in comparison to sodium stibogluconate for cutaneous infection due to *Leishmania braziliensis*. J. Am. Acad. Dermatol. 56 (4), 612–616.

World Health Organization, 2010. Control of the leishmaniases. World Health Organ. Tech. Rep. Ser. 949, xii–186.

Wortmann, G., Zapor, M., Ressner, R., et al., 2010. Lipsosomal amphotericin B for treatment of cutaneous leishmaniasis. Am. J. Trop. Med. Hyg. 83 (5), 1028–1033.

CHAPTER 40

Leprosy (Hansen's Disease)

Saba M. Lambert, Stephen L. Walker, and James P. Harnisch

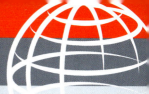

Leprosy, also known as Hansen's disease, is a chronic infectious disease predominantly affecting skin and nerves. The nerve damage occurring in leprosy may result in deformity, disability, and social stigma, creating problems for patients and their families.

The interaction between the patient's immune system and the infection is dynamic, resulting in various clinical forms of leprosy and complications.

Outside endemic areas, doctors often fail to diagnose leprosy, with unfortunate consequences for the patients. In both the United States and the United Kingdom, 40% of new cases have severe neuropathy at diagnosis, reflecting a combination of late presentation and diagnosis. Early recognition of leprosy is important, because the infection is curable and prompt treatment can reduce nerve damage and associated stigma.

ETIOLOGY

Mycobacterium leprae is an obligate intracellular pathogen, first identified in the nodules of lepromatous leprosy patients by Armauer Hansen in 1873. It is a rod-shaped, Gram-positive organism that is acid-fast when stained by the Ziehl–Nielsen or the better Fite methods. Viable organisms stain in a uniform, solid manner. With therapy, most organisms quickly lose their solid staining, appearing beaded or fragmented.

M. leprae has never been successfully grown in artificial media but can be propagated in the mouse footpad and the nine-banded armadillo, which is the only known natural reservoir of the organism. The organism has a long doubling time of 13 days at low temperatures (33-35°C), selectively invading skin macrophages and peripheral nerve Schwann cells. *M. leprae* does not produce any known toxins, and tissue injury is caused by the host's immune response or by the sheer mass of infecting bacilli.

In 2001, the genome of *M. leprae* was sequenced. The organism appears to have undergone extensive reductive evolution with considerable downsizing of its genome compared with *Mycobacterium tuberculosis*. Almost half of the genome is occupied by pseudogenes.

EPIDEMIOLOGY

In 2013, some 215,616 new cases were registered worldwide and reported to the World Health Organization (WHO) by 103 countries. Seven endemic countries reported the most new cases: India, Brazil, Indonesia, Ethiopia, Democratic Republic of the Congo, Nigeria, and Nepal. India reported 59% of the global burden of leprosy.

In the United States, 188 new cases were reported in 2013 by the Centers for Disease Control and Prevention. Immigrants from Mexico, the Philippines, Pacific Islands, and India account for the bulk of new cases. Leprosy has a long incubation period (2-10 years), so patients can present long after leaving endemic areas. However, in recent years 20-25% of new cases have occurred in those who were born in the United States, had not traveled to endemic countries, and were living in Texas, Louisiana, and Florida.

Leprosy affects adult males more than females, with ratios of 1.6:1 to 3:1 in different countries. In children the ratio is 1:1.

The exact mode of disease transmission is unknown. Studies of disease transmission have been hampered by the lack of a culture system, the absence of serologic markers, the latent period of 2-10 years before disease onset, and the high degree of natural immunity in most persons. Tuberculoid leprosy patients shed no demonstrable organisms and are regarded as noncontagious, although this is unproven. Untreated lepromatous patients shed millions of viable-appearing organisms daily, primarily in nasal and oral secretions. Bacilli may also be found in skin scales, sweat, blood, breast milk, and wound exudate. The possibility of animal-to-human transmission is supported by reports of cases in persons handling or consuming armadillos in the Americas.

Transmission is thought to occur mainly through aerosolized nasal droplets, spread when coughing or sneezing takes place. Following contact with an infective dose of *M. leprae*, most people will develop adequate protective immunity and therefore will not develop any clinically detectable signs or symptoms. Only a small percentage of individuals will develop clinical disease. Some literature suggests transmission via contact with broken skin, blood, or soil, as the mycobacteria are known to survive in the environment for up to 46 days.

CLINICAL FEATURES

Leprosy may be considered an immunologic disease. Immunity defines susceptibility to leprosy, type of clinical leprosy, pathology, and major clinical complications of leprosy. Classification of the disease is important to determine prognosis, transmission risk, and selection of treatment. There are two systems used to classify leprosy patients.

The Ridley–Jopling system uses clinical and histopathologic features and the bacteriological index (**Fig. 40.1**). Leprosy manifests in a spectrum of disease forms, ranging from the tuberculoid to the lepromatous.

The WHO classification is a simplified version depending on the number of skin lesions, which can be used in the field when slit skin smears or biopsies are not available. Patients with one to five skin lesions are classified as paucibacillary and those with six or more lesions as multibacillary. Up to 60% of patients classified as multibacillary are smear negative.

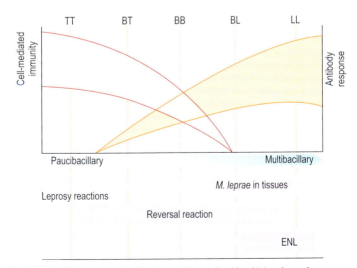

Fig. 40.1 **The Ridley–Jopling Classification and the relationship with host immunity.** *BB*, Borderline; *BL*, borderline lepromatous; *BT*, borderline tuberculoid; *ENL*, erythema nodosum leprosum; *LL*, lepromatous; *TT*, tuberculoid.

Clinical features of leprosy are a continuum between the tuberculoid and lepromatous forms of disease. There is substantial overlap in the appearance of the different forms, and careful assessment of clinical and histologic parameters is needed for accurate diagnosis. Important clinical features include (1) number of skin lesions, (2) size and morphology of skin lesions, (3) presence of neuropathy, and (4) presence of reactional states.

Indeterminate leprosy is the earliest recognizable form of the disease and may be extremely difficult to diagnose. There is typically a single hypopigmented or erythematous macule without abnormal sensation or sweating. There is no nerve enlargement. It is commonly seen in children. Biopsy is nonspecific and shows few or no organisms. Most heal without treatment, but 25% may progress to established leprosy.

Table 40.1 describes the varied clinical manifestations of leprosy. These are determined by the host's response to the leprosy bacillus: tuberculoid (TT) patients have a uniform clinical, histologic, and immunologic response manifesting as limited clinical disease, granuloma formation, and active cell-mediated immunity (**Fig. 40.2**); lepromatous leprosy (LL) patients have multiple clinical signs, a high bacterial load, and low cell-mediated immunity (**Fig. 40.3**). Between these two extremes there is a range of variations in host response; these comprise borderline cases (BT, BB, BL) (**Fig. 40.4**). Immunologically, borderline cases are unstable, while polar tuberculoid and lepromatous cases are stable.

Neural involvement in leprosy is due to selective proliferation of *M. leprae* in superficial peripheral nerves. Nerve destruction occurs either from inflammation or from infiltration by masses of infecting organisms. Inflammation in the nerves may result in nerve entrapment. Damage to peripheral nerve trunks produces sensory loss and weakness of the muscles supplied by the affected peripheral nerves. Sensory function is the earliest affected in leprosy; sensory impairment can occur alone without motor involvement. Autonomic nerve damage results in dryness of the hands and feet. The ulnar, median, posterior tibial, common peroneal, and radial nerves are most commonly involved. The central nervous system is never involved, and *M. leprae* does not usually propagate within internal organs due to high human core body temperature.

DIAGNOSIS

A clinical diagnosis of leprosy is made by considering key features associated with the disease (the presence of characteristic skin lesions with anesthesia, and thickening of one or more peripheral nerves), supported by skin smears and biopsy. A patient may present with a macular hypopigmented skin lesion, weakness or pain in the hand due to nerve involvement, facial palsy, acute foot drop, or a painless burn or ulcer in an anesthetic hand or foot. Patients may also present with painful eyes as a first indication of lepromatous leprosy. The diagnosis of leprosy should be considered in anyone from an endemic area who presents with typical skin lesions, neuropathic ulcers, or a peripheral neuropathy. In leprosy-endemic settings, a typical skin lesion that is also anesthetic is said to be 70% sensitive for the diagnosis of leprosy, and has been recommended by the WHO as sufficient for leprosy diagnosis by knowledgeable health providers. Clinicians need to have a high index of suspicion when dealing with patients from endemic areas.

Evaluation of patients should include the following:

1. A careful inspection of the skin with diagrams or photography of lesions should be carried out.
2. Areas of anhidrosis should be noted, because this correlates with loss of protective sensation.
3. Superficial nerves should be palpated for enlargement and tenderness.
4. Detailed sensory testing should be carried out to define deficits. This can be done with graded nylon monofilaments or a ball-point pen.
5. Motor testing and nerve conduction studies should be performed.
6. Examination of insensitive extremities for areas of trauma or pressure injury is important, as is assessment of the adequacy of footwear.
7. Ophthalmologic evaluation is indicated for patients with facial or ocular involvement.

TABLE 40.1 Major Clinical Features of the Disease Spectrum in Leprosy

Clinical Features		CLASSIFICATION				
	Tuberculoid (TT)	Borderline Tuberculoid (BT)	Borderline (BB)	Borderline Lepromatous (BL)	Lepromatous (LL)
	WHO PAUCIBACILLARY			WHO MULTIBACILLARY	
Skin					
Infiltrated lesions	Defined plaques, healing centers	Irregular plaques with partially raised edges	Polymorphic, "punched out centers"	Papules, nodules	Diffuse thickening
Macular lesions	Single, small, but can be large	Several, any size, "geographical"	Multiple, all sizes, bizarre	Innumerable, small	Innumerable, confluent
Nerve					
Peripheral nerve	Solitary enlarged nerves	Several nerves, asymmetrical	Many nerves, asymmetrical pattern	Late neural thickening, asymmetrical, anesthesia and paresis	Slow symmetrical loss, "glove and stocking" anesthesia
Microbiology					
Bacterial index	0-1	0-2	2-3	1-4	4-6
Histology					
Lymphocytes	+	++	+/–	++	+/–
Macrophages	–	–	+/–	–	–
Epithelioid cells	++	+/–	–	–	–
Antibody, anti-*M. leprae*	–/+	–/++	+	++	++

WHO, World Health Organization.

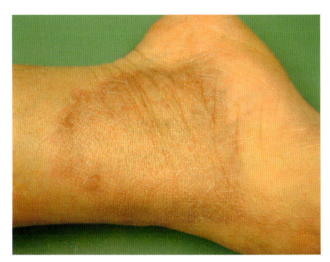

Fig. 40.2 **Tuberculoid leprosy.** Tuberculoid leprosy plaque, which is anesthetic and granulomatous, often with no bacilli on biopsy. (Courtesy of James P. Harnisch, MD.)

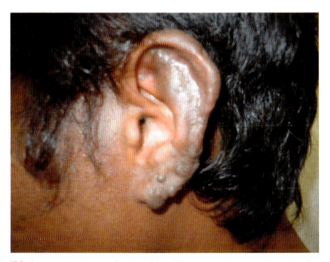

Fig. 40.3 **Lepromatous leprosy.** Classic nodules of lepromatous leprosy on the cool surface of the ear. Many bacilli seen on biopsy. (Courtesy of James P. Harnisch, MD.)

The differential diagnosis of leprosy is wide due to its protean manifestations. Individuals found to have granulomatous pathology on skin or nerve biopsy, peripheral neuropathy, mononeuritis, or mononeuritis multiplex may have leprosy. Examples of other diagnoses that may enter the differential diagnosis depending on the type of leprosy include superficial fungal infections of the skin, such as tinea corporis, pityriasis versicolor, or pityriasis alba; vitiligo; sarcoidosis; secondary and tertiary syphilis; mycosis fungoides; and psoriasis. Other

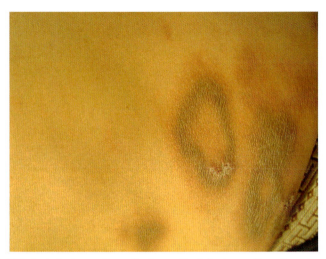

Fig. 40.4 **Borderline leprosy.** Target-like plaques of borderline leprosy. Always biopsy the peripheral border. (Courtesy of James P. Harnisch, MD.)

mycobacterial infections such as *Mycobacterium tuberculosis* and *Mycobacterium ulcerans* may also cause diagnostic confusion.

BACTERIOLOGICAL AND HISTOLOGICAL EXAMINATION

Slit skin smears should be taken to look for acid-fast bacilli. *M. leprae* on the smears are counted and the bacterial index calculated on a semi-quantitative scale. A negative result does not exclude leprosy, as TT and BT lesions may contain no detectable bacteria.

Histopathological evaluation is essential for accurate classification of leprosy lesions and is the best diagnostic test in a well-resourced setting, both for confirming and for excluding the diagnosis of leprosy. The presence of granulomata and lymphocytic infiltration of dermal nerves and skin adnexal structures such as sweat glands in skin lesions confirms the diagnosis. Biopsy should be taken from the active border of a skin lesion and stained with a Fite stain in addition to routine stains. A nerve biopsy may be required in cases with no visible skin lesions. A cutaneous sensory nerve is selected in an area of neuropathy and examined histologically for organisms and typical granulomas.

Skin smears aid in diagnosis, in assessment of bacillary load, and in following response to therapy. The bacteria should diminish within the smears or biopsies during therapy unless there is an issue of compliance or resistance. In multibacillary patients the reduction of bacilli is often slow, over many years.

SEROLOGICAL TESTS AND POLYMERASE CHAIN REACTION

Recent advances have been made in serological diagnostic testing. Antibodies to the *M. leprae*–specific PGL-1 (antiphenolic glycolipid) are present in 90% of patients with untreated lepromatous disease, but only 40-50% of patients with paucibacillary disease and 1-5 % of healthy controls. A negative test does not exclude diagnosis. This test is not available in the United States.

PCR for detection of *M. leprae* encoding specific genes or repeat sequences is potentially highly sensitive and specific, since it detects *M. leprae* DNA in 95% of multibacillary and 55% of paucibacillary patients. However, PCR is not currently used in routine clinical practice.

TABLE 40.2 Current Hansen's Disease Treatment Regimens		
Type of disease	NHDP regimen	WHO regimen
Paucibacillary	Dapsone 100 mg/day plus rifampin 600 mg/day for 12 months	Dapsone 100 mg/day (unsupervised) plus rifampin 600 mg once monthly (supervised) for 6 months
Multibacillary	Dapsone 100 mg/day plus clofazimine 50 mg/day plus rifampin 600 mg/day for 2 years (May substitute daily minocycline for clofazimine)	Dapsone 100 mg/day plus clofazimine 50 mg/day (both unsupervised) plus rifampin 600 mg and clofazimine 300 mg once monthly in supervised setting; continue regimen for 12 months of therapy

NHDP, National Hansen's Disease Program; *WHO*, World Health Organization.

TREATMENT

Multidrug therapy with a combination of dapsone, rifampicin (rifampin), and clofazimine is the current treatment for infection with *M. leprae*. Multidrug therapy is very successful, with a high cure rate, few side effects, and low relapse rates. WHO studies have reported a cumulative relapse rate of 1.1% for paucibacillary leprosy and 0.8% for multibacillary leprosy at 9 years after completion of multidrug therapy. Patients with a high initial bacillary load are thought to be at higher risk of relapse, thus treatment for at least 24 months is advocated by some.

Treatment recommendations are divided into paucibacillary or multibacillary therapy. Patients with paucibacillary leprosy require treatment for shorter periods. Treatment regimens recommended by the US National Hansen's Disease Programs and the WHO are summarized in **Table 40.2**.

Patients should be warned that rifampicin will turn their urine, sweat, semen, and tears orange/red for 48 hours post-dose. Rifampicin may decrease the efficacy of oral contraceptives and other medicines, including prednisolone. Clofazimine skin pigmentation may be very troublesome and particularly affects the actual lesions. Patients can be reassured that the pigmentation will fade after stopping multidrug therapy, but it may take many months. Dapsone is a sulfa drug that often causes mild anemia but may also cause severe hemolysis in individuals with glucose 6-phosphate dehydrogenase (G6PD) deficiency. For this reason, it is standard of care to obtain a G6PD activity level before initiating dapsone therapy. Patients should be specifically warned about dapsone allergy, which may be severe and life threatening. It usually starts 3-6 weeks after starting the drug and presents with fever, rash, and pruritus. If the drug is not stopped, the reaction may progress to an exfoliative dermatitis, hepatitis, pneumonitis, albuminuria, and death. Dapsone should be stopped immediately and medical advice sought at the first sign of any rash or unexplained fever. The role of corticosteroids in the management of severe dapsone allergy is unclear.

A number of other antibiotics are active against *M. leprae* and may be useful in combination as second-line therapy in the setting of drug intolerance or documented drug resistance. Such antimicrobials include minocycline 100 mg daily, ofloxacin 400 mg daily, and clarithromycin 500 mg daily.

LEPROSY REACTIONS

Leprosy is complicated by immunological phenomena called reactions: reversal reactions (RR), or type 1 reactions, and erythema nodosum leprosum (ENL), or type 2 reactions. Leprosy reactions are the main cause of nerve damage in leprosy. The inflammation is due to immune reactions against *M. leprae* antigens. Patients can present in reaction before multidrug therapy treatment, and a significant proportion of patients develop reactions

TABLE 40.3 Comparison of Clinical Features of Type 1 and Type 2 Leprosy Reactions

Parameter	Type 1 (RR)	Type 2 (ENL)
Patients at risk	All types but particularly BT, BB, BL	LL, BL
Onset of reaction	Usually gradual, over a few weeks but may be sudden	Sudden, "overnight"
Cutaneous lesions	Increased erythema and induration of previously existing or new lesions	Numerous erythematous, tender nodules on face, extremities, or trunk, without relationship to prior lesions
Neuritis	Frequent, often severe	Frequent, often severe
Systemic symptoms	Afebrile, mild malaise, edema	Fever, malaise, lymph node enlargement, arthritis, iritis, orchitis
Histopathological features	↑CD4 cell, granuloma edema, ↑giant cell size and numbers, dermal edema, and HLA-DR expression	Polymorphonuclear cell infiltrates in lesions <24-h old, ↑TNF-α
Treatment	Corticosteroids	Corticosteroids, thalidomide
Recurrence	30-50%	~65%

BB, Borderline; *BL*, borderline lepromatous; *BT*, borderline tuberculoid; *ENL*, erythema nodosum leprosum; *LL*, lepromatous; *RR*, reversal reactions; *TNF-α*, tumor necrosis factor α; *TT*, tuberculoid; *HLA-DR*, Human Leukocyte Antigen-antigen D related.

within the first 6 months of treatment. There is also an increase in the incidence of reactions in women during the postpartum period. However, reactions can also occur after successful multidrug therapy treatment and are probably due to persistence of *M. leprae* antigens. Patients may suffer from recurrent reactions or repeated reactions after treatment, resulting in increased suffering and disability. The clinical features of these reactions are listed in **Table 40.3**.

Management of Type 1 Reactions

The clinical manifestations of these reactions are painful, edematous, erythematous skin lesions, neuritis, and facial and peripheral edema. Acute neuritis (defined as spontaneous nerve pain, paresthesia, or tenderness with new sensory or motor impairment of recent onset) may also occur without evidence of skin inflammation. Nerve function impairment is defined as clinically detectable impairment of motor, sensory, or autonomic nerve function. Nerve function impairment may occur in the absence of symptoms and may go unnoticed by the patient—"silent neuropathy."

Type 1 reactions are treated with corticosteroids. High doses of prednisolone 40-60 mg daily should be started, depending on severity, and tapered down after clinical improvement to the minimal effective dose until the reaction subsides. Treatment should last 5-6 months

Patients seen with nerve function impairment of recent onset (within 6 months) should be given a trial of prednisolone therapy and physiotherapy. Some of these patients will recover function of the affected part.

Management of ENL Reactions

ENL reactions present as a systemic illness: a patient with ENL may be very sick with high fever, painful cutaneous and subcutaneous nodules, peripheral edema, and inflammation of the nerves, eyes, joints, muscles, bones, and testes. The onset of ENL is acute, but it may pass into a chronic or recurrent phase.

For very mild cases aspirin may be used. Severe cases require hospitalization and treatment with high doses of prednisolone (starting at 60 mg). The efficacy is variable, and some patients with chronic or recurrent ENL may need to take prednisolone for several years. These prolonged, high doses of corticosteroids are associated with adverse effects. In patients on prolonged corticosteroid courses, consider adding daily calcium carbonate and vitamin D3 for bone protection and trimethoprim-sulfamethoxazole 400/800 mg daily for *Pneumocystis jiroveci* pneumonia prophylaxis.

Thalidomide, starting at 300-400 mg daily and tapering down, is the treatment of choice for severe ENL. It has a dramatic effect in controlling ENL and preventing recurrences, but its use is strictly regulated because of teratogenicity. However, it is ineffective in the management of neuritis associated with ENL. Patients may experience sedation, and there is an increased risk of thromboembolism when used in conjunction with corticosteroids. Thalidomide has been shown to be neurotoxic when used in patients with a wide range of dermatologic conditions, but there are no studies demonstrating this in patients with leprosy. In the United States, thalidomide must now be obtained through the Celgene REMS program (1-888-423-5436).

In chronic ENL, clofazimine 100-300 mg daily may be helpful. This medication takes approximately 6 weeks to reach full efficacy. Side effects include hyperpigmentation of the skin and sclera. At prolonged high doses, nausea or intestinal obstruction can occur, which may lead to unnecessary surgical intervention.

Lucio phenomenon (erythema necroticans) is a rare reactional state seen mainly in patients from Mexico, Cuba, Brazil, or Costa Rica. This has been associated with *Mycobacterium lepromatosis*, a recently discovered acid-fast bacillus linked to diffuse lepromatous disease. Histopathologic examination reveals profound bacterial load with endovascular invasion, vasculitis, and intravascular thrombosis. The necrotic skin lesions begin as irregular or stellate macules and papules that become purpuric and ulcerate. Widespread cutaneous necrosis may occur, leading to secondary bacterial infection, sepsis, and death. Survival depends on supportive care combined with steroids and, if necessary, the addition of cyclophosphamide and treatment of the underlying infection.

MANAGEMENT OF LEPROSY

The treatment of leprosy has six main components:

- Chemotherapy
- Patient education
- Management of reactions and neuritis
- Prevention of disability
- Management of ulcers
- Social and psychological support.

All patients with leprosy need education regarding the nature of their disease. An independent interpreter may be invaluable. Fears of contagion and social rejection must be dealt with directly. Patients should be assured that *therapy will make them non-infectious* and that family and social relationships need not be altered. An attitude of openness and reassurance is important. A multidisciplinary approach is ideal, and establishing a good relationship with affected individuals and identifying and addressing their concerns is vital.

Information about mode of transmission, treatment, and complications—including the recognition and risk of leprosy reactions—is essential for patients and health providers. Patients should be taught self-examination of the hands and feet and to seek medical care immediately if signs of inflammation or trauma occur. Adequate footwear such as extra-deep shoes with a wide toe box and inserts or other protective devices should be made available to those with insensitive or deformed feet. Appropriate early physiotherapy must be instituted in cases of motor neuropathy, and patients should be referred to an appropriate specialist for evaluation and correction of ulcers and deformities. Acquired ichthyosis is common in multibacillary leprosy and with clofazimine treatment. Strong emollients such as 12% ammonium lactate lotion or 40% urea lotion should be used to prevent excessive cracking/fissuring of the skin, which can lead to secondary bacterial infection.

Having regular ophthalmic examinations will minimize the risk of visual impairment. Loss of corneal sensation and lagophthalmos from denervation are most typical of the tuberculoid end of the spectrum and can lead to exposure keratitis. Bacillary infiltration of the anterior eye occurs in borderline and lepromatous patients, causing nodular keratitis and episcleritis. ENL may cause iridocyclitis and secondary glaucoma leading to blindness. The sensory denervation of the eye results in the absence of symptoms despite progressive ocular injury, thus contributing to vision loss. Patients with corneal anesthesia need counseling and measures to prevent exposure injury such as eye covers at night and sunglasses in the day. Surgery may be useful in lagophthalmos. Inflammatory conditions associated with reactions are managed with steroids. The commonest cause of visual impairment in leprosy is cataract due to long-term steroid use.

Therapy of Contacts
No satisfactory method has been established for managing household contacts. Current practice involves a full examination of all household contacts.

Management of Complicated Cases
Consultation in the management of leprosy can be obtained by contacting the US National Hansen's Disease Program at 800-642-2477 (http://www.hrsa.gov/hansensdisease/). Additional information can be obtained through the World Health Organization website (http://www.who.int/lep/).

Availability of Clofazimine
Clofazimine is distributed worldwide though the WHO by donation of Novartis Foundation for Sustainable Development. In the United States, the drug was no longer commercially distributed as of November 2004 but is available from Novartis through the National Hansen's Disease Programs for use in treatment of leprosy under an investigational protocol. Contact the National Hansen's Disease Program for assistance in obtaining clofazimine for use in treatment of leprosy.

FURTHER READING

Britton, W.J., Lockwood, D.N., 2004. Leprosy. Lancet 363, 1209–1219.

Hartzell, J.D., Zapor, M., Peng, S., et al., 2004. Leprosy: a case series and review. South. Med. J. 97, 1252–1256.

Infolep. ILEP Learning Guide Three: How to Do a Skin Smear Examination for Leprosy. Available at <http://www.leprosy-information.org/resource/ilep-learning-guide-three-how-do-skin-smear-examination-leprosy>.

Krutzik, S.R., et al., 2005. TLR activation triggers the rapid differentiation of monocytes into macrophages and dendritic cells. Nat. Med. 11 (6), 653–660.

Lockwood, D.N.J., 1992. Contributions of laboratory research to current understanding and management of leprosy. Trop. Doct. 22, S22.

Marlowe, S.N., Lockwood, D.N., 2001. Update on leprosy. Hosp. Med. 62, 471–476.

Misch, E.A., et al., 2010. Leprosy and the human genome. Microbiol. Mol. Biol. Rev. 74, 589–620.

Moschella, S.L., 2004. An update on the diagnosis and treatment of leprosy. J. Am. Acad. Dermatol. 51, 417–426.

Rea, T.H., Levan, N.E., 1978. Lucio's phenomenon and diffuse non-nodular lepromatous leprosy. Arch. Dermatol. 114, 1023.

Ridley, D.S., 1969. Reactions in leprosy. Lepr. Rev. 40, 77–81.

Ridley, D.S., Jopling, W.H., 1966. Classification of leprosy according to immunity. A five group system. Int. J. Lepr. 34, 255–273.

Sasaki, S., Takeshita, F., Okuda, K., et al., 2001. *Mycobacterium leprae* and leprosy: a compendium. Microbiol. Immunol. 45, 729–736.

Scollard, D.M., Adams, L.B., Gillis, T.P., et al., 2006. The continuing challenges of leprosy. Clin. Microbiol. Rev. 19, 338–381.

Singh, P., et al., 2015. Insight into the evolution and origin of leprosy bacilli from the genome sequence of *Mycobacterium lepromatosis*. Proc. Natl. Acad. Sci. U.S.A. 112 (14), 4459–4464.

Truman, R.W., et al., 2011. Probable zoonotic leprosy in the southern United States. N. Engl. J. Med. 364, 1626–1633.

Walker, S.L., et al., 2014. The mortality associated with erythema nodosum leprosum in Ethiopia: a retrospective hospital-based study. PLoS Negl. Trop. Dis. 8 (3), e2690.

WHO, 2013. Global leprosy update. WHO Wkly. Epidemiol. Rec. 88 (35), 365–380.

WHO Study Group on the Chemotherapy of Leprosy, 1994. WHO Technical Report Series No. 847: Chemotherapy of Leprosy. World Health Organization, Geneva.

CHAPTER 41

Sexually Transmitted Infections and Foreign Travel

Jeanne M. Marrazzo

Because sexually transmitted infections (STIs) are defined by their transmission from one person to another during sex, travel—with its attendant opportunities for new contacts—can facilitate the transmission of STIs in several ways. The number of international travelers has increased steadily in recent years, with a trend toward areas of the world endemic for STIs not frequently seen in the United States. This allows for the exposure of travelers to relatively uncommon STIs, such as lymphogranuloma venereum (LGV). In addition, the prevalence of common STIs, such as gonorrhea and chlamydia, is higher in some destinations than in many parts of the United States. This may increase the likelihood of travelers' exposure to these pathogens within any given sexual encounter. Further, persons who purchase sex as part of a "travel experience" are often choosing partners who themselves have a higher likelihood of exposure to STIs. Finally, certain STIs, such as syphilis, are sensitive indicators of social and economic disruption; travelers to parts of the world that are experiencing wars or socioeconomic upheaval are especially vulnerable to exposure to these infections. The dynamic of STI transmission across borders has a reciprocal side: immigrants and refugees to the United States from areas with high STI prevalence may import these infections, particularly if they are clinically inapparent, as with latent syphilis.

Travelers need to be aware of the risk of STIs during travel and to understand measures to protect themselves *and* their prospective sexual partners in foreign countries.

CASUAL SEXUAL ACTIVITY AND TRAVEL

Traditionally, travelers undertaking long and frequent journeys have been recognized to be at risk for STI acquisition during travel. These groups have included long-distance truckers, seafarers, and military troops. However, as more of the population travels for recreational and business purposes, the group at risk for STI acquisition has greatly increased in size and heterogeneity, and risk stratification by occupation or reason for travel becomes less precise. In considering the relationship between international travel and exposure to STIs, the major determinant of risk is the individual's personal behavior.

Estimates of the frequency of sex associated with travel indicate that the practice occurs rather commonly, though the magnitude of such estimates depends on population surveyed and the gender of respondents. A recent meta-analysis reported a pooled prevalence of travel-associated casual sex of 20.4%, with a concomitant three-fold increased risk of acquiring an STI. Factors associated with casual sex while abroad were young age, male sex, and travel without a spouse or partner.

Several studies have examined the likelihood of sexual contacts by people living or employed in foreign or developing countries for long periods, including expatriates, overseas workers, and military personnel. In most of these studies, factors that were highly associated with these sexual contacts included not being accompanied by a partner or spouse, prior experience with purchasing sex, and history of previous STIs.

Despite the efficacy of condoms in preventing STI transmission, several studies have documented low rates of condom use in travelers (likely less than 50% use condoms consistently with casual sex). A recent meta-analysis of studies evaluating the efficacy of pre-travel counseling on incidence of STI found no difference in approaches that used standard counseling versus motivational interviewing. However, randomized trials have not been performed.

SEXUAL TOURISM

Many developing countries have actively fostered the development of tourism as an economic tonic. Particularly before the recognition of the human immunodeficiency virus (HIV) pandemic, sexual tourism was promoted by international tourist agencies, either openly or under the guise of health or "medical treatment" tours. Some of these efforts even underplayed the magnitude of the local emerging HIV epidemic. As fatalities due to acquired immunodeficiency syndrome (AIDS) accrued, the relationship between the commercial sex implied by sexual tourism and HIV acquisition became more difficult to ignore. However, many local tour agencies may still be reluctant to provide, or certainly to stress, relevant information (and attendant caution) regarding local prevalence of HIV and other STIs, for fear of discouraging potential clients.

While specific data on sexual tourism are scarce, many studies have shown that HIV-1 infection is common among commercial sex workers (CSWs): 50-85% of urban CSWs in parts of Africa and Southeast Asia are HIV infected. One tragic consequence of the increased awareness of this risk has been the promotion of child prostitution because of the belief that sex with relatively young persons is safer than with older CSWs. This assumption is false: one survey found that approximately 50% of Thai child sex workers were HIV infected. Young CSWs are quickly exposed to the same STIs and may even be more likely to become infected with STDs during sexual intercourse because of traumatic penetration.

THE INTERNATIONAL SPREAD OF HIV

The initial explosive spread of HIV-1 infection among residents of Africa and rapid spread of HIV-1 through Southeast Asia and South America over the past decades were initially attributed to the high rate of CSWs and genital ulcerative diseases (GUDs) in these areas. Other factors emerged as possible contributors, including chemokine receptors such as CCR-5, which confers relative protection to progression of HIV-1 disease and is less common in blacks relative to whites, and exceedingly high prevalence of genital infection with herpes simplex virus type-2. While HIV transmission in North America, Western Europe, Australia, and New Zealand has been predominantly among homosexual men and intravenous drug users (IDUs), heterosexual transmission accounts for up to 70% of HIV-1 infections in sub-Saharan Africa and parts of the Caribbean and Asia. In Latin America, the epidemic continues to evidence a shift from the homosexual and bisexual population to a pattern of heterosexual transmission. The heterosexual transmission of HIV-1 that is seen in developing countries has followed a consistent trend. Predominantly female CSWs become infected from infected male clients (who include IDUs and international travelers). Male partners of the infected CSWs become infected themselves, and can then infect their female spouses at home. These infected women, many of whom have only one partner—their husbands—then transmit HIV-1 to their children in subsequent pregnancies.

Industrialized countries are presently experiencing a rise in the proportion of HIV-1 transmission occurring within the heterosexual population, particularly in inner cities among IDUs, CSWs, and immigrants from high-risk areas. Men who have sex with men (MSM) continue to be at the highest risk, and many urban areas in the United States have experienced an alarming reversal of the trend toward protected sex among men who have sex with men (many of whom are HIV-1-infected already), which likely continues to sustain an endemic level of HIV-1 transmission within this group. Rates of early syphilis (primary, secondary, and early latent) are presently higher than at any time in the last two decades in many large cities globally as well.

RISKS FOR ACQUISITION OF STIS AND HIV DURING TRAVEL

Travelers should be advised that unprotected casual sex with fellow travelers is most likely to expose them to infections prevalent in their home countries: predominantly genital herpes, human papillomavirus, chlamydia, gonorrhea, and, depending on the interaction, syphilis or HIV-1. Unprotected sex with host-country nationals in the developing world may also potentially expose them to chancroid, LGV, and granuloma inguinale—diseases uncommon in Western industrialized countries.

Genital herpes, syphilis, chancroid, LGV, and granuloma inguinale are all causes of GUD. All but genital herpes are bacterial GUD and thus are curable with appropriate antibiotic treatment, and antiviral therapy can lessen the clinical symptoms and viral shedding associated with genital herpes. However, the presence of unhealed genital ulcers during intercourse increases the risk of HIV acquisition and transmission, and possibly of other viral diseases as well. In addition to HIV-1, sexual transmission of HIV-2 and other viruses (hepatitis B, hepatitis C, and human T-cell lymphotropic virus type 1) is a greater risk in parts of the developing world. While GUD is a major risk for increased transmission of HIV-1, other factors may contribute, including non-ulcerative STIs (notably, trichomoniasis), cervical ectopy, and certain sexual practices (anal intercourse, sex during menses, use of vaginal drying agents). Among men, increased HIV acquisition is strongly associated with lack of circumcision as well as the presence of GUD.

Vaginal use of the spermicide nonoxynol-9 (N-9) prevents neither HIV nor non-HIV STI transmission, and in fact, frequent use of vaginal sponges containing high doses of N-9 increased the risk of vaginal ulceration among CSWs. For these reasons, N-9 use is not recommended.

PREVENTION OF STIS AND HIV

Barrier Protection

The use of condoms is strongly recommended with every act of sexual intercourse when the status of a partner with regard to HIV infection or other STI is unknown; unfortunately, under even the best of circumstances, the protection condoms provide against STI is incomplete. For one, the normal breakage rate during vaginal intercourse with properly applied high-quality latex condoms produced in the United States is about 2%; complete slippage occurs about 1% of the time. Similar rates probably apply for anal intercourse, although failure rates as high as 5% have been reported during anal intercourse between men. Condoms manufactured abroad may have a higher breakage rate. Improper storage conditions (heat, moisture) or oil-based lubricants (mineral oil, petroleum jelly, massage oils, body lotions, shortening, cooking oil) can weaken latex condoms and contribute to a higher breakage rate. Use beyond the expiration date also increases the likelihood of breakage.

Latex condoms offer the most reliable barrier against STI. For persons with latex allergy (estimated at 1-3% of the US population), polyurethane (plastic) condoms offer an alternative; these are thinner than latex but reportedly stronger and, unlike latex, are not compromised by use with oil-based lubricants. They are, however, more costly than latex condoms and may require more lubrication. Finally, natural membrane condoms (often incorrectly called "lambskin" condoms) are generally made from lamb cecum; the membranous latticework of fibers can have pores up to 1500 nm in diameter. While this will prevent the passage of sperm, the pores are >10 times the diameter of HIV and >25 times the diameter of the hepatitis B virus. Laboratory studies suggest that viral transmission can occur with natural membrane condoms; hence, while clinical data are not available, it is generally recommended that they be avoided. They are more costly than latex as well.

The relative protection that condoms afford against STI acquisition is significant but not complete; abstinence remains the only sure method for avoiding STIs. In several studies of couples who were discordant for the presence of HIV-1 infection, use of condoms significantly reduced the risk of HIV-1 transmission to the uninfected partner (up to a 10-fold reduction).

Availability and use of the female condom has been increasing worldwide. Although its relatively high cost can present a considerable deterrent, it offers a significant advance in woman-controlled methods of barrier protection. The female condom is slightly less effective for preventing pregnancy compared with male condoms; clinical studies in small numbers of women indicate protection against trichomoniasis reinfection, implying but not yet proving similar protection against other STIs.

Travelers should also be advised that the use of alcohol or drugs can negatively affect the decision to use a condom.

HIV Pre-Exposure Prophylaxis

Daily oral pre-exposure prophylaxis with 300 mg of tenofovir disoproxil fumarate (TDF), alone or with 200 mg of emtricitabine (FTC) (TDF-FTC [Truvada], Gilead Sciences), reduces risk of HIV-1 acquisition by ≥50% among high adherers, with demonstrated efficacy in MSM, heterosexuals, and injection drug users. On this basis, the US Food and Drug Administration approved daily Truvada for prevention of HIV-1 acquisition in July 2012, and the Centers for Disease Control and Prevention has issued guidance for its use. A discussion of risk for HIV-1 acquisition as defined in this guidance should be a routine component of pre-travel assessment.

Vaccines

The US Advisory Committee on Immunization Practices (ACIP) first issued guidelines for administration of the quadrivalent human papillomavirus (HPV) vaccine to females aged 25 years and younger in 2007, and subsequently expanded that to males. Most recently, ACIP has recommended substitution of a nine-valent HPV vaccine as available, given its expanded spectrum of activity. Specific details are available at www.cdc.gov/std/hpv. The nine-valent vaccine confers protection against HPV types 6/11 (responsible for 90% of genital warts) and 16/18 (responsible for 70% of cervical cancers), as well as types 31, 33, 45, 52, and 58. In published clinical trials, the quadrivalent HPV vaccine has demonstrated efficacy for prevention of HPV-type related cervical, vaginal, anal, and vulvar cancer precursor and dysplastic lesions, and external genital warts.

Immunization against hepatitis B virus (HBV) has been routinely recommended for infants since 1991 and was subsequently recommended for adolescents. While this has been temporally associated with marked declines in HBV incidence in the United States, sexual transmission still accounts for the majority of new infections, which are especially common among unvaccinated MSM. Consequently, hepatitis B vaccination is recommended for all adults who are at risk for sexual infection, including sex partners of hepatitis B surface antigen (HBsAg)-positive persons, sexually active persons who are not in a long-term, mutually monogamous relationship, persons seeking evaluation or treatment for an STI, and MSM. Moreover, all HIV-infected persons should be immunized against hepatitis B, as the natural history of hepatitis B is accelerated in the setting of HIV, and co-infection imposes specific considerations in selection of antiretroviral agents. Hepatitis A virus (HAV) vaccine is licensed and is recommended for MSM and illicit drug users (both injecting and noninjecting). Specific details are available at http://www.cdc.gov/hepatitis. Finally, new vaccine approaches aimed at hepatitis C, including peptide, recombinant protein, DNA, and vector-based vaccines, have recently reached phase I/II human clinical trials, providing some promise for future control of this infection.

ADVICE TO TRAVELERS

As the studies alluded to above demonstrate, travelers, and especially long-term travelers, are likely to engage in casual sex, and the unfortunate reality is that condoms are used consistently by the minority during high-risk sex. Female travelers may be less likely than males to negotiate successful use of male condoms; availability of the female condom may offer a welcome alternative.

In summary, advice to travelers should include the following: (1) discuss the possibility of casual sex while abroad, (2) encourage the inclusion of high-quality latex condoms in the traveler's medical kit, (3) consider risk for sexual acquisition of HIV-1 and consider whether HIV pre-exposure prophylaxis is indicated, and (4) assure appropriate immunization status for HPV, HBV, and HAV.

Finally, travelers should be strongly encouraged to overcome reluctance to talk about personal sexual matters and to be sure to contact their personal physician or travel medicine clinic on return from travel if any unprotected sexual exposures occurred.

FURTHER READING

Bellis, M.A., Hughes, K., Thomson, R., et al., 2004. Sexual behaviour of young people in international tourist resorts. Sex. Transm. Infect. 80, 43–47.

Centers for Disease Control and Prevention, 2014. Prophylaxis for the prevention of HIV infection. MMWR 63 (19), 437.

Centers for Disease Control and Prevention, 2015. Sexually transmitted disease treatment guidelines. MMWR 64 (RR–3), 1–137.

Croughs, M., Remmen, R., Van den Ende, J., 2013. The effect of pre-travel advice on sexual risk behavior abroad: a systematic review. J. Travel Med. 21, 45–51.

Kreiss, J., Ngugi, E., Holmes, K.K., et al., 1992. Efficacy of nonoxynol-9 contraceptive sponge use in preventing heterosexual acquisition of HIV in Nairobi prostitutes. JAMA 268, 477–482.

Markowitz, L.E., et al., 2013. Reduction in human papillomavirus (HPV) prevalence among young women following HPV vaccine introduction in the United States, National Health and Nutrition Examination Surveys, 2003-2010. J. Infect. Dis. 208, 385–393.

Mast, E.E., et al., 2006. A comprehensive immunization strategy to eliminate transmission of hepatitis B virus infection in the United States: recommendations of the Advisory Committee on Immunization Practices (ACIP). Part II: immunization of adults. MMWR Recomm. Rep. 55 (RR–16), 1–33.

Matteelli, A., Carosi, G., 2001. Sexually transmitted diseases in travelers. Clin. Infect. Dis. 32, 1063–1067.

Mulhall, B.P., 1999. Sexual behaviour in travellers. Lancet 353, 595–596.

Perrin, L., Kaiser, L., Yerly, S., 2003. Travel and the spread of HIV-1 genetic variants. Lancet Infect. Dis. 3, 22–27.

Petrosky, W., Bocchini, J., Hariri, S., et al., 2015. Use of 9-valent human papillomavirus (HPV) vaccine: updated HPV vaccination recommendations of the Advisory Committee on Immunization Practices. MMWR 64 (11), 300–304.

Rogstad, K.E., 2004. Sex, sun, sea, and STIs: sexually transmitted infections acquired on holiday. BMJ 329, 214–217.

US Preventive Services Task Force, 2008. Behavioral counseling to prevent sexually transmitted infections: US Preventive Services Task Force recommendation statement. Ann. Intern. Med. 149, 491–496. W95.

Vivancos, R., Abubakar, I., Hunter, P.R., 2010. Foreign travel, casual sex, and sexually transmitted infections: systematic review and meta-analysis. Int. J. Infect. Dis. 14, e842–e851.

Wasserheit, J.N., 1994. Effect of changes in human ecology and behavior on patterns of sexually transmitted diseases, including human immunodeficiency virus infection. Proc. Natl. Acad. Sci. USA 91, 2430–2435.

Wetmore, C.M., Manhart, L.E., Wasserheit, J.N., 2010. Randomized controlled trials of interventions to prevent sexually transmitted infections: learning from the past to plan for the future. Epidemiol. Rev. 32 (1), 121–136.

World Health Organization, 2012. Global incidence and prevalence of selected curable sexually transmitted infections—2008. Available at <http://www.who.int/reproductivehealth/publications/rtis/stisestimates/en/>.

CHAPTER 42

Gonococcal and Chlamydial Genital Infections and Pelvic Inflammatory Disease

Jeanne M. Marrazzo

Infections caused by *Neisseria gonorrhoeae* and *Chlamydia trachomatis* are the most common of the bacterial sexually transmitted infections (STIs). Since 1995, genital chlamydial infections have been the most frequently reported bacterial infection in the United States; for gonorrhea, continued emergence of antimicrobial resistance remains a major threat. This chapter reviews the global epidemiology of these two pathogens, their associated clinical syndromes, and current guidelines for their management.

EPIDEMIOLOGY

While the annual incidence of gonococcal infections in the United States declined from the early 1980s to an all-time low in 2009, the rate began to creep up, and by 2013 it was 106.1 cases per 100,000. Notably, rates in men exceeded those in women for the first time in 2013, possibly representing either increased ascertainment or actual higher incidence among men who have sex with men. The highest reported rates of gonorrhea were in women 15-19 years of age and in men 20-24 years of age, with marked differences by race (higher in blacks). While gonorrhea typically infects the cervix or urethra, both rectal and pharyngeal infections occur and are an important reservoir of asymptomatic infection, which helps to promote sexual transmission.

An estimated 2 million new chlamydial infections occur annually in the United States, and 3 million in Europe. In contrast to gonorrhea, these infections are more widely geographically distributed, and peak in even younger age groups—at least in women, as the epidemiology in men has not been well defined. Biological and social factors (namely, cervical ectopy and choice of sex partners) likely play a role in placing adolescent females at highest risk for chlamydial infection. The incidence of this disease has declined dramatically in some areas, probably in response to widespread screening programs begun in the 1980s. However, these trends may be undergoing a reversal. Chlamydia prevalence also remains high in many areas of the country in which screening has not become routine, approaching or exceeding 15-25% in some adolescent populations.

The prevalence of gonorrhea and chlamydia infections, as well as other STIs, is higher in developing countries than in the United States, although surveillance data from many areas are not comprehensive. The impact of both of these diseases goes beyond the obvious clinical and economic concerns and their well-recognized sequelae for women (which include ectopic pregnancy, tubal infertility, and chronic pelvic pain). Both gonorrhea and chlamydia potentiate infectiousness for and susceptibility to HIV. Urethral infection with *N. gonorrhoeae* is associated with an eight-fold increase in the amount of HIV in semen. In a prospective study of commercial sex workers in Kenya, acquisition of cervical chlamydial infection was associated with a 2.5-fold increase in the likelihood of acquiring HIV. Thus, these infections further fuel the HIV epidemic throughout Africa, Asia, and Latin America, along with other factors such as migration of refugees, population shifts from rural to urban environments, and persistence of commercial sex and illicit drug use. The spread of HIV in developing countries is discussed in more detail in Chapter 14.

URETHRITIS

Urethritis is the most common STI-related syndrome in males throughout the world, with *N. gonorrhoeae* most commonly associated with the prototypical purulent discharge characterizing this syndrome. However, in the United States, most urethritis is nongonococcal in origin (NGU); of all NGU, 30% is caused by *C. trachomatis*, and the remainder by a variety of etiologic agents including *Mycoplasma genitalium*, *Trichomonas vaginalis*, herpes simplex virus (HSV), and adenovirus. The role of *Ureaplasma urealyticum* in causing urethritis is still unclear (see below).

The situation in many parts of the developing world is strikingly different, with *N. gonorrhoeae* accounting for up to 80% of all urethritis. The reasons for this disparity are poorly understood; inability to accurately diagnose other causes of urethritis may be partly responsible. Many studies reported from developing countries to date have utilized sub-optimal methodologies for the detection of *C. trachomatis* and have probably underestimated its true contribution. The availability of nucleic acid amplified assays (NAATs) for both gonorrhea and chlamydia (discussed below) should continue to clarify their etiologic contributions. Finally, since NGU is usually a milder disease than gonococcal urethritis, differences in the threshold for medical evaluation may exist, particularly in countries where the availability of medical care is compromised.

Most men infected with *N. gonorrhoeae* at the urethra experience purulent or mucopurulent penile discharge and dysuria, although symptomatic status is likely influenced by the duration of infection and specific strain type. Complications include epididymitis and urethral strictures; although these are rare, they are more common in developing countries. Examination of Gram-stained smears of urethral secretions reveals the Gram-negative, kidney-shaped intracellular diplococci in 98% of cases and is 99% specific for the diagnosis. NAATs, including polymerase chain reaction and transcription mediated assay, offer some increase in sensitivity (5-8%) over culture, while maintaining specificity. Perhaps most importantly, NAATs can be performed on first-catch urine (not "clean-catch" or midstream urine), obviating the need for urethral swab collection. However, gonococcal cultures should be obtained in cases of treatment failure or if there is any suspicion of antimicrobial resistance, as NAATs do not currently provide a means for antibiotic susceptibility testing.

Until recently, *C. trachomatis* caused ~30-40% of cases of NGU, particularly in heterosexual men; however, the proportion of cases due to this organism has probably declined in some populations served by effective chlamydial-control programs, and older men with urethritis appear less likely to have chlamydial infection. HSV and *T. vaginalis* each cause a small proportion of NGU cases in the United States. Recently, multiple studies have consistently implicated *M. genitalium* as a probable cause of many *Chlamydia*-negative cases. Fewer studies than in the past have implicated *Ureaplasma*; the ureaplasmas have been differentiated into *U. urealyticum* and *U. parvum*, and a few studies suggest that *U. urealyticum*—but not *U. parvum*—is associated with NGU. Coliform bacteria can cause urethritis in men who practice insertive anal intercourse. The initial diagnosis of urethritis in men currently includes specific tests only for *N. gonorrhoeae* and *C. trachomatis*; it does not yet include testing for *Mycoplasma* or *Urealyticum* species.

Diagnostic testing is required to distinguish the etiology of urethritis, and both gonorrhea and chlamydia should be specifically sought if possible. The finding of significant numbers of polymorphonuclear leukocytes (PMNs) (more than two per high power field) *without* Gram-negative intracellular diplococci is sufficient to make a presumptive diagnosis of NGU. *N. gonorrhoeae* can be easily cultured on chocolate agar; culture for *C. trachomatis*, in contrast, is not widely available due to its technical demand. NAATs are the recommended assay for chlamydia and gonorrhea. The preferred specimen for evaluation of urethritis in men is first-catch urine.

In women, *C. trachomatis* may directly infect the urethra, inducing dysuria that may simulate bacterial cystitis. This presentation is generally characterized by the presence of PMNs but not bacteria in the urine, and is often accompanied by a history of a new sex partner. Up to 50% of these women are also infected at the cervix, and all should have diagnostic cervical testing done; while the urethra can be cultured, NAATs performed on urine are particularly advantageous in this situation.

CERVICITIS

Cervical gonococcal infections are usually asymptomatic. When symptoms are present, they include vaginal discharge, intermenstrual bleeding, dyspareunia, and/or abdominal pain. Similarly, only 10% of infected cervices will evidence signs, which include mucopurulent endocervical discharge, easily induced endocervical bleeding, and cervical edema. Up to 50% of women with gonococcal cervicitis may also have gonococcal urethritis with associated dysuria, but even more will have concomitant asymptomatic colonization of the urethra. Reports of disseminated gonococcal infection (DGI) to sites such as the skin and joints (causing rash and arthritis) in the United States have declined, but isolated tenosynovitis or acute arthritis is not uncommon as a manifestation of sexually acquired gonorrhea. In developing countries, the epidemiology of DGI is less well characterized. DGI occurs more commonly in women.

Gonococcal infection of the cervix should be diagnosed by NAAT, preferably obtained with a vaginal swab or, alternatively, endocervical swab. Urine NAAT testing is sensitive for the detection of cervical infection because it not only detects concomitant gonococcal urethral infection, which occurs frequently, but also tests cervicovaginal secretions that have collected in the vulvar area. Obtaining rectal and pharyngeal specimens may increase the yield of case detection, particularly if receptive oral or anal intercourse is reported. Gram stain of endocervical discharge suggests the diagnosis of gonorrhea if intracellular Gram-negative diplococci are seen, but this occurs in only 50% of cases, making the test too insensitive to use as the sole means of diagnosis. In cases of suspected DGI, NAATs of the genital tract should be done, as well as blood and joint aspirate cultures.

Like gonorrhea, chlamydial infections in women are usually asymptomatic (90%). Because the symptoms of cervicitis are nonspecific, if at all present, chlamydial cervical infection may present like gonococcal infection. Similarly, signs occur in the minority of patients (10%) and include induced endocervical bleeding, mucopurulent endocervical discharge, and edematous ectopy. Certainly, any of these should provoke diagnostic testing with NAAT. Given the high prevalence of chlamydia in many settings, particularly in adolescent females, routine testing of young women at any presentation for STI evaluation is recommended. This is especially critical because asymptomatic untreated chlamydial infections are capable of causing tubal scarring, which can lead to infertility, ectopic pregnancy, and chronic pelvic pain.

PELVIC INFLAMMATORY DISEASE

N. gonorrhoeae and *C. trachomatis* are the causal STIs implicated most often in pelvic inflammatory disease (PID), but in recent years the role of anaerobes, Gram-negative rods, and *M. genitalium* has been stressed, emphasizing that PID is usually a polymicrobial process. Serious consequences of PID include infertility, ectopic pregnancy, tubo-ovarian abscess, chronic pelvic pain, and pelvic adhesions.

Although clinical criteria for diagnosis of PID are inexact, the diagnosis should be suspected if cervical motion, adnexal, or lower abdominal tenderness are present on bimanual pelvic exam. Women evidencing any of these signs should be tested for gonorrhea and chlamydia, and pregnancy should be ruled out. Treatment of women with presumptive PID requires broad-spectrum coverage that includes activity against *N. gonorrhoeae* and *C. trachomatis*. A complete discussion of the diagnosis and treatment of PID is beyond the scope of this chapter; however, up-to-date reviews are referenced below (see also **Table 42.1**).

TABLE 42.1 Recommendations for Treatment of Pelvic Inflammatory Disease, 2015

Intramuscular/Oral Therapy

Ceftriaxone 250 mg i.m. once

or

Cefoxitin 2 g i.m. plus probenecid 1 g orally concurrently as a single dose

or

Other third-generation parenteral cephalosporin (ceftizoxime, cefotaxime)

plus

Doxycycline 100 mg orally twice daily ×14 days

with or without

Metronidazole 500 mg orally twice daily ×7 days

Parenteral Therapy

Recommended:

Cefotetan 2 g i.v. every 12 h

or

Cefoxitin 2 g i.v. every 6 h

or

Clindamycin 900 mg i.v. every 8 h

plus

Gentamicin loading dose i.v. or i.m. (2 mg/kg), followed by maintenance dose 1.5 mg/kg every 8 h. Single daily dosing (3-5 mg/kg) can be substituted

Alternative:

Ampicillin/Sulbactam 3 g i.v. every 6 h

plus

Doxycycline 100 mg orally or i.v. every 12 h

i.m., Intramuscular; *i.v.*, intravenous.

TREATMENT OF GONORRHEA AND CHLAMYDIA

Resistant strains of *N. gonorrhoeae* originally appeared in the United States as imported infections in servicemen returning from Southeast Asia in the mid-1970s. In 1994, approximately 16% of all gonococci in the United States were resistant to penicillin on the basis of either plasmid-mediated or chromosomal resistance; they are designated penicillinase-producing *N. gonorrhoeae* (PPNG). In some urban areas, the proportion of gonococcal isolates that are PPNG may approach 60-75%. Strains of gonococci that have also acquired plasmid-mediated tetracycline resistance are designated tetracycline-resistant *N. gonorrhoeae* (TRNG) and constituted 22% of isolates in 1994. Some multidrug-resistant strains are both PPNG and TRNG. Another 10-15% of gonococci studied in the United States have chromosomally mediated resistance to multiple drugs (penicillin, tetracycline, second-generation cephalosporins, and erythromycin). Most recently, gonococci have acquired resistance to fluoroquinolones (including ciprofloxacin and ofloxacin). This has progressed worldwide to the point that the US Centers for Disease Control and Prevention (CDC) removed fluoroquinolones from its list of recommended antibiotics in April 2007. Most recently, the appearance of gonococcal strains with increasingly high-level resistance to cephalosporins, including the third-generation cephalosporin used widely to treat this infection (ceftriaxone), has been reported; these strains have been associated with treatment failure of parenteral ceftriaxone therapy. Similarly, resistance to azithromycin—an agent that has been used as an alternative in cases where cephalosporins cannot be used—has also been reported in association with treatment failure. Thus, new agents are under investigation. In the meantime, the CDC

TABLE 42.2 Treatment for Uncomplicated Gonococcal and Chlamydial Infections in Adults

Recommended:
Ceftriaxone 250 mg i.m. (single dose)
plus
Azithromycin 1 g p.o. as single dose
Alternative, *if ceftriaxone is not available:*[a]
Cefixime 400 mg p.o. as single dose
plus
Azithromycin 1 g p.o. as single dose

[a]Not recommended for gonococcal infection of the pharynx; ceftriaxone plus azithromycin should be used.
i.m., Intramuscular; *i.v.*, intravenous; *p.o.*, by mouth.

TABLE 42.3 Treatment for Gonococcal and Chlamydial Infections in Pregnant Women[a]

Treatment for uncomplicated gonococcal infection:
Ceftriaxone 250 mg i.m. (single dose)
Treatment for uncomplicated chlamydial infection:[a]
Azithromycin 1 g p.o. as single dose

[a]Test of cure should be routine (3 weeks post-initiation of therapy).
i.m., Intramuscular; *p.o.*, by mouth.

recommends that all persons with gonorrhea be treated with parenteral ceftriaxone, if tolerated. This should be accompanied by treatment with azithromycin as a single dose for the theoretical benefit of exposing the organism to two classes of antibiotics.

Approved drug regimens are given in **Tables 42.2** and **Table 42.3**. The single-dose treatment of azithromycin for chlamydia is preferred, given its obvious advantage in compliance. Azithromycin is also the recommended regimen for the treatment of chlamydia in pregnant women. Regardless of the antibiotic chosen, a test of cure at 3 weeks post-completion of therapy is essential in pregnant women; no test of cure is otherwise routinely required. With the excellent sensitivity of NAAT for chlamydia, presumptive treatment for chlamydia in the setting of gonorrhea with a negative chlamydia NAAT is no longer recommended.

Recommendations for treating rectal gonorrhea, gonorrhea in children, neonatal gonococcal infections, gonococcal ophthalmia, and complicated or disseminated gonococcal infections are covered in the CDC treatment guidelines for sexually transmitted diseases.

FURTHER READING

Brunham, R.C., Gottlieb, S.L., Paavonen, J., 2015. Pelvic inflammatory disease. N. Engl. J. Med. 372 (21), 2039–2048.

Centers for Disease Control and Prevention, 2015. Sexually transmitted disease treatment guidelines. MMWR 64 (RR-3).

Geisler, W.M., 2011. Diagnosis and management of uncomplicated *Chlamydia trachomatis* infections in adolescents and adults: summary of evidence reviewed for the 2010 Centers for Disease Control and Prevention Sexually Transmitted Diseases Treatment Guidelines. Clin. Infect. Dis. 53 (Suppl. 3), S92–S98.

Kirkcaldy, R.D., Zaidi, A., Hook, E.W., et al., 2013. *Neisseria gonorrhoeae* antimicrobial resistance among men who have sex with men and men who have sex exclusively with women: the Gonococcal Isolate Surveillance Project, 2005–2010. Ann. Intern. Med. 158, 321–328.

US Preventive Services Task Force, 2008. Behavioral counseling to prevent sexually transmitted infections: US Preventive Services Task Force recommendation statement. Ann. Intern. Med. 149, 491–496. W95.

World Health Organization, 2012. Global Incidence and Prevalence of Selected Curable Sexually Transmitted Infections—2008. Available at <http://www.who.int/reproductivehealth/publications/rtis/stisestimates/en/>.

CHAPTER 43

Syphilis

Julia C. Dombrowski, Connie Celum, and Jared Baeten

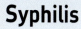

Syphilis results from infection with the spirochete *Treponema pallidum*. Transmission of syphilis occurs most often through sexual contact. Mother-to-infant transmission also occurs, and infection via blood transfusion is possible. Although *T. pallidum* induces strong humoral and cell-mediated immune responses, untreated infections can persist for decades.

EPIDEMIOLOGY

Syphilis is transmitted only through human-to-human contact; there is no animal or environmental reservoir. The World Health Organization (WHO) estimated that 10.6 million new cases of syphilis occurred among adults worldwide in 2008. Although the infection has a global distribution, 90% of syphilis cases occur in developing countries, reflecting the lack of access to treatment and prevention programs for sexually transmitted infections in resource-poor settings.

In the United States, rates of syphilis declined rapidly in the late 1940s after the introduction of penicillin therapy and accompanying public health control programs. However, a resurgence occurred in the 1980s, coincident with an epidemic of crack-cocaine use, at which time most cases occurred in heterosexuals. Medical and public health efforts substantially reduced rates of syphilis by the mid-1990s, but a second resurgence, which is ongoing, began in the late 1990s to early 2000s. In North America and Europe today, syphilis is concentrated in populations of men who have sex with men (MSM), particularly MSM infected with human immunodeficiency virus (HIV). Among HIV-negative MSM, the diagnosis of early syphilis portends a high risk for subsequent HIV infection, and MSM with syphilis represent a high priority subgroup for HIV pre-exposure prophylaxis and other HIV prevention efforts. A substantial increase in syphilis occurred in Russia, other Eastern European countries, and China beginning in the early 1990s. The majority of syphilis cases globally occur in sub-Saharan Africa and South and Southeast Asia. Rates of congenital infection and stillbirth from syphilis remain unacceptably high in many settings in these areas.

Endemic, nonvenereal treponemal infections, such as yaws and pinta, remain a source of disability in affected areas, primarily tropical regions in Africa, Latin America, and Southeast Asia. Penicillin mass treatment programs in the 1950s and 1960s significantly decreased the worldwide prevalence of these infections, but eradication was not achieved. Impoverished, remote populations are disproportionately affected.

CLINICAL PRESENTATION

Numerous monographs have been written describing the protean manifestations of syphilis, and excellent, updated reviews are available in the major medical and infectious disease texts. This discussion will be limited to specific aspects of syphilis relevant to understanding and

535

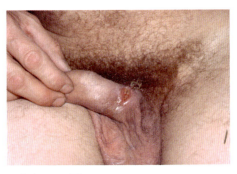

Fig. 43.1 Chancre of primary syphilis.

treating sexually transmitted infections among travelers and persons living in the developing world.

Primary Syphilis

The classic chancre of primary syphilis is a painless ulcer with an indurated margin and a clean base called a "chancre" that develops at the site of inoculation an average of 2-3 weeks post-infection (**Fig. 43.1**). Solitary lesions are typical, but multiple lesions can occur. The patient may not notice chancres, particularly in difficult-to-visualize areas such as the perianal area, labia, cervix, anus, rectum, and mouth. Secondary bacterial infection of these ulcers is rare. Unilateral or bilateral painless, nonsuppurative inguinal adenopathy follows appearance of the chancre by several days in 70-80% of cases. Spontaneous resolution of the chancre and adenopathy usually occurs within 6 weeks. Unfortunately, variation in the presentation of syphilitic ulcers makes clinical examination alone unreliable for the diagnosis of primary syphilis. Even clinicians experienced in diagnosis and management of sexually transmitted infections frequently misdiagnose the etiology of genital ulcers based on clinical examination. Use of laboratory diagnostics, when available, is crucial for appropriate etiologic diagnosis and treatment. In resource-poor settings, syndromic management of genital ulcer disease, including treatment for chancroid and syphilis, is commonly practiced.

Secondary Syphilis

Secondary syphilis is a systemic illness resulting from hematogenous dissemination of treponemes. The symptoms of secondary syphilis usually appear about 4-10 weeks after the appearance of the primary chancre. The manifestations of primary and secondary syphilis overlap in about 15% of cases. Clinical manifestations of secondary syphilis are extremely varied. The classic finding is a lacy, erythematous, maculopapular rash covering the trunk and abdomen. Palmar or plantar lesions, if present, are particularly suggestive of the diagnosis (**Fig. 43.2**). Cutaneous manifestations also include nodular, pustular, or follicular rashes, typically on the palms and soles but also more diffuse on the trunk; condylomata lata (nontender, sometimes moist, wart-like papules in the genital region), mucous patches in the mouth; and, less commonly, alopecia. The skin eruption is usually nonpruritic, but some patients complain of itching and present with excoriated lesions. Persons in the secondary stage of syphilis commonly have other manifestations of a systemic infection, including fever, generalized fatigue, and lymphadenopathy. Secondary syphilis must be considered in the differential diagnosis of *any* generalized skin eruption, particularly in MSM and pregnant women. The differential diagnosis for the rash of secondary syphilis includes viral exanthema, drug eruption, and primary HIV infection, among other etiologies. If untreated, approximately 25% of patients with secondary syphilis will have a relapse of active secondary syphilis, typically within 1 year.

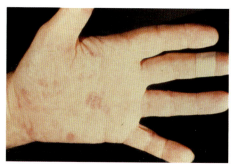

Fig. 43.2 **Palmar rash of secondary syphilis.**

Latent and Tertiary Syphilis

Untreated secondary syphilis spontaneously resolves after 3-12 weeks and is followed by latent, asymptomatic infection. Latent syphilis is defined by a positive serology in the absence of clinical disease. It is important to distinguish early latent syphilis from late latent syphilis to inform treatment decisions. Early latent syphilis is diagnosed only if the timing of infection can be confirmed as having occurred within the past year. Syphilis of unknown duration should be treated as late latent syphilis. Although syphilis is not transmitted through sexual contact during latent stages of the disease, symptoms of secondary syphilis can recur during the first year of infection. Pregnant women with latent syphilis are capable of transmitting the infection to the fetus. Elimination of congenital syphilis remains a global public health priority, and all pregnant women should be screened for syphilis at the first antenatal care visit. In the pre-antibiotic era, approximately one-third of individuals with late latent syphilis would eventually develop clinical disease, such as neurosyphilis, cardiovascular syphilis, or gummatous disease. However, the incidence of these manifestations has declined worldwide due to the widespread use of antibiotics that have some activity against latent syphilitic infection.

Neurosyphilis

Treponemal infection of the central nervous system (CNS) can occur during any stage of syphilis and is particularly common in the secondary stage. CNS infection in the setting of early syphilis (primary, secondary, and early latent) is distinct from, and much more common than, CNS manifestations in late syphilis, such as tabes dorsalis and the historic syphilis "madness" characterized by severe neurocognitive impairment. Early neurosyphilis presentations can range from subtle (e.g., headache) to severe (e.g., stroke resulting from meningovascular syphilis). All patients diagnosed with syphilis should be queried about symptoms of neurosyphilis, otosyphilis, and ocular syphilis. Changes in vision and hearing, in particular, should prompt cerebrospinal fluid (CSF) evaluation, if possible, and treatment with a neuropenetrative antibiotic regimen.

DIAGNOSIS

T. pallidum cannot be cultured. The definitive diagnostic procedure for primary and secondary syphilis is identification of spirochetes by darkfield microscopy or fluorescent monoclonal antibodies of serous exudate or scrapings obtained from lesions. Commensal spirochetes that reside in the oropharynx and intestinal tract can be difficult to differentiate from *T. pallidum* by morphologic criteria, making darkfield examination of oral and rectal lesions less reliable. However, darkfield microscopy is not widely available, requires specialized equipment and training, has limited sensitivity, and can be used only when cutaneous or

TABLE 43.1 Serologic Tests for Syphilis

Nontreponemal serologic tests

Venereal Disease Research Laboratory (VDRL) test
Rapid plasma reagin (RPR) test

Treponemal serologic tests

Enzyme immunoassay (EIA)
Chemiluminescence assay (CIA)
T. pallidum particle agglutination (TP-PA)
Fluorescent treponemal antibody absorption test (FTA-ABS)
Microhemagglutination assay for antibodies to *T. pallidum* (MHA-TP)

mucosal manifestations of syphilis are present. Thus, most cases of syphilis are diagnosed through serologic testing.

Both nontreponemal and treponemal serologic tests are used for syphilis screening and diagnosis (**Table 43.1**). The "traditional sequence" testing algorithm begins with a nontreponemal test (e.g., the Venereal Disease Research Laboratory [VDRL] and rapid plasma reagin [RPR] tests), which if positive, is followed by a treponemal test (e.g., *T. pallidum* particle agglutination [TP-PA]). Like most clinical screening activities, this algorithm begins with a highly sensitive test, which prompts follow-up with a higher specificity test if positive. In recent years, a "reverse sequence" testing algorithm has been used more commonly by some laboratories, beginning with a treponemal test (e.g., *T. pallidum* enzyme immunoassay [EIA] or chemiluminescence assay [CIA]), which, if positive, is followed by a nontreponemal test. If the results of the two tests are discordant, a second type of treponemal test is performed. Many laboratories switched to the reverse sequence algorithm as newer treponemal-specific tests became available that allow increased automation and reduced laboratory costs.

Interpretation of test results from either testing algorithm relies on recognition of two key features that differentiate treponemal-specific and nontreponemal-specific antibodies. First, nontreponemal antibodies are sensitive, but not specific, for *T. pallidum* infection. Second, treponemal-specific antibodies typically remain in the absence of active infection, either after treatment or in latent infection, whereas nontreponemal-specific antibodies decrease or disappear after resolution of clinically active syphilis.

Interpretation of test results with traditional testing is relatively straightforward (**Table 43.2**). A positive nontreponemal test with a positive treponemal test indicates syphilis; a positive nontreponemal test with a negative treponemal test indicates biologic false positivity. Numerous factors can cause biologic false positivity, including nonvenereal treponemal infections, other endemic tropical infections, and autoimmune diseases (**Table 43.3**). Interpretation of reverse sequence screening can be challenging due to the frequency of discordant test results (i.e., a positive treponemal test followed by a negative nontreponemal test). When the results of the treponemal and nontreponemal test are discordant, a second type of treponemal test is required. This is typically done reflexively in the laboratory without a clinician's order.

When the second treponemal test is negative, the results likely indicate a false positive. This can be due to either biologic or test factors, and in many instances, the false positive test reverts to negative on subsequent testing. Rarely, this pattern indicates very early infection because treponemal tests can become positive before the VDRL or RPR tests. This possibility should be considered in patients at high risk for recent syphilis infection and should prompt follow-up testing in approximately 1 month.

In the setting of discordant treponemal and nontreponemal results when the second type of treponemal-specific test is positive, additional clinical history is required to interpret the test. This pattern indicates a history of syphilis, either treated or untreated. If the patient

TABLE 43.2 Interpretation of Syphilis Testing Results

Test Results		Interpretation	Notes
Nontreponemal (RPR, VDRL)	**Treponemal-Specific (TP-PA, FTA-ABS)**		
		TRADITIONAL SEQUENCE ALGORITHM	
NR	–	No syphilis[a]	
R	R	Syphilis	Clinical history and examination required to determine stage of infection and distinguish treated from untreated infection
R	NR	False positive	See Table 43.3 for a list of possible causes.

Treponemal-Specific (EIA, CIA)	Nontreponemal (RPR, VDRL)	Treponemal-Specific (TP-PA, FTA-ABS)	Interpretation	Notes
			REVERSE SEQUENCE ALGORITHM	
NR	–	–	No syphilis[a]	
R	R	R	Syphilis	Clinical history and examination required to determine stage of infection and distinguish treated from untreated infection
R	NR	R	Past syphilis[b]	Clinical history required to distinguish successfully treated infection from untreated infection. Treat for late latent syphilis if past treatment cannot be confirmed.
R	NR	NR	False positive[b]	May be due to factors related to the test technology or biologic false positivity (see Table 43.3)

[a]All serologic tests have limitations in detection of very early syphilis (primary or incubating). Patients with clinical symptoms of syphilis or known contact with syphilis should be treated for syphilis regardless of serologic results.

[b]Because treponemal tests can become positive before nontreponemal tests, this pattern can also indicate very early syphilis infection in a patient who is at risk for acquiring syphilis.

CIA, chemiluminescence assay; *EIA*, enzyme immunoassay; *FTA-ABS*, fluorescent treponemal antibody absorption test; *NR*, nonreactive; *R*, reactive; *RPR*, rapid plasma reagin test; *TP-PA*, *T. pallidum* particle agglutination; *VDRL*, Venereal Disease Research Laboratory test; –, test not performed

TABLE 43.3   Causes of Biologically False-Positive Tests for Syphilis

Spirochetal Diseases	Other Tropical Infections	Other Infections	Other Conditions
Yaws[a]	Leprosy	Varicella (chickenpox)	Connective tissue diseases
Pinta[a]	Malaria	Rubeola (measles)	Illicit drug use
Bejel[a]	Chancroid	Infectious mononucleosis	Advanced age
Leptospirosis	Lymphogranuloma venereum	Other viruses	Pregnancy
Rat-bite fever	Trypanosomiasis	Immunizations	Malignancy
Relapsing fever	Rickettsial infections	*Mycoplasma pneumoniae*	Cirrhosis
Lyme disease	Hepatitis		

[a]Nonvenereal treponematoses.

has been previously treated, this result pattern reflects successful treatment. If the patient has not been treated for syphilis, this result indicates late latent infection (in the vast majority of cases) or very early infection (rarely). All patients who have two positive treponemal tests in the setting of a negative nontreponemal test should be treated for late latent syphilis if past treatment cannot be confirmed. In areas in which endemic treponemal infections such as pinta, yaws, and bejel are prevalent, serologic cross-reactivity may complicate interpretation of syphilis testing, making the diagnosis of latent syphilis largely presumptive. These endemic treponemal infections cannot be distinguished from syphilis with clinically available tests. Because endemic treponemes are prevalent in the same regions that syphilis is prevalent, treatment for latent syphilis is indicated even if cross-reactivity is a consideration.

Serologic tests can be negative in primary syphilis and in the incubation period before chancre development. Patients who have genital ulcers and are at risk for recent syphilis infection and patients with known contact to a sexual partner with syphilis should be empirically treated for early syphilis because serologic testing will not rule out infection. Approximately 80% of patients with primary syphilis will be seropositive by VDRL or RPR test. Virtually 100% of patients with secondary syphilis will have a reactive VDRL or RPR test, and the titers of these tests are usually higher than for other stages of syphilis (i.e., typically ≥1:32). Antibody levels detected with the nontreponemal tests fall slowly following treatment, and sequential quantitative VDRL or RPR titers are used to assess response to therapy. However, they also fall slowly with time, even in the absence of treatment, and many patients with untreated late latent syphilis are no longer seropositive with nontreponemal tests (**Table 43.4**).

Point-of-care tests for syphilis are available, most of which are treponemal tests and accordingly have the limitations of treponemal testing in the absence of nontreponemal testing. That is, a positive rapid test in isolation cannot distinguish active clinical infection from past, treated infection. A dual treponemal and nontreponemal rapid syphilis test has recently been described in the scientific literature, but it is not clinically available at the time of this writing.

Diagnosis of Central Nervous System Syphilis

No single test is definitive for the diagnosis of neurosyphilis. Lumbar puncture with CSF examination is used to detect CNS involvement in syphilis. A CSF VDRL test is highly specific but insensitive. CSF pleocytosis and elevated protein are often present; follow-up of the CSF cell count is used to monitor response to treatment for neurosyphilis. However, CSF analysis is not recommended routinely for patients with primary or secondary syphilis. CDC guidelines recommend CSF examination for patients with syphilis and any of the

TABLE 43.4 Sensitivity and Specificity of Serologic Tests for Syphilis

			SENSITIVITY BY STAGE FOR UNTREATED SYPHILIS		
	Primary	Secondary	Early Latent	Late Latent	Specificity[a]
Nontreponemal serologic tests					
VDRL	78%	100%	96%	71%	98%
RPR	86%	100%	98%	73%	98%
Treponemal serologic tests					
EIA	93%	100%	100%	unknown	NA
FTA-ABS[b]	84%	100%	100%	96%	97%
MHA-TP	76%	100%	97%	94%	99%

[a]May not apply for patients from countries with endemic nonvenereal treponemal infections due to serologic cross-reactivity.
[b]FTA-ABS and TP-PA are equally sensitive for the detection of primary syphilis
EIA, Enzyme immunoassay; *FTA-ABS*, fluorescent treponemal antibody absorption test; *MHA-TP*, microhemagglutination assay for antibodies to *T. pallidum*; *NA*, not applicable; *RPR*, rapid plasma reagin test; *VDRL*, Venereal Disease Research Laboratory test.
Adapted from Larsen, S., Hunter, E., Kraus, S. (Eds.), 1990. A Manual of Tests for Syphilis. American Public Health Association, Washington, DC, with permission.

following: (1) neurologic or ophthalmologic signs or symptoms, (2) active tertiary disease (e.g., aortitis, gumma), (3) treatment failure of non-neurologic syphilis, or (4) late latent syphilis or syphilis of unknown duration in a patient with HIV infection. The absence of clinical symptoms or signs does not rule out the possibility of CNS involvement with syphilis, although the clinical significance of asymptomatic neurosyphilis is uncertain. Some experts recommend performing a lumbar puncture on anyone with latent syphilis as well as in all HIV-infected patients regardless of syphilis stage. In addition, CSF examination should be considered for individuals with latent syphilis and high titer (≥1:32) nontreponemal serologic results or for those in whom nonpenicillin therapy is planned. Importantly, CSF testing can be normal in cases of ocular syphilis and otosyphilis. For this reason, clinicians should consider additional ophthalmologic and audiologic evaluation, when possible, and empiric treatment with a neuropenetrative antibiotic regimen for patients with syphilis who report recent changes in vision or hearing.

TREATMENT

T. pallidum has remained exquisitely sensitive to penicillin, and parenteral penicillin therapy remains the treatment of choice for all forms of syphilis. A summation of current US and WHO recommendations is provided in **Table 43.5**.

Small studies have suggested that azithromycin, provided as a single oral dose of 2 g, may be effective for treatment of primary and secondary syphilis. However, case reports of treatment failure and documented resistance to azithromycin in some areas prevent formal recommendation of use of azithromycin for treatment of early syphilis. Azithromycin treatment is not appropriate for MSM in the United States, where more than half of *T. pallidum* strains are resistant to azithromycin.

Ceftriaxone has also been used for treatment of early and latent syphilis, as well as neurosyphilis, based on small clinical studies and pharmacokinetics. For early syphilis, a dose of 1 g ceftriaxone daily, by intramuscular injection or intravenous administration, for 8-10 days, has been used. For neurosyphilis, some have recommended a dose of 2 g daily, by intramuscular injection or intravenous administration, for 10-14 days. It is important to note, however, that optimal dosing and duration of ceftriaxone therapy have not been defined in formal guidelines, have not been studied in HIV-infected patients, and can be associated with allergic reactions due to cross-reactivity in patients with penicillin allergies.

TABLE 43.5 Treatment of Syphilis in Adults

Stage	Treatment
Primary, secondary, or early latent[a]	Recommended: benzathine penicillin G 2.4 million units by intramuscular injection, single dose
	Alternative regimen for penicillin-allergic, nonpregnant patients: doxycycline 100 mg by mouth, twice daily for 14 days *or* tetracycline 500 mg by mouth, four times daily for 14 days
	Second alternative (WHO Guidelines): procaine penicillin, 1.2 million units by intramuscular injection, daily for 10 consecutive days
Late latent, syphilis of unknown duration, and tertiary disease without neurologic involvement	Recommended: benzathine penicillin G 2.4 million units by intramuscular injection, once a week for 3 consecutive weeks
	Alternative regimen for penicillin-allergic, nonpregnant patients: doxycycline 100 mg by mouth, twice daily for 28-30 days *or* tetracycline 500 mg by mouth, four times daily for 28-30 days
	Second alternative (WHO Guidelines): procaine penicillin, 1.2 million units by intramuscular injection, daily for 20 consecutive days
Neurosyphilis[c]	Recommended: aqueous crystalline penicillin G 18-24 million units per day, administered intravenously in divided doses every 4 h or by continuous infusion, for 10-14 days
	Alternative: procaine penicillin G 1.2-2.4 million units by intramuscular injection daily *plus* probenecid[b] 500 mg by mouth, four times daily. Both for 10-14 days.
	Penicillin-allergic patients, including allergic pregnant patients, should undergo penicillin desensitization, followed by treatment with one of the above regimens.
	WHO guidelines suggest that doxycycline 200 mg by mouth, twice daily for 30 days or tetracycline 500 mg, by mouth, four times daily for 30 days may be considered alternatives for penicillin-allergic, nonpregnant patients, although these regimens have not been evaluated in systematic studies. Many experts do not endorse these regimens for neurosyphilis due to limited clinical experience and concerns about compliance.

[a]Latent syphilis is defined by seroreactivity without clinical evidence of disease. Early latent syphilis (defined as infection within 1 year by CDC guidelines and 2 years by WHO guidelines) requires at least one of the following: (1) documented seroconversion within the defined time period, (2) unequivocal symptoms of primary or secondary syphilis within the time period, or (3) a sex partner with primary, secondary, or early latent syphilis within the time period.
[b]Patients with serious allergies to sulfonamides should not be treated with a probenecid-containing regimen.
[c]Of note, some experts recommend treating patients with cardiovascular syphilis with a neurosyphilis regimen.

The optimal management strategies for late latent syphilis, neurosyphilis, and cardiovascular syphilis continue to be debated, and recommendations are based on clinical experience rather than controlled trials. In general, penicillin-based regimens for the appropriate stage of syphilis are recommended for treatment of pregnant women. WHO guidelines offer erythromycin-based regimens for penicillin-allergic, pregnant patients with syphilis without CNS involvement; however, erythromycin does not reliably cure infection in the fetus. Penicillin desensitization should be attempted, if possible. Infants born to mothers who have to be treated with erythromycin should receive penicillin after birth. The reader is encouraged to consult available experts and the Further Reading section for further details related to syphilis in pregnancy and management of congenital disease.

Finally, all patients treated for syphilis should be tested for HIV and other sexually transmitted diseases (e.g., gonorrhea and chlamydial infections).

ASSESSING THERAPEUTIC RESPONSE

Treatment failure can occur with any regimen given for any syphilis stage. All patients treated for syphilis require clinical and serologic follow-up at 6, 12, and, for those treated for latent syphilis, 24 months. Treatment failure is defined as persistent symptoms or signs or a sustained four-fold increase or failure to achieve a four-fold decrease in those with high-titer initial results (equivalent to a two-dilution change) in nontreponemal test titer. A lumbar puncture to evaluate for neurosyphilis should be considered when initial treatment is unsuccessful. Approximately 5-15% of patients with primary or secondary syphilis will not achieve an adequate serologic decline after initial therapy and require retreatment despite adequate serologic response to appropriate treatment. The same regimens recommended for initial treatment should be used for retreatment, unless the CSF is abnormal.

Many patients with latent syphilis, whether early or late, remain reactive by VDRL or RPR testing at a persistent low titer (1:1 to 1:8) for several years. These patients require careful follow-up with periodic testing: a four-fold (i.e., two dilution) increase in titer indicates treatment failure or reinfection.

As detailed above, lumbar puncture with CSF examination is recommended for patients with treated early syphilis whose titers do not fall adequately. Those treated for neurosyphilis should have repeat CSF examination at 3-6 months after therapy, and then 6-monthly thereafter until normalization of CSF findings. Failure to normalize CSF cell count by 2 years should prompt consideration of retreatment.

MANAGEMENT OF SEX PARTNERS

Sexual transmission of syphilis occurs when mucocutaneous lesions are present; the risk of sexual transmission is low from patients with untreated syphilis of >1 year duration. Nonetheless, sex partners of patients with syphilis of any stage should be evaluated clinically and serologically for syphilis. Presumptive treatment is recommended for those exposed within 90 days preceding a diagnosis of primary, secondary, or early latent syphilis in a sex partner, as serologic results may not yet become positive in such individuals.

HIV AND SYPHILIS

Persons with syphilis are at risk for HIV infection due to factors related to sexual behavior and biology. Ulcerative sexually transmitted infections such as syphilis appear to facilitate the acquisition and transmission of HIV. All persons with suspected or confirmed syphilis should be tested for HIV infection, and MSM with syphilis are a priority population for HIV pre-exposure prophylaxis. In patients with early syphilis and concurrent immunosuppression from HIV infection, aggressive or atypical manifestations may occur. HIV infection increases the risk of early or persistent CNS invasion. In general, syphilis in HIV-infected persons should be treated according to the standard guidelines for HIV-uninfected populations. Some specialists extend therapy for early syphilis in persons with HIV by providing weekly benzathine penicillin for 3 weeks, rather than just a single dose; this practice is controversial and is not endorsed in guidelines. HIV-infected patients with syphilis should be monitored closely for clinical and serologic response after treatment—CDC guidelines recommend follow-up at 3, 6, 9, 12, and 24 months after therapy.

FURTHER READING

Causer, L.M., Kaldor, J.M., Conway, D.P., et al., 2015. An evaluation of a novel dual treponemal/nontreponemal point-of-care test for syphilis as a tool to distinguish active from past treated infection. Clin. Infect. Dis. 61 (2), 184–191. Epub ahead of print.

Centers for Disease Control and Prevention, 2011. Discordant results from reverse sequence syphilis screening—five laboratories, United States, 2006–2010. MMWR 60, 133–137.

Chen, Z.Q., Zhang, G.C., Gong, X.D., et al., 2007. Syphilis in China: results of a national surveillance programme. Lancet 369, 132–138.

Golden, M.R., Marra, C.M., Holmes, K.K., 2003. Update on syphilis: resurgence of an old problem. JAMA 290, 1510–1514.

Larsen, S., Hunter, E., Kraus, S. (Eds.), 1990. A Manual of Tests for Syphilis. American Public Health Association, Washington, DC.

Lukehart, S.A., Hook, E.W., III, Baker-Zander, S.A., et al., 1988. Invasion of the central nervous system by *Treponema pallidum*. Ann. Intern. Med. 109, 855–862.

Lukehart, S.A., Godornes, C., Molini, B.J., et al., 2004. Macrolide resistance in *Treponema pallidum* in the United States and Ireland. N. Engl. J. Med. 351, 154–158.

Musher, D.M., 1999. Early syphilis. In: Holmes, K.K., Sparlin, P.F.Märdh, P.-A. (Eds.), Sexually Transmitted Diseases, third ed. McGraw-Hill, New York, pp. 479–485.

Park, I.U., Chow, J.M., Bolan, G., et al., 2011. Screening for syphilis with the treponemal immunoassay: analysis of discordant serology results and implications for clinical management. J. Infect. Dis. 204, 1297–1304.

Pathela, P., Braunstein, S.L., Blank, S., et al., 2015. The high risk of an HIV diagnosis following a diagnosis of syphilis: a population-level analysis of New York City men. Clin. Infect. Dis. 61 (2), 281–287. Epub ahead of print.

Patton, M.E., Su, J.R., Nelson, R., et al., 2014. Primary and secondary syphilis—United States, 2005–2013. MMWR 9, 402–406.

Rolfs, R.T., Joesoef, M.R., Hendershoot, E.F., et al., 1997. A randomized trial of enhanced therapy for early syphilis in patients with and without human immunodeficiency virus infection. N. Engl. J. Med. 337, 307–314.

Sparling, P.F., 1999. Natural history of syphilis. In: Holmes, K.K., Sparlin, P.F.Märdh, P.-A. (Eds.), Sexually Transmitted Diseases, third ed. McGraw-Hill, New York, pp. 473–478.

Stoner, B.P., 2007. Current controversies in the management of adult syphilis. Clin. Infect. Dis. 44, S130–S146.

Swartz, M.N., Healy, B.P., Musher, D.M., 1999. Late syphilis. In: Holmes, K.K., Sparlin, P.F., Märdh, P.-A. (Eds.), Sexually Transmitted Diseases, third ed. McGraw-Hill, New York, pp. 487–509.

Tichinova, L., Bonshenko, K., Ward, H., et al., 1997. Epidemics of syphilis in the Russian Federation: trends, origins and priorities for control. Lancet 350, 210–213.

Wasserheit, J., 1992. Epidemiological synergy. Interrelationships between human immunodeficiency virus and other sexually transmitted diseases. Sex. Transm. Dis. 19, 61–77.

Workowski, K.A., Berman, S., 2010. Sexually transmitted diseases treatment guidelines, 2010. MMWR 17, 1–110.

WHO. Global incidence and prevalence of selected curable sexually transmitted infections—2008. Available at <http://apps.who.int/iris/bitstream/10665/75181/1/9789241503839_eng.pdf> (accessed April 23, 2015).

Zetela, N.M., Klausner, J.D., 2007. Syphilis and HIV infection: an update. Clin. Infect. Dis. 44, 1222–1228.

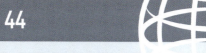

CHAPTER 44

Genital Ulcer Disease

Aliza Monroe-Wise, R. Scott McClelland, and Carey Farquhar

A genital ulcer is defined as a discrete mucosal or cutaneous discontinuity involving the genitals, perineum, or surrounding tissues. Genital ulcer disease (GUD) is an important risk factor for sexual acquisition and transmission of human immunodeficiency virus (HIV), and serious long-term sequelae can result from all causes of GUD. The etiologies of GUD vary geographically and are strongly associated with behavioral, demographic, and socioeconomic factors, in addition to the prevalence of HIV infection. Genital herpes is the most common cause of GUD worldwide, followed by syphilis, chancroid, lymphogranuloma venereum (LGV), and granuloma inguinale (also known as donovanosis). These causes of sexually transmitted GUD will be discussed here, with the exception of syphilis, which is described in detail in Chapter 43. Nonsexually transmitted causes of GUD such as systemic viral illnesses, aphthous ulcers, autoimmune disease, and *Schistosoma hematobium* infection are less common and are associated with specific risk factors, including geographic location, medical comorbidities, demographics, and behavioral factors.

Herpes simplex virus type 2 (HSV-2) is recognized as the leading global cause of GUD, with seropositivity up 50% in certain populations in the United States and over 70% among sexually active adults in many regions of sub-Saharan Africa. While syphilis and chancroid remain important contributors to GUD in some resource-limited settings, these are now significantly less prevalent than they were a decade ago. This important shift from bacterial to viral causes of GUD may be secondary to improved syndromic management, increased antibiotic use, and behavioral change. Additionally, advances in laboratory testing facilitate the detection of viral pathogens that might previously have gone undetected.

In returning travelers and recent immigrants with GUD who have engaged in unprotected sex, one must consider HSV, as well as causes of genital ulceration rarely observed in developed countries. The classic presentation of genital herpes is with multiple vesicles or ulcerative lesions on examination. The presence of a single ulcer should prompt work-up for other causes of GUD in addition to HSV. A careful history, including the timing and geographic location of the encounter, may also suggest a specific etiology. Incubation periods vary from several days in the case of chancroid and HSV to several weeks with LGV, and certain ulcerative diseases such as donovanosis are highly prevalent in certain parts of the world and rarely reported in others (**Table 44.1**). Systemic symptoms, such as fever and general malaise, may be present with primary HSV, syphilis, chancroid, LGV, and donovanosis but are observed most frequently in individuals with genital herpes and secondary syphilis. Inguinal adenopathy can also be observed with any of the GUD syndromes discussed in this chapter, as well as with primary syphilis. Additionally, the duration of symptoms may provide clues to diagnosis. While the clinical course of bacterial GUD is measured in weeks to months, genital herpes typically resolves spontaneously within days to weeks and recurs weeks to months later (**Table 44.1**).

545

TABLE 44.1 Overview of Characteristics of Genital Ulcer Disease (excluding syphilis; see Chapter 43)

	Geographic Region	Incubation Period	Appearance of Genital Lesions	Systemic Symptoms	Duration of Symptoms
Herpes simplex virus (HSV)	Worldwide	3-5 days	Multiple small, vesicles, pustules or ulcers; large ulcer after small lesions coalesce; adenopathy usually in primary	Yes (primary, not recurrent)	Lifetime recurrence of episodes lasting 5-10 days; primary infection lasts 2-6 weeks
Chancroid	Sub-Saharan Africa, Asia	3-5 days for papules 1-2 weeks for ulcers	Single or multiple ulcers	Yes	Several weeks for ulcers; adenopathy may last 1-3 months
Lymphogranuloma venereum (LGV)	Africa, Southeast Asia, South America, Caribbean; Europe and North America among MSM	3-12 days for ulcers; 10-30 days for adenopathy	Painless blister (single or multiple) that ulcerates; tender inguinal adenopathy; proctitis/proctocolitis	Yes	Several weeks to months
Granuloma inguinale (donovanosis)	Papua New Guinea, Southern Africa, India, Brazil, Caribbean	4-6 weeks	Single or multiple tender and vascular ulcers; inguinal inflammation may occur	Rarely	Several months

MSM, Men who have sex with men.

TABLE 44.2 Laboratory Evaluation of Sexually Active Patients with Genital Ulcer Disease

Lesions typical of genital herpes[a]

PCR, direct FA, or culture for HSV

Screening tests for other STDs (syphilis, HIV, chlamydia, and gonorrhea)

Other genital ulcers

PCR, DFA, or culture for HSV

Type-specific HSV serology

Darkfield microscopy or direct FA test for *Treponema pallidum*

Syphilis serology

Selected cases

Culture or PCR for *Haemophilus ducreyi* (if available)

PCR and serology for *Chlamydia trachomatis* (LGV) (if available)

Culture for pyogenic bacteria

[a]For example, a cluster of vesicular or pustular lesions, or multiple superficial ulcers.
DFA, Direct fluorescent antibody test; *HIV*, human immunodeficiency virus; *HSV*, herpes simplex virus; *LGV*, lymphogranuloma venereum; *PCR*, polymerase chain reaction; *STDs*, sexually transmitted diseases.

Since presentations of GUD vary and have substantial overlap, clinical diagnosis is both insensitive and nonspecific, making it important to supplement the clinical history and examination with diagnostic laboratory testing, especially among HIV-1-infected individuals (**Table 44.2**). However, even with an extensive evaluation, a definitive diagnosis will not be made in as many as 25% of cases due to the lack of sensitive and specific laboratory testing. As the dominant risk factors for acquisition of GUD are those associated with all sexually transmitted infections (STIs) (multiple sex partners, intercourse with a new partner or high-risk partner, and failure to use condoms), laboratory testing for other STIs should be incorporated into routine work-up of GUD. HIV testing is particularly important to incorporate into the STI work-up; higher rates of chancroid and HSV-2 infection are observed in HIV-1-infected individuals, and these two infections have been strongly associated with HIV-1 transmission and acquisition.

HERPES SIMPLEX VIRUS (HSV)

Epidemiology

Genital herpes, which can be caused by either of the herpes simplex viruses (HSV-1 and HSV-2), is now the most prevalent cause of GUD worldwide. HSV is a lifelong, incurable infection, believed to be indefinitely contagious to sex partners. Genital HSV increases the risk of acquiring HIV almost three-fold, likely due to the mucosal and epithelial disruption and recruitment of CD4$^+$ T cells to the genital area that result from HSV infection. Globally, HSV-2 is the most common cause of genital herpes, with seroprevalence ranging from ~20% among adults in the general population in the United States and parts of Western Europe to 50-70% in sub-Saharan Africa. Among commercial sex workers in parts of Africa and Southeast Asia, rates may be as high as 90%, and around 60% of HIV-negative men who have sex with men (MSM) in South America may be HSV-2-seropositive.

HSV-1, which also causes orolabial herpes (cold sores), is an increasingly common cause of genital herpes, most notably in the United States and Northern Europe, perhaps as a result of the declining rates of HSV-1 acquisition in childhood. In some populations HSV-1 now causes the majority of primary genital herpes. While the seroprevalence of HSV-1 ranges from >50% in developed countries to nearly 100% in developing countries, the frequency of genital HSV-1 infection in most parts of the world is not known, as serology does not reveal the anatomic location of HSV-1 infection.

Most people with genital herpes are unaware of their infection. The proportion of HSV-2-seropositive individuals who report being aware of a history of genital herpes has ranged from only 9% in the general population up to 34% among women attending a sexually transmitted diseases clinic in the United States. As a result, most cases of genital herpes are acquired from sex partners who are unaware of being infected themselves. Women have a higher risk of genital HSV acquisition than men, likely due to greater mucosal surface area in women and the fact that younger women frequently have male sexual partners who are older and thus more likely to be infected with HSV-2.

Pathogenesis
HSV entry occurs via the genital mucosa or a break in the genital skin. During primary infection, the virus enters sensory neurons and migrates to the sacral dorsal root ganglion, where it establishes latency. Primary infection is controlled, and viral dissemination may be prevented, by a cytotoxic T lymphocyte response. During HSV reactivation, which can be triggered by immunosuppression, ultraviolet light, trauma, fever, and possibly stress, the virus travels down the axon and multiplies within epithelial cells, producing similar but less severe lesions to those found during primary infection.

Clinical Manifestations and Diagnosis
There are three types of genital HSV infection: primary, nonprimary first episode, and recurrent. Primary infection is defined by the presence of HSV (of either type) in the genital tract of an individual seronegative for both HSV-1 and HSV-2. Nonprimary first episode is defined by the presence of HSV-2 in the genital tract of an individual with only HSV-1 antibodies or, rarely, the presence of HSV-1 in an individual with only HSV-2 antibodies. Recurrent infection is defined as the presence of either type of HSV in the genital tract of an individual with antibodies autologous to the genital type. Prior HSV-1 antibodies do not significantly reduce the risk of infection with HSV-2 but do reduce the likelihood of symptomatic HSV-2 infection.

Primary genital HSV infection is characterized by bilateral multiple small vesicular or pustular lesions that may coalesce into large ulcerated areas, which persist for 4-15 days and then crust over. Over 75% of patients experience a second crop of lesions during primary infection, which begin between day 4 and day 10. Complete healing of all lesions takes a mean of 16.5 days in men and 19.5 days in women. Local symptoms, including itching, pain, dysuria, tender inguinal lymphadenopathy, and urethral and/or vaginal discharge, occur frequently. Among women, 70-90% have HSV cervicitis during primary infection. Nearly 70% of women and 40% of men report systemic symptoms, including fever, malaise, myalgias, and headache, during primary infection. Less commonly, aseptic meningitis and/or disseminated HSV infection can occur, including HSV hepatitis. HSV proctitis and anorectal infection may also occur, especially among MSM.

Manifestations of recurrent genital herpes are generally confined to the mucosa or skin. Most people with HSV recurrence experience some degree of prodromal symptoms, which may include tingling, burning, and/or pain. During recurrence, lesions are generally unilateral, cover a much smaller area than those of primary infection, and last 4-5 days. The median number of recurrences in the first year of infection is five in men and four in women. Recurrence rates decrease by a median of one episode per year. Recurrence of genital HSV-1 is much less frequent, averaging only one episode per year, and only 60% of patients with genital HSV-1 have a recurrence within the first year.

"Atypical" presentations of genital HSV are common. Vesicles and ulcers may be absent, with fissures, furuncles, erythema, or pain instead. Lesions caused by HSV may be mistakenly attributed to other infectious agents (e.g., *Candida*), trauma, insect bites, allergic reaction, "irritation," or hemorrhoids, or may appear in an atypical location such as the thigh. Thus, all genital lesions, especially recurrent lesions present in the S2 or S3 dermatomes, should be evaluated for HSV.

Since clinical diagnosis of genital herpes is neither sensitive nor specific, patients presenting with genital lesions should undergo virologic testing to determine the diagnosis (**Table 44.2**). In patients presenting with multiple vesicular lesions and/or history consistent with genital herpes, initiation of presumptive therapy while awaiting laboratory results is advisable. Polymerase chain reaction (PCR) is four times more sensitive than viral culture and has become the standard of care in the developed world. Antigen detection via direct fluorescent antibody testing is also sensitive and specific for identifying HSV on a smear taken from vesicular fluid or an ulcer base. Viral culture is another option, but the sensitivity declines rapidly within a few days of onset, as lesions begin to heal. A Tzanck test to look for cytopathic changes associated with herpetic lesions is unreliable and not advised. Since antibodies to HSV generally appear within several weeks after infection and persist indefinitely, type-specific serologic tests can be useful in confirming a diagnosis of HSV but cannot distinguish between new and pre-existing infection. All patients with new genital herpes infection should be tested for HIV; testing for other STIs should also be considered.

Treatment and Prevention

All patients with first-episode genital herpes should be treated with oral antivirals to reduce the risk of severe local spread as well as the likelihood and severity of systemic symptoms (**Table 44.3**). Episodic antiviral therapy shortens the duration of symptoms, while suppressive therapy can reduce the recurrence rates by 70-80% among patients with frequent outbreaks. Treatment of recurrences should be initiated within 24–48 hours of symptom development, as efficacy declines after that window. See **Table 44.3** for details on treatment of genital HSV infection.

TABLE 44.3 Treatment of Genital HSV Infection

First episode of genital herpes
Acyclovir 400 mg orally three times a day (or 200 mg orally five times a day) for 7-10 days
or
Famciclovir 250 mg orally three times a day for 7-10 days
or
Valacyclovir 1.0 g orally twice a day for 7-10 days

Severe infection that requires parental therapy
Acyclovir 5-10 mg/kg body weight i.v. every 8 h for 2-7 days or until clinical improvement is observed, followed by oral antiviral therapy to complete at least 10 days total therapy

Episodic treatment of recurrent herpes
Acyclovir 400 mg orally three times a day for 5 days (or 800 mg orally twice a day for 5 days, or 800 mg three times a day for 2 days)
or
Famciclovir 125 mg orally twice a day for 5 days (or 1 g orally twice a day for 1 day, or 500 mg orally once followed by 250 mg twice daily for 2 days)
or
Valacyclovir 500 mg orally twice a day for 3 days (or 1 g orally once a day for 5 days)

Suppressive therapy[a]
Acyclovir 400 mg orally twice a day
or
Famciclovir 250 mg orally twice a day
or
Valacyclovir 500 mg (<10 episodes/year) or 1000 mg (>10 episodes/year) orally once a day

[a]The need to continue suppressive therapy should be discussed periodically (e.g., annually).
Adapted from specific product package inserts; standard guidelines for therapy of genital herpes in otherwise healthy adults (not pregnant); and Centers for Control and Prevention, 2010. Sexually transmitted diseases treatment guidelines 2010. MMWR 51(RR-06):11–12.

Methods of preventing genital HSV infection include condoms and use of suppressive antiviral therapy in the infected partner. For both men and women, the use of condoms is associated with ~50% decrease in HSV-2 acquisition, and daily suppressive antiviral therapy administered to the HSV-2 infected partner can reduce risk of HSV-2 transmission among monogamous couples by approximately one-half. Patients with genital herpes should be counseled that viral shedding, which can result in transmission to sex partners, is common even in the absence of symptoms.

CHANCROID

Epidemiology

The global prevalence of chancroid has decreased dramatically during the last decade. Nonetheless, chancroid remains an important cause of genital ulcers in certain resource-limited areas. Sentinel surveillance in various parts of sub-Saharan Africa and Asia has reported decreases in prevalence from 48 to 95% throughout the 1980s and 1990s, leading to discussion of the feasibility of eradication. Chancroid is uncommon in developed countries. For example, only 85 cases were reported from 2009 to 2013 in the United States. In developed countries, chancroid occurs in localized epidemics in populations having high sex-partner change rates. Chancroid is closely linked to commercial sex work, substance abuse, and economic deprivation, relying heavily on core groups for transmission and persistence within populations. Other risk factors include male gender, lack of circumcision, and HIV-1 seropositivity. HIV-1 infected individuals have longer duration of symptoms and may not respond well to treatment, further increasing their risk of transmitting HIV-1, chancroid, or both.

Pathogenesis

Haemophilus ducreyi, the cause of chancroid, is a small, Gram-negative bacillus. The organism is nutritionally fastidious, slow growing, and difficult to isolate. Bacteria enter genital mucosa via superficial abrasions that occur during sexual intercourse, and infect epithelial cells. This results in an inflammatory papule that rapidly evolves into a pustule and later ulcerates. The predominant immune response to *H. ducreyi* is a Th1 cell-mediated response, with CD4 T-cell infiltration of ulcers. Although antibodies are produced to several outer membrane proteins, their specificity and contribution to acquired immunity is not known.

Clinical Manifestations and Diagnosis

Symptoms usually appear 3-5 days after exposure but can occur up to 2 weeks after sexual contact. A tender papule or pustule characterizes the first stage and precedes ulcer formation by several days to up to 2 weeks. Individuals may be infectious during this period. Ulcers may be single or multiple, erythematous, and usually 1-2 cm in diameter, although the appearance can vary, especially in the setting of HIV infection. Chancroid was historically called the "soft chancre," reflecting the fact that the edges of ulcers are not indurated when compared with syphilis. The ulcer shape may be round, oval, or irregular, and the base is typically covered with purulent exudate. Some cases are mild, with nonspecific-appearing lesions. Most ulcers occur on the penis, especially under the foreskin in uncircumcised men, and near the introitus in women. Sores can also develop in the perianal area or rectum. Infection with *H. ducreyi* is usually painful but may be asymptomatic or painless in women, which may delay diagnosis and treatment.

Approximately 50% of male patients with untreated chancroid will also have inguinal lymphadenopathy, which is more commonly unilateral than bilateral and develops 1-2 weeks after the appearance of ulcers. Overlying cutaneous erythema and fluctuance are often present and help to distinguish chancroid from syphilis or herpes, which do not present with the characteristic "bubo." If untreated, lymph nodes may rupture and drain spontaneously, leaving open, ulcerated sores. Despite the locally aggressive nature of the infection, fever and disseminated infection rarely occur. Ulcerative lesions may persist for several weeks in the absence of treatment, and adenopathy can persist for 1-3 months. Complications from

TABLE 44.4   Recommended Regimens for Treatment of Chancroid
Azithromycin 1.0 g orally in a single dose
Ceftriaxone 250 mg intramuscularly in single dose
Ciprofloxacin 500 mg orally twice a day for 3 days
Erythromycin 500 mg orally 3 times a day for 7 days

From: Centers for Control and Prevention, 2010. Sexually transmitted diseases treatment guidelines 2010. MMWR 51 (RR-06), 11–12.

genital ulcers and buboes include phimosis, inguinal scarring, superinfection, and development of fistulas after bubo rupture.

The diagnosis of chancroid can be challenging, since culturing *H. ducreyi* requires special culture medium and assay sensitivity is <75%. Multiplex PCR has been developed to test specimens for *H. ducreyi*, syphilis, and HSV, but it is primarily available for surveillance and research purposes. Gram-stain sensitivity ranges from 10 to 90% and shows small, pleomorphic, Gram-negative rods. Serology is not helpful in most cases, because it is unable to distinguish past from present infection and is usually not available.

Treatment and Prevention

Several studies in the last decade have documented the efficacy of single-dose treatment of chancroid with ceftriaxone or azithromycin and with 3-day regimens of ciprofloxacin or other fluoroquinolones. The 2010 Centers for Disease Control and Prevention recommendations are shown in **Table 44.4**. Resistance has been documented against penicillin, ampicillin, and tetracycline; all regimens have somewhat reduced efficacy in HIV-infected persons. Fluctuant lymph nodes should be aspirated as often as necessary to prevent spontaneous rupture, and an examination should be carried out 7 days after starting treatment. If there is no obvious improvement, it is important to consider other diagnoses. Testing for syphilis and HIV-1 at time of ulcer and 3 months later is recommended in all cases. Condom use and good personal hygiene, including washing with soap and water after sexual exposure, have been shown to reduce transmission of chancroid. However, condoms do not cover all areas that may be affected by chancroid and may not ensure complete protection. Partners of persons with chancroid should be treated, regardless of whether they have symptoms, if there has been sexual contact within the 10 days preceding onset of symptoms.

LYMPHOGRANULOMA VENEREUM (LGV)

Epidemiology

LGV is a systemic, chronic, sexually transmitted infection that is endemic in parts of Africa, Southeast Asia, South America, and the Caribbean. It disproportionately affects individuals in lower socioeconomic strata and those with multiple sexual partners. Although historically considered rare in North America, Europe, and Australia, several recent outbreaks of LGV proctitis have been described among MSM on these continents, specifically among populations with high HIV prevalence. Additionally, there is increasing evidence that LGV is often asymptomatic. As a result, it is frequently underdiagnosed in high-risk populations.

Pathogenesis

LGV is caused by *Chlamydia trachomatis* serovars L1, L2, L3, and recently discovered L2b, thought to be responsible for many of the recent outbreaks in Europe. Compared with the more prevalent oculogenital strains (Chapter 42), these serovars grow rapidly and are more cytolytic in cell culture. While both humoral and cellular immune responses occur, past infection does not confer immunity. Delayed hypersensitivity is considered to be responsible for the chronic, relapsing lymphadenopathy and lymphatic obstructions that are the hallmarks of untreated infection.

Clinical Manifestations and Diagnosis

LGV has both acute and chronic manifestations. One week to several months after the initial exposure, small blisters or papules appear on the mucous membranes and skin around the genital area. These may spread to involve the groin or anus and can develop into ulcerative lesions similar to those caused by chancroid, syphilis, or herpes. Although discomfort increases as the infection progresses, the sores are not usually painful and may go unnoticed. Primary infection may also include urethritis or cervicitis, similar to infection with other *C. trachomatis* serovars. Systemic spread results in regional lymphadenopathy that is usually erythematous, tender, and fluctuant and may be associated with fever and other systemic symptoms that evolve over 2-4 weeks. In MSM and women, this stage may also present as acute hemorrhagic proctocolitis, and symptoms may include fever, rectal pain, tenesmus, rectal discharge, and bleeding.

The majority of individuals recover spontaneously. However, some will develop chronic inflammation if not treated with antibiotics. Late complications include indurated, matted nodes with sinus tracts, nonhealing genital ulcers, abscesses, and rectal strictures. Rarely, squamous cell carcinoma or lymphatic obstruction occurs, with elephantiasis of the genitals or lower extremities. Although PCR of urine, bubo pus, or rectal discharge for chlamydia species can aid in the diagnosis, a positive test does not distinguish serovars L1, L2, L3, and L2b from other chlamydia strains. As such, a clinical diagnosis is often made after exclusion of other causes of inguinal adenopathy.

Treatment and Prevention

The recommended regimen for LGV is doxycycline 100 mg orally twice a day for 3 weeks. Alternate regimens include erythromycin 500 mg four times daily for 3 weeks or possibly azithromycin once weekly for 3 weeks, although clinical data in support of azithromycin are lacking. Ulcers should begin to clear within 1 week after initiating treatment and heal completely within 3-5 weeks. Partners with whom a patient has had sexual contact in the 30 days prior to onset of symptoms should be examined, tested for chlamydial urethritis and cervicitis, and treated appropriately.

GRANULOMA INGUINALE

Epidemiology

Granuloma inguinale, also known as donovanosis, is a rare STI that is most commonly diagnosed in the Indian subcontinent, Papua New Guinea, isolated areas of Australia, Southern Africa, Brazil, and parts of the Caribbean. Most cases in the United States are imported from such endemic areas, and a mean of only 11 cases was reported annually in the 1990s.

Pathogenesis

Klebsiella granulomatis, the cause of granuloma inguinale, is a small, pleomorphic, Gram-negative coccobacillus that typically appears intracellularly in macrophages ("Donovan bodies"). The histologic picture and course suggest that the clinical manifestations are due largely to a cell-mediated immune response.

Clinical Manifestations and Diagnosis

Granuloma inguinale presents with one or more indolent, mildly tender ulcerative lesions in the inguinal region. Lesions typically appear vascular with hypertrophic granulation-like tissue and may bleed on contact. Inguinal masses are due more frequently to subcutaneous extension of inflammatory tissue than to lymphadenopathy. Rarely, lesions spread with an appearance similar to that of squamous cell carcinoma and lead to penile autoamputation. Although systemic symptoms do not occur, disseminated osteolytic lesions have been described. Diagnosis is made by visualization of dark-staining Donovan bodies in biopsied tissue. *K. granulomatis* recently has been sustained in culture for the first time, which may lead to improved characterization of the organism.

Treatment and Prevention

A 3-week course of doxycyclne or trimethoprim-sulfamethoxazole is the recommended treatment for donovanosis. Alternative regimens include 3-week courses of ciprofloxacin, erythromycin, or azithromycin. Since relapse can occur months after therapy is completed, longer durations may be indicated in severe cases, and patients should be monitored for resolution of clinical symptoms. While the utility of treating sexual partners has not been established, it is recommended that individuals who have had sexual contact within 60 days prior to symptomatic disease be examined and offered treatment.

FURTHER READING

Ashley, R.L., Wald, A., 1999. Genital herpes: review of the epidemic and potential use of type-specific serology. Clin. Microbiol. Rev. 12, 1–8.

Bom, R.J., van der Helm, J.J., Schim van der Loeff, M.F., et al., 2013. Distinct transmission networks of *Chlamydia trachomatis* in men who have sex with men and heterosexual adults in Amsterdam, The Netherlands. PLoS ONE 8, e53869.

Centers for Disease Control and Prevention, 2010. Sexually transmitted diseases treatment guidelines, 2010. MMWR 59 (RR–12), 1–110.

Centers for Disease Control and Prevention, 2014. Sexually Transmitted Disease Surveillance 2013. U.S. Department of Health and Human Services, Atlanta, GA.

Corey, L., Wald, A., Celum, C.L., et al., 2004. The effects of herpes simplex virus-2 on HIV-1 acquisition and transmission: a review of two overlapping epidemics. J. Acquir. Immune Defic. Syndr. 35, 435–445.

Corey, L., Wald, A., Patel, R., et al., 2004. Once-daily valacyclovir to reduce the risk of transmission of genital herpes. N. Engl. J. Med. 350, 11–20.

De Vrieze, N.H., van Rooijen, M., Schim van der Loeff, M.F., et al., 2013. Anorectal and inguinal lymphogranuloma venereum among men who have sex with men in Amsterdam, The Netherlands. Trends over time, symptomatology and concurrent infections. Sex. Transmit. Infect. 89, 548–552.

Gupta, R., Warren, T., Wald, A., 2007. Genital herpes. Lancet 370 (9605), 2127–2137.

Holmes, K.K. (Ed.), 2007. Sexually Transmitted Diseases, fourth ed. McGraw Hill, New York.

Lewis, D.A., 2003. Chancroid: clinical manifestations, diagnosis, and management. Sex. Transmit. Infect. 79, 68–71.

Looker, K.J., Margaret, A.S., Turner, K.M.E., et al., 2015. Global estimates of prevalence and incidence of herpes simplex virus type 2 infections in 2012. PLoS ONE 10 (1), e114989.

O'Farrell, N., 2002. Donovanosis. Sex. Transmit. Infect. 78, 452–457.

Steen, R., 2001. Eradicating chancroid. Bull. World Health Organ. 79, 818–826.

Wald, A., Langenberg, A.G., Krantz, E., et al., 2005. The relationship between condom use and herpes simplex virus acquisition. Ann. Intern. Med. 143, 707–713.

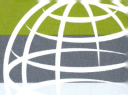

CHAPTER 45

Common Intestinal Roundworms

Paul S. Pottinger and Elaine C. Jong

The worms crawl in,
The worms crawl out,
The worms play pinochle on your snout.
Anonymous (children's song)

GENERAL CONSIDERATIONS

Medically important worms belonging to the phylum Nematoda (roundworms) parasitize the gastrointestinal tract of humans. It is estimated that 60% of the world population is infected with at least one intestinal helminth. The worms are commonly acquired through ingestion of contaminated food (especially raw or undercooked vegetables), through skin contact with contaminated soil, or, in some instances, from direct contact with infected persons or their fomites.

Individuals most likely to be infected with intestinal nematodes will frequently give a history of one of the following: (1) travel or residence in the developing world, (2) emigration from the developing world, (3) residence in a rural farming community, (4) ingestion of organically grown vegetables, (5) the use of untreated wastewater for agriculture, or (6) pica. In low-resource tropical countries, environmental sanitation may be substandard or absent. However, unsanitary conditions may be found in isolated rural areas and in farming communities in high-resource countries as well.

Fresh vegetables can serve as a major source of food-borne parasitic disease. A study performed by Duedu et al. (2014) in Ghana showed that vegetables (cabbage, sweet bell pepper, carrot, lettuce, tomato, and onion) sold at open-aired markets in Accra were more heavily contaminated than those sold at supermarkets. Lettuce (61%) and cabbage were the most contaminated, and the least was tomato (18%). The most prevalent parasites were *Strongyloides stercoralis* larvae (43%) and *Cryptosporidium parvum* oocysts (16%). Helminth eggs detected included those of hookworm nematodes (*Ancylostoma duodenale, Necator americanus*), *Trichuris trichiura, Enterobius vermicularis*, and the trematode *Fasciolopsis buski*. Other pathogens contaminating the vegetables included *Entamoeba histolytica, Giardia lamblia, Cyclospora cayetanensis, Entamoeba coli*, and *Isospora belli*.

In rural El Salvador, the use of solar urine-diverting desiccating latrines was found to be associated with a lower risk of intestinal helminths relative to use of pit latrines, or the absence of any type of latrine, presumably because the solid waste dries out more quickly in such a system, and eggs require a certain amount of time in moist soil to embryonate. In Mexico, intestinal helminth prevalence rises in children from low-income families and unemployed or less educated mothers. In Alexandria, Egypt, the risk of vegetable-transmitted parasites including *Ascaris lumbricoides* was found to be reduced by soaking leafy vegetables in water with an added substance such as vinegar, lemon juice, or salt; however, only 9.6% of households did this.

In general, the prevalence of intestinal parasites is higher in rural regions. For example, in a study of Bangladeshi men seeking work abroad, geohelminth infection rates were found to be 5.2% in those from urban areas and 27.6% in those residing in rural areas. However, in a study performed in India that looked at intestinal parasite rates in slum, rural, and urban populations, the highest prevalence (19%) was found in those residing in slums. Thus, insufficient access to sanitation of solid human waste is a key factor in transmission of these pathogens.

Pica, or geophagy, is not rare: in one study in Kenya, 77% of children ate soil daily, presumably triggered by iron-deficiency anemia. Intestinal roundworms transmitted by contact with contaminated soil are known collectively as "geohelminths" or "soil-transmitted helminths" (STHs).

ETIOLOGY

Species of geohelminths causing infections in humans include *A. lumbricoides* ("common roundworm"), *Ascaris suum* ("pig roundworm"), *Ancylostoma duodenale* and *Necator americanus* ("human hookworms"), *T. trichiura* ("whipworm"), *S. stercoralis*, and *E. vermicularis* ("threadworm" or "pinworm"). Human intestinal infection with the marine roundworm *Anisakis* will also be considered in this chapter.

CLINICAL FEATURES

1. Patients with intestinal nematodes will frequently be asymptomatic.
2. Returned travelers should be reassured that, with the exception of *Strongyloides*, these parasites cannot complete their life cycle within the human host, and even without treatment they will die of old age, often within a year of infection.
3. Vague abdominal complaints are sometimes the only symptoms reported with light to moderate infections.
4. Chronic, heavy infections are associated with growth stunting in children.
5. Occasionally, asymptomatic patients will pass a recognizable worm, and this will be the first sign that they have acquired an intestinal parasite.
6. At other times, the diagnosis is suspected or made on finding eosinophilia on a routine white blood cell differential analysis or on finding ova or parasites in a stool examination done for screening purposes.

In general, the severity of signs and symptoms will be related to the intensity of the infection (worm burden). Young children, possibly because of unsanitary habits (a tendency to put dirty fingers and objects into their mouths, play outdoors without shoes, etc.) and possibly because of immature host defense mechanisms, tend to acquire heavier parasite loads than adults living in the same area.

These infections are remarkably prevalent. Ascariasis is commonly associated with diarrhea in the developing world. In a study performed in rural south Mozambique, *A. lumbricoides* was the second most common pathogen isolated from stool, following diarrheogenic *E. coli* (9.3% and 22.6%, respectively). Almost one billion people are infected with hookworm. The hallmark of human hookworm infection is iron-deficiency anemia. For salient features of infection with intestinal nematodes, see **Table 45.1**.

PREVENTION

General food safety practices should dramatically reduce the incidence of ascariasis and trichuriasis, which are spread via contaminated foods (see Chapter 8). Wearing shoes should also afford some protection against hookworm infection and strongyloidiasis, which are spread via skin contact with infested soil. There now exists a vaccine for canine hookworm; an antihookworm human vaccine is under clinical investigation.

DIAGNOSIS

Hematology

The absolute eosinophil count is usually normal when infection is established with *Ascaris*, *Trichuris*, hookworms, and *Enterobius*, because the adult worms live in the intestines and reveal few antigens to the gut-associated lymphatic tissue. Thus normal eosinophil counts do not rule out geohelminth infection. On the other hand, eosinophilia (>450/mm^3) may

TABLE 45.1 Intestinal Nematode Infections

Infection	Agent	Geographic Distribution	Mode of Infection	Clinical Features	Diagnosis	Indication for Treatment
Common roundworm Pig roundworm	Ascaris lumbricoides Ascaris suum	Worldwide	Raw fruits and vegetables, or contact with contaminated soil	Pneumonitis, colicky epigastric pain, nausea and vomiting, passage of a mature pencil-sized worm[a]	Ova in stool or identification of mature worm	A single retained worm, multiple worms, obstruction of a viscus, or presence of other parasites requiring treatment
Hookworm (Old World) Hookworm (New World)	Ancylostoma duodenale Necator americanus	Worldwide	Percutaneous or perioral infections from contaminated soil or vegetation	"Ground itch" (rash), pneumonitis, abdominal pain, diarrhea, anemia (with large worm burdens and iron-deficient diet)[b]	Ova in stool	Heavy infection (>2000 eggs/g of stool) Anemia Malnutrition
Strongyloides	Strongyloides stercoralis	Worldwide	Skin contact with wet, infected soil	Rash on buttocks or thighs, abdominal pain, nausea and vomiting, weight loss, eosinophilia, recurrent bacterial systemic infections with gastrointestinal flora in immunocompromised patients	Rhabditiform larvae in stool or jejunal aspirate Serology available	Documented infection
Whipworm	Trichuris trichiura	Worldwide	Raw fruits and vegetables, soil contact, flies on food	Mild anemia, bloody diarrhea, rectal prolapse in heavy infections	Ova in stool	Symptoms associated with heavy infection (>3000 eggs/g of stool) Not necessary to treat patients with low egg counts
Pinworm	Enterobius vermicularis	Worldwide	Anus–finger–mouth cycle, or from clothing, bedding, dust	Perianal itching, irritation, restlessness, sleeplessness	Ova from perianal skin seen on cellophane tape swab	Symptomatic disease, psychosocial reasons

[a]Rare: bile duct obstruction, acute pancreatitis, appendicitis.
[b]A. duodenale causes a more severe anemia than does N. americanus.

happen during lung migration in early infection due to *Ascaris* or hookworms or at any time during chronic autoinfection due to *Strongyloides*.

Microbiology

Examination for ova and parasites of up to three different stool specimens collected on three different days at 2- to 3-day intervals should be sufficient for diagnosis. It is not uncommon for stool examinations to be negative for diagnostic forms of *Strongyloides* or *Enterobius* (pinworm).

An epidemiologic study of geohelminth prevalence in Zanzibar, Tanzania, found that when used alone, Wisconsin flotation and simple gravity sedimentation yielded sensitivities for detecting geohelminth eggs of approximately 90%. When two methods were used in combination, either Kato-Katz plus simple gravity sedimentation or Wisconsin flotation plus simple gravity sedimentation, sensitivity improved to 99.0%. Thus, if clinical suspicion remains high in spite of negative fecal ova and parasite preparations, request that the laboratory perform two techniques.

Serology

Because *Strongyloides* autoinfection exposes the immune system to worm significant antigen load, serology may be helpful for diagnosing this condition. Both immunofluorescence assay and enzyme-linked immunosorbent assay (ELISA) serologic tests for *Strongyloides* (available through commercial laboratories or arranged through state health departments and performed by the Parasite Serology Laboratory at the Centers for Disease Control and Prevention, Atlanta, GA) can be helpful in making the diagnosis in a patient with an appropriate geographic history, peripheral blood eosinophilia, and negative stool examinations for ova and parasites. ELISA sensitivity and specificity are improved if used in conjunction with Western blot. All serologic diagnostic tests for *Strongyloides* are limited by the patient's ability to mount an immune response to the worm, and complicated by cross-reactivity with filarial antigens, meaning neither the positive nor the negative predictive value is perfect.

The String Test

The "Entero-Test" method for sampling proximal jejunal secretions may be a useful diagnostic procedure for *Strongyloides* diagnosis (see Chapter 32, under Giardia, Diagnosis).

Adhesive Tape Test

The diagnosis of *Enterobius* is best made from microscopic examination of adhesive tape pressed adhesive side down on the perianal skin (preferably in the morning on a patient who has been instructed not to bathe before the examination), and then directly mounted, adhesive side down, on a glass microscope slide. The distinctive dome-shaped eggs are rarely found in the stool.

Baermann Funnel Gauze Method

Strongyloides larvae do not float in hypertonic saline, which is used to concentrate other parasites. The Baermann method utilizes gauze, warm water, and larval sedimentation in the neck of a funnel.

TREATMENT

For treatment of common intestinal nematodes in patients without severe underlying health problems, see **Table 45.2**.

If *Ascaris* is present, this parasite generally should be treated during the first round of antiparasitic therapy, even if other drugs will be used subsequently to treat other parasites that are present. The reason for this is the propensity for mature *Ascaris* worms to migrate into unpredictable ectopic sites when they are irritated but not killed by drugs, fever, or even starvation in the host. Migrating worms may cause perforation of an abdominal viscus, appendicitis, biliary obstruction, pancreatitis, or intestinal obstruction. Antiparasitic therapy directed at *Ascaris* may be administered concurrently with antibiotics for other infections.

TABLE 45.2 Antihelminthic Drugs

Helminth	Primary Treatment (Adults)	Alternate Treatment (Adults)
Ascaris lumbricoides	Albendazole[a] 400 mg PO once; *or* mebendazole 100 mg bid PO × 3 days	Ivermectin[a] 150-200 mcg/kg PO once
Hookworm (*Ancylostoma duodenale* and *Necator americanus*)	Albendazole[a] 400 mg PO once; *or* mebendazole 100 mg bid PO × 3 days	Pyrantel pamoate[a] × 11 mg/kg base (max. 1 gram) PO daily × 3 days
Trichuris trichiura	Albendazole[a] 400 mg PO × 3 days	Mebendazole 100 mg b.i.d PO × 3 days; *or* ivermectin[a] 200 mcg/kg/day PO × 3 days
Strongyloides stercoralis	Ivermectin 200 mcg/kg/day PO × 2 days	Albendazole[a] 400 mg b.i.d. PO × 7 days
Enterobius vermicularis	Albendazole[a] 400 mg PO once, repeat dose in 2 weeks; *or* mebendazole 100 mg PO once, repeat dose in 2 weeks	Pyrantel pamoate 11 mg/kg base (max 1 g) once, repeat dose in 2 weeks
Anisakis simplex	Physical removal	Albendazole[a] 400 mg b.i.d. PO × 6-21 days.

[a]Not FDA-approved for this indication.
b.i.d., Twice per day; *PO*, by mouth.

Special Therapeutic Considerations

Intestinal Obstruction Due to Ascaris

A gastrointestinal tube should be placed, retained fluids aspirated, and an appropriate dose of piperazine citrate instilled (Antepar 75 mg/kg per day, not to exceed 3.5 g). The piperazine will paralyze the worms, allowing them to be passed out by the intestinal peristalsis of the host. If relief of the obstruction is not obtained within 1-2 days, a surgical procedure may be necessary, as in the other complications caused by migratory *Ascaris* worms. Approximately 20,000 people die from *Ascaris* infection each year, but given that one-quarter of the world, or 1.5 billion people are infected, the case-fatality rate is only 0.000013.

Surgery

If a person with an *Ascaris* infection needs anesthesia prior to treatment, the anesthesiologist should be informed because of the remote possibility that the anesthetic agent could cause ectopic worm migration into the trachea, causing respiratory obstruction.

Pregnant and Lactating Women

There are very few controlled data on the use of antiparasitic drugs in pregnancy and lactation. Both mebendazole and albendazole have been shown to have teratogenic potential in animal models. It would be prudent to withhold therapy during the first trimester and to delay therapy as long as possible, ideally until after delivery. There is no evidence for transplacental transmission of roundworm infections in humans. If antiparasitic therapy is inadvertently given during the first trimester of pregnancy, the patient should be advised that there is no consensus on the possible effects of therapy on fetal outcome. These medications have been administered countless times in mass drug administration settings overseas without confirmed harm. Thus, adverse fetal outcome directly related to antiparasitic drugs given during pregnancy is thought to be a very rare but possible occurrence.

If therapy of a lactating woman is contemplated, asking the patient to use mechanical means for milk expression during, and for 48 hours following, antiparasitic therapy would be prudent. In addition to teratogenic considerations, side effects including nausea, vomiting, malaise, and rare cases of Stevens–Johnson syndrome have been associated with the use of some of the drugs mentioned in this section.

Infants

There are very few controlled data on the use of antiparasitic drugs in infants <2 years of age. In a severely ill infant, in whom the presence of parasites is thought to contribute to the disease process (intestinal obstruction due to ascarids, severe anemia due to hookworm, etc.), the possible risks of antiparasitic therapy must be weighed against the effects of the untreated infection, and the dosage of the appropriate drug adjusted for weight.

Altered Immune States

Disseminated strongyloidiasis ("strongyloides hyperinfection syndrome"), a potentially untreatable and fatal development, has been reported in patients with chronic underlying illnesses (diabetes, alcoholism, and human T-lymphotropic virus type 1 infection), in patients being treated with immunosuppressive drugs (corticosteroids, transplant immunosuppressants, cancer chemotherapeutic agents) or radiation therapy, and in patients with malignancy, particularly lymphoma and leukemia. The tiny strongyloides worms can disseminate to all the major internal organs, including the liver, lungs, heart, and central nervous system. Along with consideration of *Pneumocystis* and *Toxoplasma* infections, disseminated *Strongyloides* infection should be considered, especially in the case of immunocompromised patients who develop bilateral pulmonary infiltrates, sepsis, or polymicrobial bacteremia with gastrointestinal bacteria.

It is important to consider the diagnosis in asymptomatic patients from high-risk geographic areas and to immediately treat those who have positive stool examinations or unexplained hypereosinophilia and positive *Strongyloides* serologies. Serology is not entirely reliable; thus, regardless of results, high-risk patients should be treated empirically for *Strongyloides* with ivermectin before corticosteroid therapy, cancer chemotherapy, or radiation therapy is instituted. Frustratingly, many patients with *Strongyloides* hyperinfection do not have peripheral eosinophilia, and results of serology may take days to return; examination of sputum or bronchial lavage fluid may reveal larvae much more quickly. If parasite dissemination in a compromised host is believed to have occurred (usually diagnosed on the basis of tissue biopsy or sputum specimens), treatment with the appropriate dosage of ivermectin may be extended to ≥5 days. Subcutaneous ivermectin has been used for hyperinfection, although the evidence for this practice is poor and there is no form of this drug approved by the US Food and Drug Administration.

Another phenomenon described in immunocompromised patients and associated with disseminated *Strongyloides* infections is recurrent polymicrobial bacteremia with enteric bacteria. The bacteria are thought to stick to the cuticle of worm and to gain access to the circulation when *Strongyloides* larvae migrate out of the gut.

Chronic Strongyloides Infections

Infections persisting for >30 years are possible because of an autoinfective cycle, in which eggs laid by mature worms in the proximal small intestine hatch in transit with the fecal stream. The resulting rhabditiform larvae undergo maturational changes, becoming infective filariform larvae by the time they reach the rectum. These are capable of exiting from the anus and perforating the skin in the perianal area, buttocks, and upper thighs, thus initiating a new cycle of infection. Local rashes (larva currens) and perianal itching may be the presenting complaints. Among former Allied prisoners of war who worked on the Burma–Thailand railroad during the Second World War, rates of infection were found 30-40 years later to be 21-37%. Two-thirds of these former POWs had episodic, recurring symptoms. Diagnosis and treatment are the same as for more acute infections with *Strongyloides*.

Pinworm

Pinworm is probably the most common worm infection in the United States, occurring mainly in school-aged children (via anus–finger–mouth transmission) and their families (via

TABLE 45.3 Prevalence of Intestinal Nematodes in Rural Regions (%)

	Ascaris lumbricoides	*Trichuris trichiura*	Hookworm
China	63	60	87
Vietnam	83	94	59
Ethiopia	29-38	13	7-24
Madagascar	93	55	27
Mali			53 (*Necator americanus*)
Brazil	41	40	
Paraguay			59
Venezuela	27	33	6

Note: Additionally, studies on Pemba Island, Tanzania, and Barru district, Sulawesi, Indonesia, showed that 58% and 17.4%, respectively, of inhabitants were infected with all three of the above parasites.

household environmental transmission through dust and fomites). Pinworm infections have been linked to increased risk of urinary tract infection in young girls. Rarely, pinworm infection may cause appendicitis or peritonitis. In addition to antiparasitic therapy (**Table 45.3**), keeping fingernails trim and scrubbed, stopping thumb-sucking, thorough house cleaning, and washing of underclothes and bedclothes in hot soapy water will contribute to breaking the transmission cycle.

Other Roundworms

A. suum, the roundworm of pigs, is infective for humans and is grossly indistinguishable from the roundworm of humans, *A. lumbricoides*. Environmental contamination with pig excrement may account for acquisition of the common roundworm in patients who report no significant travel history. Anisakiasis (caused by marine roundworm) will be covered separately below.

Other Hookworm Species

Hookworm species other than *A. duodenale* and *N. americanus* (most commonly *Ancylostoma braziliense* and *Ancylostoma caninum*) can infest human skin but cannot penetrate deeper to continue their life cycle in humans. This aggravating condition, a leading dermatosis transmitted in the developing world, is called cutaneous larva migrans. It is discussed in Chapter 37.

Mass Drug Administration

In situations where solving sanitation problems is not feasible, scheduled treatment of whole populations may be appropriate. A study in a highly endemic area in Bangladesh found that mass chemotherapy with albendazole at 18-month intervals was superior to two regimens that involved health education. However, the cost/benefit analysis of targeted community mass drug programs is still an active topic of analysis and discussion. There are numerous published studies trying to assess the association of mass drug administration programs with markers of pediatric growth and development: stunting, cognitive performance, and micronutrient deficiencies (e.g., iron deficiency, vitamin A deficiency). Multivariate analysis of published studies suggests that future studies need to be done with an attempt to standardize age groups studied, measure pre-intervention parameters, ascertain the intensity of STH infection and efficacy of the antihelminthic drug(s) used, and standardize environmental factors (e.g., diet, tap water, latrines, maternal education) so valid comparisons and conclusions may be made.

ANISAKIASIS

Anisakiasis is a gastrointestinal illness occurring when humans are infected with larval forms of marine ascarids, or roundworms belonging to the family Anisakidae, most commonly

Anisakis simplex and *Pseudoterranova decipiens*. The larvae are present in the flesh of many market fish, including salmon, chum, mackerel, cod, pollock, herring, whiting, bonito, sole, pike, and squid. Man becomes infected by eating raw, pickled, or lightly salted fish. The larvae (third stage) are present in the muscles and visceral organs of the fish and can survive 51 days in vinegar, 50 days at 2°C, 6 days in 10% formalin at room temperature, and about 2 hours at −20°C. The larvae are killed in seconds at 60°C. The larvae are 18-36 mm in length and 0.24-0.69 mm in width.

Epidemiology

The disease was first recognized in the 1950s in Holland among people eating raw (green) or lightly pickled herring and was called "green-herring" disease. Thousands of cases have been reported from Japan, where raw or pickled marine fish dishes are consumed (e.g., sushi, sashimi, sunomono, and vinegared salads). Fewer cases have been reported from the United States and other countries. Gastric anisakiasis is the most common presentation in Japan, whereas in Europe and elsewhere, intestinal anisakiasis is the most common form.

The parasite's definitive hosts are marine mammals: *Anisakis* spp. infect Cetacea (whales, dolphins) and *Pseudoterranova* infects Pinnipedia (seals, sea lions, walruses). The adult parasites living in the stomach of these animals lay eggs, which exit in the feces and hatch in seawater. The larvae are eaten by squid, crustaceans, and other macro-invertebrates, which in turn are eaten by fish. Marine mammals then eat the fish, completing the life cycle. If man eats the fish or squid, the larvae cannot reach sexual maturity, and they never lay eggs.

Clinical Presentation

1. *Gastric anisakiasis* is an acute illness occurring 1-12 hours after the ingestion of raw seafood, with the sudden onset of severe stomach pain, nausea, and vomiting. In >50% of cases, there is a peripheral blood eosinophilia of up to 40% without a marked leukocytosis; in 70% of cases, occult blood is found in gastric juices and stools. Anaphylactoid reactions are common; arthralgia and arthritis occur rarely. Untreated infections usually become chronic, with similar manifestations lasting for >1 year. Penetrating lesions, abscess formation, or granulation may occur at the site of larval attachment to the stomach.
2. *Intestinal anisakiasis* is a more chronic disease. Severe pain in the lower abdomen, nausea, vomiting, fever, diarrhea, and occult blood in the stools begin about 1-5 days after ingestion of raw seafood. Marked leukocytosis with no or mild eosinophilia may be present. Over months, occasionally for years, infiltrative and mass lesions of the intestinal tract occur, with continued cramping, abdominal pain, diarrhea, and dysmotility. Perforation of the intestine, abscess formation, and granulation may occur at the site of the infection.

Diagnosis

The history of eating raw fish is the most important historic finding. While immunologic methods of detecting specific antibodies against *Anisakis* (cutaneous skin prick with *A. simplex* extract, and ELISA) may support the diagnosis of anisakiasis, usually the diagnosis is made by upper endoscopy. The histology of lesions in specimens from biopsy or resection is characterized by an eosinophilic granulomatous inflammation; the finding of characteristic larvae in cross section within the tissue confirms the diagnosis.

The gastric form is often misdiagnosed as ulcer, cancer, tumor, polyp, or food poisoning, while the intestinal form has been misdiagnosed as regional enteritis or appendicitis.

Treatment

Antiparasitic drugs appear to be ineffective. If the larva is seen during gastroscopy, it can be removed during the procedure. In chronic disease, surgical resection of the affected part may be necessary.

Prevention

Reinfections with additional larvae can occur in acute or chronic *Anisakis* infections. The best prevention is to avoid raw, undercooked, or lightly pickled marine fish and squid. If raw fish is eaten, it should be frozen at −20°C for at least 24 hours; otherwise, it should be thoroughly cooked to a temperature of 60°C.

FURTHER READING

Behnke, J.M., De Clercq, D., Behnke, J.M., et al., 2000. The epidemiology of human hookworm infections in the southern region of Mali. Trop. Med. Int. Health 5, 343–354.

Booth, M., Bundy, D.A., Albonico, M., et al., 1998. Associations among multiple geohelminth species infections in schoolchildren from Pemba Island. Parasitology 116, 85–93.

Changhua, L., Xiaorong, Z., Dongchuan, Q., et al., 1999. Epidemiology of human hookworm infections among adult villagers in Hejiang and Santai Counties, Sichuan Province, China. Acta Trop. 73, 243–249.

Corrales, L.F., Izurieta, R., Moe, C.L., 2006. Association between intestinal parasitic infections and type of sanitation system in rural El Salvador. Trop. Med. Int. Health 11, 1821–1831.
Community sanitation methods can affect the prevalence of geohelminths.

Duedu, K.O., Yarnie, E.A., Tetteh-Quarcoo, P.B., et al., 2014. A comparative survey of the prevalence of human parasites found in fresh vegetables sold in supermarkets and open-aired markets in Accra, Ghana. BMC Research Notes 7, 836. Available at <http://www.biomedcentral.com/756-0500/7/836>.
Fresh vegetables sold in the open-aired markets in Accra were contaminated with multiple infective parasite forms and were more contaminated than vegetables sold in supermarkets.

Fawzi, M., El-Sahn, A.A., Ibrahim, H.F., et al., 2004. Vegetable-transmitted parasites among inhabitants of El-Prince, Alexandria and its relation to housewives' knowledge and practices. J. Egypt. Public Health Assoc. 79, 13–29.
A minority of housewives in Alexandria employed methods to wash vegetables that would decrease parasite contamination.

Geisslet, P.W., Mwaniki, D., Thiong'o, F., et al., 1998. Geophagy as a risk factor for geohelminth infections: a longitudinal study of Kenyan primary schoolchildren. Trans. R. Soc. Trop. Med. Hyg. 92, 7–11.
Among the Kenyan children studied, 77% of them ingested soil daily.

Jemaneh, L., 1998. Comparative prevalences of some common intestinal helminth infections in different altitudinal regions in Ethiopia. Ethiop. Med. J. 36, 1–8.

Khatun, M., Naher, A., 2006. Prevalence of soil transmitted helminth infections among Bangladeshi males seeking jobs abroad. Mymensingh Med. J. 15, 159–162.
In this population, residents from rural agricultural areas had a greater prevalence of intestinal parasites compared with urban dwellers.

Khurana, S., Aggarwal, A., Malla, N., 2005. Comparative analysis of intestinal parasitic infections in slum, rural and urban populations in and around union Territory, Chandigarh. J. Commun. Dis. 37, 239–243.
In this study, inhabitants of slums had the highest rate of intestinal parasitic infections, illustrating that crowding with unsanitary conditions and lack of access to sanitary disposal of feces serve as significant risk factors in parasite transmission.

Kightliner, L.K., Seed, J.R., Kightlinger, M.B., 1998. *Ascaris lumbricoides* intensity in relation to environmental, socioeconomic, and behavioral determinants of exposure to infection in children from southeast Madagascar. J. Parasitol. 84, 480–484.

Labiano Abello, N., Canese, J., Velazquez, M.E., et al., 1999. Epidemiology of hookworm infection in Itagua, Paraguay: a cross sectional study. Mem. Inst. Oswaldo Cruz 94, 583–586.

Morales, G., Pino, L.A., Artega, C., et al., 1998. Relationships in the prevalence of geohelminth infections in humans from Venezuela. Bol. Child. Parasitol. 53, 84–87.

Needham, C., Kim, H.T., Hoa, N.V., et al., 1998. Epidemiology of soil transmitted nematode infections in Ha Nam Province, Vietnam. Trop. Med. Int. Health 3, 904–912.

Pelletier, L.L., Jr., 1984. Chronic strongyloidiasis in World War II Far East ex-prisoners of war. Am. J. Trop. Med. Hyg. 33, 55–61.
Fascinating report on strongyloidiasis persisting for decades in veterans after exposure in an endemic area.

Pham-Duc, P., Nguyen-Viet, H., Hattendorf, J., et al., 2013. *Ascaris lumbricoides* and *Trichuris trichiura* infections associated with wastewater and human excreta use in agriculture in Vietnam. Parasitol. Int. 62, 172–180.
Contact with polluted river water and the use of human excreta as a fertilizer were associated with increased risk of helminth infections. Access to tap water in households was associated with a significant decrease in infection with both A. lumbricoides *and* T. trichiura.

Pinkus, G.S., Coolidge, C., Little, M.D., 1975. Intestinal anisakiasis. First case report from North America. Am. J. Med. 59, 114–120.
Provides a brief history of the recognition of human disease due to anisakiasis; eating raw or undercooked salmon was the risk factor in North America.

Quihui, L., Valencia, M.E., Crompton, D.W., et al., 2006. Role of the employment status and education of mothers in the prevalence of intestinal parasitic infections in Mexican rural schoolchildren. BMC Public Health 6, 225.
Children of employed and educated mothers had fewer intestinal parasites in rural Mexico.

Salam, R.A., Haider, B.A., Humayun, Q., 2015. Effect of administration of antihelminthics for soil-transmitted helminths during pregnancy. Cochrane Database Syst. Rev. (6), CD005547, doi: 10.1002/14651858.XD5547.pub3.
Multivariate analysis showing there is not enough evidence at the time of the study to demonstrate benefit resulting from the administration of anthelmintic drugs during pregnancy.

Saldiva, S.R., Silveira, S.A., Philippi, S.1., et al., 1999. *Ascaris–Trichuris* association and malnutrition in Brazilian children. Paediatr. Perinat. Epidemiol. 13, 89–98.

Suchdev, P.S., Davis, S.M., Bartoces, M., et al., 2014. Soil-transmitted helminth infection and nutritional status among urban slum children in Kenya. Am. J. Trop. Med. Hyg. 90, 299–305.
A cross-sectional survey of pre-school and school-aged children, of whom approximately 40% were infected with soil-transmitted helminths (STH), primarily Ascaris *and* Trichuris. *Multivariate analysis showed no significant association between STH and anemia and stunting in both study groups but did show a significant association between STH and iron-deficiency anemia and vitamin A deficiency in the pre-school children. This suggests that community treatment programs against STH and provision of micronutrient supplementation might be more advantageous in the pre-school population.*

Taylor-Robinson, D.C., Maayan, N., Soares-Weiser, K., et al., 2015. Deworming drugs for soil-transmitted intestinal worms in children: effects on nutritional indicators, haemoglobin, and school performance. Cochrane Database Syst. Rev. (7), CD000371.
Challenges the common belief that administration of deworming drugs is solely responsible for significant improvements in nutritional indicators, haemoglobin, and school performance. Observed benefits among children studied in mass drug administration programs against soil-transmitted helminths are multifactorial and may involve nutrient supplementation, maternal education, improved sanitation practices, and addressing concurrent infectious diseases in the community (e.g., diarrheal diseases and vaccine-preventable diseases), as well as antihelminthic drugs.

Toma, A., Miyagi, I., Kamimura, K., et al., 1999. Questionnaire survey and prevalence of intestinal helminthic infections in Barru, Sulawesi, Indonesia. Southeast Asian J. Trop. Med. Public Health 30, 68–77.

CHAPTER 46

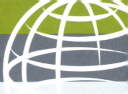

Cestodes: Intestinal and Extraintestinal Tapeworm Infections, Including Echinococcosis and Cysticercosis

Douglas W. MacPherson

Man is the only animal which esteems itself rich in proportion to the number and voracity of its parasites.
George Bernard Shaw (1856-1950)

Infections by cestodes (tapeworms, or flat, segmented worms) in the United States, Canada, and other affluent countries are rare but do occur in specific at-risk populations related to geographic, behavioral, or migration risk characteristics. Clinical suspicion is needed to detect quiescent infections or asymptomatic disease.

Some of the tapeworms affecting humans are endemic in the United States, Canada, and other developed nations. Practically, these can be divided clinically into tapeworm infections that are purely intestinal-dwelling (*Taenia saginata*, beef tapeworm; *Taenia solium*, pork tapeworm; and *Diphyllobothrium latum*, fish tapeworm), purely tissue invasive (echinococcosis), or with both phases (pork tapeworm and cysticercosis). All other human tapeworm infections are usually not clinically significant but reflect poor socioeconomic or immigration status. Rarely, transmission of tapeworm infections introduced by means of infected food handlers under unhygienic circumstances (a public health issue) has been reported. **Table 46.1** shows the common tapeworm infections affecting humans, their usual distribution, and clinical significance.

Humans acquire infective tapeworm larvae or eggs through ingestion of contaminated soil or infected food or by accidentally swallowing the intermediate vectors such as the flea or beetle. *Echinococcus* spp. are tapeworms of carnivorous mammals, usually dogs, that serve as the definitive hosts for the parasite. The extraintestinal larval stages of *Echinococcus* spp. cause cystic mass lesions, most often in the liver of sheep, deer, or moose, but can affect virtually all other organs as well. Humans are an inadvertent and usually "dead-end" intermediate host.

EPIDEMIOLOGY AND DEMOGRAPHICS OF HUMAN TAPEWORM INFECTIONS IN DEVELOPED NATIONS

Intestinal Tapeworms

In the United States and other developed nations, tapeworm infections are uncommon in the general population and are found more frequently in defined migrant, ethnic, and certain cultural groups with specific risks, such as exposures in endemic regions of the world, dietary practices, food choices, and methods of food preparation. Occupational risk exposures include certain animal contacts, veterinary care, and animal control. Humans act as the definitive host for the beef, pork, and fish tapeworm, becoming infected through the

TABLE 46.1   Distribution and Usual Clinical Significance of Tapeworms Affecting Humans

Parasite	Distribution	Usual Clinical Significance
Taenia saginata (beef tapeworm)	*T. saginata* is common in cattle-breeding regions worldwide with humans being a definitive host and cattle the intermediate host. Areas with the highest (i.e., >10%) prevalence are Central Asia, the Near East, and Central and Eastern Africa. Areas with low (i.e., 1%) prevalence are Southeast Asia, Europe, and Central and South America. Pre-patent period: 3-5 months Life span: up to 25 years Length of worms: 4-8 m	Adult tapeworms live in the gastrointestinal tract of the human host. Eggs are excreted in the stools, and motile tapeworm segments can also be expelled from the bowels. The beef tapeworm does not cause invasive disease in humans, but in regions where distribution overlaps with pork tapeworm, must be distinguished from the latter, which does cause tissue infections in people. All ages, races, and genders are susceptible to infection that is acquired by eating larvae-infected undercooked beef meat.
Taenia solium (pork tapeworm)	*T. solium* is endemic in Central and South America, Southeast Asia, India, the Philippines, Africa, Eastern Europe, and China, with humans being a definitive host and pigs the intermediate host. Areas of highest prevalence include Latin America and Africa. In some regions of Mexico, prevalence of infection may reach 3.6% of the general population. Pre-patent period: 3-5 months Life span: up to 25 years Length of worms: 3-5 m	Adult tapeworms live in the gastrointestinal tract of the human host. Eggs are excreted in the stools, and motile tapeworm segments can also be expelled from the bowels. The pork tapeworm larvae causes invasive disease in humans affecting soft tissues and the brain (cysticercosis). All ages, races, and genders are susceptible to infection that is acquired by eating larvae-infected undercooked pork meat or by ingestion of pork tapeworm eggs.

Continued

TABLE 46.1 Distribution and Usual Clinical Significance of Tapeworms Affecting Humans—cont'd

Parasite	Distribution	Usual Clinical Significance
Diphyllobothrium latum (fish tapeworm)	In North America, *D. latum* infections have been previously reported in fish from the Great Lakes. There are six *Diphyllobothrium* species known to reside in Alaskan lakes and rivers, and some saltwater species may also be seen in North America. *Diphyllobothrium* infections are not species specific, and widespread reports describe infection in North American fish-eating birds and mammals. Humans are a definitive host, and crustaceans, followed by fish, are intermediate hosts. The incidence in the USA has been declining recently. Pike, perch, and salmon are among the fish most commonly infected. Reports are commonly made of *D. latum* infection in humans residing in Europe, Africa, and the Far East. Pre-patent period: 3-5 weeks Life span: up to 25 years Length of worms: 4-10 m	Adult tapeworms live in the gastrointestinal tract of the human host. Eggs are excreted in the stools, and motile tapeworm segments can also be expelled from the bowels. The fish tapeworm does not cause invasive disease but due to its length and potential to interfere with vitamin B12 absorption can cause a number of nonspecific symptoms. All ages, races, and genders are susceptible to infection that is acquired by eating undercooked, infected fish flesh. People preparing fresh fish, implements used to prepare fish (e.g., knives and cutting boards), and raw or undercooked fish meals (e.g., sushi, sashimi, ceviche) may be associated with a higher risk of infection.
Dipylidium caninum	*D. caninum* is a cosmopolitan tapeworm infection of dogs with inadvertent human infections occurring through ingestion of the intermediate host, a flea that has fed on the tapeworm eggs contaminating the animal's fur or dog feces. Human infections have been reported in Europe, the Philippines, China, Japan, Argentina, and North America. Pre-patent period: 3-4 weeks Life span: <1 year Length of worms: 10-70 cm	Adult tapeworms live in the gastrointestinal tract of the inadvertent human host, usually a child. Perianal irritation may occur with the passage of motile segments of the tapeworm; small "grain of rice-like" motile segments may be seen in the stools. The proglottids are motile when passed and may be mistaken for maggots or fly larvae.
Hymenolepis nana (dwarf tapeworm)	*H. nana* is a cosmopolitan intestinal tapeworm usually infecting rodents (mice or rats). The intermediate host, a beetle, is not required to complete its lifecycle in definitive hosts. Ingestion of tapeworm eggs by a definitive host, including humans, can reestablish an adult tapeworm infection. Pre-patent period: 2-3 weeks Life span: many years due to autoinfection Length of worms: 2.5-4 cm	Often associated with environments with poor sanitation, the dwarf tapeworm causes few clinical problems with nonspecific abdominal complaints, loosening of the stools, perianal irritation, and the possible presence of small motile segments visible in the stool or on undergarments.

Hymenolepis diminuta

The rat tapeworm requires a grain beetle as an intermediate host, so is most common in grain-producing areas of the world or where grain or other dry foods are stored. Human infections are uncommon.

Pre-patent period: 3 weeks

Life span: <1 year

Length of worms: 20-60 cm

Often associated with environments with poor sanitation, the rat tapeworm rarely infects humans and causes few clinical problems with nonspecific abdominal complaints, loosening of the stools, and perianal irritation and the possible presence of small motile segments visible in the stool or on undergarments.

Echinococcus granulosis and Echinococcus vogeli

E. granulosis is a tapeworm of canines (dogs) with other vertebrates, most commonly sheep, as the intermedia te host. Ingesting tapeworm eggs passed in the stools of infected dogs infects humans. Once common in all sheep-raising areas of the world (Asia, Europe, the Americas, Africa, and Ocea nia), animal husbandry practices are resulting in effective disease control in most affected areas.

The larval tapeworm infection in humans causes hydatid disease with large, complex cystic masses occurring most commonly in the liver, but any organ can be affected, presenting with mass effects. Cysts can rupture, causing allergic reactions and anaphylactic shock. Cysts can also present with secondary bacterial infection. Pulmonary cysts can spontaneously rupture and be expelled through the mouth. If intraperitoneal rupture of a primary cyst occurs, multiple secondary cysts can develop in the peritoneal cavity.

Echinococcus multilocularis

E. multilocularis is a tapeworm of canines, with foxes and wolves being particularly important definitive hosts with other vertebrates (small rodents such as voles, lemmings, and mice) as intermediate hosts. Humans become infected by ingesting tapeworm eggs passed in the stools of infected canines. This is a rare form of echinococcosis that occurs predominantly in Arctic regions of Europe and North America. It can be prevented by carefully washing strawberries, cranberries, blueberries and other foods that may be contaminated with canine feces.

The larval tapeworm infection in humans causes alveolar hydatid disease with large, complex externally budding cystic masses, occurring most commonly in the liver. Due to its rapid growth and budding characteristics, this form of echinococcosis behaves more like a malignancy displacing liver tissue than an indolent infection, such as cystic hydrosis.

ingestion of encysted larvae in the muscles of various animals. Humans can also be infected by ingesting tapeworm eggs of *T. solium* and *Echinococcus* spp., both leading to cystic tissue disease, or *Hymenolepis nana*, leading to development of an adult worm and patent infection.

In the typical lifecycle of tapeworm infection, ingesting the cyst-infected meat releases the larval forms in the gastrointestinal tract. The larvae attach to the mucosal lining of the small intestine by the head, or scolex. The tapeworm grows from each scolex, forming proglottids containing both male and female reproductive organs. Adult tapeworms (beef, pork, and fish) may reach lengths of 4.5-10 m. The proglottids may detach from each other, forming a short chain of segments (strobila) containing fertilized eggs. These segments and eggs are passed in the stool. If the scolex and neck of the tapeworm remain attached to the host gut mucosa, it can continue to produce proglottids for many years.

The beef tapeworm (*T. saginata*) infection is most common in people who eat raw or undercooked beef dishes. Recent immigrant groups from areas endemic to *T. saginata* in cattle-rearing Africa (i.e., Ethiopia), cattle and llama-rearing areas in Latin America, and reindeer-rearing areas in the Northern Hemisphere are at greatest risk.

The adult pork tapeworms and cystic forms of the infection (cysticercosis) are found among people exposed to undercooked pork or in contact with the excreted eggs of *T. solium*. This is most common in immigrants and refugees from endemic areas in the developing world.

Infection with the fish tapeworm, *D. latum* and other *Diphyllobothrium* species, occurs when eating raw, smoked, pickled, or undercooked fish. Those at risk are the Inuit, fishermen, Jewish home cooks (uncooked gefilte fish), and consumers of sushi and sashimi, ceviche, or caviar made from infected fresh water fish and roe. The highest risk fish are raw salmon and other anadromous fish (fish ascending rivers to spawn): American shad, blueback herring, short-nose sturgeon, striped bass, and steelhead trout. In Europe, these fish include pike, perch, and turbot.

H. nana and *Hymenolepis diminuta* are rodent tapeworms with rare human infections in developed nations. Human infections are through accidental ingestion of rodent feces containing the tapeworm egg (*H. nana*), or larvae-containing fleas and grain beetles (*H. nana* and *H. diminuta*). Young children in rodent-infested environments are at risk of *H. nana*. Person-to-person transmission of *H. nana* occurs through fecal-oral contamination.

Dipylidium caninum infection usually occurs in children living in households with exposures to a dog, where accidental ingestion of an infected flea can result in a human infection.

Tissue Tapeworms

In the United States, areas endemic to *Echinococcus granulosus* exist in sheep-raising areas of California, Utah, and in Alaska, where dogs, wolves, and other canines are frequently infected. Immigrants from the Mediterranean region, the Middle East, and South America are also at greater risk. Alveolar hydatid disease caused by *Echinococcus multilocularis* is endemic in Alaska and the Arctic regions, central North America involving some parts of Canada, the United States, central Europe, Siberia, and northern Japan.

Cysticercus cellulosae are the tissue lesions caused by larval dissemination of *T. solium*. This disease occurs in Mexico, Central and South America, Africa, India, China, Eastern Europe, and Indonesia. Cysticercosis infection of the central nervous system is a common cause of seizures among immigrants from Latin America to the United States.

People are usually infected with *T. solium* when the eggs passed in the stool are ingested in contaminated food or water. Person-to-person transmission in household settings has been documented in non-endemic areas. Autoinfection by refluxing *T. solium* eggs within the human gut may be a means of larval infection. The larvae are found in subcutaneous connective tissue. The second most common site is the eye, followed by the brain, muscle, heart, liver, and lungs. Cysts may cause irreparable damage to the eye.

Sparganosis has been reported from many countries of the world but is most common in eastern Asia and rarely elsewhere. It is almost impossible to identify spargana to the species level, making it unclear as to which species actually infect humans. Infection in humans is caused by swallowing the first intermediate infected copepod hosts in contaminated drinking water or eating raw or undercooked amphibians, reptiles, or mammals, which are second intermediate hosts in endemic areas. The spargana can migrate to virtually any part of the body and grow up to 6 cm in length. Asymptomatic soft tissue or internal organ infection is most common in humans. Surgical removal, if necessary, is the usual treatment.

Clinical Presentation of Tapeworm Infections

Intestinal tapeworm infections usually asymptomatic. Nonspecific abdominal pain, cramps, and diarrhea have been described. Discovery of infection occurs when a motile segment or a "tape" of proglottids is passed during a bowel movement or spontaneously appears in the undergarments. Perianal or vaginal irritation may also occur. Chronic *D. latum* infection may rarely cause vitamin B12 deficiency and megaloblastic anemia.

Tapeworm infections are confirmed by the presence of eggs or segments found in stool specimens during parasitological examination.

Tissue infection with *Echinococcus* spp. (*E. granulosis* or *E. vogeli*) causes hydatid disease and most commonly presents with a mass effect of the slow-growing cystic lesions, usually in the liver, taking decades to reach symptomatic size. Primary cysts may reach 25 cm or more in diameter. Rupture of a cyst can release antigenic material, causing an acute allergic or anaphylactic reaction. Secondary bacterial infection of liver cysts can present as a liver abscess. Previous leakage of a liver cyst into the peritoneal cavity may cause multiple secondary cystic growths throughout the abdominal cavity. Pulmonary echinococcal cysts are usually asymptomatic, but if they rupture into the bronchial tree they can cause hemoptysis and coughing out of daughter cysts that look like grape skins. Echinococcal cysts in other organs (e.g., skin, bone, brain, eye, and visceral organs) have been described. Alveolar echinococcal infections (*E. multilocularis*) present as a rapidly progressive solid tumor mass in the liver. Due to their aggressive presentations, these infections clinically behave like a malignancy.

Tissue infection with cysticerci of *T. solium* infection is usually asymptomatic, even when the cysts are in the brain. Neurocysticercosis is a common cause of seizure disorder in Mexico, Central and South America, Africa, India, China, Eastern Europe, and Indonesia. A rare form of central nervous infection, called racemose cysticercosis, is associated with grape-like cystic growths in the brain causing obstructive hydrocephalus, arachnoiditis, and cerebellitis.

Diagnosis

A clinical diagnosis to the species level cannot be made from general history, physical examination of the patient, or the gross examination of expelled tapeworm segments in the stool. Patient demographics can be very suggestive of a specific adult tapeworm or tissue cystic presentation, but definitive diagnosis requires expert parasitologic laboratory testing, radiographic imaging, and, on occasion, pathologic specimen examination for parasitic elements.

Parasitologic Testing

Note: tapeworm segments or proglottids containing eggs of *T. solium* are infectious.

1. *Stool specimens*: eggs of *Taenia* spp., *Diphyllobothrium* spp., *D. caninum*, and *Hymenolepis nana* may be found in concentrated stool preparations made from fresh or preserved stool samples. The eggs of *T. saginata* and *T. solium* are morphologically indistinguishable; identification depends on examination of proglottids and scolices, if available. *Taenia* eggs may also be found on adhesive tape preparations taken near the anus. A copro-antigen enzyme-linked immunosorbent assay (ELISA) has been developed to detect *Taenia* species antigens from feces. Polymerase chain reaction is highly sensitive, specific, and an easy technique to detect *T. saginata*.

2. *Tapeworm segments*: tapeworm segments may be found in the fresh or preserved stool by macroscopic examination or directly as a segment in formalin. If the head of the tapeworm is found, the species can be identified by the scolex.

   The tapeworm species can also be identified by the characteristics of the proglottid seen on staining in the parasitology laboratory with India ink. The proglottid can also be stained with hematoxylin-eosin (H&E).

3. *Cystic fluid*: cystic fluid obtained during surgery or by aspiration can be examined for the hydatid "sand" of *Echinococcus* hooklets or protoscolices. Microscopic wet mounts and smears are stained by an acid-fast procedure. Microscopic examination of H&E-stained smears of the hydatid cyst shows a wall surrounded by host tissue capsule, a laminated acellular layer, and an inner, nucleated, germinal layer that gives rise to brood capsules. These capsules can degenerate or form "daughter" cysts containing many viable protoscolices.

4. *Parasite serology*: serologic testing for tissue infection with *T. solium* and *Echinococcus* spp. is performed by the Centers for Disease Control and Prevention (http://www.cdc.gov/dpdx/).

   For hydatid disease, specific immunoglobulin G (IgG) ELISA is the most sensitive test (83.5% sensitivity in one study). The CDC's immunoblot assay with purified *T. solium* antigen is the test of choice by the World Health Organization and the Pan American Health Organization. It has 100% specificity and a high sensitivity. These tests do not differentiate between active and inactive infections and cannot be used to evaluate the outcome and prognosis of medically treated patients.

Radiology

Barium contrast studies of the bowel can show filling defects of the long ribbon-like bodies of adult tapeworms. Any radiologic imaging technique (ultrasound, computed tomography, or magnetic resonance) will demonstrate the classical features of hydatid disease with primary cyst and multiple daughter cysts. Hydatid cysts in the lung may not have discernible daughter cysts, and they rarely calcify in the outer membrane. Alveolar echinococcal disease of the liver appears as a solid mass with external extensions that spread to adjacent organs, making it difficult to distinguish from other invasive tumors in the liver. Cysticerci in the soft tissues appear as small calcifications. Neuroradiology of cysticerci in the brain will show typical lesions very suggestive of the diagnosis in the cystic form of the disease. Racemose cysticercosis of the brain can be very challenging to diagnose with radiology alone.

Pathology

Pathologic examination is not indicated in intestinal tapeworm infections. In tissue examinations of an echinococcal cyst and its contents, cysts tend to be round or oval. The wall consists of a fibrous capsule of host tissue; a tough, elastic, laminated, acellular layer; and an inner nucleated germinal layer from which arises the brood capsule. The fluid or "sand" in the cysts contains protoscolices, daughter cysts, and degenerated brood capsules that have liberated protoscolices and hooklets. In alveolar hydatid disease, the laminated layer is invasive and diffusely spread in the tissue; brood capsules are not produced.

Brain or muscle tissue examination for cysticerci is generally not required for a diagnosis of disseminated *T. solium* infection.

Clinical Management

Treatment

Antihelminthic drugs and their dosages for treatment of tapeworm infections are listed in **Table 46.2**. Praziquantel and albendazole are the drugs of choice for most intestinal infections. Niclosamide tablets must be taken on an empty stomach and thoroughly chewed and swallowed. Niclosamide kills the parasite by direct contact with the tapeworms. If the scolex is protected from contact with the drug, the adult tapeworm infection may survive

TABLE 46.2   Treatment for Human Tapeworm Infections

Parasite	Drug	Dosage
Taenia saginata	Praziquantel	Single dose of 5-10 mg/kg
	Alternative: niclosamide	2.0 g once (50 mg/kg once)
Taenia solium (intestinal)	Praziquantel	Single dose of 5-10 mg/kg
	Alternative: niclosamide	2.0 g once (50 mg/kg once)
T. solium (tissue larval)	Seizure control	See specific anticonvulsants or seek specialist's consultation
	Alternatives:	
	Albendazole	400 mg p.o. (15 mg/kg, max. 400 mg b.i.d.) b.i.d. × 8-30 days (repeat if necessary)
	or	
	Praziquantel	50-100 mg/kg per day in three divided doses ×30 days
Diphyllobothrium latum	Praziquantel	Single dose of 5-10 mg/kg
	Alternative: niclosamide	2.0 g once (50 mg/kg once)
Dipylidium caninum	Praziquantel	Single dose of 5-10 mg/kg
	Alternative: niclosamide	2.0 g once (50 mg/kg once)
Echinococcus granulosis	See indications for surgery or percutaneous drainage. Albendazole	400 mg b.i.d. × 1-6 months (15 mg/kg per day; max. 400 mg b.i.d.)
Echinococcus multilocularis	See indications for excisional surgery	Albendazole or mebendazole may be adjunctive to curative surgery or, if inoperable, supportive therapy
Hymenolepis nana	Praziquantel	Adults and children: single dose of 25 mg/kg
	Alternative: nitazoxanide	500 mg × 3 days (1-3 years old: 100 mg b.i.d. × 3 days; 4-11 years old: 200 mg b.i.d. × 3 days)
Hymenolepis diminuta	Praziquantel	Adults and children: single dose of 5-10 mg/kg
	or	
	Nitazoxanide	500 mg × 3 days (1-3 years old: 100 mg b.i.d. × 3 days; 4-11 years old: 200 mg b.i.d. × 3 days)

b.i.d., Twice per day; p.o., by mouth.

treatment. Drinking orange juice, lemonade, or similar acidic, mucolytic beverage 30 min before taking the tablets is recommended.

Presumptive mass treatment may be chosen over individual assessment in some settings.

Surgical excision is the only reliable means of cure of hydatid disease and is the primary therapy for alveolar echinococcal disease. In nonresectable cases, treatment with albendazole may stabilize and sometimes cure infection. Hydatid cysts may be treated with albendazole for an extended period of time (1-6 months) with good clinical outcomes. Affected patients may also benefit from surgical resection or percutaneous drainage of cysts. Percutaneous aspiration–injection–reaspiration with ultrasound guidance plus albendazole or mebendazole therapy has been effective for management of hepatic hydatid cyst disease. Praziquantel is indicated preoperatively or in case of surgical spillage of cyst contents.

Initial therapy for patients with inflamed central nervous system parenchymal cysticercosis should focus on symptomatic treatment with antiseizure medication. Treatment of central nervous system parenchymal cysticerci with antiparasitic drugs (albendazole or praziquantel) remains controversial due to the potential of an exacerbated inflammatory response in the brain to dead and dying parasites. If treatment is undertaken, patients with live parenchymal cysts and seizures should be treated with combination drug therapy, for example, albendazole together with steroids (6 mg dexamethasone or 40-60 mg prednisone daily) and an antiseizure medication.

Public Health and the Role of Screening

An identified index case of intestinal tapeworm infection may have community or public health implications, depending on the species of tapeworm, the socioeconomic and geographic setting, and whether institutionalized care is a potential co-factor. Gastrointestinal infection with *T. solium* has been associated with larval infection in communities not usually associated with the consumption of pork meat products. The diagnosing clinician may wish to consult with the regional public health officials on recommendations for reporting, surveillance, or investigation of unusual parasitologic findings.

Prognosis

Untreated intestinal and tissue tapeworm infections may persist for years and may be associated with mild eosinophilia. Megaloblastic anemia is rare in chronic *D. latum* infection. *T. solium* infections may result in a disseminated extraintestinal larval infection called cysticercosis.

Management of associated seizure disorders in neurocysticercosis is generally all that is required for affected patients. Very rarely is a persistent adult *T. solium* tapeworm infection found, but this diagnosis should prompt consultation with a specialist before antiparasitic treatment is initiated, due to the possibility of exacerbating adverse consequences of undiagnosed larval infection of the central nervous system, as noted previously.

The prognosis of both hydatid and alveolar echinococcal disease has very much improved with modern surgical, percutaneous, and therapeutic management. Long-term follow-up is required to monitor clinical improvement and to observe for recurrences.

FURTHER READING

Andreassen, J., 1998. Intestinal tapeworms. In: Cox, F.E., Kreier, J.P., Wakelin, D. (Eds.), Topley and Wilson's Microbiology and Microbial Infections—Parasitology, vol. 5, ninth ed. Arnold, London, pp. 521–537.
Excellent reference text on parasite diagnostics.

Desowitz, R.S., 1987. New Guinea Tapeworms and Jewish Grandmothers: Tales of Parasites and People. W. W. Norton & Company, New York.
A novel narrative of humans and their parasites.

Koneman, E.W. (Ed.), 2006. Koneman's Color Atlas and Textbook of Diagnostic Microbiology, sixth ed. Lippincott Williams & Wilkins, Baltimore, MD.
Excellent text on parasite microbiology and graphic depictions of lifecycles.

Medical Letter, 2013. Drugs for Parasitic Infections, third ed. Available at <http://www.medicalletter.org/parasitic>.
Excellent reference for the medical treatment of parasitic infections.

Miller, J.M., Boyd, H.A., Ostrowski, S.R., et al., 2000. Malaria, intestinal parasites, and schistosomiasis among Barawan Somali refugees resettling to the United States: a strategy to reduce morbidity and decrease the risk of imported infections. Am. J. Trop. Med. Hyg. 62, 115–121.
Very nice epidemiological report of the burden of parasitic diseases in migrants to the United States and means to reduce the clinical and social impacts of these infections.

Moore, A.C., Lutwick, L.I., Schantz, P.M., et al., 1995. Seroprevalence of cysticercosis in an Orthodox Jewish community. Am. J. Trop. Med. Hyg. 53, 439–442.
An interesting public health investigation of a virulent presentation of parasitic disease in an epidemiologically low-risk population.

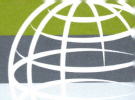

CHAPTER 47

Filarial Infections

Thomas B. Nutman

Filarial worms are nematodes or roundworms that dwell in the subcutaneous tissues and the lymphatics. Although eight filarial species commonly infect humans, four are responsible for most of the pathology associated with these infections. These are (1) *Brugia malayi*, (2) *Wuchereria bancrofti*, (3) *Onchocerca volvulus*, and (4) *Loa loa*. The distribution and vectors of all the filarial parasites of humans are given in **Table 47.1**.

In general, each of the parasites is transmitted by biting arthropods. Each goes through a complex life cycle that includes an infective larval stage carried by the insects and an adult worm stage that resides in humans, either in the lymph nodes or adjacent lymphatics or in the subcutaneous tissue. The offspring of the adults, the *microfilariae* (200-250 μm long and 5-7 μm wide), either circulate in the blood or migrate through the skin. The microfilariae then can be ingested by the appropriate biting arthropod and develop over 1-2 weeks into infective larvae, which are capable of initiating the life cycle over again. A generalized schematic is shown in **Figure 47.1**.

Adult worms are long lived, whereas the lifespans of microfilariae range from 3 months to 3 years depending on the filarial species. Infection is generally not established unless exposure to infective larvae is intense and prolonged. Furthermore, clinical manifestations of these diseases develop rather slowly.

There are significant differences in the clinical manifestations of filariasis, or at least in the time course over which these infections are acquired, in patients native to the endemic areas and those who are travelers or recent arrivals in these same areas. Characteristically, the disease in previously unexposed individuals is more acute and intense than that found in natives of the endemic region; also, early removal of newly infected individuals tends to speed the end of clinical symptomatology or at least halt the progression of the disease.

LYMPHATIC FILARIASIS

There are three lymphatic-dwelling filarial parasites of humans: *B. malayi*, *Brugia timori*, and *W. bancrofti*. Adult worms usually reside in either the afferent lymphatic channels or the lymph nodes. These adult parasites may remain viable in the human host for decades.

Epidemiology

B. malayi *and* B. timori

The distribution of brugian filariasis is limited primarily to China, India, Indonesia, Korea, Japan, Malaysia, and the Philippines. In both brugian species, two forms of the parasite can be distinguished by the periodicity of their microfilariae. *Nocturnally periodic forms* have microfilariae present in the peripheral blood primarily at night, whereas the *sub-periodic forms* have microfilariae present in the blood at all times, but with maximal levels in the afternoon.

TABLE 47.1   Filarial Parasites of Humans

Species	Distribution	Vector	Primary Pathology
Brugia malayi	Southeast Asia	Mosquito	Lymphatic, pulmonary
Brugia timori	Indonesia	Mosquito	Lymphatic
Wuchereria bancrofti	Tropics	Mosquito	Lymphatic, pulmonary
Onchocerca volvulus	Africa and Central and South America	Blackfly	Dermal, ocular, lymphatic
Mansonella streptocerca	Africa	Midge	Dermal
Loa loa	Africa	Deerfly	Allergic
Mansonella perstans	Africa and South America	Midge	Probably allergic
Mansonella ozzardi	Central and South America	Midge	?

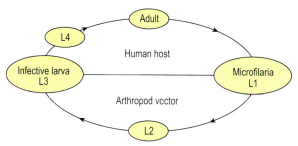

Fig. 47.1   **General life cycle of the filarial parasites in humans. Microfilariae (*L1*) are produced by the adult worms. *L2* and *L3* are larval development stages in the arthropod vector. *L3* larval forms are infective for humans. *L4* develop from the newly arrived infective larval forms.**

   The nocturnal form of brugian filariasis is more common and is transmitted in areas of coastal rice fields (by *Mansonia* and *Anopheles* mosquitoes), whereas the subperiodic form is found in the swamp forests (*Mansonia* vector). Although humans are the common host, *B. malayi* can be a natural infection of cats. *B. timori* has been described only on two islands of the Indonesian archipelago (including East Timor).

W. bancrofti

Bancroftian filariasis is found throughout the tropics and subtropics, including Asia and the Pacific islands, Africa, areas of South America, and the Caribbean basin. Humans are the only definitive host for this parasite and are therefore the natural reservoir for infection. Like brugian filariasis, there is both a periodic and a sub-periodic form of the parasite. Generally, the sub-periodic form is found only in the Pacific Islands (including Cook and Ellis Islands, Fiji, New Caledonia, the Marquesas, Samoa, and the Society Islands); elsewhere, *W. bancrofti* is nocturnally periodic. The natural vectors are *Culex fatigans* mosquitoes in urban settings and usually *Anopheles* or *Aedes* mosquitoes in rural areas.

Pathology

Most of the pathology associated with bancroftian and brugian filariasis is localized to the lymphatics. Damaged lymphatics first lead to reversible lymphedema and then to chronic obstructive changes (in the limbs, breasts, or genitalia or to chyluria). The location of the lymphatic damage determines the type and site of the pathology.

Although the underlying mechanisms of pathology in this form of the disease are not yet known with certainty, it is thought that adult worms residing in the lymph nodes or neighboring lymphatics induce local inflammatory reactions and/or changes in lymphatic function. These reactions result in dilation of the lymphatics and hypertrophy of the vessel walls, although as long as the adult worm remains viable, the vessel is said to remain patent. Death of the worm, however, leads to local necrosis and a granulomatous reaction around the parasite. Fibrosis occurs and lymphatic obstruction develops. Although some recanalization and collateralization of the lymphatics takes place, lymphatic function remains compromised.

Clinical Manifestations in Those Native to the Endemic Region

The three most common presentations of the lymphatic filariases are asymptomatic (or subclinical) microfilaremia, adenolymphangitis (ADL), and lymphatic obstruction.

1. Patients with *asymptomatic microfilaremia* rarely come to the attention of medical personnel except through the incidental finding of microfilariae in the peripheral blood during surveys in endemic regions or when blood eosinophilia leads to a diagnostic evaluation for lymphatic filariasis. Such asymptomatic persons are clinically unaffected by the parasites, although lymphoscintigraphic evaluation of these individuals suggests that lymphatic dysfunction (and tortuosity) is common, as is scrotal lymphangiectasia (detectable by ultrasound) in men with *W. bancrofti* infection.

2. Acute *filarial* ADL is characterized by high fever (and shaking chills), lymphatic inflammation (lymphangitis and lymphadenitis), and transient local edema. The lymphangitis is retrograde, extending peripherally from the lymph node draining the area where the adult parasites reside. Regional lymph nodes are often enlarged, and the entire lymphatic channel can become indurated and inflamed. Concomitant local thrombophlebitis can occur as well. In brugian filariasis, a single local abscess may form along the involved lymphatic tract and subsequently rupture to the surface. The lymphadenitis and lymphangitis occur in both the upper and the lower extremities in both bancroftian and brugian filariasis, but involvement of the genital lymphatics occurs almost exclusively with *W. bancrofti* infection. Genital involvement can be manifested by funiculitis, epididymitis, scrotal pain, and tenderness.

3. Chronic manifestations of lymphatic filariasis develop in only a small proportion of the filarial-infected population. If lymphatic damage progresses, transient lymphedema can develop into *lymphatic obstruction* and the permanent changes associated with elephantiasis. Brawny edema follows the early pitting edema, and thickening of the subcutaneous tissues and hyperkeratosis occur. Fissuring of the skin develops, as do hyperplastic changes. Superinfection of these poorly vascularized tissues becomes a problem. In bancroftian filariasis, when genital involvement is evident, scrotal lymphedema or hydrocele formation occurs. Furthermore, if there is obstruction of the retroperitoneal lymphatics, renal lymphatic pressure can increase to the point at which they rupture into the renal pelvis or tubules so that chyluria is seen. The chyluria is characteristically intermittent and is often prominent in the morning just after the patient arises.

Clinical Manifestations in New Arrivals to Endemic Areas

As mentioned previously, there are significant differences in the clinical manifestations of filarial infection, or at least in the time course over which they appear, between individuals who have recently entered the endemic areas (travelers or "transmigrants") and those who are native to these areas.

Given sufficient exposure to the vector (generally 3-6 months), patients often present with the signs and symptoms of acute lymphatic or scrotal inflammation. Urticaria and localized angioedema are common. Lymphadenitis of the epitrochlear, axillary, femoral, or inguinal nodes is often followed by lymphangitis, which is retrograde.

Acute attacks are short lived and, in contradistinction to filarial ADL, patients, are generally not accompanied by fever. If allowed to continue (by chronic exposure to infected mosquitoes), these attacks become increasingly severe and quickly (compared with the indigenous population) lead to permanent lymphatic inflammation and obstruction. Important to note, however, is that early removal of the patients from continued reexposure seems to hasten the end of the clinical syndrome.

Diagnosis

Diagnosis of filarial diseases can be problematic, because these infections most often require parasitologic techniques to demonstrate the offending organisms. In addition, satisfactory methods for the definitive diagnosis in amicrofilaremic states can be extremely difficult. The diagnostic procedures, however, should take advantage of the periodicity of each organism as well as its characteristic morphologic appearance. **Table 47.2** and **Figure 47.2** address

TABLE 47.2 Characteristics of Microfilariae in Humans

Species	Location	Periodicity	Presence of Sheath
Brugia malayi	Blood	Nocturnal, subperiodic	+
Brugia timori	Blood	Nocturnal	+
Wuchereria bancrofti	Blood, hydrocele fluid	Nocturnal, subperiodic	+
Onchocerca volvulus	Skin	None	−
Mansonella streptocerca	Skin	None	−
Loa loa	Blood	Diurnal	+
Mansonella perstans	Blood	None	−
Mansonella ozzardi	Blood	None	−

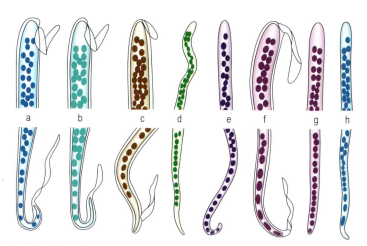

Fig. 47.2 **Differential characterizations of the microfilariae. (a)** Brugia malayi, **(b)** Brugia timori, **(c)** Wuchereria bancrofti, **(d)** Onchocerca volvulus, **(e)** Mansonella streptocerca, **(f)** Loa loa, **(g)** Mansonella perstans, **(h)** Mansonella ozzardi. (Adapted from Craig, C.F., Faust, E.C., 1964. Clinical Parasitology, seventh ed. Lea & Febiger, Philadelphia.)

these issues specifically. The following techniques may be used for examining blood or other fluids, such as chyle, urine, and hydrocele fluid.

Direct Examination

A small volume of fluid is spread on a clean slide. The slide is then air dried, stained with Giemsa stain, and examined microscopically.

Nuclepore™ filtration

A known volume of anticoagulated blood is passed through a polycarbonate (Nuclepore) filter with a 3-μm pore. A large volume (50 mL) of distilled (or filtered) water is passed through (the water will lyse or break open the red cells, leaving the microfilariae intact and more easily visible). The filter is then air dried, stained with Wright's or Giemsa stain, and examined by microscopy. For studies in the field, 1 mL of anticoagulated blood can be added to 9 mL of a solution of 2% formalin/10% Teepol and stored for up to 9 months before performing filtration.

Knott's concentration technique

In this technique, 1 mL of anticoagulated blood is placed in 9 mL of 2% formalin. The tube is centrifuged at 1500 rpm for 1 min. The sediment is spread on a slide and dried thoroughly. The slide is then stained with Wright's or Giemsa stain and examined microscopically.

Indirect Measures

Detection of circulating parasite antigen

Assays for circulating antigens of *W. bancrofti* permit the diagnosis of microfilaremic and cryptic (amicrofilaremic) infection. There are currently two commercially available tests, one in an enzyme-linked immunosorbent assay format (Trop-Ag *W. bancrofti*, manufactured by JCU Tropical Biotechnology, Townsville, Queensland, Australia), and the other a rapid-format card test (marketed by Allere, Scarborough, ME). Both assays have reported sensitivities that range from 96 to 100% and specificities that approach 100%. There are currently no tests for circulating antigens in brugian filariasis.

Serodiagnosis using parasite extract

Development of serodiagnostic assays of sufficient sensitivity and specificity for routine use has proven difficult, primarily because of their poor specificity. As is the case for serodiagnosis of most infectious diseases, it is difficult to differentiate previous infection or exposure to the parasite (aborted infection) from current active infection. Indeed, most residents of filariasis-endemic regions are antibody positive. Nevertheless, such serologic assays have a definite place in diagnosis, as a negative assay result effectively excludes past or present infection.

Molecular diagnostics

Polymerase chain reaction (PCR)-based assays for DNA of *W. bancrofti* and *B. malayi* in blood have also been developed. In a number of studies evaluating PCR-based diagnosis, the method is of equivalent or greater sensitivity compared with parasitologic methods, detecting patent infection in almost all infected subjects.

Imaging studies

In cases of suspected lymphatic filariasis, examination of the scrotum or female breast using high-frequency ultrasound in conjunction with Doppler techniques may result in the identification of motile adult worms within dilated lymphatics. Worms may be visualized in the lymphatics of the spermatic cord in up to 80% of infected men with *W. bancrofti*. Live adult worms have a distinctive pattern of movement within the lymphatic vessels (termed the "filaria dance sign"). This technique may be useful to monitor the success of antifilarial chemotherapy, by observing for the disappearance of the dance sign.

Radionuclide lymphoscintigraphic imaging of the limbs reliably demonstrates widespread lymphatic abnormalities both in asymptomatic microfilaremic persons and in those with clinical manifestations of lymphatic pathology. While of potential utility in the delineation of anatomic changes associated with infection, lymphoscintigraphy is unlikely to assume primacy in the diagnostic evaluation of individuals with suspected infection.

Differential Diagnosis

The diagnosis of filariasis often must be made clinically, because many patients with lymphatic filariasis are not microfilaremic. In acute episodes, the differential diagnosis includes thrombophlebitis, infection, and trauma. Edema and changes associated with chronic filariasis must be distinguished from the similar changes that are seen to occur with malignancy, post-surgical scarring, trauma, and congestive heart failure, along with the less common congenital or idiopathic lymphatic system abnormalities. The many disorders associated with eosinophil and serum immunoglobulin E elevations must be considered as well.

Treatment

With newer definitions of clinical syndromes in lymphatic filariasis and new tools to assess clinical status (e.g., ultrasound, lymphoscintigraphy, circulating filarial antigen assays), approaches to treatment based on infection status and pathogenesis have been proposed.

Microfilaria-Positive Individuals

A growing body of evidence indicates that although they may be asymptomatic, virtually all persons with *W. bancrofti* or *B. malayi* microfilaremia have some degree of sub-clinical disease (hematuria, proteinuria, abnormalities on lymphoscintigraphy). Thus, early treatment of asymptomatic persons is recommended to prevent further lymphatic damage. Diethylcarbamazine (DEC), which has both macrofilaricidal and microfilaricidal properties, is the drug of choice.

Microfilaria-negative antigen-positive individuals

Because lymphatic disease is associated with the adult worm, treatment with DEC is recommended for microfilaria-negative adult worm carriers (i.e., persons who are microfilaria negative but filaria antigen or ultrasound positive).

Acute Manifestations of Lymphatic Filariasis

Filarial Adenolymphangitis (ADL)

Supportive treatment is recommended, including rest; postural drainage, particularly if the lower limb is affected; cold compresses at the site of inflammation; and antipyretics and analgesics for symptomatic relief. During the acute episode, treatment with antifilarial drugs is not recommended, because it may provoke additional adult worm death and exacerbate the inflammatory response. After the acute attack has resolved, if the patient remains microfilaria or antigen positive, DEC can be given to kill the remaining adult worms.

For patients with ADL secondary to bacterial or fungal infections, cold compresses, antipyretics, and analgesics are recommended. The patient should remain at rest, with the affected limb elevated. Antibiotic therapy must be initiated while awaiting results of cultures of blood or tissue aspirates. The bacteria isolated during these attacks are sensitive to most systemic antibiotics, including penicillin.

Chronic Manifestations of Lymphatic Filariasis

Chronic manifestations of lymphatic filariasis include lymphedema and urogenital disease. Although antifilarial drug therapy is rarely, if ever, the "definitive" treatment for these conditions, such treatment is indicated if the patient has evidence of active infection (e.g., detection of microfilaria or filarial antigen in the blood or of the "filaria dance sign" on ultrasound examination). Not infrequently, the inflammatory response secondary to treatment-induced death of the adult worm exacerbates manifestations of chronic disease.

Lymphedema

Careful attention must be paid to the management of lymphedema once it has occurred. Elevation of the affected limb, elastic stockings, and local foot care will ameliorate some of the symptoms associated with lymphedema. Data indicate that filarial elephantiasis and lymphedema of the leg may be partially reversible with a treatment regimen that emphasizes hygiene, prevention of secondary bacterial infections, and physiotherapy. This regimen is similar to that now recommended for treatment of lymphedema of most nonfilarial causes where it is known by a variety of names, including complex decongestive physiotherapy and complex lymphedema therapy. A six week course of doxycycline has been shown to improve (but not reverse) filarial-associated lymphedema in a single study in Ghana. Surgical decompression using a nodovenous shunt may provide improvement in extreme cases. Hydroceles can be drained repeatedly or managed surgically.

Treatment Options and Dosage

The recommended course of DEC treatment (12 days; total dose 72 mg/kg) has remained standard for many years; however, data indicate that single-dose DEC treatment with 6 mg/kg may be equally efficacious. The 12-day course provides more rapid short-term microfilarial suppression.

Regimens that utilize combinations of single doses of albendazole and either DEC or ivermectin have all been demonstrated to have a sustained microfilaricidal effect. Interestingly, 6 weeks of daily doxycycline (200 mg/day)—a regimen that targets the intracellular *Wolbachia* endosymbiont—or a 7-day course of DEC/albendazole has both significant macrofilaricidal activity and sustained microfilaricidal activity.

Side effects of DEC treatment include fever, chills, arthralgias, headaches, nausea, and vomiting. Both the development and severity of these reactions are directly related to the number of microfilariae circulating in the bloodstream and may represent an acute hypersensitivity reaction to the antigens being released by dead and dying parasites. To avoid these side effects, one can either initiate treatment with a very small dose of DEC and increase the dose to the full level over a few days or premedicate the patient with corticosteroids. Ivermectin has a side-effect profile similar to that of DEC when used in lymphatic filariasis. Albendazole (when used in single-dose regimens) has relatively few side effects associated with its use in lymphatic filariasis.

DEC is not commercially available in the United States and must be obtained from the Centers for Disease Control and Prevention. Albendazole, ivermectin, and doxycycline are all available commercially.

PREVENTION AND CONTROL

Avoidance of mosquito bites is usually not feasible for residents of endemic areas, but visitors should make use of insect repellent and mosquito nets. Impregnated bed nets have been shown to have a salutary effect. DEC can kill developing forms of filarial parasites and has been shown to be useful as a prophylactic agent in humans.

Mass drug administration is the current approach to elimination of lymphatic filariasis. The underlying tenet of this approach is that mass annual distribution of antimicrofilarial chemotherapy—albendazole with either DEC (for all areas except those where onchocerciasis is co-endemic) or ivermectin—will profoundly suppress microfilaremia. If the suppression is sustained, then transmission can be interrupted. As an added benefit, these combinations have secondary effects on gastrointestinal helminths. Community education and clinical care for persons already suffering from the chronic sequelae of lymphatic filariasis are important components of morbidity management that is currently part of the lymphatic filariasis elimination programs.

TROPICAL EOSINOPHILIA SYNDROME

Tropical eosinophilia syndrome, or tropical pulmonary eosinophilia (TPE), was recognized as being of filarial etiology only in the late 1950s or early 1960s, when it was noted that the antifilarial drug DEC was effective in this syndrome and that patients with TPE had extraordinarily high levels of antifilarial antibodies in their blood. Although circulating microfilariae were rarely found, lung and lymph node biopsies occasionally revealed trapped microfilariae.

Patients with this syndrome are primarily male (4:1 predominance). Characteristically, those with this form of the disease are in their third or fourth decade of life. A majority of cases have been reported from India, Pakistan, Sri Lanka, Southeast Asia, Guyana, and Brazil.

Clinical Features
The main features of this syndrome, besides a history of residence in a filarial-endemic region, include paroxysmal cough and wheezing (usually nocturnal), occasional weight loss, low-grade fever, adenopathy, and extreme peripheral blood eosinophilia (>3000/mm^3). Chest radiographs may be normal but generally show increased bronchovascular markings, diffuse miliary lesions, or mottled opacities primarily involving the mid and lower lung fields. Pulmonary function testing often shows restrictive abnormalities, which may be accompanied by obstructive defects.

This syndrome is associated with marked elevations of antifilarial antibodies, as well as extremely elevated levels of total serum IgE (10,000-100,000 ng/mL). Furthermore, in the absence of successful treatment, permanent pulmonary damage (interstitial fibrosis) can develop.

Pathology
Tropical eosinophilia is now considered to be a form of *occult filariasis* in which rapid clearance of the microfilariae occurs, presumably on the basis of host immunologic hyperresponsiveness to the parasite. This clearance takes place in the lung, and the clinical symptoms are probably the result of allergic and inflammatory reactions elicited by the cleared parasites. In some subjects, the microfilarial trapping occurs in other organs of the reticuloendothelial system (liver, spleen, lymph nodes), in which case hepatomegaly, splenomegaly, or lymphadenopathy occurs.

Differential Diagnosis
Tropical eosinophilia must be distinguished from Löffler syndrome, chronic eosinophilic pneumonia, allergic bronchopulmonary aspergillosis, some of the vasculitides, the idiopathic hypereosinophilic syndrome, drug allergies, and some other helminth infections. Although there is no single clinical or laboratory criterion that aids in distinguishing tropical eosinophilia from these diseases, residence in the tropics, the presence of high levels of antifilarial antibodies, and a rapid clinical response to DEC favor the diagnosis of tropical eosinophilia.

Treatment
DEC is the drug of choice for treatment of TPE, the dose typically being 6 mg/kg per day for 14 days. Symptoms usually resolve between days 4 and 7 of therapy. Characteristically, respiratory symptoms rapidly resolve after treatment with DEC. Despite dramatic initial improvement after conventional treatment with DEC, symptoms recur in approximately 20% of patients 12-24 months after treatment, and a majority of patients continue to have subtle clinical, radiographic, and functional abnormalities. Repeat treatment may be necessary to prevent pulmonary fibrosis, a serious sequela of TPE if left untreated.

ONCHOCERCIASIS

Epidemiology
Onchocerciasis, sometimes called river blindness, is caused by infection with *Onchocerca volvulus*, a subcutaneous-dwelling filarial worm. Approximately 18 million people are infected, mostly in equatorial Africa, the Sahara, and Yemen, with only a few remaining foci in Central and South America (Venezuela and Brazil). The infection is transmitted to humans through the bites of black flies of the genus *Simulium*, which breed along fast-flowing rivers in the previously mentioned tropical areas.

Pathology

The pathology of onchocerciasis is limited primarily to the skin, lymphatic system, and eyes.

Onchocerciasis is a *cumulative* infection. Intense infections, which lead to the disease's severest complications, are believed to reflect repeated inoculation of infective larvae.

Skin

In the skin, granulomatous and fibrous reactions tend to occur in response to the adult worm. Similarly, dead microfilariae in the skin tend to produce small granulomata with eosinophilic infiltrates. Over a period of years, adult worms are encased by host tissue, thereby forming the characteristic subcutaneous nodules (onchocercomata).

Lymph Nodes

The pathology of the lymph nodes consists of scarring of the lymphoid areas (*O. volvulus* infection in Africa) or follicular hyperplasia (*O. volvulus* infection in Yemen). Histologically the lymph nodes draining areas of onchodermatitis show capsular fibrosis, atrophic follicles, and dilation of the subcapsular sinusoids and lymphatics.

Eyes

The pathologic processes that occur in the ocular tissues are not yet well elucidated. The conjunctiva can show an infiltrate with plasma cells, eosinophils, and mast cells. Punctate keratitis occurs and is believed to reflect inflammation around degenerating microfilariae. Anterior uveitis and chorioretinitis may occur and are thought to be a result of a low-grade inflammation, although autoimmune reactions may play a role.

Clinical Features

The major disease manifestations of onchocerciasis are localized to the skin, lymph nodes and lymphatics, and eyes.

Skin

Pruritus is the most frequent manifestation of onchocercal dermatitis. This pruritus may be accompanied by the appearance of localized areas of edema and erythema that is characteristically evanescent. If the infection is prolonged, lichenification and pigment changes (either hypopigmentation or hyperpigmentation) can occur; these often lead to atrophy, "lizard skin," and mottling of the skin. The skin can also become superinfected, particularly in the presence of excoriation or trauma. An immunologically hyperreactive form of dermatitis (commonly termed "sowda," or localized onchodermatitis) can occur with the affected skin becoming darker as a consequence of the profound inflammation that occurs as microfilariae in the skin are being cleared.

The subcutaneous nodules contain the adult worm. In Africa, the onchocercomata tend to be found over bony prominences, such as the coccyx, femoral trochanter, iliac crests, lateral aspects of the knee and elbow, and head. Interestingly, it is thought that for every palpable nodule, there are probably at least five deeper nodules.

Lymph Nodes

Lymphadenopathy is frequently found, particularly in the inguinal and femoral areas. As the glands enlarge, they can come to lie within areas of loose skin (so-called hanging groin), which predisposes the affected patients to hernias. Scarring in lymph nodes may lead to regional lymphedema.

Eyes

Onchocercal eye disease can take many forms, and most can lead to severe visual loss or blindness. Usually seen in persons with moderate or heavy infections, the ocular disease spares no part of the eye. Conjunctivitis, anterior uveitis, iridocyclitis leading to secondary glaucoma, sclerosing keratitis, optic atrophy, and chorioretinal lesions can be found.

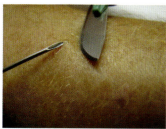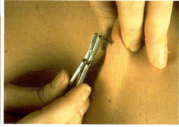

Fig. 47.3 *Left panel*: Skin snips being removed with needle and scalpel. Note the small tent of skin that is lifted up the needle. *Right panel*: Skin snip being performed using a corneoscleral punch.

Diagnosis

Definitive diagnosis depends on finding an adult worm in an excised nodule or, more commonly, microfilariae in a skin snip.

Skin Snip

A small piece of skin is elevated by the tip of a needle or skin hook held parallel to the surface, and a razor or scalpel blade is used to shave off the skin area stretched across the top surface of the needle (**Fig. 47.3**). Alternatively, a sclerocorneal punch can be used to obtain a blood-free circular skin specimen.

Skin snips are generally obtained from an area of affected skin or from the scapular, gluteal, and calf areas. Once obtained, the skin snips are incubated in a physiologic solution (such as normal saline); the emergent microfilariae can be seen under a microscope after 2-4 hours. Occasionally, in light infections, overnight incubation is necessary.

Serodiagnosis

A variety of serodiagnostic and antigenic skin tests have been described. Recently, recombinant onchocercal-specific antigens have been produced, one of which has been developed into a rapid format card test.

Molecular Diagnosis

Highly specific and sensitive PCR-based assays have been developed for the detection of *O. volvulus* DNA in skin snips that are microscopically negative. This has proved useful in the detection of very low infection levels but requires expensive equipment and reagents, as well as rigorous training and quality control.

Differential Diagnosis

Onchocerciasis must be differentiated from scabies, contact dermatitis, and, rarely, streptocerciasis (see the following section).

Treatment

The major goals of therapy are to prevent irreversible lesions and to alleviate bothersome symptoms. Surgical excision of nodules is recommended when the nodules are located on the head because of the proximity of the microfilaria-producing adult worms to the eye, but chemotherapy is the mainstay of treatment.

Ivermectin, a semisynthetic macrocyclic lactone, is considered first-line therapy for onchocerciasis. It is given orally in a single dose of 150 μg/kg. It is characteristically given yearly or semiannually. With treatment, most patients have a mild or no reaction. Pruritus, cutaneous edema, and/or a maculopapular rash occur in approximately 1–10% of treated individuals. Significant ocular complications are extremely rare, as is hypotension (1 in

10,000). Contraindications to treatment include pregnancy, breastfeeding, age <5 years, and central nervous system (CNS) disorders that might increase the penetration of ivermectin into the CNS (e.g., meningitis).

Although treatment with ivermectin results in a marked drop in microfilarial density, its effect can be short lived (much less than 6 months in some cases). Thus, it is occasionally necessary to give ivermectin more frequently for persistent symptoms.

STREPTOCERCIASIS

Mansonella streptocerca (formerly *Dipetalonema streptocerca*, *Tetrapetalonema streptocerca*) is largely found in the tropical forest belt of Africa from Ghana to Zaire. It is transmitted to the human host by biting midges (*Culicoides* spp.).

The pathology of streptocerciasis is both dermal and lymphatic. In the skin, there are hypopigmented macules (and occasionally papular rashes) that are thought to be secondary to inflammatory reactions around microfilariae. The distribution of the parasite in the skin of the human host tends to be across the shoulders and upper torso. Lymph nodes of affected individuals may show chronic lymphadenitis with scarring.

The major clinical manifestations are related to the skin: pruritus, papular rashes, and pigmentation changes. Most infected individuals also show inguinal lymphadenopathy; however, many patients are completely asymptomatic.

The diagnosis is made after finding the characteristic microfilariae on skin-snip examination. Leprosy and granuloma multiforme are the two other diseases that must be distinguished from streptocerciasis.

DEC is particularly effective in treating infection by both the microfilarial and the adult form of the parasite. The recommended dosage is 6 mg/kg per day in divided doses for 21 days. After treatment, as in onchocerciasis, one can often see urticaria, arthralgias, myalgias, headaches, and abdominal discomfort. Ivermectin at a dose of 150 μg/kg appears to have a salutary microfilaricidal effect that can be sustained at least a year following therapy.

LOIASIS

The distribution of *Loa loa* is limited to the rain forests of West and Central Africa. Tabanid flies (deer flies) of the genus *Chrysops* are the intermediate hosts. The adult parasite lives in the subcutaneous tissues in humans; then microfilariae circulate in the bloodstream with a diurnal periodicity.

Pathology

The pathology associated with loiasis includes: (1) the classic "Calabar swelling" (localized areas of transient angioedema), found predominantly on the extremities; (2) peripheral (entrapment) neuropathy; (3) nephropathy presumed to be immune complex mediated; (4) encephalopathy thought to be secondary to either an acute cerebral edema or a chronic, subacute encephalitis; and (5) cardiomyopathy presumably related to the marked hypereosinophilia that these patients may have.

Clinical Manifestations

Loa loa infection may be present as asymptomatic microfilaremia, with the infection being recognized only after subconjunctival migration of an adult worm (the so-called eye worm). Other patients have episodic Calabar swellings. If the associated inflammation extends to the nearby joints or peripheral nerves, corresponding symptoms (such as entrapment neuropathy or arthritis) can develop. Nephropathy, encephalopathy, and cardiomyopathy can occur, but rarely.

There appears to be a difference between the presentation of loiasis in those native to the endemic area and those who are visitors. The latter tend to have a greater predominance of allergic symptomatology. The episodes of Calabar swellings tend to be more frequent and debilitating, and such patients rarely have microfilaremia. In addition, those who are not native to the endemic area have extreme elevation of eosinophils in the blood, as well as marked increases in antifilarial antibody titers.

Diagnosis

Definitive diagnosis is made through parasitologic examination, either by finding microfilariae in the peripheral blood or by isolating the adult worm from the eye or in subcutaneous biopsy material following treatment. Molecular diagnostics (PCR) can be used for definitive diagnosis as well. However, the diagnosis must often be made on clinical grounds, particularly in travelers (usually amicrofilaremic) to the endemic region.

Treatment

DEC, 8-10 mg/kg per day for 21 days, is the recommended treatment. The drug is effective against both the adult and microfilarial forms of the parasite, but multiple courses of therapy are necessary before there is complete resolution of the disease. In cases of heavy microfilaremia, allergic or other inflammatory reactions can occur; in the most severe cases, there may be CNS involvement, with coma and encephalitis. Heavy infections can be managed initially with low doses of DEC (0.5-1.0 mg/kg per day) and the simultaneous administration of corticosteroids.

Albendazole or ivermectin (although neither is approved for this use by the US Food and Drug Administration) has been shown to be effective in reducing microfilarial loads, although ivermectin has been implicated in serious (and life-threatening) adverse events in heavily loa-microfilaremic individuals. DEC (300 mg weekly) is an effective prophylactic regimen for loiasis.

PERSTANS FILARIASIS

Mansonella perstans is distributed across the center of Africa and in northeastern South America. The infection is transmitted to humans through the bites of midges (*Culicoides* spp.). The adult worms reside in the body cavities (pericardial, pleural, peritoneal) as well as in the mesentery and the perirenal and retroperitoneal tissues. The microfilariae circulate in the blood without periodicity. As with *Mansonella ozzardi* (see the following discussion), the pathology relating to this infection is ill-defined.

Although most patients appear to be asymptomatic, clinical manifestations of this infection include transient angioedematous swellings of the arms, face, or other body parts (not unlike the Calabar swellings of *Loa loa* infection); pruritus; fever; headache; arthralgias; neurologic or psychologic symptoms; and right upper quadrant pain. Occasionally, pericarditis and hepatitis occur.

The diagnosis is made through parasitologic evaluation by finding the microfilariae in the blood or in other body fluids (serosal effusions). Perstans filariasis is often associated with peripheral blood eosinophilia and antifilarial antibody elevations. Although DEC, ivermectin, and albendazole have all been tried in this infection, none has proven to be of significant benefit. With the discovery of a *Wolbachia* endosymbiont specific to *M. perstans*, targeted therapy with doxycycline (200 mg daily for 6 weeks) has been shown to be effective.

MANSONELLA OZZARDI INFECTION

The distribution of *Mansonella ozzardi* is restricted to Central and South America, as well as certain Caribbean islands. The parasite is transmitted to the human host by biting midges (*Culicoides furens*) and black flies (*Simulium amazonicum*). Although adult worms have only twice been recovered from humans, studies on the microfilariae show that they circulate in the bloodstream with little periodicity. The pathology of *M. ozzardi* infection is poorly characterized. Furthermore, many consider this organism to be nonpathogenic. However, headache, articular pain, fever, pulmonary symptoms, adenopathy, hepatomegaly, and pruritus have been ascribed to infection with this organism. Eosinophilia accompanies *M. ozzardi* infection as well. Diagnosis is made by demonstrating the characteristic microfilariae in the peripheral blood. DEC has little or no effect on this infection, but ivermectin has been shown to be effective in reducing symptoms and circulating microfilariae. Like *M. perstans*, *M. ozzardi* also has a *Wolbachia* endosymbiont, suggesting that a 6-week course of doxycycline should be effective.

FURTHER READING

Babu, S., Nutman, T.B., 2012. Immunopathogenesis of lymphatic filarial disease. Semin. Immunopathol. 34 (6), 847–861.

Coulibaly, Y.I., Dembele, B., Diallo, A.A., et al., 2009. A randomized trial of doxycycline for *Mansonella perstans* infection. N. Engl. J. Med. 361 (15), 1448–1458.

Based on the finding of a specific Wolbachia *endosymbiont in* Mansonella perstans, *this study demonstrates that* M. perstans *can be effectively treated with doxycycline and provides the possibility that* M. perstans *can be targeted for effective therapy.*

Herrick, J.A., Metenou, S., Makiya, M.A., et al., 2015. Eosinophil-associated processes underlie differences in clinical presentation of loiasis between temporary residents and those indigenous to Loa-endemic areas. Clin. Infect. Dis. 60 (1), 55–63.

Hoerauf, A., Mand, S., Adjei, O., et al., 2001. Depletion of *Wolbachia* endobacteria in *Onchocerca volvulus* by doxycycline and microfilaridermia after ivermectin treatment. Lancet 357 (9266), 1415–1416.

Lipner, E.M., Law, M.A., Barnett, E., et al., 2007. Filariasis in travelers presenting to the GeoSentinel Surveillance Network. PLoS Negl. Trop. Dis. 1 (3), e88.

Using a large multinational reporting system used by sentinel tropical medicine and travel clinics, this study identifies some of the risks associated with the development of pathologic filarial infections.

McCarthy, J.S., Ottesen, E.A., Nutman, T.B., 1994. Onchocerciasis in endemic and nonendemic populations: differences in clinical presentation and immunologic findings. J. Infect. Dis. 170 (3), 736–741.

Meyers, W.M., Connor, D.H., Harman, L.E., et al., 1972. Human streptocerciasis: a clinico-pathologic study of 40 Africans (Zairians) including identification of the adult filaria. Am. J. Trop. Med. Hyg. 21 (5), 528–545.

Mullerpattan, J.B., Udwadia, Z.F., Udwadia, F.E., 2013. Tropical pulmonary eosinophilia—a review. Indian J. Med. Res. 138 (3), 295–302.

An important review of the tropical pulmonary eosinophilia syndromeco-authored by one of the pre-eminent experts in this field, who was able to clearly demonstrate the filarial etiology underlying this syndrome.

Nutman, T.B., Miller, K.D., Mulligan, M., et al., 1988. Diethylcarbamazine prophylaxis for human loiasis: results of a double-blind study. N. Engl. J. Med. 319 (12), 752–756.

Omura, S., Crump, A., 2014. Ivermectin: panacea for resource-poor communities? Trends Parasitol. 30 (9), 445–455.

A perspective on the use of ivermectin for a variety of infections including the filariae.

Raccurt, C.P., Brasseur, P., Boncy, J., 2014. Mansonelliasis, a neglected parasitic disease in Haiti. Mem. Inst. Oswaldo Cruz 109 (6), 709–711.

Ramaiah, K.D., Ottesen, E.A., 2014. Progress and impact of 13 years of the global programme to eliminate lymphatic filariasis on reducing the burden of filarial disease. PLoS Negl Trop Dis. 8 (11), e3319.

Simonsen, P.E., Onapa, A.W., Asio, S.M., 2011. *Mansonella perstans* filariasis in Africa. Acta Trop. 120 (Suppl. 1), S109–S120.

Taylor, M.J., Hoerauf, A., Bockarie, M., 2010. Lymphatic filariasis and onchocerciasis. Lancet 376 (9747), 1175–1185.

Taylor, M.J., Hoerauf, A., Townson, S., et al., 2014. Anti-*Wolbachia* drug discovery and development: safe macrofilaricides for onchocerciasis and lymphatic filariasis. Parasitology 141 (1), 119–127.

*An important treatise on the use of anti-*Wolbachia *agents to target the adult filarial worms that are responsible for onchocerciasis and lymphatic filariasis.*

Taylor, M.J., Makunde, W.H., McGarry, H.F., et al., 2005. Macrofilaricidal activity after doxycycline treatment of *Wuchereria bancrofti*: a double-blind, randomised placebo-controlled trial. Lancet 365 (9477), 2116–2121.

Vijayan, V.K., 2007. Tropical pulmonary eosinophilia: pathogenesis, diagnosis and management. Curr. Opin. Pulm. Med. 13 (5), 428–433.

Walker, M., Specht, S., Churcher, T.S., et al., 2015. Therapeutic efficacy and macrofilaricidal activity of doxycycline for the treatment of river blindness. Clin. Infect. Dis. 60 (8), 1199–1207.

Walther, M., Muller, R., 2003. Diagnosis of human filariases (except onchocerciasis). Adv. Parasitol. 53, 149–193.

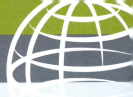

CHAPTER 48

Trematodes

Paul S. Pottinger and Elaine C. Jong

The flukes, or trematodes, are long-lived parasites that can cause human disease by mechanical obstruction and by inciting local inflammatory responses in affected organs (**Table 48.1**). Blood flukes (*Schistosoma* spp.), hepatobiliary flukes (*Clonorchis sinensis*, *Opisthorchis* spp., and *Fasciola hepatica*), and lung flukes (*Paragonimus* spp.) can be associated with major systemic pathology, whereas intestinal flukes (*Metagonimus yokogawai*, *Heterophyes heterophyes*, *Fasciolopsis buski*, and *Echinostoma* spp.) usually cause gastrointestinal symptoms such as diarrhea, anorexia, and abdominal pain only in heavy infections.

SCHISTOSOMIASIS

Schistosomiasis is a trematode infection caused by blood flukes. In Africa, schistosomiasis is often called "Bilharzia" after Theodore Bilharz, the German physician who first described the parasitic origin of the clinical disease. Species pathogenic for man include *S. mansoni*, *S. japonicum*, *S. mekongi*, and *S. haematobium*. Acute infection of humans with nonpathogenic avian species of schistosomes can result in an allergic skin reaction called swimmers' itch (see below and Chapter 37).

Schistosomiasis affects approximately 200 million people worldwide and is an important cause of morbidity and mortality in rural tropical and semitropical areas. *S. japonicum* is endemic in the Philippines and the People's Republic of China (but no longer Japan, in spite of its name); *S. mekongi* along the Mekong River valley; *S. mansoni* in the Middle East, Africa, eastern South America, and parts of the Caribbean; and *S. haematobium* in the Middle East and Africa.

Transmission

Microscopic cercariae penetrate wet human skin during contact or immersion in fresh water inhabited by infected snails, the obligate intermediate host in the parasite lifecycle. After infection, the cercariae transform into schistosomula, which develop into adult worms over a 4- to 6-week period. During maturation, the schistosomula migrate through the patient's lungs to specific sites, depending on the species. Adult females find their way into the gynecophoric groove, or "schist," of a male, and the pair enters a lifelong state of copulation. The mated pair begin to produce hundreds to thousands of eggs per day. Migration in the patient appears to be a species-specific phenomenon. *S. japonicum* and *S. mekongi* worm pairs migrate to the superior mesenteric vein, *S. mansoni* to the inferior mesenteric vein, and *S. haematobium* to the venous plexus surrounding the bladder.

The eggs deposited by the female worms on the peritoneal side of the intestines or bladder work their way through the walls of these organs and are passed outside the body in the feces or urine. When stool or urine from infected humans is deposited into fresh water, the eggs hatch, and motile miracidia emerge and infect snails of certain species, thus completing the lifecycle.

TABLE 48.1 Location, Source of Infection, and Clinical Features of Trematode Infections

Species	Location	Source of Infection	Clinical Features
Blood flukes			
Schistosoma mansoni	Africa, Caribbean, South America, and Middle East	Fresh water, penetration of skin by cercaria from infected snails	Dermatitis, abdominal pain, hematochezia, and portal hypertension
S. japonicum	China and Southeast Asia		Same
S. mekongi	Cambodia and Laos		Same
S. haematobium	Africa and Middle East		Hematuria
Hepatobiliary flukes			
Opisthorchis viverrini	Thailand and Laos	Freshwater fish	Asymptomatic or abdominal pain
O. felineus	Eastern Europe and Vietnam		
Clonorchis sinensis	Far East		
Fasciola hepatica	Worldwide, sheep- and cattle-raising areas	Raw vegetables, especially watercress	Asymptomatic or abdominal pain, hepatomegaly, and fever
Lung flukes			
Paragonimus westermani	Worldwide	Freshwater crustaceans such as crabs or crawfish	Hemoptysis, cough, ± extrapulmonary involvement
P. heterotremus	Thailand, Laos, and China		
P. skrjabini (P. szechuanensis)	China	Same	Same but also with cutaneous nodules
Intestinal flukes			
Metagonimus yokogawai	Asia, Russia, and Spain	Freshwater fish	Asymptomatic or diarrhea with abdominal pain
Heterophyes heterophyes	Middle East, Egypt	Freshwater fish	
Echinostoma spp.	Asia	Freshwater snails, fish, or vegetables	
Fasciolopsis buski	Asia	Freshwater plants	

The adult worms can persist in the human host for decades; thus, infections acquired in endemic tropical areas can present as puzzling diagnostic problems years later if infected individuals emigrate to non-endemic areas where these infections are rarely encountered by clinicians.

Clinical Features

Asymptomatic Infections

Patients with a low worm burden (light infections) resulting from limited exposure to freshwater environments in areas of transmission may be completely asymptomatic.

Katayama Fever

At the time of initial parasite egg laying (oviposition), about 4-6 weeks after infection, the patient sometimes presents with a severe febrile illness called Katayama fever. The etiology of this systemic reaction is probably a hypersensitivity to egg-associated antigens; it has been mainly associated with *S. mansoni* and *S. japonicum* infections. This febrile syndrome presents with fevers, headache, cough, urticaria, lymphadenopathy, tender hepatosplenomegaly, and hypereosinophilia of the peripheral blood. This syndrome typically settles spontaneously in a matter of days or weeks, although severe and even fatal cases have been reported.

Bloody Diarrhea and Obstipation

Eggs deposited by the female *S. mansoni*, *S. japonicum*, and *S. mekongi* worms on the peritoneal side of the colon work their way through the bowel wall and cause tissue inflammation and lesions on the luminal side. This acute process can produce cramping, abdominal pain, and bloody diarrhea.

As the infection progresses, some eggs are retained in the bowel wall, inciting a granulomatous response with eventual fibrosis. As increasing fibrosis displaces normal bowel wall tissue, the contractile dysfunction of the colon can result in obstipation.

Hepatosplenic Disease

In chronic infections, usually due to *S. mansoni*, *S. japonicum*, and *S. mekongi*, some eggs fail to penetrate the intestine walls but instead are carried via the portal blood to the liver. Egg granulomas in the portal triad area progress to extensive hepatic fibrosis (pipestem fibrosis). The result is development of portal hypertension and its sequelae of passive splenic congestion, ascites, and esophageal varices. In endemic areas, death by exsanguination from bleeding esophageal varices is not uncommon in heavily infected individuals in the second and third decades of life. Interestingly, hepatocellular function is usually preserved, so aminotransferase levels in the blood may be normal even during severe portal hypertension.

Urinary Tract Disease

The passage of eggs through the bladder wall in *S. haematobium* infections can result in microscopic or gross hematuria. Granulomatous lesions of the urinary bladder, especially in the trigone area, contribute to the development of ureteral obstruction, with subsequent reflux, hydroureter, and chronic bacterial pyelonephritis. In endemic areas, chronic *S. haematobium* infections are associated with the development of squamous cell carcinoma of the bladder. If eggs penetrate the seminal vesicles, hematospermia may develop; in women egg expulsion may lead to lesions of the vagina or Bartholin glands.

Lung Disease

Eosinophilic pneumonitis results when eggs reaching the general circulation are trapped in the alveolar capillaries.

Skin Disease

Acute penetration of the skin by cercarial forms may cause a short-lived pruritic rash. In chronic infections, *S. mansoni* eggs reaching the general circulation may lodge in the skin and cause chronic egg dermatitis. In northern regions, patients may develop a rash when they become infected with avian schistosomiasis. Here, species of *Schistosoma* that have evolved to infect birds accidentally enter the skin of human bathers in freshwater lakes or ponds; they elicit an intensely pruritic rash ("swimmer's itch"), a condition discussed in Chapter 37.

Central Nervous System (CNS) Disease

Cases of acute transverse myelitis occurring after the initial 4- to 6-week incubation period have been reported in patients infected with *S. mansoni* and *S. haematobium*. Presumably, eggs or worm pairs gain access to the spinal cord through the venous drainage system of the lower abdomen, resulting in an acute inflammatory reaction where they lodge in the spinal cord. *S. japonicum* eggs carried in the circulation to the brain may be a significant cause of seizure disorders in the Far East.

Bacteremia

For reasons that are unclear, patients with schistosomiasis are at increased risk of recurrent bloodstream infection with bacteria in the *Salmonella enterica* family. Thus, schistosomiasis should always be considered in patients who present with this condition, starting with an exposure history.

Schistosomiasis in Pregnancy

Eggs lodging in the placenta may cause poor placental development and premature placental separation (Chapter 14).

Laboratory Studies

A definitive diagnosis can be made by identifying the schistosome eggs in samples of stool or urine submitted to the laboratory. The egg of each schistosome species has its own characteristic morphologic appearance and can be readily differentiated from the others. *S. mansoni* has a prominent lateral spine, *S. haematobium* has a terminal spine, and both *S. japonicum* and *S. mekongi* have a rudimentary lateral spine.

Eosinophilia of the peripheral blood may be present during the initial stages of clinical disease but is not a constant finding in late chronic infections.

Expatriates and travelers returning from schistosomiasis-endemic areas with CNS abnormalities should be studied by computed tomography (CT) or magnetic resonance imaging scan, and a diagnosis of neuroschistosomiasis should be considered, even in the absence of typical clinical features of acute schistosomiasis, and even if urine and stool examinations are negative.

Serologic testing with sensitive tests for schistosomiasis (Falcon assay screening test–enzyme-linked immunosorbent assay) and specific tests (immunoblot) for schistosomiasis is available from the Centers for Disease Control and Prevention (CDC) Parasitic Diseases Branch. Specimens for testing are submitted to the CDC through the state public health department, accompanied by a CDC medical history and request form (so that the correct immunoblot test can be performed based on the most likely species involved). The tests may be helpful to detect low-intensity infections in travelers, expatriates, and immigrants with a history of freshwater exposure in schistosomiasis-endemic areas who have negative stool and urine examinations. If the clinical picture and geographic history are strongly suggestive of schistosomiasis, but the stool or urine samples are negative for eggs, biopsies of inflamed areas of rectum or colon (via sigmoidoscopy or colonoscopy) or bladder (via cystoscopy) may reveal schistosome eggs retained in the tissues. The eggs may be seen in wet mounts of crushed tissue or histologically stained preparations of the biopsy specimens.

Treatment

Praziquantel is an oral drug and the only drug that is efficacious against all forms of schistosomiasis. Oxamniquine is an oral drug that has efficacy against *S. mansoni* infections only. It is contraindicated in patients with a history of seizures. Metrifonate is an oral drug that has efficacy against *S. haematobium* infections. Neither oxamniquine nor metrifonate is available in the United States.

Artemisinins exhibit antischistosomal properties as well as antimalarial activity. In preclinical studies, artemether administered at therapeutic doses for malaria in research mice infected with *S. mansoni* showed significantly lower worm burdens. Further epidemiologic studies in areas where malaria and schistosomiasis co-exist, and where artemisinin-based combination therapy (ACT) is being used for malaria control, may show that ACT has ancillary benefits against schistosomiasis and other trematode infections in humans.

Treatment of acute hypersensitivity syndromes (Katayama fever, acute transverse myelitis) is directed toward general systemic support of severely ill patients. Corticosteroids to decrease the inflammatory reaction to parasite antigens may be indicated.

Potentially exposed individuals should be counseled to watch for influenza-like symptoms 4-6 weeks following water exposure, because this could represent Katayama fever and should trigger prompt medical evaluation. Some travelers choose to treat themselves presumptively following return from endemic regions. If this is considered, it should be limited to those with symptoms or those who had a true freshwater exposure (swimming, rafting) and should be administered at least 6 weeks after the last exposure, because praziquantel is most effective against the adult worms, not their immature forms.

Prevention

Prevention consists of avoiding water contact or immersion in areas known to be endemic for schistosomiasis. If accidental water contact occurs, travelers should be counseled that rapid toweling to dry the skin may prevent parasite penetration but that this technique is far from perfect.

In endemic areas where water contact is unavoidable, annual mass drug administration (MDA) programs using praziquantel combined with environmental measures to control the snails and promote sanitary disposal of human waste must proceed concurrently to decrease the incidence and prevalence of the disease. In areas of overlapping disease endemicity, efforts to integrate schistosomiasis into other MDA programs against onchocerciasis and lymphatic filariasis by simultaneous administration of safe oral antihelminthic drugs (praziquantel, ivermectin, and albendazole) will promote optimal use of health services infrastructure in resource-poor economies.

For travelers, as noted above, a vaccine against schistosomiasis in humans is not available at the time of writing, although an irradiated cercarial vaccine against a bovine strain of schistosomiasis has been used in cattle in Africa with some success.

HEPATOBILIARY FLUKES: *CLONORCHIS* AND *OPISTHORCHIS*

Biliary fluke infections with *Clonorchis sinensis* or *Opisthorchis* species are common among people from Laos, Cambodia, Thailand, the southern People's Republic of China, Hong Kong, Korea, Japan, and the far-eastern regions of the Soviet Union.

Transmission

Humans acquire liver fluke infections from eating raw, undercooked, pickled, or smoked fish. Parasite eggs, passed in the feces, hatch in fresh water. The first intermediate hosts, snails, become infected and shed free-swimming cercariae into the water, which then infect fish and encyst in the muscles. After humans eat infected undercooked fish, the larvae (metacercariae) migrate up the bile duct and mature into adult worms. In addition to humans, definitive hosts for the liver flukes may be dogs, cats, pigs, badgers, and ducks, thus serving as reservoirs of infection in endemic areas.

Liver flukes mature in the hepatic biliary radicles, and the infection may be silent, although parasite adults induce ductal hyperplasia and fibrosis. The eggs in the bile exit the body via the fecal stream.

Clinical Features

The majority of chronically infected individuals are asymptomatic. For patients with heavy worm burdens, right upper quadrant abdominal pain and jaundice may be present.

Acute Biliary Obstruction

This is a surgical emergency occurring in late infections characterized by heavy parasite loads. Physical obstruction by numerous flukes and narrowed bile duct lumen secondary to fibrosis probably contribute to the condition. As with all kinds of acute biliary obstruction, restoration of bile flow may be important. However, in minor cases where acute surgical or endoscopic decompression is not necessary, treatment with praziquantel may be effective.

Acute Pancreatitis

Occasionally, the flukes migrate into the pancreatic ducts and cause obstruction and inflammation.

Recurrent Pyogenic Cholangitis

This is a clinical syndrome with fever, right upper quadrant pain, jaundice, and intrahepatic biliary gallstones. This infectious process is thought to be secondary to bacterial infection in the presence of fibrosis and foreign bodies in the biliary tree. While recurrent pyogenic cholangitis has not conclusively been shown to be caused by *C. sinensis* or *Opisthorchis* species, there is some epidemiologic and anatomic evidence to suggest that these flukes may be associated with this syndrome.

Cholangiocarcinoma

Primary biliary carcinoma is a relatively rare form of malignancy. However, an increased incidence has been found among people living in endemic areas for biliary fluke infection and may be related to chronic inflammation of the biliary tree.

Laboratory Studies

Infections are detected by finding the characteristic eggs in stool specimens. The eggs are among the smallest of parasite eggs and are more easily detected by stool concentration techniques.

The eggs of intestinal flukes *Metagonimus* and *Heterophyes* are relatively difficult to differentiate from the *Clonorchis* and *Opisthorchis* eggs. Fortunately, the drug of choice for biliary fluke infections is also the recommended treatment for intestinal fluke infections (**Table 48.2**).

In difficult cases of biliary obstruction, endoscopic retrograde cholangiopancreatography may be performed, with adult flukes and eggs recovered directly from the bile during the procedure.

TABLE 48.2   Drug Treatment of Human Fluke Infections

Parasite	Drug of Choice	Alternative Drugs
Blood flukes		
S. japonicum	Praziquantel: 60 mg/kg given orally in three divided doses 4-6 h apart on a single day	
S. mansoni	Praziquantel: 40 mg/kg given in two divided doses on a single day	
S. haematobium	Praziquantel: 40 mg/kg in two divided doses on a single day	
Hepatobiliary flukes		
Clonorchis sinensis, *Opisthorchis viverrini*	Praziquantel: 75 mg/kg given orally in three divided doses 4-6 h apart	Albendazole: 10 mg/kg × 7 days
Fasciola hepatica	Bithionol: 30-50 mg/kg per day given orally alternate days for 10-15 total doses	Triclabendazole: 10 mg/kg once or twice[a]
Lung flukes		
Paragonimus spp. (*P. westermani*, *P. heterotremus*, *P. skrjabini*)	Praziquantel: 75 mg/kg per day given orally in three divided doses 4-6 h apart on two consecutive days	
Intestinal flukes		
Metagonimus yokogawai, *Heterophyes heterophyes*, *Echinostoma* spp., *Fasciolopsis buski*	Praziquantel: 75 mg/kg given orally in three divided doses 4-6 h apart on a single day[b]	

[a]Not available for human use in the United States.
[b]Considered an investigational drug for this purpose.

Treatment

In light of the potentially serious consequences of long-term infection with liver flukes, even asymptomatic infections should be treated when they are detected. Praziquantel is the drug of choice and has been known to cure over 90% of infections after a single therapeutic dose (**Table 48.2**). Acute biliary obstruction due to liver flukes requires surgical decompression and drainage. Prevention of infection consists of eating only well-cooked fish. No vaccine is available, and reinfection is possible.

HEPATOBILIARY FLUKES: *FASCIOLA HEPATICA*

Fasciola hepatica is a large liver fluke that lives in the bile ducts of its mammalian hosts, which commonly include sheep and cattle. It is endemic in more than 40 countries, including those in Europe, North Africa, Asia, South America, and the Western Pacific.

Transmission

Parasite eggs passed in the feces hatch into miracidia, which infect freshwater snails. Cercaria emerge from the snails after 6-7 weeks and attach to aquatic plants where they encyst as metacercaria. Humans become infected from ingestion of contaminated aquatic plants, such as watercress, in sheep- and cattle-raising areas. After ingestion, the metacercaria penetrate the intestinal wall, enter the peritoneal cavity, and then penetrate through Glisson capsule into the liver.

Clinical Features

Acute Phase

This phase occurs during parasite migration from the duodenum to the liver via the peritoneal cavity. The classic symptoms and signs include right upper quadrant abdominal pain, fever, and hepatomegaly.

Chronic Phase

After reaching the hepatobiliary system, the chronic phase of the disease begins. Patients can develop cholangitis and cholecystitis, although it is not clear what percentage of patients progress to these complications. There is no association of *F. hepatica* with cholangiocarcinoma, as there is with *Clonorchis* and *Opisthorchis*, presumably because its smooth tegument elicits less inflammation of the biliary lining, but this is not certain.

Laboratory Studies

Diagnosis is made by finding the characteristic eggs in stool or duodenal aspirates. The sensitivity ranges widely depending on the microscopy technique, intensity of infection, and phase of infection (no egg secretion during the acute migration phase). Serologic tests are also available. Ultrasound and CT scan findings include linear hepatic tracks and a subcapsular location.

Treatment

Bithionol has been the first-line agent for fascioliasis at a dose of 30-50 mg/kg on alternate days for 10-15 doses (**Table 48.2**). It is considered an investigational drug in the United States and must be obtained from the CDC. Unfortunately, it is no longer manufactured, and only limited supplies are currently available. While praziquantel is effective for most trematode infections, treatment of fascioliasis has been only partially successful. Investigational alternatives to bithionol include triclabendazole, nitazoxanide, emetine (cardiac toxicity), niclofolan, metronidazole, and albendazole. Triclabendazole has become the drug of choice in many regions of the world but is not commercially available in the United States.

LUNG FLUKES

Chronic pulmonary infection with *Paragonimus westermani* and related species can mimic pulmonary tuberculosis, and the diagnosis should be considered in "atypical" cases of tuberculosis that do not seem to respond to standard chemotherapy (Chapter 25).

Paragonimiasis is endemic in areas where freshwater crab, crawfish, or shrimp are eaten raw, pickled, or undercooked. The infection is worldwide in distribution, with cases reported from Asia, South America, and Africa. A lung fluke infection acquired in California was documented in a man who ate "drunken" crab (dunked live in alcohol then swallowed); however, most cases seen in North America are imported infections among immigrant and refugee populations from Asia and Southeast Asia.

Transmission
Adult flukes live in the lungs of humans and other mammals, such as cats, dogs, minks, and opossums. The worms lay eggs that are coughed up in the sputum or swallowed and then passed in the feces. The eggs hatch in fresh water and develop into miracidia that infect freshwater snails. The infection in snails produces cercariae, which then infect freshwater crabs, crawfish, or prawns. The encysted parasites at this stage are called metacercariae and are in the muscle, viscera, and gills. When raw or inadequately cooked crabs, crawfish, or prawns are eaten by humans and other mammals, the parasites excyst in the small intestine, penetrate the bowel wall, and migrate through the peritoneum, diaphragm, and pleura until they reach the lung parenchyma. In the lungs, the larvae mature into adult flukes and start the lifecycle over again.

Clinical Features

Pulmonary Paragonimiasis
While hemoptysis, dyspnea, and chest pain are the classic presenting symptoms, light pulmonary infections may be completely asymptomatic. Symptoms often develop 6 months to several years after infection. On chest radiography, parenchymal lesions of the lung, including segmental or diffuse infiltrates, nodules, cavities, or "ring" cysts, may be seen. Less frequently, the radiographic appearance is that of a pleural effusion. Peripheral eosinophilia is commonly present.

Extrapulmonary Paragonimiasis
Around 30% of patients present with extrapulmonary features thought to result from ectopic migration of excysted larvae from the bowel. Involved locations include the skin, liver, kidney, peritoneum, epididymis, spinal cord, and brain. The most serious complications from lesions involving the brain include seizures, headache, motor deficits, and visual disturbances. Subcutaneous nodules are a distinct feature of *Paragonimus skrjabini* infections found in China. The nodules range in size from a few millimeters to several centimeters and are often migratory.

Laboratory Studies
The diagnosis of paragonimiasis can be made by identification of the characteristic operculated eggs in specimens of sputum or stool. Sputum concentration techniques on 24-hour sputum specimen collections may be helpful in recovering eggs when random sputum specimens are negative. Eggs present in sputum specimens may be destroyed by Gram stain or acid-fast staining techniques, so the microbiology laboratory must be alerted when specimens are being submitted for parasitologic examination.

If the sputum or stool specimen is submitted to a laboratory that does not regularly do parasitologic examinations, the eggs of *Paragonimus* species may be misinterpreted as *Diphyllobothrium latum* eggs. If *D. latum* is reported in a specimen from an immigrant or refugee patient, the clinician should ask for a review of the specimen by a consulting parasitologist. Complement fixation and immunoblot tests are available and may be helpful in establishing the diagnosis in patients from endemic areas with radiographic lesions and nondiagnostic sputum studies.

Treatment
The drug of choice in the treatment of this infection is praziquantel, a total of 150 mg/kg given orally in divided doses over two consecutive days (75 mg/kg per day) (**Table 48.1**).

Adverse effects associated with drug treatment include nausea on the days of medication and urticaria during the week following medication (presumed to be a hypersensitivity reaction to antigen released by dead and dying parasites). Bithionol was previously used for the treatment of paragonimiasis (**Table 48.2**) but is considered an investigational drug in the United States and can be obtained only from the CDC. In addition, bithionol treatment failures have been noted in Southeast Asians with lung fluke infections.

INTESTINAL FLUKES

Endemic areas for the intestinal flukes *Metagonimus yokogawai* and *Heterophyes heterophyes* include countries in the Far East (Japan, China, Taiwan, eastern Siberia, Korea, the Philippines, and Thailand), where humans acquire infections from eating raw or undercooked fish. *Metagonimus* infections have also been reported from Israel, Romania, and Spain, and *Heterophyes* infections from India, Egypt, and Tunisia. The lifecycle of the organism is similar to that of *Clonorchis sinensis* and *Opisthorchis* species, except for the anatomic residence of the adult flukes in the intestines instead of the biliary tract.

Fasciolopsis buski is a relatively large intestinal fluke that is acquired in the Far East from ingestion of parasite cysts attached to aquatic plants, such as water chestnuts, contaminated by feces from infected mammals (pigs, humans). Human infection with *Echinostoma* species can be found in Indonesia, the Philippines, Taiwan, and Thailand. Transmission occurs via ingestion of infected snails, fish, or vegetables.

Clinical Features

Light infections with intestinal flukes are often asymptomatic. Persons with heavy infections may present with abdominal pain, chronic diarrhea, anorexia, nausea, and weight loss. Rarely, extraintestinal lesions may result from ectopic migration of larvae or from eggs gaining access to the circulation and being deposited in ectopic sites.

Laboratory Studies

Diagnosis can be made by finding the characteristic parasite eggs in submitted stool samples. No diagnostic serologic tests are available.

Treatment

The treatment of choice is praziquantel (**Table 48.2**). Tetrachloroethylene, a drug not available for human use in the United States, is often used in developing countries because of its low cost.

FURTHER READING

Harinasuta, T., Pungpak, S., Keystone, J., 1993. Trematode infections: opisthorchiasis, clonorchiasis, fascioliasis, and paragonimiasis. Inf. Dis. Clin. N. Am. 7, 699–716.
A comprehensive review of liver and lung fluke infections by authors with extensive clinical experience.

Kilpatrick, M.E., Farid, Z., Bassily, S., et al., 1981. Treatment of *Schistosomiasis mansoni* with oxamniquine—five years' experience. Am. J. Trop. Med. Hyg. 30, 1219–1222.
Oxamniquine is a drug that is not commonly used outside schistosomiasis-endemic areas.

Nagayasu, E., Yoshida, A., Hombu, A., et al., 2015. Paragonimiasis in Japan: a twelve year retrospective case review (2001–2012). Intern. Med. 54, 179–186.
Paragonimiasis in Japan decreased in the 1970s, possibly as a result of increased public awareness of food-borne risks, but reemerged in the 1980s. Immigrants from other parts of Asia (China, Thailand, Korea) accounted for one-fourth of the cases in this retrospective case review and acquired their infections from eating raw freshwater crabs. Cases in resident Japanese citizens tended to be from one region and were acquired by eating fresh wild boar meat or freshwater crabs.

Olsen, A., 2007. Efficacy and safety of drug combinations in the treatment of schistosomiasis, soil-transmitted helminthiasis, lymphatic filariasis and onchocerciasis. Trans. R. Soc. Trop. Med. Hyg. 101, 747–758.
Co-infection with multiple parasites is common in tropical rural environments; efficacy and safety of drug combinations against multiple parasites is an important consideration for treatment programs where access to health care is limited.

Schwartz, D.A., 1986. Cholangiocarcinoma associated with liver fluke infection: a preventable source of morbidity in Asian immigrants. Am. J. Gastroenterol. 81, 76–79.
Liver flukes can live for a decade or two (or more) in human hosts, so it is worthwhile to screen for liver fluke infection among Asian immigrants from endemic areas, even if they left years before, and to treat all infections detected.

Sharma, O.P., 1989. The man who loved drunken crabs: a case of pulmonary paragonimiasis. Chest 953, 670–672.
Paragonimiasis acquired in the United States by a Los Angeles dock worker who loved to eat drunken crabs with his international co-workers.

Utzinger, J., Xiao, S.H., Tanner, M., et al., 2007. Artemisinins for schistosomiasis and beyond. Curr. Opin. Investig. Drugs 8, 105–116.
A relatively limited menu of drugs available to treat parasitic infections and emerging drug resistance among parasites fuels the search for new combinations and new uses for antiparasitic drugs already in use. This article explores the use of artemesinins in the treatment of malaria and schistosomiasis.

Wright, R.S., Jean, M., Rochelle, K., et al., 2011. Chylothorax caused by *Paragonimus westermani* in a native Californian. Chest 140, 1064–1066.
The patient acquired P. westermani by eating imported live raw crabs from Asia in California sushi restaurants. Food-borne trematode infections in non-endemic areas will become an increasing problem in the future due to the growth of international seafood markets.

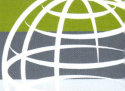

CHAPTER 49

The Eosinophilic Patient with Suspected Parasitic Infection

Martin S. Wolfe

Elevations of the peripheral blood absolute eosinophil count (>450 eosinophils/mm³) can occur in a wide variety of clinical situations, including parasitic infections, allergic states, collagen vascular diseases, hypereosinophilic syndromes, and other miscellaneous disorders (**Table 49.1**). The immunobiology of eosinophils is thoroughly described in Weller (1997). The absolute eosinophil count is a more reliable indicator of the presence of eosinophilia than is the relative eosinophil count (percentage of eosinophils), the normal level of which is less than 6%. For example, a person with a total white blood cell count of 4000 and a relative eosinophil count of 9% has an absolute eosinophil count of 360, which is not elevated.

CLINICAL FEATURES

Eosinophilia in a traveler returning from long-term residence or visit to the developing world or in an immigrant or refugee from a tropical area should first suggest the possible presence of a helminthic infection. Although eosinophilia particularly suggests presence of a helminth, the absence of eosinophilia cannot exclude these parasites. With a few notable exceptions, protozoan and other infections are seldom associated with eosinophilia, and as noted above, non-infectious etiologies must always be considered.

Eosinophil counts are generally higher in the early acute invasive phase than in chronic helminthic infections, particularly during initial infection with the parasite in a non-immune individual, and there may be considerable variation in the person-to-person response to the same helminth. Eosinophilia in the presence of a helminthic infection may be considered to be an adaptive increase in the number of eosinophilic cells available to damage the parasite. In addition, eosinophilia under these circumstances may be associated with qualitative changes in the eosinophils themselves.

The greatest number of tissue and blood eosinophils are found in infections in which the association of the parasite with host tissue is closest, that is, those with migrating larvae or extended retention of parasite lifecycle stages in tissue. Especially high eosinophil levels may be found in *Ascaris* pneumonia, strongyloidiasis, filariasis, tropical pulmonary eosinophilia, and acute schistosomiasis. Another situation leading to high eosinophilia is when humans become accidentally infected with parasites whose definitive host (host in which sexual maturity and reproduction of the parasite takes place) is in another animal species. The "lost" larval stages wander in the tissues until they die or become encysted; examples of such infections are trichinosis and visceral larva migrans (toxocariasis caused by dog and cat roundworm species). Intestinal helminths that remain in the bowel lumen and do not invade the intestinal mucosa (e.g., adult *Ascaris* and tapeworms) cause minor or no eosinophilia. Increased eosinophilia can develop after drug treatment of helminths, and it may take several months for elevated eosinophil levels to return to normal after initial parasite destruction.

TABLE 49.1   Less Common Causes of Eosinophilia

Rare Parasites
  Capillaria hepatica
  Fasciolopsis buski
  Spirometra (sparganosis)
  Anisakiasis
Skin Diseases
  Eczema
  Dermatitis herpetiformis
  Eosinophilic cellulitis (Wells syndrome)
Malignancy
  Eosinophilic leukemia
  Myelogenous leukemia
  Hodgkins disease and other lymphomas
  Carcinoma of the bowel, ovary, lung, pancreas, and other solid organs
Collagen Vascular Disease
  Polyarteritis nodosa
  Dermatomyositis
  Rheumatoid arthritis
Hypereosinophilic Syndromes
  Löffler eosinophilic endomyocarditis
  Löffler pulmonary syndrome
  Pulmonary infiltration with eosinophilia
  Eosinophilic gastroenteritis
  Eosinophilic granuloma
Other
  Drug reactions
  Allergic disorders
  Hypersensitivity pneumonitis
  Wegener granulomatosis
  Inflammatory bowel disease
  Pernicious anemia
  Eosinophilia-myalgia syndrome
  Sarcoidosis
  Hypoadrenalism

Reprinted from: Jong, E.C. (Ed.), 1999. Medical Clinics of North America: Travel Medicine. W.B. Saunders, Philadelphia, 83, p. 4.

DIAGNOSIS

The diagnosis of common intestinal helminths is usually made by finding the characteristic egg or larva in stool specimens submitted for microscopic examination. Clinical recognition and diagnosis of extraintestinal or disseminated parasites may be more difficult. If the stool examinations do not suggest a likely diagnosis, the following approach is suggested in the work-up of the patient with suspected parasite infection.

1. The *geographic or travel history* of the patient with eosinophilia may indicate a past exposure to parasites. Because the patient with tissue stage parasites can have either multiple systemic symptoms or few clinical symptoms to report, and often will have negative stool examinations for ova and parasites, the geographic history is of prime importance. For instance, the history of swimming in freshwater lakes or rivers in endemic areas of Africa, South America, or Asia should suggest the possibility of schistosomiasis.

2. In the immunocompromised patient with fever, pneumonia, or central nervous system (CNS) signs, *Strongyloides* should be considered even in the absence of eosinophilia.
3. The history of exposure to pets, livestock, and wild animals or mosquito bites in rural areas may provide valuable clues to potential parasite exposure (e.g., filariasis, toxocariasis, cutaneous larva migrans, echinococcosis).
4. The history of eating exotic or raw, smoked, pickled, or undercooked food may provide additional clues to past opportunities for parasite exposure (e.g., liver and intestinal flukes, paragonimiasis, trichinosis, cysticercosis, anisakiasis, angiostrongyliasis, gnathostomiasis).

The diagnosis of a parasitic etiology for hypereosinophilia in a given patient is important for the following reasons:

1. Specific antiparasitic treatment may be indicated.
2. Prolonged hypereosinophilia can have uncomfortable and potentially life-threatening sequelae (pruritic skin rashes, painful subcutaneous swellings, endomyocardial fibrosis, and so forth).
3. The prompt search for other etiologies of hypereosinophilia may be indicated (e.g., allergy, occult tumor, leukemia, connective tissue disease, sarcoidosis, hypereosinophilic syndrome).

LABORATORY STUDIES IN EOSINOPHILIA

It is important to consider the long prepatent period of many helminth infections before the appearance of eggs or larvae in the stool or other body fluids or tissue. For intestinal helminths and protozoa, a series of three stool examinations (one every other day) should be collected in a preservative and examined by direct, concentration, and stained slide methods. Examinations of small bowel fluid taken via nasogastric tube or endoscopy, the string test (Enterotest), or small bowel biopsy may be required to confirm infection with *Strongyloides stercoralis*, hookworms, liver flukes, *Trichostrongylus* species, or the protozoan *Isospora belli*. Rectal biopsy has been used to diagnose cryptic cases of schistosomiasis species, including *Schistosoma haematobium*.

Filariasis infections of the blood can be diagnosed by concentration or microfilter examinations of blood taken at midday for all species except *Wuchereria bancrofti*, whose nocturnal periodicity makes midnight blood specimens optimal. A provocative challenge with a daytime dose of 100 mg of diethylcarbamazine and drawing blood 1 hour later can increase the number of *W. bancrofti* microfilariae to approximate midnight blood levels. For skin filariae, skin snips or biopsy specimens often reveal microfilariae (Chapter 47).

Sputum examination is useful in the detection of *Paragonimus* eggs and occasionally *Strongyloides* or *Ascaris* larvae. Eosinophils and Charcot-Leyden crystals in the sputum can suggest a pulmonary helminth larval migration, asthma and other nonparasitic allergic disorders, or a hypereosoniphilic syndrome. Eosinophilic pleural effusion can signify a pulmonary parasitic infection and various other causes of systemic and pulmonary eosinophilia.

The presence of eosinophils in the cerebrospinal fluid (CSF) is such an uncommon finding that it is most often the result of certain helminthic infections of the CNS. Parasitic infections to be considered in a returnee from the tropics with this finding include gnathostomiasis, cerebral cysticercosis, schistosomiasis, paragonimiasis, echinococcosis, and angiostrongyliasis. On the other hand, the absence of eosinophils in the CSF cannot rule out a CNS helminthic infection. Nonparasitic causes of CSF eosinophilia include tuberculosis, syphilis, coccidioidomycosis, viral infection, malignancy, and drug hypersensitivity, among others.

Charcot-Leyden crystals in the stool can be seen with a range of parasitic and noninfectious causes of bowel diseases. These crystals are hallmarks of eosinophil involvement in some tissue reactions. They are seen in amebic dysentery, and although not necessarily diagnostic, they may constitute a useful indicator. Charcot-Leyden crystals are also seen in the stool of patients with *Trichuris trichiura* and *I. belli* infections as well as in those with ulcerative colitis and carcinoma of the colon. They may also be seen in granulomas associated with tissue-invading helminths.

TABLE 49.2   Parasite Serologic Tests Useful in Evaluation of Eosinophilia

Disease	Test	Test Laboratory[a]
Toxocariasis	ELISA	CDC
Strongyloidiasis	ELISA	CDC
Filariasis	ELISA	NIH
Trichinosis	BFT, CIE, ELISA	State public health department
Cysticercosis	ELISA, Immunoblot	CDC
Schistosomiasis	ELISA, Immunoblot	CDC
Paragonimiasis	ELISA	CDC
Fascioliasis	ELISA	University of Puerto School of Medicine, Department of Pathology and Laboratory Medicine, Dr. George Hillyer
Gnathostomiasis	Immunoblot	Faculty of Tropical Medicine, Mahidol University, Bangkok, Thailand (Dr. Wanpen Chaicunpa, e-mail: tmwcc@mahidol.ac.th)

[a]Serum specimens are sent to the Centers for Disease Control (CDC) via the state public health department. Before serum specimens will be accepted for testing by the CDC, the clinician must furnish sufficient clinical and epidemiologic data to justify the request for the test. Depending on the suspected diagnosis, attempts must be made to make the diagnosis by prior laboratory testing, including (1) complete blood counts, (2) stool and/or urine specimens for ova and parasite examinations (strongyloidiasis, cysticercosis, schistosomiasis, paragonimiasis), (3) skin or tissue biopsies as appropriate (filariasis, trichinosis, cysticercosis), and (4) isolation of the parasite from blood by filtration or concentration techniques (filariasis). Similar serologic tests may be offered by commercial laboratories.
BFT, Bentonite flocculation; CDC, Centers for Disease Control and Prevention; CIE, counter immunoelectrophoresis; ELISA, enzyme-linked immunosorbent assay; NIH, National Institutes of Health.

Radiologic examinations are useful diagnostic aids. Chest radiographs can give evidence for pulmonary invasive infections such as migrating *Ascaris* and *Strongyloides* larvae, paragonimiasis, acute schistosomiasis, hydatid cyst, and tropical pulmonary eosinophilia. Ultrasound studies or computed tomography scans of the liver can identify lesions that are suggestive of early prepatent liver fluke infections or hydatid cyst. Soft tissue radiographs can identify calcified cysticerci. Radiographic imaging studies (computed tomography, magnetic resonance imaging) of the brain can reveal the presence of lesions compatible with invasive cerebral parasites such as cysticercosis, hydatid cyst, paragonimiasis, and schistosomiasis.

Serologic tests, not all commercially available, can provide evidence for the presence of particular helminth infections. Serologic tests are available from the Centers for Disease Control and Prevention (CDC) for strongyloidiasis, trichinosis, cysticercosis, schistosomiasis, paragonimiasis, toxocariasis, and echinococcosis. Serum and tissue specimens are submitted to the CDC through the state public health department or through direct consultation with CDC parasitology consultants (http://www.cdc.gov). Filariasis serology may be obtained from the Laboratory of Parasitic Diseases of the National Institutes of Health. *Fasciola hepatica* serology is performed at the University of Puerto Rico. A reliable gnathostomiasis test is available at the Department of Tropical Medicine, Mahidol University, Bangkok, Thailand (**Table 49.2**).

SPECIFIC INFECTIONS

Helminths

Ascariasis

In the early stage of *Ascaris* infection, before eggs are present in the stool, larvae migrate through the lungs. Although often unrecognized clinically, the larvae can cause a Löffler-like pneumonia, characterized by hypereosinophilia and pulmonary infiltrates and presenting with cough, dyspnea, and malaise. The pathogenesis is believed to be a hypersensitivity response to highly allergenic components of *Ascaris* larvae. The most reliable diagnostic criterion is the finding of typical third-stage larvae in the sputum or gastric aspirate of suspected patients.

Most patients with established intestinal ascariasis are asymptomatic. Young children with heavy infections may develop intestinal obstruction. *Ascaris* infections produce a higher blood eosinophil count in children than in adults, in whom infections are associated with a mild eosinophilia. Infection is usually self-limited within 3 years. Diagnosis is by finding typical eggs on stool examination. Treatment is with mebendazole or albendazole (Chapter 48).

Strongyloidiasis

Infection with *Strongyloides stercoralis* is primarily from penetration of the exposed skin by infective stage larvae. Developing larvae migrate through the lungs and eventually reach the small bowel where they mature. Female worms invade the intestinal mucosa and deposit eggs, which hatch and liberate rhabdoid larvae. These larvae may then be passed in the feces, or they may develop within the lumen of the bowel into infective larvae that can autoinfect the carrier. Infections may therefore be long lived, 40 years or more in some cases.

Some infections are asymptomatic, but others may cause abdominal pain, intermittent diarrhea, asthma, or patchy pneumonitis. Urticaria may occur primarily on the buttocks and thighs, and creeping eruption may be present. Debilitated or immunocompromised patients may develop a lethal hyperinfection syndrome. Eosinophilia is often strikingly high in the earlier years of infection, although in long-established infections eosinophilia may be normal. Patients with the hyperinfection syndrome usually have a normal level of eosinophils. Diagnosis is by finding larvae in the stool, and often repeated special larval concentration tests are required. When strongyloidiasis is suspected and larvae cannot be found in the stool, duodenal fluid should be examined. An enzyme-linked immunosorbent assay (ELISA) serologic test (available at the CDC) is useful in making a presumptive diagnosis. Treatment is with ivermectin (Chapter 48).

Hookworm

Hookworm infection was the most common cause of eosinophilia in returned Vietnam veterans. It was also the most common intestinal helminthic cause of eosinophilia in Caucasians returning from the tropics to the United Kingdom. In 128 Indochinese refugees in the United States with persistent eosinophilia greater than $500/mm^3$ for whom initial comprehensive routine screening had failed to yield an explanation, hookworm and *S. stercoralis* were among the potentially pathogenic intestinal parasites most frequently implicated (55% and 38%, respectively).

In the early stage of hookworm infection, pulmonary symptoms and hypereosinophilia may be present. Most established imported hookworm infections seen in temperate areas are with relatively few worms, and anemia does not occur. But vague upper abdominal pain and nausea may be present. Heavy infections are required to cause hookworm anemia. Eosinophilia is usually less than $1500/mm^3$ but may reach $2500-3000/mm^3$. Infections are self-limited within 3 years. Diagnosis is by finding eggs in the stool. Treatment is with mebendazole or albendazole (Chapter 48).

Whipworm (Trichuris trichiura)

Whipworm is a relatively commonly diagnosed intestinal helminth in travelers, most of whom have light, asymptomatic infections. Heavily infected children who are natives of endemic areas may have diarrhea, anemia, or rectal prolapse. The majority of cases in travelers have normal eosinophil counts, but levels of up to $1500/mm^3$ may occur. This worm does not have a pulmonary migration stage, and infections seldom last more than 2 or 3 years. Diagnosis is by finding typical eggs on stool examination. Treatment is with mebendazole or albendazole (Chapter 48).

Trichostrongyliasis

Trichostrongyliasis, caused by various *Trichostrongylus* species, is particularly common in the Far East and Near East. Infections are usually light, and symptoms are unusual. Rarely, hypereosinophilia may be present, but in most cases infection is light, and eosinophils may be normal. Some infections may last for up to 8 years. Diagnosis is by finding typical eggs, which resemble but are larger than hookworms, either in the stool or in duodenal contents. Treatment is with pyrantel pamoate, mebendazole, or albendazole.

Pinworms

Infections with *Enterobius vermicularis* is more commonly present in young children, and prevalence is higher in temperate than in tropical climates. It is not well appreciated that pinworms may cause a low-grade eosinophilia. Diagnosis is by the examination of cellophane tape applied to the anus on arising in the morning and before bathing; the tape is placed sticky-side down on a glass slide and a search is made for eggs. Only 10-15% of those with pinworms pass eggs in stool. Treatment is with mebendazole, albendazole, or pyrantel pamoate (Chapter 48).

Trichinosis

Trichinosis infection usually occurs from ingestion of raw or undercooked pork products or from undercooked bear or walrus meat. Trichinosis has a worldwide distribution but is more frequently acquired in temperate than in tropical climates, and it is a rarely reported imported infection in the United States. Two outbreaks were reported in immigrant Thais in New York City. Thais can safely eat raw pork in Thailand where pigs are relatively trichinosis-free, but they probably lacked knowledge of the danger of eating raw pork in the United States.

Initial symptoms of trichinosis infection during the immediate period after ingestion are primarily diarrhea and abdominal pain, which usually precede the appearance of eosinophilia. In the second or third week after infection, penetration of muscle by larvae occurs, and the classic clinical picture of high eosinophilia (which can reach $\geq 7000/mm^3$), myalgias, peri-orbital edema, and fever appears. Definitive diagnosis is by biopsy of an involved muscle, pressing the tissue specimen between two glass slides, and microscopic examination to identify the larvae. Indirect evidence of infection can be made by specific serologic tests, but these may not become positive until about 4 weeks after infection. Severe infection can be treated with steroids and mebendazole or albendazole.

Visceral Larva Migrans

Infection occurs from ingestion of eggs of the dog or cat roundworms, *Toxocara canis* and *Toxocara cati*, usually in children who eat dirt contaminated by the feces of these domestic animals. Most cases seen in the United States are acquired domestically, although the risk of infection is present worldwide. The disease syndrome, visceral larva migrans, can then develop with the prolonged migration of parasitic larval forms in the internal organs. A child with a history of pica presenting hepatomegaly and pneumonitis must be considered to possibly have this syndrome. Infections are often self-limited, but deaths have been reported. Rarely, larvae may localize in the eye, and consideration must be given to their presence in the differential diagnosis of malignant tumor of the eye in young children, to avoid needless enucleation. Specific diagnosis requires identification of larvae from sputum or hepatic granulomas; an ELISA serologic test is also available. Drugs of choice are meben-dazole or albendazole.

Gnathostomiasis

Gnathostoma spinigerum and other *Gnathostoma* species cause illnesses similar to visceral larva migrans and creeping eruption. Gnathostomiasis in humans occurs in Thailand, Japan, China, Vietnam, and East Africa. The definitive hosts for *Gnathostoma* species include dogs, cats, tigers, lions, leopards, minks, and raccoons. Humans are accidentally infected with interme-diate larval forms of this animal nematode by eating infected raw undercooked freshwater fish, eels, frogs, and snakes. If chicken and pigs have eaten infected fish, humans can acquire the infection from eating undercooked chicken and pork.

If intermediate hosts of *Gnathostoma* are eaten, encysted larvae in the muscle or connective tissue undergo excystation in the stomach of the new animal. The larvae then migrate in the internal organs or subcutaneous tissues. Symptoms of disease depend on the route of the larval migrations. Acute larval migration is accompanied by nausea, vomiting, pruritus, urticaria, and abdominal discomfort. Peripheral blood eosinophilia may be as high as 90%. The larval migrations usually go to the subcutaneous tissues after the acute phase, causing transitory subcutaneous swelling accompanied by local erythema, pruritus, and discomfort. Larval migration into the CNS is a serious complication and is in the differential diagnosis of eosinophilic myeloencephalitis. Diagnosis is made by identification of the parasite in biopsy specimens. A serological test may be available through consultation with medical scientists at Mahidol University in Bangkok, Thailand. Albendazole, 400 mg twice a day for 21 days, has been used as an effective tissue larvicidal agent for cutaneous gnathostomiasis.

Cerebral Angiostrongyliasis

In April 2000, 10 tourists from Chicago and other US cities developed symptoms and signs of meningitis a median of 10 days after leaving Jamaica, West Indies. Serology indicated that *Angiostrongylus cantonensis* was the etiologic agent. Eight of the tourists required hospitalization.

In the last 50 years, *Angiostrongylus cantonensis*, the rat lungworm, which is the most common cause of eosinophilic meningitis, has spread from Southeast Asia to the South Pacific, Africa, India, the Caribbean, and recently to Australia and North America. The primary mode of spread has been via rats on cargo ships. Infection in humans is acquired by eating snails or food items (prawns, crabs, vegetables) contaminated by the mucus of infected slugs, land snails, aquatic snails, or planarians. The definitive host is the rat, where the adult rat lungworms live in the pulmonary arteries and the right heart.

When humans become accidentally infected through contaminated food, the larvae migrate to the CNS and cause eosinophilic meningitis. The eyes also may be involved. The severe illness, lasting 2-4 weeks, either ends in death or becomes dormant with residual CNS findings (focal neurologic defects, cognitive impairment, blindness). People with light infections may spontaneously recover without neurologic residua. Diagnosis is made by identifying the parasite in the CSF or brain tissue.

There is no specific drug treatment recommended for this infection. Cautious removal of CSF at 3- to 7-day intervals, which causes marked improvement of headache, is advised until there is clinical and laboratory improvement. In severe cases, corticosteroids are used to reduce cerebral pressure. Although *A. cantonensis* is susceptible to multiple antihelmintic agents, including thiabendazole and mebendazole, these agents should not be used, since they can cause clinical deterioration or death from inflammation due to dead or dying worms in the brain.

Filariasis

The most common diagnosed blood filaria infection in returnees to North America and the United Kingdom from Africa is caused by *Loa loa*. This parasite is present primarily in the rain forests of West and Central Africa. The incubation period is 12 months or longer, and adult worms can live for 15 years or more. Classic symptoms are recurrent swellings (Calabar swellings) on the dorsa of the hands and forearms and on the lower limbs, which last 2-3 days, and movement of the adult worm across the conjunctiva. Eosinophilia may reach 5000-8000/mm^3, but the level may vary from time to time.

Mansonella perstans is also present throughout tropical Africa and has been one of the most frequently diagnosed filarial infections in the United Kingdom. There is some controversy regarding the pathogenicity of this parasite; symptoms associated with infection include abdominal pain, allergic symptoms, fever, headache, and exhaustion. Significant eosinophilia is frequently present in *M. perstans* infections.

The most common filaria infection worldwide is bancroftian filariasis, caused by *Wuchereria bancrofti*. Expatriates are rarely infected; the few cases seen are usually in longer-term expatriate residents or in natives of endemic areas, who have the prolonged, heavy exposure necessary for infection. In the acute stage of infection, symptoms are related to allergic inflammatory reactions to adult worms in the lymphatics and include recurrent swelling and tenderness of the genital organs and extremities, fever, chills, malaise, and headaches. After many years of infection, chronic elephantiasis of the limb or scrotum can occur, but it is virtually unheard of for an expatriate to develop these gross deformities. Eosinophilia in the range of 1000-2500/mm^3 or higher is a prominent characteristic in the acute stage of infection, but eosinophils may well be normal in chronic infections.

Brugia malayi occurs only in Asia, and symptoms are similar to those of *W. bancrofti*. *B. malayi* is rarely diagnosed in expatriates. Eosinophilia is common in the acute stage. *Mansonella ozzardi* occurs in tropical areas of Central and South America and on some Caribbean islands. Only a few cases of this infection have been documented in expatriates. Infections are usually asymptomatic, but eosinophilia commonly occurs.

Diagnosis of all forms of blood filariasis is by finding typical microfilariae in blood concentration tests. Most cases also have a positive filariasis serologic test. Treatment of all species of blood filariae is with diethylcarbamazine except for *M. perstans*, for which albendazole or mebendazole is recommended (Chapter 47).

Two species that cause filariasis, *Onchocerca volvulus* and *Mansonella streptocerca*, are parasites of the skin. The former occurs throughout tropical Africa, in a small area of the Yemen, and in parts of Central and South America and is, along with *Loa loa*, the most commonly diagnosed form of filariasis in North America and the United Kingdom. Only a few cases of *M. streptocerca* have been described in expatriates. Symptoms of both parasites include maculopapular pruritic rash, occurring most commonly on the buttocks, thighs, and trunk, and, less commonly, unilateral limb swelling. *O. volvulus* may also cause subcutaneous nodules and, in long-standing heavy infections in natives, may cause blindness. Blindness from this infection is almost unheard of in expatriates. Significant eosinophilia, often exceeding 5000/mm^3, is common with these parasites; in expatriates eosinophilia may be present with only minimal cutaneous lesions. Diagnosis is by finding microfilaria in skin snips or biopsy specimens taken from affected areas. The filariasis serologic test is usually positive. In suspected cases in which microfilariae cannot be found, administration of 50-100 mg of diethylcarbamazine (the Mazzotti test) almost invariably leads to an exacerbation of cutaneous symptoms and a rise in eosinophilia, strongly suggesting infection. Treatment is with ivermectin, which does not destroy adult worms and must be administered approximately yearly for the lifespan of the worms (12-14 years) (Chapter 47).

Tropical pulmonary eosinophilia is a disease syndrome related to occult infection with animal or human filariae and is most prevalent in South and Southeast Asia. It is particularly common in Indians, even outside India. The syndrome results when adult worms produce microfilariae, which are destroyed primarily in the lungs by an intense tissue reaction; this hypersensitive immune reaction leads to pulmonary symptoms, radiologic changes, lymphadenopathy, a positive filariasis serology test, and hypereosinophilia with leukocytosis. Characteristic symptoms are a nocturnal paroxysmal cough, asthma, fatigue, and low-grade fever. Diagnostic differentiation from other forms of eosinophilia present in the tropics is made on the basis of several major criteria: typical pulmonary symptoms, peripheral eosinophilia of 3000/mm^3 or greater, positive filarial serology, and response of the symptoms to diethylcarbamazine.

Cestode (Tapeworm) Infections

Intestinal cestode infections give rise to eosinophilia less commonly than nematode or trematode infections. Perhaps the most commonly diagnosed cestode is *Taenia saginata*, the beef tapeworm, contracted from eating raw or undercooked beef. Infection is particularly common in Africa but occurs worldwide. Patients are usually asymptomatic but may occasionally describe vague abdominal discomfort. Infection is often initially manifested by the spontaneous passage per anus of motile tapeworm segments. *Taenia solium*, the pork tapeworm, also has a worldwide distribution wherever raw or undercooked pork is eaten. The mature intestinal tapeworm usually causes no symptoms, and intact segments are usually not passed. When humans ingest viable *T. solium* eggs or, more rarely, regurgitate eggs into the stomach after vomiting, however, cysticercosis of the muscles and brain can occur. *Hymenolepis nana*, or dwarf tapeworm, is common in drier parts of the world; humans become infected by ingesting eggs. Most infections are asymptomatic, but abdominal pain and diarrhea may result. *Diphyllobothrium latum*, the fish tapeworm, occurs primarily in northern climates, and infection results from eating certain fish raw or undercooked. Infections are usually asymptomatic.

Diagnosis of all these tapeworm infections is by finding eggs in the stool or by identification of gravid proglottids in the stool or passed spontaneously. Characteristic calcified cysticerci can be seen on radiographic film in cysticercosis, but these do not occur before 5-10 years after infection. Eosinophilia of up to $1000/mm^3$ occurs in about half of *T. saginata* infections. A mild eosinophilia is also common in *H. nana*, *D. latum*, and intestinal *T. solium* infections. Eosinophilia has been described in the invasive stage of cysticercosis, and in cerebral cysticercosis with meningeal inflammation, eosinophils are commonly found in the CSF. Treatment of intestinal tapeworm infections is with praziquantel. Cysticercosis can be treated with praziquantel or albendazole (Chapter 46).

Echinococcosis (Hydatid Cyst)

Echinococcosis infection is common in sheep-raising countries where humans are closely associated with heavily infected sheepdogs and can ingest the eggs. Autochthonous cases are rare in North America, and most cases seen are contracted abroad, in areas such as the Mediterranean littoral, the Middle East, or South America. Symptoms may not present for 10 or more years after infection, because the cysts are slow growing. The usual cyst location is in the liver or lung. Eosinophilia does not usually occur with an intact cyst, and when it is present, it is usually related to some leakage of fluid. Approximately one-quarter of cases seen in North America had an eosinophilia of $>500/mm^3$. Cysts are often initially recognized with radiographic imaging studies, and confirmation can be made serologically. Depending on cyst location and complexity, treatment may include drug therapy (albendazole, mebendazole, praziquantel), surgery, and/or percutaneous aspiration–injection–reaspiration (Chapter 46).

Schistosomiasis

The acute stage of schistosomiasis may not be recognized in many of those infected, but in some cases, 4-8 weeks after infection the so-called Katayama syndrome may occur. This syndrome coincides with the initial deposition of eggs by recently matured worms and can include fever, chills, headache, diarrhea, hepatosplenomegaly, urticaria, pulmonary infiltrates, cough, wheezing, and eosinophilia, which may reach levels of $6000/mm^3$ or greater. This syndrome occurs most frequently with *Schistosoma japonicum* infections contracted in the Far East; less frequently with *Schistosoma mansoni* infections contracted in Latin America or the Caribbean, Africa, or Southwest Asia; and least commonly with *S. haematobium* contracted in Africa or the Middle East. Acute schistosomiasis symptoms are usually self-limited, but some severely affected individuals may require praziquantel therapy with steroids.

Most established schistosomiasis infections in travelers and natives of endemic areas are asymptomatic, although some people may have gastrointestinal or urinary complaints, fatigue, or weight loss. Hematuria is the most typical presentation of *S. haematobium* infections. In established infections, eosinophilia is variable. In 173 white expatriates returning to Britain with the sole diagnosis of schistosomiasis, eosinophilia was found in 48% of those with *S. mansoni* and in 24% of those with *S. haematobium*. A history of freshwater exposure in an endemic area is necessary to make the presence of schistosomiasis tenable.

Diagnosis of the intestinal forms—*S. japonicum* or the related *Schistosoma mekongi* from Southeast Asia and *S. mansoni*—is by finding typical eggs in the stool. *S. haematobium* is found by examination of urine sediment. When eggs cannot be found after concentration examination of stool or urine, a rectal biopsy specimen may show the presence of eggs of all the species; a rectal snip pressed out between two glass slides can give a rapid diagnosis. Fluorescent antibody, FAST (Falcon assay screening test)–ELISA, and specific *S. mansoni* and *S. haematobium* immunoblot tests can be used to serologically screen people with suspected cases and other travelers with a history of exposure to infections. Attempts can then be made to find eggs in stool or urine. Because eggs may be difficult to find in early infection or in lightly infected persons, praziquantel treatment in a 1-day, usually well-tolerated and effective course, can be considered for positive serologic reactors with an exposure history (Chapter 48).

Liver and Lung Flukes

Clonorchis sinensis and *Opisthorchis viverrini* are the most common liver flukes diagnosed in returnees to temperate areas, and eosinophilia frequently occurs in these infections. The former is not uncommon in Chinese immigrants, and both can occasionally be seen in returned expatriates. *O. viverrini* is commonly seen in Southeast Asian refugees, particularly those from Laos and Thailand. *Fasciola hepatica* is rarely seen in North America but is found in Europe and Latin America. Many liver fluke infections are relatively light, and patients may be asymptomatic. In more heavily infected individuals, manifestations can include low grade fever, diarrhea, and liver pain. In the acute stage, a high eosinophilia may be present, but eosinophilia is usually mild in established infections. Diagnosis is by finding typical eggs in the stool or in duodenal contents. *Paragonimus westermani*, the lung fluke, is usually seen in Asian immigrants, rarely in West African immigrants, and rarely in expatriates. Clinical manifestations can resemble tuberculosis, with fever, weight loss, blood-tinged sputum, cough, chest pain, and pulmonary nodules and cavities. Eosinophilia is often present. Diagnosis is by finding typical eggs in the sputum or occasionally in the feces when eggs are coughed up and swallowed. Praziquantel is the treatment of choice for all these flukes except *F. hepatica*, which is best treated with bithionol or triclabendazole. However, both of these latter drugs are investigational in the United States.

Protozoan Infections

The more common intestinal protozoa, *Giardia lamblia* and *Entamoeba histolytica*, are not a cause of eosinophilia. *Dientamoeba fragilis*, an increasingly recognized flagellate parasite of the large bowel, may cause diarrhea, cramps, and gas. Infections appear to be somewhat more common in children. In one report, significant peripheral eosinophilia was found in 53% of adults with *D. fragilis* and chronic eosinophilia. Reports on eosinophilia in patients with *D. fragilis* have not been uncommon when a differential white blood cell count has been performed. There is some evidence that eosinophilia in children with *D. fragilis* infections may be associated with pinworms, but this is certainly not always the case. *Isospora belli*, a rarely diagnosed small bowel coccidial parasite, may occasionally cause long-lasting infections leading to chronic diarrhea, malabsorption, and fever. Eosinophilia, occasionally profound, has been associated with *I. belli* infections. Diagnosis of these infections is by finding parasites in the stool, and with *I. belli* also in duodenal contents or biopsy specimen. Patients with malaria who have eosinophilia are usually found also to have other parasitic infections as the cause.

Bacterial and Fungal Infections

Eosinophilia is not usually associated with bacterial, viral, rickettsial, and fungal infections. It has been irregularly described in late scarlet fever and chronic indolent tuberculosis. In primary coccidioidomycosis (which occurs not only in the southwestern United States, but also in parts of Central and South America), eosinophilia occurs in as many as 88% of patients. Eosinophils may also appear in the CSF in *Coccidioides immitis* meningitis. *Aspergillus fumigatus*, causing allergic bronchopulmonary aspergillosis, is associated with eosinophilia. Imported infections with these fungi are distinctly uncommon in the United States. Eosinophilia has been reported with human immunodeficiency virus infection.

Drug Reactions

Many drugs can cause eosinophilia as a feature of a hypersensitivity reaction. Products containing sulfa drugs, such as trimethoprim/sulfamethoxazole and the antimalarial Fansidar (pyrimethamine and sulfadoxine) should be considered as the cause of eosinophilia in patients taking these products. The initiation of treatment for helminthic infections such as schistosomiasis and filariasis may lead to an acute exacerbation of eosinophilia related to rapid destruction of parasites.

Endomyocardial Fibrosis

Endomyocardial fibrosis has been described primarily in tropical Africa and South America, especially in natives. There have also been convincing reports of endomyocardial fibrosis in Europeans who have lived for long periods in West and Central Africa. In most of them, filariasis was present, and there was marked eosinophilia. There are many hypotheses concerning endomyocardial fibrosis besides an association with filariasis, however, and the exact cause has not yet been established.

Other Diseases with Eosinophils

Other less common entities that can be considered in the cause of eosinophilia, although not all necessarily related to tropical exposure in returned travelers or immigrants from tropical areas, are listed in **Table 49.1**.

FURTHER READING

Biggs, B.-A., Caruana, S., Mihrshahi, S., et al., 2009. Short report: management of chronic strongyloidiasis in immigrants and refugees: is serologic testing useful? Am. J. Trop. Med. Hyg. 80, 788–791.
Serologic testing should be carried out 6-12 months, or possibly longer, after treatment to ensure a downward trend suggesting cure.

Harries, A., Myers, B., Bhattacharrya, D., 1986. Eosinophilia in Caucasians returning from the tropics Trans. Roy. Soc. Trop. Med. Hyg. 80, 327–328.
In 38.7% of 119 Caucasians, a definite parasitological diagnosis was made, and in all those followed up eosinophilia decreased with appropriate chemotherapy.

Kim, Y.-J., Nutman, T.B., 2006. Eosinophilia: causes and pathology in persons with prior exposures in tropical areas with an emphasis on parasite infections. Curr. Infect. Dis. Rep. 8, 43–50.
Eosinophilia in patients exposed to tropical environments caused most commonly by helminth infections.

Medical Letter, 2013. Drugs for Parasitic Infections.
Tables listing first-choice and alternative drugs for most parasitic infections.

Nutman, T.B., 2006. Asymptomatic peripheral blood eosinophilia redux: common parasitic infections presenting frequently in refugees and immigrants. Clin. Infect. Dis. 42, 368–369.
Eosinophilia in refugees and immigrants from many areas of the world is most often due to helminth infection.

Nutman, T.B., Ottesen, E.A., Sackoson, I., et al., 1987. Eosinophilia in Southeast Asian refugees: evaluation at a referral center. J. Infect. Dis. 155, 309–313.
A study at the National Institutes of Health of 128 Indochinese refugees. Intestinal parasites were the cause of the eosinophilia in all but six of these patients.

Price, T.A., Tuazon, C.U., Simon, G.L., 1993. Fascioliasis: case reports and reviews. Clin. Infect. Dis. 17, 426–430.
Two imported cases and a good review of this relatively uncommon liver fluke in the United States.

Schulte, C., Krebs, T., Jelinek, T., et al., 2002. Diagnostic significance of blood eosinophilia in returning travelers. Clin. Infect. Dis. 34, 407–411.
A study from Germany in 14,298 returnees from developing countries, 689 of whom had blood eosinophilia.

Seybolt, L.M., Christiansen, D., Barnett, E.D., 2006. Diagnostic evaluation of newly arrived asymptomatic refugees with eosinophilia. Clin. Infect. Dis. 42, 363–367.
A study of 2224 refugees to determine the prevalence of eosinophilia and develop a standardized approach to evaluate those with eosinophilia.

Spencer, M.J., Chapin, M.R., Garcia, L.S., 1982. *Dientamoeba fragilis*: a gastrointestinal protozoan infection in adults. Am. J. Gastroenterol. 77, 565–569.
Eight of 15 (53%) adults with D. fragilis and chronic symptoms had peripheral eosinophilia.

Weller, P.F., 1997. Human eosinophils. J. Allergy Clin. Immunol. 100, 283–287.
A thorough discussion of immunobiology of eosinophilia.

APPENDIX

TABLE A.1   Global Health Information Resources

Centers for Disease Control and Prevention (CDC)
    website: www.cdc.gov
World Health Organization (WHO)
    website: www.who.org
Association for Safe International Road Travel (ASIRT)
    11769 Gainsborough Rd
    Potomac, MD 20854
    Tel. 301-983-5252
    website: www.asirt.org
    (Information for travelers on road safety conditions throughout the world; road travel reports for
        150 countries)
Bureau on Consular Affairs
    US State Department
    website: www.travel.state.gov
    (Country-by-country information on document requirements, health issues, road safety information,
        and tips for travel abroad)
International Association for Medical Assistance to Travelers (IAMAT)
    40 Regal Rd
    Guelph, Ontario N1K 1B5
    Tel. 519-836-0102
    website: www.iamat.org
    (Nonprofit organization that provides medical information about countries around the world as well
        as associated English-speaking doctors)
i.Jet Intelligent Risk Systems
    910F Bestgate Rd
    Annapolis, MD 21401
    Tel. 410-573-3860
    website: www.ijet.com
    (Health and security information for international businesses, by subscription)
Travax
    Shoreland, Inc.
    O Box 13795
    Milwaukee, WI 53213-0795
    website: www.shoreland.com
    (Information services for travel health professionals, by subscription)
Travel Medicine Advisor
    AHC Media LLC
    3525 Piedmont Rd
    Atlanta, GA 30305
    Tel. 404-262-7436
    website: www.travelmedicineadvisor.com
    (Monthly newsletter for travel health professionals, by subscription)

TABLE A.2   CDC Sources for Malaria Prophylaxis, Diagnosis, and Treatment Recommendations

Type of Information	Source	Availability	Telephone Number, Website, or Email Address
Prophylaxis	CDC's voice information system	24 h/day	877-394-8747 (877-FYI-TRIP)
Prophylaxis	CDC's Traveler's Healthfax information service	24 h/day	888-232-3299
Prophylaxis	CDC's Traveler's Health website (includes online access to Health Information for International Travel)	24 h/day	http://www.cdc.gov/travel
Prophylaxis	Health Information for International Travel (*The Yellow Book*)	Order from Public Health Publication Sales, PO Box 753, Waldorf, MD 20604	877-252-1200 or 301-645-7773 or http://www.phf.org
Diagnosis	CDC's Division of Parasitic Diseases diagnostic website (DPDx)	24 h/day	http://www.dpd.cdc.gov/dpdx
Diagnosis	CDC's Division of Parasitic Diseases diagnostic website (DPDx)	Order by electronic mail from the CDC Division of Parasitic Diseases	dpdx@cdc.gov
Treatment	CDC's Malaria Branch	0800–1630 Eastern time, Monday to Friday	770-488-7788*
Treatment	CDC's Malaria Branch	1630–0800 Eastern time, evenings, weekends, and holidays	770-488-7100* (*This is the number for the CDC's Emergency Operations Center. Ask the staff member to page the person on call for the Malaria Branch.) http://www.cdc.gov/malaria/diagnosis_treatment/treatment.htm

CDC, Centers for Disease Control and Prevention.

TABLE A.3 Professional Organizations with Publications and Educational Programs of Interest to Practitioners of Travel and Tropical Medicine

American College of Emergency Medicine (ACEP)
  website: www.acep.org
American Public Health Association (APHA)
  website: www.apha.org
American Society of Tropical Medicine and Hygiene (ASTMH)
  website: www.astmh.org (Membership directory of clinical travel and tropical medicine providers; certificate examination offered)
Infectious Diseases Society of America (IDSA)
  website: www.idsa.org (Membership directory of infectious diseases specialists)
International Society of Travel Medicine (ISTM)
  website: www.istm.org (Membership directory of travel health providers; certificate examination offered)
Wilderness Medical Society (WMS)
  website: www.wms.org

TABLE A.4 Emergency Medical Assistance for Travelers

MEDEX Insurance Services, Inc.
  PO Box 19056
  Baltimore, MD 21284
  Tel. 1-800-732-5309, 0800–1700 Eastern Standard Time, Monday to Friday
  website: www.medexassist.com
International SOS Pte Ltd
  Worldwide Headquarters
  331 North Bridge Road #17-00 Odean Towers
  Singapore 188720
  Tel. 65-6338-2311
  website: www.internationalsos.com

TABLE A.5   Vendors of Travel Accessories and Gear

Chinook Medical Gear, Inc.
120 Rock Point Drive, Unit C
Durango, CO 81301
Tel. 800-766-1365
website: www.chinookmed.com
(Custom medical solutions for the harshest environments on Earth; gear for adventure travel,
    expeditions, and scientific explorations)

Magellan's Travel Gear
110 W. Sola Street
Santa Barbara, CA 93101
Tel. 800-962-4943
website: www.magellans.com
(Travel accessories, supplies, clothing, and luggage)

Recreational Equipment Inc. (REI)
Sumner, WA 98352-0001
Tel. 800-426-4840
website: www.rei.com
(Clothing, supplies, and gear for outdoor adventure travel)

Travel Smith Outfitters
60 Leveroni Court
Novato, CA 94949
Tel. 800-950-1600
website: www.travelmith.com
(Clothing and supplies for travel)

TABLE A.6 Celsius to Fahrenheit Conversion Table

Celsius	Fahrenheit	Celsius	Fahrenheit	Celsius	Fahrenheit
0	32	31	87.8	72	161.6
0.1	32.18	32	89.6	73	163.4
0.2	32.36	33	91.4	74	165.2
0.3	32.54	34	93.2	75	167
0.4	32.72	35	95	76	168.8
0.5	32.9	36	96.8	77	170.6
0.6	33.08	37	98.6	78	172.4
0.7	33.26	38	100.4	79	174.2
0.8	33.44	39	102.2	80	176
0.9	33.62	40	104	81	177.8
		41	105.8	82	179.6
1	33.8	42	107.6	83	181.4
2	35.6	43	109.4	84	183.2
3	37.4	44	111.2	85	185
4	39.2	45	113	86	186.8
5	41	46	114.8	87	188.6
6	42.8	47	116.6	88	190.4
7	44.6	48	118.4	89	192.2
8	46.4	49	120.2	90	194
9	48.2	50	122	91	195.8
10	50	51	123.8	92	197.6
11	51.8	52	125.6	93	199.4
12	53.6	53	127.4	94	201.2
13	55.4	54	129.2	95	203
14	57.2	55	131	96	204.8
15	59	56	132.8	97	206.6
16	60.8	57	134.6	98	208.4
17	62.6	58	136.4	99	210.2
18	64.4	59	138.2	100	212
19	66.2	60	140	200	392
20	68	61	141.8	300	572
21	69.8	62	143.6	400	752
22	71.6	63	145.4	500	932
23	73.4	64	147.2	600	1112
24	75.2	65	149	700	1292
25	77	66	150.8	800	1472
26	78.8	67	152.6	900	1652
27	80.6	68	154.4	1000	1832
28	82.4	69	156.2		
29	84.2	70	158		
30	86	71	159.8		

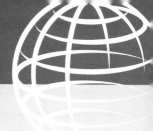

Index

Page numbers followed by "*f*" indicate figures, "*t*" indicate tables, and "*b*" indicate boxes.

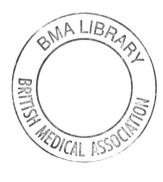